Industrial Applications for Bioprocessing and Biomanufacturing

Ayush Madan
People's University, India

Mohd Tariq
Parul University, India

Mantosh Kumar Satapathy
Taipei Medical University, Taiwan

Yousef Rasmi
Urmia University of Medical Sciences, Iran

IGI Global
Scientific Publishing
Publishing Tomorrow's Research Today

Vice President of Editorial	Melissa Wagner
Director of Acquisitions	Mikaela Felty
Director of Book Development	Jocelynn Hessler
Production Manager	Mike Brehm
Cover Design	Jose Rosado

Published in the United States of America by
IGI Global Scientific Publishing
701 East Chocolate Avenue
Hershey, PA, 17033, USA
Tel: 717-533-8845 | Fax: 717-533-7115
Website: https://www.igi-global.com E-mail: cust@igi-global.com

Library of Congress Cataloging-in-Publication Data

LCCN: 2025027400 (CIP Data Pending)
ISBN13: 979-8-3373-2873-7
Isbn13Softcover: 979-8-3373-2874-4
EISBN13: 979-8-3373-2875-1

British Cataloguing in Publication Data
A Cataloguing in Publication record for this book is available from the British Library.

Table of Contents

Detailed Table of Contents

This chapter highlights the transformative potential of bioprocessing and biomanufacturing as central forces in biotechnology, ecology, and medicine. Bioprocessing is the foundation of modern biotechnology because it actively employs biological systems to produce valuable compounds while simultaneously addressing urgent global challenges. Through carefully designed processes, bioprocessing mitigates climate change, strengthens ecosystem resilience, and responds to the escalating demands of global population growth by enabling sustainable production of food, medicines, and renewable energy. Emphasize that bioprocessing not only creates bio-based products but also reshapes industrial practices by reducing dependence on fossil resources and promoting environmentally responsible alternatives demonstrate that bioprocessing and biomanufacturing serve as vital engines of innovation in biotechnology, ecology, and medicine.

Bio-manufacturing is a potential area for production of biologically active products for the welfare of human beings using biological systems in the bioreactors industrially. It is well known that microbial or cell culture systems play vital role in bio-manufacturing industry. Bio-manufacturing is an interdisciplinary approach with a combination of Microbiology, Biochemistry and Chemical Engineering. Recent developments in science introduced a variety of biological systems for the production of important molecules/products. Initially, bio-manufacturing was carried out with recombinant microbial systems, later with mammalian cell cultures. This chapter emphasizes the evolution of bio-manufacturing systems, microbial and cell culture systems in producing various biological products through industrial bioreactors with special focus on wild to genetically modified cell culture systems and the challenges in quality improvement of the bio-products.

Metabolic engineering and synthetic biology are enhancing the design and production of microbial cells with scaled capabilities for producing high-demand bio-based products, such as biofuels, enzymes, nutraceuticals, and food industry products. Metabolic engineering provides cellular metabolism to maximize product yields and minimize wastages. Synthetic biology further modifies and enables the production of complex molecules that are difficult to synthesize through other methods. This chapter provides an in-depth exploration and study of the latest innovations and developments, highlighting their transformative impact on optimized biomanufacturing processes. It also highlights the advanced genetic tools, genome-scale modelling, etc. Additionally, it discusses prospects, challenges, and potential solutions for next-generation biomanufacturing, emphasizing the role of Artificial Intelligence (AI) and Machine Learning (ML) in system metabolic engineering.

A bioreactor is a specialized vessel designed to facilitate biological reactions, harnessing the capabilities of microorganisms, mammalian cells, or other biological systems to convert raw materials into valuable products. Bioreactor systems serve as the central hub of bioprocessing, from laboratory-scale experiments to pilot and industrial-scale manufacturing, bridging upstream and downstream operations. Their design and optimization are critical for achieving high productivity, maintaining process efficiency, and ensuring cost-effectiveness. This chapter provides a comprehensive overview of advanced bioreactor systems, including stirred-tank, airlift, perfusion, and single-use bioreactors, highlighting their advantages, limitations, and applications. It explores key design principles such as oxygen transfer, mixing dynamics, shear stress minimization, and real-time process monitoring.

The bioprocess monitoring market, valued at \$12.3 billion in 2023, is expected to grow at a CAGR of 9.1% to reach \$20.5 billion by 2030. This growth is driven by biosensors, machine learning, and Industry 4.0. Innovations like Raman spectroscopy and NMR have improved metabolite profiling accuracy, leading to enhanced process control. Artificial intelligence-driven models have reduced batch variability by 20%, while digital twin technologies have reduced process development time by 25%. Automated fed-batch strategies have increased recombinant protein yields by 15-25%, while microfluidic bioreactors enable high-throughput screening with a 5-fold reduction in reagent costs. Soft-sensor technologies have adjusted metabolic flux projections by 35%, reducing process variation. IoT-enabled bioprocessing has reduced manual interventions by 40%, improving operational effectiveness.

Effective monitoring and control of bioprocesses in the biotechnology and pharmaceutical sectors helps to maximize both biopharmaceutical manufacture and enzyme production of bio-based chemical outputs. Real-time tracking of significant elements including regulatory controls of temperature and pH and nutritional parameters with biomass concentration follows through regulatory controls. Modern technologies combining sensors, data analytics, automaton, ion, and data analysis improve yield, process efficiency, and product quality and maintenance. Through these techniques, nutraceuticals, food and beverage sectors as well as pharmaceuticals items have industrial-scale bioprocessing. Different sectors have developed to demand sophisticated process monitoring and control systems; so, enhanced process control becomes indispensable for maximizing yields and improving processes. Innovations in healthcare engineering such as automated living materials and stem cell production open new opportunities but also demand solutions to technological challenges and operational constraints.

With the increasing global demand for biopharmaceuticals and industrial biologics, optimizing biomanufacturing processes become imperative. The optimization of bioprocesses aims to maximize the efficiency and yield in biomanufacturing while maintaining cost-effectiveness. This chapter discusses the key strategies employed for bioprocess optimization and scale-up for the efficient production of biological products. It also discusses the importance of bioreactor configuration refinements, dynamic media optimization, process parameter refinement and real-time monitoring via advanced PAT. The integration of AI and ML in predictive modelling, efficiency enhancement and minimizing operational risks are also presented. Furthermore, the transition from batch to continuous manufacturing and the implementation of QbD as key drivers of efficiency and consistency are emphasized. Optimizing downstream processing are equally crucial to enable higher product recovery. Finally, addressing key bottlenecks such as scale-up and regulatory constraints are also reviewed.

Biotechnology in the food and beverage industry has revolutionized production by enhancing nutritional value, sustainability, and waste valorization. Plant-based beverages, agro-industrial by-products, and food waste are utilized in microbial fermentation, enzyme technologies, and genetic engineering to produce high-value products such as bioactive compounds, organic acids, bioplastics, and nutraceuticals. Microbial enzymes improve texture, taste, shelf life, and economic efficiency in food processing. Enzyme functionality is further enhanced through immobilization and protein engineering. However, biotechnology faces challenges in safety, regulation, ethics, and consumer acceptance. Regulatory systems, like GRAS norms in the U.S. and EU pre-market assessments, vary globally. Ethical concerns include environmental risks, socio-economic factors, and cultural sensitivities. Transparency, labeling, and risk management are crucial in building trust and balancing innovation with responsibility.

Bioplastics are derived from renewable resources, such as microorganisms, biowaste, or plants, rather than non-renewable resources like fossil fuels or petroleum. Algal bioplastics provide a renewable alternative to Petroleum-based polymers. Various microalgae strains grown in different environments can produce a wide range of

This chapter comprehensively explores the principles, technologies, applications, economic considerations and future directions of green biomanufacturing. It covers biological production platforms, waste valorization, sustainable materials, regulatory dynamics, analyze core principles; waste minimization, energy efficiency & lifecycle assessment. Evaluating enabling technologies; microbial fermentation, enzyme catalysis, synthetic biology, plant/algae-based systems. It reviews industrial applications in pharmaceuticals, biofuels, biomaterials, waste management and explore economic viability, policy incentives and challenges in scalability. The study finds that green biomanufacturing offers significant environmental and economic benefits, including reduced emissions, enhanced resource efficiency and new value chains from waste streams. Future research should focus on optimizing process control through AI, next-gen bioreactors, expanding public-private partnerships for scale-up infrastructure and harmonizing global regulatory frameworks.

Rising global demand for waste-to-wealth generation has caught a lot of attention towards the biological remediation methods with human interventions to enhance capabilities to detoxify pollutants. This comprehensive book chapter aims to focus on

separation phases, this chapter illustrates the diverse array of ongoing bioprocess intensification initiatives.

Preface

INTRODUCTION

Bioprocessing and biomanufacturing have become foundational pillars in the advancement of modern biotechnology. What began as traditional fermentation and microbial cultivation has now evolved into a dynamic, interdisciplinary field at the intersection of biology, engineering, and computational science. The convergence of synthetic biology, automation, and artificial intelligence is rapidly reshaping how we design, optimize, and scale bioprocesses—offering innovative solutions to some of the most pressing global challenges, from sustainable energy and food production to cutting-edge biopharmaceuticals.

In this context, we are pleased to present *Industrial Applications for Bioprocessing and Biomanufacturing*, an edited volume that reflects the latest developments and industrial practices shaping this transformative field. This book was conceived with the intent to bridge the gap between fundamental bioprocessing principles and their real-world implementation in industrial settings. It provides an in-depth and accessible exploration of core topics including microbial and mammalian cell culture, bioreactor engineering, downstream processing, and regulatory compliance.

What distinguishes this volume is its emphasis on both foundational concepts and forward-looking technologies. Readers will find chapters addressing innovations in continuous biomanufacturing, AI-driven process optimization, and the growing role of bioprocessing in the circular bioeconomy. We believe that integrating these perspectives is essential for fostering a new generation of scalable, sustainable, and high-precision manufacturing systems.

This book is designed for a diverse and multidisciplinary audience. Whether you are a researcher seeking to advance the frontiers of bioprocess engineering, an industry professional working to optimize production systems, a policymaker shaping regulatory frameworks, or an entrepreneur exploring bio-based product development, we trust this book will serve as a valuable reference and practical guide.

We are deeply grateful to the contributing authors whose expertise and insights have made this volume possible. Their contributions not only illuminate current best practices but also chart a path forward for future innovations. We also extend our appreciation to the academic and industrial communities that continue to drive this field with their creativity, collaboration, and commitment to solving complex global challenges through biotechnology.

It is our hope that this book will inspire further inquiry, support cross-sector collaboration, and contribute meaningfully to the continued evolution of bioprocessing and biomanufacturing.

ORGANIZATION OF THE BOOK

This volume, *Industrial Applications for Bioprocessing and Biomanufacturing*, brings together cutting-edge research, technological innovation, and industrial insights across 15 chapters. Together, they form a comprehensive roadmap through the foundations, current advances, and future directions of bioprocessing and biomanufacturing. Below is an overview of each chapter, written from the perspective of the editors, to guide readers through the book's structure and thematic flow.

Chapter 1: An Introduction to Bioprocessing and Industrial Biomanufacturing – Foundations and Evolution

This opening chapter sets the stage by positioning bioprocessing and biomanufacturing as transformative forces in biotechnology, ecology, and medicine. It frames bioprocessing not merely as a method for producing bio-based products, but as a catalyst for systemic industrial change—one that reduces fossil fuel dependency, supports climate resilience, and advances sustainable development. The chapter underscores how these technologies are foundational to modern biotech, simultaneously responding to global challenges and driving innovation.

Chapter 2: Advanced Bioreactor Systems and Design Principles for Scalable Biomanufacturing

Bioreactors are the physical and functional cores of bioprocessing operations. This chapter presents a comprehensive examination of various bioreactor types—including stirred-tank, airlift, perfusion, and single-use systems—and the design considerations that impact scale, efficiency, and product quality. Key engineering principles like oxygen transfer rates, mixing dynamics, and shear stress management are unpacked with practical industrial relevance.

Chapter 3: Bioprocess Optimization Strategies – Enhancing Efficiency and Yield in Biomanufacturing

The demand for biologics and biopharmaceuticals necessitates constant process refinement. This chapter reviews strategies for optimizing upstream and downstream processes, including bioreactor configuration, media formulation, and the use of predictive AI models. Special attention is given to process analytical technology (PAT), continuous manufacturing, and Quality by Design (QbD) frameworks—all of which contribute to higher yield, reduced variability, and improved regulatory compliance.

Chapter 4: Microbial and Cell Culture Systems for Biomanufacturing

This chapter dives into the biological systems at the heart of biomanufacturing, particularly microbial and mammalian cell cultures. It tracks the evolution of industrial bio-production from wild-type microbes to genetically engineered strains, and from microbial fermentation to complex mammalian cell culture platforms. Emphasis is placed on the interdisciplinary nature of biomanufacturing and the technical challenges involved in improving product quality and consistency at scale.

Chapter 5: Metabolic Engineering and Synthetic Biology – Pioneering Innovations for Optimized Biomanufacturing

Here, the reader is introduced to two of the most powerful tools for advancing biomanufacturing: metabolic engineering and synthetic biology. This chapter provides an in-depth look at how cellular pathways are redesigned to boost yield, reduce waste, and enable the production of complex molecules. Innovations such as genome-scale modeling, advanced genetic editing, and AI/ML integration are explored, with a forward-looking lens on next-generation biomanufacturing systems.

Chapter 6: Automation and Advanced Control Systems in Biomanufacturing – Ensuring Precision and Consistency

Automation is crucial for achieving consistency and scalability in biomanufacturing. This chapter explores how modern sensors, robotics, and data analytics have enhanced regulatory control over critical parameters like pH, temperature, and nutrient feed. It emphasizes how automation enables industrial-scale production of biopharmaceuticals, nutraceuticals, and food products—while also introducing new challenges in system integration and workforce adaptation.

Chapter 7: Sustainable Biomanufacturing – Green Technologies for Environmental and Economic Benefits

Green biomanufacturing is not only an environmental imperative but an economic opportunity. This chapter outlines sustainable production platforms, waste valorization strategies, and energy-efficient technologies. It evaluates policy incentives, industrial applications, and economic models that support green transitions. The role of AI, next-generation bioreactors, and international collaboration in scaling these technologies is also emphasized.

Chapter 8: Advances in Bioprocess Monitoring and Control Systems

Focusing on real-time process intelligence, this chapter showcases the rapid evolution of bioprocess monitoring, driven by technologies such as biosensors, Raman spectroscopy, and digital twin models. The integration of AI and IoT into process control has resulted in significant gains in yield, efficiency, and reproducibility. Through detailed industry data, the chapter outlines how smart monitoring tools are transforming process development and manufacturing precision.

Chapter 9: Biopharmaceutical Manufacturing – Challenges and Solutions

Biopharmaceuticals are among the most complex and valuable outputs of biomanufacturing. This chapter examines the industry's challenges, including high production costs, regulatory hurdles, and scalability issues. Solutions such as single-use technologies, continuous processing, AI-driven analytics, and sustainable feedstocks are discussed as enablers of a more agile, cost-effective, and environmentally responsible biopharma sector.

Chapter 10: Biomanufacturing of Biofuels and Bioplastics – Innovations for a Sustainable Future

A key driver of the circular bioeconomy, this chapter delves into the production of biofuels and bioplastics from renewable biological sources. It highlights the growing importance of algal bioplastics and microbial fermentation in reducing reliance on petroleum-based materials. The discussion emphasizes sustainability, innovation, and the role of biomanufacturing in climate change mitigation and waste reduction.

Chapter 11: Biotechnology in the Food and Beverage Industry – Fermentation and Beyond

This chapter explores the role of bioprocessing in revolutionizing food and beverage manufacturing. From microbial fermentation to enzyme engineering, the use of biotechnology has improved nutritional profiles, reduced food waste, and enabled novel product development. It also examines the regulatory and ethical considerations that accompany innovations in this consumer-facing sector, underscoring the need for transparency and responsible innovation.

Chapter 12: Regulatory Frameworks and Quality Assurance in Biomanufacturing – Ensuring Compliance and Safety

The regulatory landscape is foundational to the safe, effective, and ethical practice of biomanufacturing. This chapter provides a global overview of regulatory frameworks, biosafety classifications, and quality assurance protocols. It covers risk management, compliance auditing, and the growing importance of adaptive regulatory science in balancing innovation with public health and safety.

Chapter 13: Future Trends and Innovations in Bioprocessing and Biomanufacturing

Concluding the volume, this chapter looks ahead to the future of smart, sustainable, and intensified biomanufacturing. It examines the integration of nature-inspired biocatalysts, modular production systems, and digital technologies to create more efficient and environmentally friendly processes. With a focus on process intensification across upstream and downstream stages, this chapter maps the trajectory of bioprocessing toward meeting the rising global demand for bio-based products.

Chapter 14: Biomanufacturing for Environmental Sustainability and Remediation

Biomanufacturing is increasingly recognized as a tool for environmental remediation. This chapter focuses on the biological treatment of pollutants, e-waste, and plastics using engineered microbes and biosystems. It details how metabolic engineering and circular economy strategies enhance detoxification processes, reduce waste, and generate bioelectricity—presenting a holistic view of bioprocessing for ecological restoration.

Chapter 15: Biomanufacturing Challenges in Developing Economies

This chapter brings critical attention to the unique barriers faced by developing nations in advancing biomanufacturing. From infrastructure limitations and funding gaps to regulatory constraints and skill shortages, the challenges are numerous—but not insurmountable. Policy reform, investment in capacity-building, and international partnerships are presented as key strategies to unlock the full potential of bio-based industries in the Global South.

Together, these chapters form a cohesive and multidimensional reference, offering both foundational knowledge and visionary perspectives. Whether readers are navigating technical challenges, exploring new markets, or shaping policy, *Industrial Applications for Bioprocessing and Biomanufacturing* offers a timely and authoritative resource for advancing the next era of biotechnology.

CONCLUSION

As we conclude this preface to *Industrial Applications for Bioprocessing and Biomanufacturing*, we reflect on the breadth and depth of topics explored throughout the chapters of this volume. Collectively, they illustrate not only the remarkable progress that has been achieved in bioprocessing and biomanufacturing but also the vast potential that lies ahead. From foundational principles to frontier technologies, this book captures a critical moment in the evolution of biotechnology—one where biology, engineering, and digital innovation converge to address some of the most pressing global challenges.

Our aim in curating this collection has been to provide a comprehensive and accessible resource for diverse stakeholders across academia, industry, government, and entrepreneurial ecosystems. Whether optimizing microbial cell factories, implementing advanced bioreactor systems, or navigating regulatory landscapes, the chapters herein provide both conceptual clarity and practical insights to support real-world applications.

Importantly, this volume emphasizes a forward-looking perspective. The future of biomanufacturing will be shaped not only by technological advancements but also by global efforts to promote sustainability, equity, and resilience. The integration of AI-driven optimization, the transition to continuous and green manufacturing, and the democratization of biotechnologies in developing economies will play defining roles in shaping the bioeconomy of tomorrow.

We extend our sincere gratitude to the contributing authors whose expertise has brought this book to life. Their diverse perspectives and shared commitment to scientific and industrial advancement are evident in every chapter. We also thank the broader scientific and professional community, whose ongoing work continues to push the boundaries of what is possible.

It is our hope that this book serves not just as a reference, but as a catalyst—for learning, for innovation, and for collaborative progress across disciplines and sectors. As bioprocessing and biomanufacturing continue to evolve, so too must our collective efforts to ensure that these technologies are harnessed responsibly, sustainably, and inclusively—for the benefit of people and the planet.

Chapter 1

An Introduction to Bioprocessing and Industrial Bio-Manufacturing Foundation and Evolution

Rabin Debnath
NEPEDS College of Pharmaceutical Sciences, India

Mohd Aftab Siddiqui
Integral University, India

Tapoban Bordoloi
NEPEDS College of Pharmaceutical Sciences, India

Izaz Hussain
Independent Researcher, India

Sneha Parbin
Arunachal University of Studies, India

Mostafa Khursid Alam
USTM, India

Sachin Kumar
Delhi Pharmaceutical Sciences and Research University, India

Shriyansh Srivastava
https://orcid.org/0000-0002-3738-4381
Galgotias University, India

Rakesh Sahu
Ben Gurion University of the Negev, Israel

ABSTRACT

This chapter highlights the transformative potential of bioprocessing and biomanufacturing as central forces in biotechnology, ecology, and medicine. Bioprocessing is the foundation of modern biotechnology because it actively employs biological systems to produce valuable compounds while simultaneously addressing urgent global challenges. Through carefully designed processes, bioprocessing mitigates climate change, strengthens ecosystem resilience, and responds to the escalating demands of global population growth by enabling sustainable production of food, medicines, and renewable energy. Emphasize that bioprocessing not only creates bio-based

DOI: 10.4018/979-8-3373-2873-7.ch001

products but also reshapes industrial practices by reducing dependence on fossil resources and promoting environmentally responsible alternatives demonstrate that bioprocessing and biomanufacturing serve as vital engines of innovation in biotechnology, ecology, and medicine.

INTRODUCTION

Bio-processing is the multidisciplinary science that encompasses technology, engineering, and biology in order to develop products using biological systems. It plays a vital role in businesses such as environmental management, food production, agriculture, and pharmaceuticals.

Definition and Scope of Bioprocessing

Bioprocessing is defined as the process that uses biological systems, such as microorganisms, enzymes, plant or animal cells, and their components to produce valuable products or to induce predetermined biochemical changes, (Abu, Gundersen, & Woodley, 2015). Fundamentally, it integrates biology with engineering to develop, optimize, and scale processes that transform feedstock into a valuable product. Biotechnology applications are interdisciplinary and include upstream processing (i.e. growth and cultivation of biological materials), downstream processing (i.e. recovery, purification, and formulation of products), and process optimization (i.e. efficiency, scalability, and regulations), (Azubuike, Chikere, & Okpokwasili, 2016). The most impact it has had is within the pharmaceutical industry allowing for the mass production of therapeutic proteins, monoclonal antibodies, recombinant therapies and therapies based on gene and cell treatment, (Bailey & Ollis, 2018). Bioprocessing also has applications other than in healthcare. For instance, in the bioenergy sector, it promotes the manufacture of advanced biofuels, such as bioethanol, biodiesel, and biogas, so as to mitigate the dependence on fossil fuels, (Barrangou & Doudna, 2016). In the food and beverage sector, fermentation processes form the basis for the production of essential foodstuffs like bread, cheese, yoghurt, beer, among other modern probiotics and functional foods that promote the health of the gut, (Bhardwaj et al., 2014). Bioprocessing also leads to new bioproducts such as bioplastics, biosensors, and artificial biomolecules with broad applications. Recent innovations in bioengineering and genetic engineering have made it possible to develop stable, high-yield microbial and mammalian cell "factories", whereas synthetic biology is providing new opportunities for the manufacture of sustainable bio-based materials. It further enables speedy process development, real-time process optimization and quality control, and as a result, bioprocesses are becoming a core technology shaping medicine, food, energy and sustainable industries, (Buchner & Rapp, 1899; Bud, 1994).

History and Evolution of Bioprocessing

Bioprocessing dates back millennia, with early applications of fermentation by ancient societies such as Mesopotamia and Egypt to preserve food, bake bread, and create alcohol, (Butler, 2005). At the time, the important part played by microorganisms was not yet known, but these early processes paved the way for the use of microbes in today's biotechnological food production. The industrial revolution of the 19th century led to a revolution in human microbiology, with Louis Pasteur putting science on a new path when he eventually showed that microbes were involved in the biochemical transformations in life, laying the foundations for microbiology and the science of fermentation, (Cappia, 2004). His methods now describe contemporary brewing, dairy fermentation, and probiotic processes in which carefully chosen strains of microorganisms are used to control flavour, safety, and nutritional properties. Meanwhile, Eduard Buchner's finding of cell-free fermentation with yeast extracts (Chen et al., 2013) laid the idea of enzymatic catalysis, which led to whole industries for large-scale enzyme manufacturing development. Enzymes such as amylases and proteases of industrial significance today are used in detergents, textile and food industries. The 20th century saw the dawn of the golden age of bioprocessing, in particular, towards the end of World War II, when submerged fermentation was exploited for the large-scale production of penicillin, which saved innumerable lives, (DeLisa, Kargi, & Shuler, 2017). This breakthrough led the biopharmaceutical industry to the designs of engineered microbial and mammalian cell culture systems for the production of recombinant proteins, monoclonal antibodies, and vaccines at a industrial scale. Additional developments in bioreactor design, aeration, and process control in the mid-20th century (Demain & Elander, 1999) allowed for the today's large-scale single use and continuous systems, enhancing sterility, scalability, and cost effectiveness. Another earth-shifting turning point occurred in the 1970s when recombinant DNA technology was introduced. The synthesis of human insulin via recombinant Escherichia coli (Doran, 1995) highlighted the supremacy of genetic engineering and served as a template for developing biosimilars, gene therapy, and biologics. This was followed by the development and utilization of mammalian cell culture systems which facilitated the production of more complex biologics, as monoclonal antibodies, (Dragosits & Mattanovich, 2013). One of the obligated biologicals is trastuzumab (Herceptin®), made in CHO (Chinese Hamster Ovary) cells, and that is still considered a typical course of therapy in breast cancer. Bioprocessing has evolved into a multidisciplinary field that combines biotechnology, chemical engineering and informatics. Recent trends including process analytical technology (PAT), automation, high-throughput experimentation and continuous manufacturing (Ecker, Jones, & Levine, 2014) have precedence in the historical evolution of process monitoring and control. In addition, emerging technologies in synthetic biology and CRISPR genome editing (Eibl & Eibl, 2019), are pushing Pasteur's heritage into new areas, such as sustainable production of biofuels, bioplastics, and chemical specialities.

Applications of Bioprocessing in Various Industries

Pharmaceutical Industry

Bringing therapeutic proteins, monoclonal antibodies, and vaccines to large-scale production, the opportunity in bioprocessing has revolutionized the pharmaceutical industry. Mammalian cell cultures, the most used mammalian cell line being Chinese Hamster Ovary (CHO), can be used to produce complex biologics that require proper upstream processing to produce the correct folding and post-translational modifications of proteins. Such a fine example is the applications of monoclonal antibodies (mAbs), such as trastuzumab (Herceptin), which are the recommended therapies for diseases such as breast cancer and significantly improve the patient outcome, (Food and Drug Administration, 2004). Also, bioprocessing can provide the consistency of quality, efficacy, and safety through the development of advanced therapies like gene therapies and recombinant vaccines.

Food and Beverage Industry

In its traditional and modern applications, the food and beverage industry heavily relies on bioprocesses, particularly fermentation. Fermentation in microbes has a long history, with the production of commodities such as cheese and beer, as well as yogurt. Moreover, there has been an increased focus on the use of probiotics in the industry that enhances digestion and gastrointestinal microbiomes and also increases the value of products. To meet the demand of consumers regarding functional foods, advancements in fermentation technologies are being made to provide product flavour, texture, and shelf life, (Garcia-Ochoa & Gomez, 2009).

Biofuel Production

Biofuel production relies heavily on the technique of bioprocessing, which is necessitated by the increased need for renewable energy in the market. Micro-organisms such as yeast and Clostridium species are either produced or occur naturally to provide the biofuels that can be used through biomass like lignocellulosic waste, and agricultural residues converted into fuel products like ethanol, butanol, and biodiesel. These processes reduce the dependence on non-renewable energy sources and overall emissions of greenhouse gases by providing feasible alternatives to fossil fuels. Another advancement of biofuel production systems that has boosted their yield and efficiency is the development of metabolic activities and subjecting the process to engineering work, (Goeddel et al., 1979).

Environmental Biotechnology

One common example of bioprocessing as applied in environmental biotechnology is bioremediation, where microorganisms degrade pollutants into less toxic substances. These are some of the applications of the heavy metal detoxification of polluted zones, treating wastewater in an industrial context, and cleaning up oil spills. Environmental bioprocessing helps in ecological restoration and sustainable waste management through functional design of the consortia of microbes as well as their optimum conditions, (Guieysse, Govantes, & Torre, 2011).

Agriculture

Microbial fermentation to generate biopesticides and biofertilizers can be used in the agriculture sector using bioprocessing. Biofertilizers, including biofertilizers containing the nitrogen-fixing bacteria, Rhizobium, and Azotobacter, assist sustainable agriculture through fertilization of the soil and reduction in dependence on chemical fertilizers. In a similar manner, genetically engineered strains or microbial metabolites produce biopesticides that provide alternatives to the use of chemical pesticides on crops and boost their yield and reduce their environmental toxicity, (Seenivasagan & Babalola, 2021). A schematic representation of the various application of bioprocessing have been represented in the figure given below in Figure 1.

Figure 1. Various application of bioprocessing

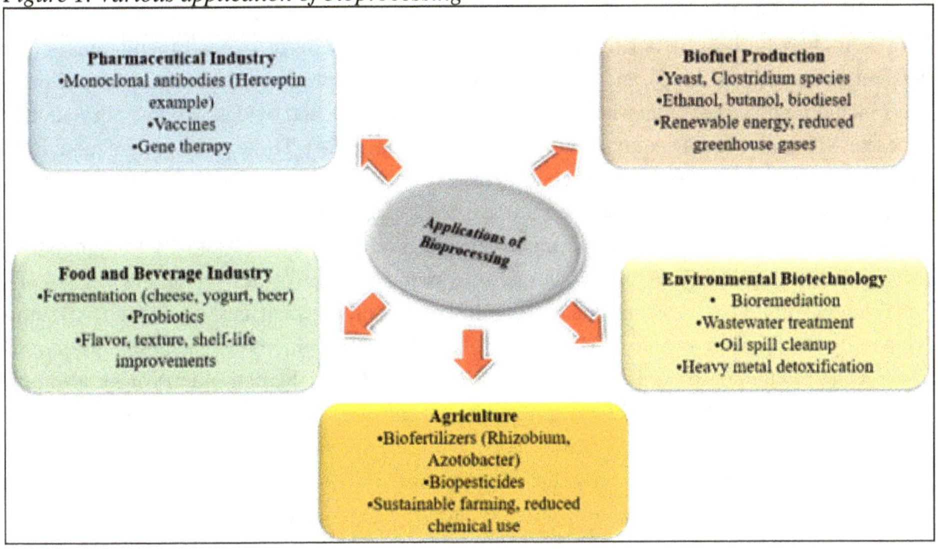

PRINCIPLES OF BIOPROCESSING

Bioprocessing is the employment of biological systems, which entail commercially desirable products. It is efficient based on basic principles such as the physiology of the microbes, the design of the bioreactor, and the management of contamination. The section discusses the main principles of the operation of bioprocessing.

Bioprocess Fundamentals

Microbial Physiology in Bioprocessing

The bioprocess fundamentals are the fundamental scientific principles that have led to the use of biological systems in industry for the production of useful products. They give the basis for developing, optimising, and scaling up processes from the bench to industrial scale. Understanding these fundamentals properly will mean the processes are efficient (high yields), scalable (working at small and large volumes), reproducible (produce the same quality every time to a high level) and sustainable (using a minimal amount of resources and minimising waste). The fundamentals of bioprocesses stand on three major poles; these are microbial physiology, microbial growth and product formation kinetics, and biochemical reaction thermodynamics. These principles enable scientists and engineers to predict process performance, optimize culture conditions, and troubleshoot manufacturing problems. Microbial physiology studies how the microbial cell carries out its functions, how a cell grows, divides, responds to environmental changes, and forms products. Its growth is highly dependent on environmental factors, including pH, oxygen and temperature, (Jagschies et al., 2018). Well-studied industrial microbes are, e.g., Escherichia coli and Saccharomyces cerevisiae (Parapouli et al., 2020) (selected from species with well-characterised metabolic networks). Transport systems at the cell membrane uptake nutrients, (Wang et al., 2025), and once intracellular, they are processed through metabolic pathways including glycolysis, the tricarboxylic acid (TCA) cycle, and oxidative phosphorylation to generate ATP and reducing equivalents, (Trejo-Solís et al., 2024). These pathways are modulated to keep homeostasis under different conditions, (Marcello, 2024; Lee, 1996). *Escherichia coli* is an optimal strain for recombinant protein expression for practical reasons, as it is a fast and genetically manipulable growing organism, despite problems with endotoxin contamination, (Madigan et al., 2021). *S. cerevisiae* is the most popular organism for producing ethanol and heterologous protein expressions due to its ability to fold proteins correctly and its GRAS status (Generally Recognised as Safe), (Madigan et al., 2018). Other microbes, including *Streptomyces* (for the production of antibiotics) and *Bacillus subtilis* (production of enzymes), also play significant roles, (McDonnell, 2020). In the era of systems and synthetic biology that microbial physiology can now see strain improvements toward higher yield, robustness and biosynthesis of new products, (Monod, 2012). Kinetics of microbial growth and metabolite formation govern the rate of growth and production of a metabolite in a given condition. Growth rates may be described by the Monod equation, (Munro, 2017).

μ=μmax[S]Ks+[S]\mu = \frac{\mu_{\text{max}} [S]}{K_s + [S]}μ=Ks+[S]μmax[S]

Where:

- μ = specific growth rate
- μmax = maximum growth rate
- [S] = substrate concentration
- Ks = half-saturation constant

Product formation can be either growth-associated (e.g., ethanol fermentation, where product is formed alongside microbial growth) or non-growth-associated (e.g., antibiotic production, where product accumulates mainly after growth slows), (Naik et al., 2010). In industry, these concepts guide strategies: ethanol production benefits from optimizing sugar feeding during growth, while antibiotics are harvested later for maximum yield.

Thermodynamics in bioprocessing determines whether a biochemical reaction is possible and how efficiently cells use energy. The feasibility of reactions is explained by Gibbs free energy (ΔG), (Neidhardt, Ingraham, & Schaechter, 1990):

ΔG=ΔG∘+RTlnQ\Delta G = \Delta G^\circ + RT \ln QΔG=ΔG∘+RTlnQ

Where:

- ΔG° = standard free energy change
- R = gas constant
- T = temperature
- Q = reaction quotient

The energy efficiency of microbial metabolism is optimized. Aerobic respiration generates more ATP per molecule of substrate, but anaerobic fermentation is less productive but faster, for anoxic environments. Thermodynamic principles are important in the context of metabolic engineering to balance ATP and NADH requirements, and can drive pathways towards a specific product. For instance, yields in biofuel and bioplastic production are raised. In brief, the microbiological (physiology, kinetics, and thermodynamics) aspects of processing comprise the basis of the bioprocessing. Physiology describes how microbes grow and metabolize, kinetics how fast they grow and produce end products, and thermodynamics whether or not the reaction is favoured and efficient. These basics inform the selection of the proper organisms for a product, the right culture conditions, and whether a metabolic pathway will be successful. Together, they make the earlier predictability, scalability, and sustainability, and allow biotechnology to continue to solve the industry problems across pharma, food, fuel, and materials.

Bioreactor Design and Operation

Types of Bioreactors

Stirred-Tank Bioreactors (STRs). The most popular systems for laboratory and industrial-scale bioprocesses are stirred-tank bioreactors. To guarantee adequate mixing of nutrients, gases, and microbial or cell cultures, they are outfitted with a mechanical agitation system, typically made up of impellers. The agitation keeps the environment uniform throughout the vessel and facilitates effective oxygen transfer. Because of this, STRs are very adaptable and appropriate for enzymatic reactions, mammalian cell culture, and microbial fermentation. Their usefulness in food biotechnology, biofuels, and pharmaceuticals is further increased by their scalability and adaptability to various operating conditions, (Nielsen & Keasling, 2016). One drawback, though, is the possibility of shear stress, which can harm delicate plant or mammalian cells.

Airlift Bioreactors. To create circulation and mixing, airlift bioreactors use gas sparging rather than mechanical agitation. The system usually has a riser and a downcomer area. The culture medium circulates naturally in the riser as a result of the sparged gas lowering the liquid density there. Airlift bioreactors are especially well-suited for shear-sensitive cells, including plant, animal, and filamentous microorganism cells, because of their design, which minimizes shear stress while ensuring effective gas-liquid mass transfer. Furthermore, compared to mechanically agitated systems, their comparatively simple design leads to lower operating and maintenance costs, (Nienow, 2006). Notwithstanding these benefits, airlift systems may not be as effective at transferring oxygen at very high cell densities, which would limit their use in some large-scale applications.

Packed-Bed Bioreactors. Because packed-bed bioreactors have a solid support matrix, immobilized cells or enzymes can stay in the system while the culture medium passes through the bed. This arrangement permits continuous operation for prolonged periods of time and improves cell stability and product yield. When recovering products from free-floating cells is difficult or when stabilizing enzymes for catalytic reactions is necessary, packed-bed reactors are especially useful. They have been widely employed in immobilized enzyme applications, wastewater treatment, and the synthesis of valuable metabolites, (Pasteur, 1857). However, there are drawbacks, particularly in large-scale operations, such as potential clogging, irregular flow distribution, and mass transfer restrictions.

Key Design Parameters. The design parameters of bioreactor are essential to the success of a bioprocess, as they will define the environment in which the cells are growing, mixing efficiency and the scalability of the process from laboratory to industrial scale. These are of importance, as they determine not only the performance of a process but also the uniformity of product quality and the repeatability over batches during large production runs. The key parameters that need to be properly controlled in a design are OTR, mixing efficiency and scale-up issues.

In aerobic cultures, usually the less soluble nutrient is oxygen. Oxygen transfer rate (OTR) is a measure of how efficiently oxygen (O_2) can be transferred from the gaseous take-phase to the liquid fermentation medium, where it becomes available to cells through the Process of oxidative phosphorylation. OTR is dependent on factors including bubble size, agitation rate, and type of impeller. Small bubbles offer more surface area for oxygen to diffuse, and greater agitation for mixing and dispersion, but both factors need to be balanced and controlled in a way that cells are not damaged. For instance, mammalian cell cultures for the production of monoclonal antibodies are severely hampered by inadequate oxygen supply, which lessens cell viability and forces cells to switch to anaerobic metabolism. This metabolic byproduct increases the level of lactate that acidifies the culture medium and decreases product formation, (Pirt, 1975). Therefore, it is critical to preserve the health of the cells and enforce high productivity in large pharmaceutical operations by controlling the OTR.

The other important aspect is mixing efficiency, which ensures that every part of the reactor gets a proper supply of nutrients, dissolved gases, as well as required pH. Insufficient mixing can cause gradients of various species to arise in different areas of the reactor, leading to "dead zones" where cells may be depleted of nutrients or laden with toxic byproducts. This leads to non-uniform growth and non-uniform product formation. But, too much mixing is just as bad, especially for sensitive cells. Products are subject to high shear forces during aggressive conditions, which may rupture sensitive mammalian or hybridoma cells. As an example, the agitation parameters, such as specific impeller type, rotation speed and power input, must be specially optimized in order to preserve the minimum level of homogeneity of nutrients and gases whilst avoiding excessive shear stress on cells for cultures of hybridoma and stem cells. This means that bioreactor designs have to constantly weigh the tradeoff between mixing efficiency while maintaining cell integrity, which often involves selecting a careful impeller and agitation strategies.

The third important feature of design parameters is scale-up. Bioprocesses that are successful at the laboratory scale frequently struggle to overcome significant hurdles during the transfer to industrial-scale bioreactors. Alterations in oxygen transfer, mixology, and heat removal can cause unforeseen performance challenges. To solve these problems, engineers use dimensionless numbers like the Reynolds number, power input per volume, and oxygen mass transfer coefficient (kLa) between systems in order to have a relative measure where comparisons across scales will lead to predictable performance of the system. These principles were most historically well documented as they relate to penicillin fermentation. As the process was scaled to industrial $100m^3$ fermenters from the lab, engineers carefully tuned aeration and oxygen transfer to retain antibiotic titres, (Rathore, Bhambure, & Ghare, 2010). This shows that scale-up is not only an increase of the vessel volume but entails a complete redesign of process parameters to maintain cellular performance and productivity at industrial scales.

Sterilization and Contamination Control

Though design criteria guarantee an optimal growth of cells, sterility is also an equally essential consideration in industrial bioprocessing. Due to the fact that bioprocesses use living systems, they are susceptible to contamination by undesired bacteria, fungi, or viruses. This type of contamination is not only responsible for reducing yields, but also can present a safety issue, which may result in a complete batch loss and severe economic damage. It is for this reason that sterilization and contamination control are central to the implementation of industrial bioprocesses.

Different materials or sterilizers can use different methods for sterilization. Among these methods, heat sterilization is the most commonly used. In lab environments, a key feature of any technology is its ability to be autoclaved to rid process contaminants, and on the industrial front, steam-in-place (SIP) technology becomes a necessity. SIP circulates steam under pressure through pipes, valves, and fermenter vessels to sterilize the vessels prior to inoculation. For example, antibiotic fermentation plants at the industrial scale rely largely on SIP to preserve the aseptic condition between production batches, thereby avoiding contamination and ensuring that the process can be reproduced, (Sandle, 2012; Shintani, 2016).

Alternatively, heat-labile substances such as vaccines, sera and culture medium components are sterile filtered. This procedure filters the solution through membranes with pores (0.1–0.2 μm) that physically capture the microorganisms without causing damage to these sensitive biomolecules. In vaccine production, filtration also fulfils a vital function by ridding virus suspensions of bacterial contamination and preserving their efficacy, (Shukla & Gottschalk, 2013). Another technique, chemical sterilization, is used when objects or instruments don't tolerate heat or pressure. Agents like ethylene oxide and hydrogen peroxide vapours are very efficient in eradicating microorganisms, but they are very hazardous and should be dealt with using proper safety measures and clothing because of their toxic status. An example of chemical sterilization in practice can be found in the manufacture of medical devices, where devices are sterilized with ethylene oxide prior to introduction into biomanufacturing facilities, (Shukla & Hinckley, 2008). Apart from sterilization, the measures of continuous prevention of contamination are required during the whole production process. Aseptic measures, e.g. closed systems, sterile connectors or laminar flow benches, during culture manipulations reduce the risk of culture contamination. The growing use of single-use technologies, such as commodity bags and tubing, has further minimised risks due to the fact that there is no expensive, repeatable cleaning and sterilization between runs and fewer opportunities for contamination, (Shukla & Thömmes, 2010). Antibiotics or antifungal agents are sometimes included in cultures as an additional protective measure against contamination by microorganisms, but the routine employment is not recommended due to the possibility of selecting resistant strains, (Simpson & Sastry, 2013). Environmental surveillance finally constitutes an essential part of the prevention of contamination. Through ongoing sampling of air, surfaces and water in production areas, contaminants can be detected at an earlier stage. Corrective actions, such as cleaning, stopping production, or discarding implicated lots, would be taken in response to contamination signals to maintain product safety and quality, (Singh et al., 2016).

INDUSTRIAL BIOMANUFACTURING

Using living cells to produce pharmaceuticals, biofuels, enzymes, and other high-value bioproducts on a large scale is known as industrial biomanufacturing. An outline of industrial biomanufacturing's main procedures and quality assurance methods is given in this section.

Overview of Industrial Biomanufacturing

Under strictly regulated circumstances, industrial biomanufacturing uses biological systems such as microbial, mammalian, or plant cells to create valuable commercial goods. To provide reliable, scalable, and sustainable manufacturing solutions, it combines developments in genetic engineering, biotechnology, and process engineering, (Tamime, 2009). This area has revolutionized the development and production of industrial materials, food products, energy sources, and pharmaceuticals.

Pharmaceuticals

Since the introduction of recombinant DNA technology and improvements in cell culture, pharmaceutical biomanufacturing has expanded rapidly. These days, mammalian cell lines such as CHO (Chinese hamster ovary) cells are used on an industrial scale to produce monoclonal antibodies, vaccines, gene therapies, and recombinant proteins. For treatments aimed at infectious, autoimmune, and cancerous conditions, biomanufacturing guarantees stringent process control, scalability, and product consistency. Single-use bioreactor systems and continuous bioprocessing are two innovations that further increase production efficiency and lower costs, (Tangyu et al., 2019).

Biofuels

A key component of the production of renewable energy is biomanufacturing. Ethanol and biodiesel are environmentally friendly substitutes for fossil fuels that are produced by microbial fermentation of agricultural feedstocks like corn, sugarcane, and lignocellulosic biomass. Next-generation biofuels that can be easily incorporated into current energy infrastructures, such as biobutanol, algal biofuels, and drop-in hydrocarbons, are the subject of increased research. Biofuels help lower carbon emissions and improve energy security, but there are still issues with scalability and feedstock constraints, (Van Dijl & Hecker, 2013).

Food & Beverages

Industrial biomanufacturing helps the food industry produce a variety of fermented foods, probiotics, and enzymes. Amylases, proteases, and lactases are examples of enzymes that enhance the nutritional value, texture, and efficiency of food processing. Probiotic cultures, which provide health advantages like enhanced gut microbiota and immune modulation, are added to functional foods and dietary supplements. Beer, cheese, yogurt, and other staple foods can be consistently produced on a large scale through the use of modern bioprocessing techniques in conjunction with traditional fermentation techniques, (Walsh, 2013).

Industrial Enzymes

One of the most important products of biomanufacturing is industrial enzymes. Enzymes like cellulases, lipases, and proteases are produced mostly by microbial fermentation and are used extensively in the pulp and paper, detergent, textile, and bio-based chemical industries. By increasing efficiency and reducing energy consumption, these biocatalysts offer environmentally friendly substitutes for harsh chemical processes. Recent developments in directed evolution and enzyme engineering have increased the stability and activity of enzymes, increasing their industrial uses, (Zeng & Sabra, 2011).

Biomanufacturing Processes

Upstream Processing (USP)

Upstream processing involves cell cultivation and biomass production under optimized conditions.

Steps in USP

1. **Strain Development:** To increase cell productivity, boost yields, and facilitate the creation of new biomolecules, genetic engineering methods like CRISPR and recombinant DNA technology are used, (Singh et al., 2025).
2. **Inoculum Preparation:** It involves increasing the size of a seed train bioreactor from a small laboratory culture to increasingly larger ones in order to guarantee steady growth and metabolic activity prior to large-scale production, (Ben Yahia et al., 2023).
3. **Fermentation/Bioreactor Cultivation:** Batch, fed-batch, and continuous modes are among the cultivation strategies; each offers unique benefits in terms of cost-effectiveness and productivity, (Kittler et al., 2025). To maintain ideal conditions for cell growth and metabolite production, critical process parameters like pH, dissolved oxygen (DO), temperature, and agitation are closely monitored and controlled, (Yang et al., 2024).

Challenges in USP

- Heterogeneous growth environments caused by oxygen limitation in large-scale bioreactors frequently result in decreased efficiency, (Arulrajah et al., 2025).
- Aeration and agitation-induced shear stress can harm sensitive cell lines, especially mammalian cultures used to produce therapeutic proteins. To lessen these difficulties, sophisticated bioreactor designs and computational fluid dynamics are being used more and more, (Kwon et al., 2024).

Downstream Processing (DSP)

After fermentation or cell culture, downstream processing (DSP) includes the recovery, separation, purification, and formulation of bioproducts. It is an important step in the bioprocessing process because it establishes the quality, safety, and effectiveness of the finished product, especially when producing therapeutic proteins, monoclonal antibodies, and vaccines. DSP seeks to guarantee purity and adherence to regulatory standards like those set forth by the FDA and EMA, in contrast to upstream processing, which is concentrated on optimizing yield. The entire cost of producing biopharmaceuticals is greatly increased by the resource-intensive DSP steps.

Steps in DSP

Harvesting & Cell Separation. Separating the desired biomolecules from the cellular biomass is the first stage in the DSP process. In order to rid the culture broth of cells, cell debris, and other particulate contaminants, this step is crucial. Typical methods include:

- **Centrifugation:** This method uses the density differences between the cells and the culture medium to separate them. It is frequently used in large-scale processes involving mammalian cells and microbial cultures.
- **Microfiltration:** This method effectively removes cells and large particles by using membranes with pore sizes that are usually between 0.1 and 0.5 μm. In comparison to centrifugation, this approach is especially beneficial because it is scalable and causes less shear stress, (Zhu et al., 2025).

Primary Purification. The target protein needs to be isolated from a complex mixture of host cell proteins, DNA, endotoxins, and other contaminants after the cell has been removed. Important strategies consist of:

- **Affinity chromatography:** This method is very effective for purifying monoclonal antibodies because it depends on interactions, such as Protein A binding to antibodies.
- **Ion-exchange chromatography:** This method allows for the enrichment of the target protein and the removal of charged contaminants by separating proteins according to net surface charge, (Mortensen & Williams, 2016).

Polishing & Formulation. Following the removal of the majority of impurities, further actions are necessary to stabilize the product and attain clinical-grade purity:

- **Ultrafiltration/diafiltration:** Membrane-based techniques for protein concentration, buffer exchange, and the elimination of impurities with low molecular weights.
- **Lyophilization (freeze-drying):** A formulation process that produces a stable powder by eliminating water at low pressure and temperature, improving the long-term stability of protein therapeutics.

Challenges in DSP

Downstream processing continues to be a significant production bottleneck for biopharmaceuticals despite technological advancements:

High Cost Contribution. DSP can make up between 60 and 80 percent of the total cost of production, mostly because it requires sterile conditions and costly chromatography resins and membranes, (Chitnis et al., 2024). Because of this, cost-cutting techniques like continuous DSP and substitute resin technologies are a top area of study.

Protein Instability. During purification and formulation, recombinant proteins—especially monoclonal antibodies and enzymes—are susceptible to denaturation, aggregation, or proteolytic degradation. These stability problems necessitate careful buffer, additive, and processing condition optimization because they impair product yield and efficacy, (Elsayed et al., 2023).

Quality Control and Assurance in Biomanufacturing

Quality Control (QC) in Biomanufacturing

QC ensures product consistency through analytical testing:

Identification Testing. SDS-PAGE and mass spectrometry methods verify that the generated biomolecule is molecularly identical to the intended product, (Gillespie et al., 2024).

Purity Testing. Purity testing guarantees that the finished product is devoid of endotoxins, DNA, host cell proteins, and other contaminants. Product-related and process-related contaminants are frequently separated and quantified using high-performance liquid chromatography (HPLC), whereas ELISA provides sensitive detection of contaminants like leftover proteins or viral particles, (Hernández-Longoria et al., 2021).

Potency Testing. To ensure the therapeutic product's clinical efficacy, potency assays quantify its biological activity. Functional activity and receptor binding are frequently assessed using cell-based assays, (Jia et al., 2021).

Quality Assurance (QA) Systems

Instead of depending only on testing the finished product, QA frameworks are intended to incorporate quality into the process and guarantee adherence to regulatory standards. Error prevention, consistency, and guaranteeing that biopharmaceutical products fulfil redetermined safety, efficacy, and quality standards are the main goals of these systems.

Good Manufacturing Practices (GMP). GMP is both the foundation of quality assurance in biomanufacturing and of comprehensive documentation, validated processes, and competent workers. Regulatory agencies (European Medicines Agency (EU GMP Annex 1), and the U.S. FDA (21 CFR Part 210/211)) define strict guidelines on the manufacturing of sterile products and on the qualification of equipment, facility design and control of raw materials. Having to achieve GMP compliance ensures that there is a traceability, minimizes the chances of contamination and increases regulatory confidence in the eventual end product, (Patel, Koç, & Otegbeye, 2025).

Process Validation. One vital QA method that ensures stability in the manufacturing process in terms of performance over multiple manufacturing cycles is process validation. Its three main phases are process design, process qualification and the continuous process verification. Manufacturers ensure robustness and reproducibility through the evaluation of such factors as consistency of yields, critical processes controls, and the performance of equipment. Besides enhancing production, it prevents the costly failures of a batch in production, (Ouranidis et al., 2021).

Environmental Monitoring. Quality assurance requires environmental monitoring particularly in aseptic processing environments where there is a high-level risk of contamination. This would include the frequent sampling of manufacturing surfaces, water systems and cleanroom air to locate microbiological and particulate contaminants. To provide sterility, such mechanisms as molecular assays, settle plates, and active air sampling are commonly used. The monitoring program also fixes alert and action limits that, in case of deviations, trigger corrective actions ensure the safety of products and regulatory compliance, and therefore, induce corrective actions, (Krämer & Federici, 2020).

Emerging Trends in QA/QC

Process Analytical Technology (PAT). Process Analytical Technology (PAT), that integrate advanced in-process analytical technologies into manufacturing process, is proactive ingredient to quality control. PAT also allows real-time monitoring and control of critical quality attributes (CQAs), such as pH, dissolved oxygen, nutrient concentrations, metabolite concentrations, and others, as an alternative to relying only on end-product testing. In the manufacturing process, one often applies the use of multi-parametric sensors, Raman spectroscopy and near-infrared (NIR) spectroscopy to determine the quality of the end product. This ensures that there is conformance with the Quality by Design (QbD), reduces failure of the batches and production variability, (Gibbons et al., 2023).

Single-Use Technologies. Disposable bioreactors, tubing, filters, and sampling systems are examples of single-use technologies (SUTs) that have grown in popularity in biomanufacturing because of their capacity to lower the risk of cross-contamination, lessen cleaning validation work, and increase operational flexibility. These systems are especially useful for small-batch personalized therapies and multiproduct facilities where quick process transitions are necessary. Additionally, SUTs support sustainable biomanufacturing practices by using less energy and water than conventional stainless-steel systems, (Barone et al., 2019).

EVALUATION OF BIOPROCESSES

Bioprocessing, as it is widely known, is the use of biological systems, including microbes, enzymes and cell cultures to manufacture drugs, chemicals and materials. Encompassing renewable feedstocks, modelling, and process optimisations ensure they are both economically and environmentally sustainable. Evaluation frameworks integrate techno-economic assessment (TEA) and life cycle assessment (LCA) as cost-effectiveness must be balanced with low environmental impact. It provides functionality for simulation, real-time monitoring and integrated design tools that enable scale-up, optimisation of resources, and compliance with sustainability requirements. This creates the building blocks of an innovative and future-proof bio-manufacturing sector, buttressed by sustainability through bioprocessing design and implementation, (Fu et al., 2023).

Process Optimisation and Scale-Up

In bioprocess evaluation, process optimisation and scale-up are key steps that allow transferring fermentations from the lab scale to production scale while optimising the yield, titer and productivity. The aforementioned integrated approach by Xia et al. integrates kinetic modelling, including the Monod equations, with CFD to incorporate microbial metabolism, oxygen transfer, mixing behaviour as well as shear stress. This approach relies on small-scale experiments to obtain relevant growth and metabolic parameters and phenomenological data, and CFD simulations to estimate flow patterns, volumetric mass transfer coefficients (kLa), and power input per unit vessel volume. Here, scale-up is directed by preserving dimensionless similarity (with parametric ellipses e.g. Reynolds and Power numbers) in order to ensure that local hydrodynamic features over scales are maintained while minimising oxygen or pH gradients that may inhibit cell function, (Bao, Ye, & Zhong, 2016). Complementary to this, Zhang, Hou, and Bao (2016) multi-scale analysis links online process variables such as dissolved oxygen, pH, temperature, oxygen uptake rate (OUR), carbon dioxide evolution rate (CER), and respiratory quotient (RQ) to environmental shifts, enabling real-time adjustment of feeding strategies. In *Bacillus subtilis* guanosine production, shifts in metabolic flux were identified that permitted redirection toward product synthesis; in *Pichia pastoris* fermentations, dissolved oxygen depletion was prevented by optimising medium composition and feeding profiles and in antibiotic fermentations, yields were improved by up to 30% through CFD-informed adjustments. The report further stated that scale-up of this strategy to 100 m^3 has been demonstrated at the industrial scale for the production of guanosine, recombinant proteins, penicillin, erythromycin, and avermectin. These approaches are aspirational because biological variability and computational challenges are significant hurdles to overcome, yet the combination of CFD, kinetic modelling, and multi-scale monitoring can benefit process predictability and scalability while minimising trial-and-error experimentation, ultimately leading to rapid commercialisation of sustainable biomanufacturing, (de Mello et al., 2024).

Both process optimisation and scale-up of the process are key aspects in bioprocess evaluation, central to translating laboratory discovery to successful industrial production, which has been covered in several reviews on bioreactor scale-up strategies in general. In the case of optimisation, this is commonly done at bench scale in 1–15 L bioreactors or shake flasks where parameters such as nutrient composition, pH, temperature, agitation rate, aeration and operational mode (batch, fed-batch or continuous) are optimised to maximise biomass yield and product titer while minimising overall cost. Owing to the nature of experimental design methodologies, as well as kinetic modelling, these optimised parameters are later validated with independent experiments for reproducibility. The next stage of scale-up is pilot-scale bioreactors (50 – 500 L) and then the fully implemented industrial systems to mirror their bench-scale performance while addressing a number of common engineering constraints, including mass and heat transfer limitations, delivering oxygen, as well as enhanced viscosity, (Du et al., 2022). Ways to achieve successful scale-up are by having geometric similarity such as constant height-to-diameter ratios (H:D), and retaining important process parameters. In these comparisons, the aerated reactors are characterised by kLa values that are kept constant throughout all aerobic process conditions; non-aerated systems by power/volume (P/V) net value and stirred tank reactors by adequate Re numbers to ensure similar mixing efficiencies. The pneumatic bioreactors are in favour of higher gas holdup and better bubble dynamics, whereas photobioreactors put more emphasis on surface to volume ratios and optimum light irradiance. The requirements change in the case of solid-state fermentations, which include but are not limited to air flow and porosity control owing to low moisture. Examples range from scaling itaconic acid production from 5 L to 50 L at constant kLa for equivalent biomass yields of (12–12.2 g/L), to scaling biohydrogen production from molasses across scales of 50-10,000L reactors with consistent trends in gas production. When we combine iterated scaling with CFD-based hydrodynamic simulations, these integrated high-quality methods to accommodate cell requirements to engineering constraints reduce risks and also promote sustainable biomanufacturing, (Clementschitsch & Bayer, 2006).

Mathematical modeling is vital for process optimization and scale-up, which improves the efficiency and productivity of industrial bio-manufacturing. Mechanistic modeling strategies like unstructured Monod kinetics for microbial growth, constraintbased modeling (CBM), flux balance analysis (FBA) and metabolic flux analysis (MFA) help gain an understanding of cellular metabolism and prediction of fermentation parameters namely, optimal medium formulation, pH, temperature, and substrate uptake rates. For example, FBA provides theoretical maximum yields and MFA can determine metabolic flux distributions for given process conditions which can then be used to optimize bioethanol or antibiotic production. In contrast to mechanistic models that rely on fundamental principles, data-driven methods based on machine learning (ML) such as support vector machines and artificial neural networks analyze large datasets to predict process outputs and optimize parameters without previous mechanistic knowledge of the system. ML, as either a complement or alternative to traditional CBM, results in enhanced prediction accuracy and applicability in CNCS, so there is a growing interest in hybrid approaches. These modelling strategies, which help to factor in observed environmental gradients typically developed during scale-up evaluation in larger bioreactors that influence cell functional fitness and product quality. The integration of biological models with CFD facilitates the simulation of hydrodynamics, mass transfer, and metabolic response; employing either Euler-Lagrange or Euler–Euler computational frameworks, which are used to predict heterogeneity, shear stress effects, and the loss of yield. The integrated modelling provides a rational basis for process design, reduces experimental burden and aids in a sustainable and reliable scale-up, (Rathore et al., 2021). In conclusion, process optimization and scale-up are key steps in bioprocess assessment in order to validate that the laboratory method can be transferred to a production scale without loss of product quality, product yield, or process stability. Optimization is thus the fine-tuning of operating parameters like mixing, mass and heat transfer, pH control, nutrient and oxygen delivery, to attain the highest productivity at minimum cost. This requires a thorough knowledge of microbial or cell culture physiology since minor perturbations in conditions can greatly alter growth kinetics, product synthesis and process robustness. Scale-up takes these parameters, developed at the small, laboratory bioreactor level, to pilot and industrial units, but introduces large-scale issues that have to be solved, e.g. Scale-up of chemical engineering unit operations involves some complicated process such as homogeneous mixing, shear damage and various volumetric oxygen transfer rates due to larger volume. On the other hand, scale-down models are used to simulate industrial conditions in the lab for the purpose of troubleshooting, risk prediction, and process optimisation on a small scale without the costs of full-size trials. This combined optimization and scale-up demands an interdisciplinary approach, encompassing bioprocess engineering, real-time analytical monitoring, and compliance with regulatory metrics, notably in the manufacture of pharmaceutical and high-value bio-based products. These stages help to minimise operational risks, enhance regulatory approval processes, and better economic viability, hence environmental sustainability if executed efficiently, thus forming the cornerstone for commercialisation of a bioproduct, (Lisci, Grosso, & Tronci, 2020).

Bioprocess Monitoring and Control

Bioprocess monitoring and control are crucial aspects of bioprocessing and industrial biomanufacturing providing production efficiency, product quality assurance, and compliance with various regulatory frameworks including the Process Analytical Technology (PAT) initiative. Recombinant protein production in microbial systems is complex due to the coupling of host cell metabolism with expression of the heterologous gene and requires improved monitoring strategies to develop the protein process faster and more economically. Most of the traditional monitoring approaches depend on a small set of online sensors that measure these physical and chemical parameters like temperature, pH, dissolved oxygen, and substrate concentration. Nevertheless, these parameters mostly overlook biologically meaningful variables such as biomass density, cell viability status, metabolic load, and PCN (ratio of recombinant gene to genome content). Selective, shape-preserving, non-invasive measurements by state-of-the-art sensor technologies, such as dielectric spectroscopy (e.g., Biomass Monitor for viable cell capacitance), 2D-fluorescence spectrometry (e.g., BioView for intracellular fluorophores like NAD(P)H), infrared spectrometry (e.g., FossNIR-Systems for cellular constituents), mass spectrometry (e.g., PTR-MS for volatile compounds), and metal oxide field effect transistors (e.g., ALPHA M.O.S for sensor arrays) with responder (RS) arrays and the device reading mathematical modelling to correlate their readings with offline data points. These state-of-the-art devices have disadvantages like drift and a need for recalibration and indirect measurement. Employing innovative methods that combine online measurements with predictive modelling has demonstrated the possibility of tracking offline variables continuously, thus providing a tool for early detection of critical conditions. Abstract: An example of the use of readily accessible online data to predict a complex biological variable in this case, the recombinant *E. coli* fed-batch cultivation processes to improve monitoring capabilities, ultimately providing baseline information for model-based processes supervision and control, (Brignoli et al., 2020). Biological systems, which are innately variable and susceptible to environmental disturbances, could benefit from proper control strategies to sustain essential operational conditions for bioprocesses. Although basic control methods including open loop methods and proportion–integral–derivative (PID) controllers are still in use, more dynamic and complex control strategies have also developed, cascade control, model predictive approaches (MPC), fuzzy logic, artificial neural networks (ANN), and hybrid model-based systems to rank among others. Such techniques facilitate controlled and efficient management of process variability, perhaps due to the non-linear dynamics of the system behaviours that is essential for maximising process performance. Incorporating soft sensors, AI-based analytics and automation improve the mixing environment allowing for drug disturbance prediction, real-time adaptability, and reproducibility enhancement. Successfully controlling bioprocesses not only lessens the likelihood of batch failure, reduces cost of goods sold but also allows for rapid and consistent scale-up through replicating lab-optimized conditions at industrial scale. This enables the manufacturing process to be economically viable and environmentally sustainable while adhering to the current regulatory requirements as outlined under Quality by Design (QbD) and Process Analytical Technologies (PAT) initiatives, (Butler, 2005). Bioprocess monitoring and control applications range from biopharmaceuticals, enzymes, bio-based chemicals to biofuels. Monitoring refers to capturing of a continuous or at least periodic measurement of crucial quality attributes (CQAs) and critical process parameters (CPPs) including nutrient concentrations, biomass density, pH temperature over production cycles in bioreactors and fermentation tanks. Real-time sensors, data analytics, and automated control systems allow for rapid detection of process deviations and immediate correction, preserving product yield and quality. Not only do they help to comply with regulations, but at the same time lower costs and increase efficiency while speeding up innovative product formulations such as vaccines, antibiotics and sustainable fuels. The use of these products in manufacturing leads to better health outcomes, better pharmaceutical competitiveness, and environmental sustainability, (Abo-Zaid et al., 2020). Although bioprocessing has been utilized for centuries, for example in the fermentation of dough, the complexity of contemporary three-phase systems (containing a liquid, gas, and solid) makes them particularly difficult to monitor and control. Many essential biological variables have limited on-line measurement tools available, which complicates precise control. New methods, like the adjustable-structure geometric observer, which is a model-based soft sensor, have recently been developed and appear to perform better than extended Kalman filters in the presence of noise. For instance, Lisci, Grosso, and Tronci (2020) used these methods to estimate bioreactor variables, while Brignoli et al. (2020) implemented feedforward–feedback controller with dielectric spectroscopy as the control input to control specific growth rates in *Kluyveromyces marxianus* fed-batch cultures and cope up with the noise and exponential growth nature of the process. Similar cases exist for scaling up and optimising; for example, Abo-Zaid et al. (2020) upscaled siderophore production from fluorescent Pseudomonas using exponential fed-batch fermentation, resulting in higher yields and an effective biocontrol against plants fungal diseases, and Zhang et al. (2020) with a bactericide secretion optimisation from *Bacillus subtilisnatto*, resulting in confirmed antimicrobial activity against pathogens. In sequencing batch reactors, Kim, Hong, and Choi (2020) developed a method of enriching selenate-reducing bacteria which allowed potassium selenate to be reduced at the same time with nitrate. In case of analytical monitoring, Feidl et al. (2019) improved monoclonal antibody tracking from chromatography through Raman Spectroscopy coupled with a Kalman filter for signal noise reduction. Additionally, Youssef et al. designed zoned IR heating-based model predictive controllers for bird egg incubation and HVAC systems with model-based prediction of human thermal sensation via support vector machines. Conjugated macromolecules for biological sample biosensing have been summarised by Krywko-Cendrowska, Szweda, and Szweda (2020), (Krause et al., 2011; Jiménez-González & Woodley, 2010).

In specific applications like brewing technology, efficient yeast propagation is essential for the quality of subsequent processes, so bioprocess monitoring and control are invaluable. In this context, a major challenge has been the unavailability of online detection tools for the key characteristics of yeast and an inability to build effective temporal control systems. To cope these problems intelligent approaches based on right parameter identification combined with expert linguistic steering by means of fuzzy logic or state observers have been proposed in literature. Ultrasonic-based devices show promise for monitoring key process parameters, but cannot be used inline because they are affected by fluctuations in temperature and gas bubbles. Adaptive sensor calibration approaches, based on the temperature dependencies of the time-of-flight and frequency characteristics of ultrasonic waves, have been implemented to address these challenges. Using offline data, maximum prediction errors for solute concentrations (maltose and ethanol) in aqueous solutions of 0.48 g/100 g have been achieved with multivariate models. In addition, literature-derived mechanistic models of growth were also used to model yeast based on temperature, and included simulations for biomass production, ethanol yield, and substrate uptake. Such developments allow the regulation of aeration and temperature in a more flexible way contributing to yeast maintenance, boosting transparency on the process and prompting the operations closer to the principles of the PAT for real-time validation and efficiency, (Petrides, 2000).

Economic and Environmental Evaluation of Bioprocesses

Assessing bioprocesses for use in bioprocessing and industrial bio-manufacture is central to supporting sustainable development, whereby economic and environmental considerations are given equivalent significance. Fermentation, microbial catalysis and enzyme-mediated processes are used in the development of bioprocesses comprising low-value chemicals along with pharmaceuticals based on renewable feedstocks. Consequently, sustainability in these systems needs sophisticated modelling for an objective evaluation of processes. Simulation & optimisation Process systems engineering is essential for an assessment of new process options and the design of biorefineries at a more integrated level. The existing databases (e.g., EPA DSSTox) do not cover all of the compounds considered here, so new property models are needed to provide more accurate assessments. The use of life cycle assessment (LCA) and life cycle inventory methodologies substantially advances the ability to quantify global environmental footprints, laying a cornerstone that combines sustainability metrics together with economic feasibility to guide innovation. The next generation of engineers will need to have the skills necessary to design cost-effective, ecologically responsible bioprocesses. Mechanistic modelling, data driven techniques and their hybridisations, like proposed in "Optimization and Scale-Up of Fermentation Processes Driven by Model", can aid in gaining important insights on scaling challenges, yield prediction and optimisation. Despite focusing on different aspects of bioprocesses, "Improvement of Bioprocess Monitoring" stresses the need for real-time monitoring, allowing to shortening development cycles, while "Bioprocesses: Modeling Needs" emphasises that various types of modelling are essential to adhere to principles related to sustainability, (Krömer et al., 2020). Economic and environmental evaluations form the crux of the design optimization and sustainability of bioprocesses for industrial bio-manufacturing. Petrides et al., describe modeling methodologies of bioprocess simulation and scheduling, which provide an organised approach to process model and resource allocation with respect to economic feasibility. This is especially applicable in process manufacturing industries such as pharmaceutical and chemical production, where operational efficiency and cost-effectiveness are critical. Utilising modern simulation and scheduling tools like those developed by Intelligen, Inc. helps reduce the development time and costs. Simultaneously in, wise ecological aspects help towards LCA, where it compares planned practices not only in terms of output and industrial performance, but also footprint so that green manufacturing would not be at the expense of losing the green of the environment, (Ögmundarson et al., 2020). Integrating economic and environmental performance within a joint evaluation framework is important for minimizing the overall cost and environmental impact of biochemical production and supports the development of a sustainable bioeconomy. We propose an effort to assess economic/techno-economic assessment (TEA) and LCA indicators through their integration in a single score, to help in the clear demarcation of trade-offs over the biochemical life cycle. This approach solves two of the most significant issues of our time, economic barriers, like poor cost-competitiveness driven by erratic fossil-based chemical and biofeedstock markets, and sustainability risks, where prioritising economic savings in first-of-a-kind biofuel plants, for example, could lead to increased environmental damage by embracing cost-saving shortcuts. The objective of early-stage optimisation is critical to alleviating technical and economic barriers as integrally highlighted by the growth trajectory of the biochemical industry, wherein production doubled from 2011 to 2018 and the biochemicals producing over 20% of the global market by 2025 are projected. This framework improves early-stage decision-making by establishing consistent system boundaries and adopting quantitative metrics of sustainability that ensure that biochemicals are economically viable and environmentally sustainable. This comprehensive method enables hotspots to be identified, and resources to be optimised and footprint reduction, consistent with the global shift away from fossil-derived chemicals and chemistries towards sustainable alternatives, (Cristofoli et al., 2023). While the two aspects are justified as independent and are often assessed separately, economic and environmental assessments are equally important for the purpose of integrating and optimising fermentation processes in industrial bio-manufacturing. This recent work, demonstrates the benefit of simulation tools for not only outsized process efficiency, but also economic performance. Such tools allow for detailed process modelling, which is invaluable for cost estimation, resource management, and operational planning, critical elements for cost-effective scale-up. Despite not going into detail on metrics of environmental performance, as these are hardly covered in the literature, the implicit drive for cost reduction by means of simulation links again to the bigger sustainability picture. Simulation tools serve the dual purposes of ensuring that the designs are economically viable while simultaneously minimising environmental impacts in modern industrial bio-manufacturing by uncovering strategies that are cost-effective and designs that are optimal, (Ali et al., 2024). The production of bio-aromatics, such as para-hydroxybenzoic acid (pHBA), stand out the most from a focus on economic process evaluation and environmental LCA. The study by Krömer et al. gives an combined analysis of the production costs along with environmental impacts considering parameters, including culture pH, carbon source and process scale. As one of the most lucrative derivatives available, fuel and chemical users are less focused on valuing bio-based aromatics against petrochemical-derived alternatives for all but criterial applications where sustainability or health safety might be key discriminators. Most of the synthetic biology and metabolic engineering strategies target to improve yields/productivities to be comparable to well-established bulk bioprocesses as demonstrated in amino acid production. The LCA part of this study highlights environmental trade-offs, sensitivity to fermentation parameters determining impacts, while the economic aspect demonstrates that it is challenging to reach cost competitive scale vs. production based on fossils. Finally, the study stresses that early-stage optimization is well placed to spot cost and environmental hotspots to unlock a transition from bio-aromatics as niche products to serious market players. This paper is an integrated assessment of a frequently neglected aspect of biocatalyst development: the connection between strain engineering and overall process economics & sustainability, (Khang & Akhai, 2024).

Viewed from these different angles, evaluating the industrial bio-manufacturing processes of biotechnology calls for an assessment on two levels: economic performance and environmental impact. When coupled with life cycle and techno-economic assessments, advanced simulation, optimisation and monitoring tools facilitate the development of bioprocesses that are competitive but also sustainable. By understanding model-based journalism, metrics of sustainability and insight into the real-time processes, we can design systems more effectively without sacrificing environmental integrity. Industry will find that employing both economic and environmental frameworks gives weight to decision making at early development stages--while at mean time attracting new trade circles with the globe's increased emphasis on sustainability studies as a complete solution for all. However, both at national and international levels, it is obvious nowadays that an ecological framework for sustainable development gives considerable support in the face of the cutthroat competition of bio-based industries.

FUTURE PERSPECTIVES AND CHALLENGES

The field of bioprocessing and industrial bio-manufacturing is being revolutionized, enabling biological products ranging from therapeutic proteins to sustainable biofuels to be developed, optimized, and scaled for worldwide markets, (Jenzsch et al., 2018). This is a transition of the industry from mostly empirical, trial-and-error practices towards data-driven, model-based, and completely integrated production systems. The change is motivated by technological improvements across fields of synthetic biology, high-throughput analytics, automation and artificial intelligence (AI) that jointly are expected to accelerate the pace of product development and enhance quality while reducing costs, (Isoko et al., 2024). With further development combining some of the most advanced technologies across sectors, the future view is of even more networked, smart, and sustainable manufacturing platforms able to address increasing global needs for pharmaceuticals, speciality chemicals, food ingredients and renewable energy carriers. This evolution will provide both opportunities and challenges as the increased technical complexity, regulatory burden, cost containment, along with the resolve to have a lean workforce skill, will necessitate a balanced approach between innovation and operational excellence, (Turanli et al., 2024).

Emerging Trends in Bioprocessing and Biomanufacturing

One of the most prominent trends in the field is the growing adoption of continuous bioprocessing. Continuous systems provide stable product output, improved process control, and increased manufacturing flexibility compared to classic batch operations. If these systems are integrated with real-time monitoring under the Process Analytical Technology (PAT) framework, they can be adjusted for changes in the quality of raw materials or environmental conditions so that the product quality is maintained, (Samaras, Micheletti, & Ding, 2022). In conjunction with the Quality by Design (QbD) principles, continuous bioprocessing allows a move to more efficient and predictable manufacturing streams, (Morgado et al., 2018). The other exciting avenue is the application of high-level modeling technologies, such as mechanistic kinetic models, genome-scale metabolic models, and computational fluid dynamics (CFD), integrated with AI/Machine Learning analytics. This would enable a manufacturer to predict and mimic bioreactor performance in different conditions or feeding strategies, or determine bottlenecks that may not be apparent before they occur, (Chen et al., 2020). This predictive capability enables rapid process development before scaling-up from lab and for industrial manufacturing. These kinds of developments in single-use technologies have also been influencing the way (mostly biopharmaceutical) facilities are now being designed. This strategy decreases cleaning and sterilization as well as turnaround times and contamination risks through the use of disposable bioreactors, mixers and filtration units, (Tawo & Mbamalu, 2025). The modular nature of the systems allows for quick changeover between products, useful in personalized medicine where production runs may be smaller and different from one another. Furthermore, the rise of synthetic biology and cell-free systems is an opportunity. Recent developments in synthetic biology have made it possible to use engineered microorganisms and cascades of in vitro enzymes that biosynthesize many complex molecules for which there had been impractical (or too costly) traditional chemical synthesis, (Qadir, 2023). This trend both broadens the spectrum of conceivable products and offers more sustainable manufacturing options replacing petrochemical processes by biochemical ones. As already mentioned, industrial scales of process integration will be made possible by digital transformation, i.e., Industry for biomanufacturing. Progress in cloud-based data platforms, digital twins, and advanced process control systems will harmonize research, development, and manufacturing operations in the areas of real-time visibility and decision-making, (Zhao et al., 2024). This integration enables enterprises to build and maintain transparency, increase compliance with regulations and respond quickly to changes in the market or disruptions in the supply chain. As it is; sustainability becomes an integral driver of innovation. Process design will now be incorporating renewable feedstocks, energy efficient operations and waste valorization right from inception. Recent metabolic engineering developments are no longer restricted to the use of traditional substrates but instead allow bio-production from unusual non-traditional substrates including lignocellulosic biomass, industrial off-gases and food waste for production of bio-based fuels, chemicals and materials. This brings biomanufacturing in line with wider environmental and circular economy ambitions.

Challenges and Opportunities in the Field

There are also significant challenges that the field faces, despite these advances. Technical complexity is a significant challenge as the multi-technology integration between biological, chemical, mechanical and digital elements require extensive interdisciplinary knowledge, (Vegineni, 2025). For example, continuous processes require advanced process control systems that are able to manage large numbers of interacting variables in real time and while AI can be beneficial in this context the training of models relies on good quality, robust datasets which can be hard to come by Filippi, Mekkattu, and Katzschmann (2025). Compliance with regulation is another challenge to overcome, which becomes even more difficult for products destined for the pharmaceutical markets. In the case of novel production methods, such as continuous manufacturing or synthetic biology-based platforms, which may sit outside existing regulatory frameworks this can mean a lack of stability in terms of approval processes. Interlocking of industry and regulatory agencies ensures innovation is disarmed by clawing, safety, efficacy breathes in no menacing shadows. However, one recurring issue is how to scale up the technology especially for processes containing mammalian cells, sophisticated metabolic pathways or large-scale microbial fermentations. Despite the developed models and CFD, unforeseen environmental gradients or shear stress effects can appear at industrial levels, (Chien et al., 2021), and lead to oxygen limitation issues, affecting yield and quality. Such opportunities can be realized through the development of more robust scale-down models that match large-scale conditions and permit early troubleshooting and optimization at laboratory scale. Of course, economic matters do not stay behind in this case. Although single-use bioreactors, real-time sensors, and automation provide advanced technologies to increase efficiencies, they are expensive to purchase and install. The main challenge might be that small- and medium-sized enterprises (SMEs) will find it hard to invest in such infrastructure without a well-defined return on investment, (Ullah et al., 2023). This can be possible with innovative business models, common manufacturing facilities, and public–private partnerships.

In the future, continuous bioprocessing, in silico modelling, AI-driven analytics, and sustainable design principles will likely form the backbone of industrial biomanufacturing going forward. The new facilities will be smarter, suppler and cleaner with the ability to produce more different types of products in better quality and at a lower cost. The road ahead is fraught with significant technical, regulatory and economic challenges, but the abundance of opportunities contributes to the continued maturation of bioprocessing/bio-manufacturing as a field driven by real-world need for healthcare, energy, materials and environmental remediation.

CONCLUSION

Bioprocessing and industrial bio-manufacturing are the core technologies for current sustainable production systems, enabling conversion of renewable feedstocks to value-added products like pharmaceuticals, speciality chemicals, biofuels and biopolymers. In order to support not only the operational efficiency but also the inherently sustainable operation of these processes, it is necessary to evaluate optimisation and scale-up, monitoring and control as well as economic and environmental assessment. Optimisation and scale-up processes help to maximise the benefits of laboratory research on an industrial scale, adopting computational tools, mechanistic or hybrid modelling techniques, and integrating real-time data to ensure product quality and yield scalability. Monitoring and control strategies, combined with high-level sensors, automation and predictive algorithms, allow adjustments to be proactive & implemented in biological systems that are ever changing maintaining process stability for regulatory compliance. Therefore, economic and environmental evaluations are necessary to use techno-economic assessment (TEA) and life cycle assessment (LCA) models that consolidate a cradle-to-gate methodology. They look at trade-offs and balances between cost and environmental impact, which can help design processes that are competitive and sustainable. Integrating these assessments early on allows for innovations to be market-viable and environmentally sustainable. These include on the one hand, modern technologies such as continuous bioprocessing, single-use technologies, AI-driven analytics and digital twins, and on the other, small to large-scale manufacturing platforms. Nevertheless, many challenges remain to address scale-up complexity, regulatory evolution, high capital costs and interdisciplinary labour upskilling, which will require a sustained effort from the entire community. In this book, the development and assessment of bioprocesses is considered in its totality, combining engineering excellence with data-driven understanding in tandem with principles of sustainability. With an approach of systematic operations optimisation, performance monitoring and economic/environmental trade-offs, the bio-factory sector can address market-driven demand for the next generation of industrial solutions, greener and more resistant bioproducts available from innovative design. This systemic approach gives a competitive advantage and is necessary to move us beyond the circular bioeconomy.

REFERENCES

Abo-Zaid, G. A., Soliman, N. A., Abdullah, A. S., El-Sharouny, E. E., Matar, S. M., & Sabry, S. A. (2020). Maximization of siderophores production from biocontrol agents, *Pseudomonas aeruginosa* F2 and *Pseudomonas fluorescens* JY3 using batch and exponential fed-batch fermentation. *Processes (Basel, Switzerland)*, *8*(4), 455. Advance online publication. DOI: 10.3390/pr8040455

Abu, R., Gundersen, M. T., & Woodley, J. M. (2015). Thermodynamic calculations for systems biocatalysis. In *Computer aided chemical engineering* (Vol. 37, pp. 233–238). Elsevier., DOI: 10.1016/B978-0-444-63576-1.50037-6

Ali, M., Shabbir, K., Ali, S., Mohsin, M., Kumar, A., Aziz, M., Zubair, M., & Sultan, H. M. (2024). A new era of discovery: How artificial intelligence has revolutionized biotechnology. *Nepal Journal of Biotechnology*, *12*(1), 1–1. DOI: 10.3126/njb.v12i1.67165

Arulrajah, P., Lievonen, A. E., Subaşı, D., Pagal, S., Weuster-Botz, D., & Heins, A. L. (2025). Scale-down bioreactors—Comparative analysis of configurations. *Bioprocess and Biosystems Engineering*. Advance online publication. DOI: 10.1007/s00449-025-03158-4

Azubuike, C. C., Chikere, C. B., & Okpokwasili, G. C. (2016). Bioremediation techniques—Classification based on site of application: Principles, advantages, limitations and prospects. *World Journal of Microbiology & Biotechnology*, *32*(11), 180. Advance online publication. DOI: 10.1007/s11274-016-2137-x

Bailey, J. E., & Ollis, D. F. (2018). *Biochemical engineering fundamentals* (2nd ed.). McGraw-Hill.

Bao, J., Ye, Q., & Zhong, J. J. (Eds.). (2016). *Bioreactor engineering research and industrial applications II*. Springer., DOI: 10.1007/978-3-662-48347-3

Barone, P. W., Avgerinos, S., Ballard, R., Brussel, A., Clark, P., Dowd, C., Gerentes, L., Hart, I., Keumurian, F. J., Kindermann, J., & Leung, J. C. (2019). Biopharmaceutical industry approaches to facility segregation for viral safety: An effort from the consortium on adventitious agent contamination in biomanufacturing. *PDA Journal of Pharmaceutical Science and Technology*, *73*(2), 191–203. DOI: 10.5731/pdajpst.2018.009118

Barrangou, R., & Doudna, J. A. (2016). Applications of CRISPR technologies in research and beyond. *Nature Biotechnology*, *34*(9), 933–941. DOI: 10.1038/nbt.3659

Ben Yahia, B., Piednoir, A., Dahomais, T., Eggermont, S., & Paul, W. (2023). "Organized stress" for robust scale-up of intensified production process with fed-batch seed bioreactor. *Biotechnology and Bioengineering*, *120*(9), 2509–2522. DOI: 10.1002/bit.28487

Bhardwaj, D., Ansari, M. W., Sahoo, R. K., & Tuteja, N. (2014). Biofertilizers function as key player in sustainable agriculture by improving soil fertility, plant tolerance and crop productivity. *Microbial Cell Factories*, *13*, 66. Advance online publication. DOI: 10.1186/1475-2859-13-66

Brignoli, Y., Freeland, B., Cunningham, D., & Dabros, M. (2020). Control of specific growth rate in fed-batch bioprocesses: Novel controller design for improved noise management. *Processes (Basel, Switzerland)*, *8*(6), 679. Advance online publication. DOI: 10.3390/pr8060679

Buchner, E., & Rapp, R. (1899). Alkoholische gährung ohne hefezellen. *Berichte der Deutschen Chemischen Gesellschaft*, *32*(1), 127–137. DOI: 10.1002/cber.18990320120

Bud, R. (1994). *The uses of life: A history of biotechnology*. Cambridge University Press.

Butler, M. (2005). Animal cell cultures: Recent achievements and perspectives in the production of biopharmaceuticals. *Applied Microbiology and Biotechnology*, *68*(3), 283–291. DOI: 10.1007/s00253-005-1980-8

Cappia, J. M. (2004). Principles of steam-in-place. *Pharmaceutical Technology*, *24*(Suppl.), S40.

Chandrababu, K. B., Kannan, A., Savage, J. R., Stadmiller, S., Ryle, A. E., Cheung, C., Kelley, R. F., Maa, Y. F., Saggu, M., & Bitterfield, D. L. (2024). Stability comparison between microglassification and lyophilization using a monoclonal antibody. *Journal of Pharmaceutical Sciences*, *113*(4), 1054–1060. DOI: 10.1016/j.xphs.2023.11.022

Chen, X., Zhou, L., Tian, K., Kumar, A., Singh, S., Prior, B. A., & Wang, Z. (2013). Metabolic engineering of *Escherichia coli*: A sustainable industrial platform for bio-based chemical production. *Biotechnology Advances*, *31*(8), 1200–1223. DOI: 10.1016/j.biotechadv.2013.08.009

Chen, Y., Yang, O., Sampat, C., Bhalode, P., Ramachandran, R., & Ierapetritou, M. (2020). Digital twins in pharmaceutical and biopharmaceutical manufacturing: A literature review. *Processes (Basel, Switzerland)*, *8*(9), 1088. Advance online publication. DOI: 10.3390/pr8091088

Chien, F., Ngo, Q. T., Hsu, C. C., Chau, K. Y., & Iram, R. (2021). Assessing the mechanism of barriers towards green finance and public spending in small and medium enterprises from developed countries. *Environmental Science and Pollution Research International*, *28*(43), 60495–60510. DOI: 10.1007/s11356-021-14907-1

Chitnis, A. V., Nair, L. L., Gupta, D., & Dhoble, A. S. (2024). Non-sterile cultivation of oleaginous organisms. *Trends in Biotechnology*, *42*(12), 1583–1587. DOI: 10.1016/j.tibtech.2024.06.004

Clementschitsch, F., & Bayer, K. (2006). Improvement of bioprocess monitoring: Development of novel concepts. *Microbial Cell Factories*, *5*, 19. Advance online publication. DOI: 10.1186/1475-2859-5-19

Cristofoli, N. L., Lima, A. R., Tchonkouang, R. D., Quintino, A. C., & Vieira, M. C. (2023). Advances in the food packaging production from agri-food waste and by-products: Market trends for a sustainable development. *Sustainability*, *15*(7), 6153. Advance online publication. DOI: 10.3390/su15076153

de Mello, A. F., de Souza Vandenberghe, L. P., Herrmann, L. W., Letti, L. A., Burgos, W. J., Scapini, T., Manzoki, M. C., de Oliveira, P. Z., & Soccol, C. R. (2024). Strategies and engineering aspects on the scale-up of bioreactors for different bioprocesses. *Systems Microbiology and Biomanufacturing*, *4*(2), 365–385. DOI: 10.1007/s43393-023-00230-9

DeLisa, M., Kargi, F., & Shuler, M. (2017). *Bioprocess engineering: Basic concepts* (3rd ed.). Pearson.

Delvigne, F., Takors, R., Mudde, R., van Gulik, W., & Noorman, H. (2017). Bioprocess scale-up/down as integrative enabling technology: From fluid mechanics to systems biology and beyond. *Microbial Biotechnology, 10*(5), 1267–1274. DOI: 10.1111/1751-7915.12782

Demain, A. L., & Elander, R. P. (1999). The β-lactam antibiotics: Past, present, and future. *Antonie van Leeuwenhoek, 75*(1), 5–19. DOI: 10.1023/A:1001790109552

Doran, P. M. (1995). *Bioprocess engineering principles.* Elsevier.

Dragosits, M., & Mattanovich, D. (2013). Adaptive laboratory evolution—Principles and applications for biotechnology. *Microbial Cell Factories, 12*, 64. Advance online publication. DOI: 10.1186/1475-2859-12-64

Du, Y. H., Wang, M. Y., Yang, L. H., Tong, L. L., Guo, D. S., & Ji, X. J. (2022). Optimization and scale-up of fermentation processes driven by models. *Bioengineering (Basel, Switzerland), 9*(9), 473. Advance online publication. DOI: 10.3390/bioengineering9090473

Ecker, D. M., Jones, S. D., & Levine, H. L. (2015). The therapeutic monoclonal antibody market. *mAbs, 7*(1), 9–14. DOI: 10.4161/19420862.2014.989042

Eibl, R., & Eibl, D. (Eds.). (2019). *Single-use technology in biopharmaceutical manufacture* (2nd ed.). John Wiley & Sons.

Elsayed, A., Jaber, N., Al-Remawi, M., & Abu-Salah, K. (2023). From cell factories to patients: Stability challenges in biopharmaceuticals manufacturing and administration with mitigation strategies. *International Journal of Pharmaceutics, 645*, 123360. Advance online publication. DOI: 10.1016/j.ijpharm.2023.123360

Feidl, F., Garbellini, S., Luna, M. F., Vogg, S., Souquet, J., Broly, H., Morbidelli, M., & Butté, A. (2019). Combining mechanistic modeling and Raman spectroscopy for monitoring antibody chromatographic purification. *Processes (Basel, Switzerland), 7*(10), 683. Advance online publication. DOI: 10.3390/pr7100683

Filippi, M., Mekkattu, M., & Katzschmann, R. K. (2025). Sustainable biofabrication: From bioprinting to AI-driven predictive methods. *Trends in Biotechnology, 43*(2), 290–303. DOI: 10.1016/j.tibtech.2024.07.008

Food and Drug Administration. (2004). *PAT—A framework for innovative pharmaceutical development, manufacturing, and quality assurance.* U.S. Food and Drug Administration. https://www.fda.gov/regulatory-information/search-fda-guidance-documents/pat-framework-innovative-pharmaceutical-development-manufacturing-and-quality-assurance

Fu, R., Kang, L., Zhang, C., & Fei, Q. (2023). Application and progress of techno-economic analysis and life cycle assessment in biomanufacturing of fuels and chemicals. *Green Chemical Engineering, 4*(2), 189–198. DOI: 10.1016/j.gce.2022.06.002

Garcia-Ochoa, F., & Gomez, E. (2009). Bioreactor scale-up and oxygen transfer rate in microbial processes: An overview. *Biotechnology Advances, 27*(2), 153–176. DOI: 10.1016/j.biotechadv.2008.10.006

Gibbons, L., Maslanka, F., Le, N., Magill, A., Singh, P., Mclaughlin, J., Madden, F., Hayes, R., McCarthy, B., Rode, C., & O'Mahony, J. (2023). An assessment of the impact of Raman-based glucose feedback control on CHO cell bioreactor process development. *Biotechnology Progress, 39*(5), e3371. Advance online publication. DOI: 10.1002/btpr.3371

Gillespie, P. F., Wang, Y., Yin, K., Groegler, E., Cunningham, N., Stiving, A. Q., Raffaele, J., Marusa, N., Tubbs, C. M., Loughney, J. W., & Winters, M. A. (2024). Automated, quantitative capillary Western blots to analyze host cell proteins in COVID-19 vaccine produced in Vero cell line. *Vaccines, 12*(12), 1373. Advance online publication. DOI: 10.3390/vaccines12121373

Goeddel, D. V., Kleid, D. G., Bolivar, F., Heyneker, H. L., Yansura, D. G., Crea, R., Hirose, T., Kraszewski, A., Itakura, K., & Riggs, A. D. (1979). Expression in *Escherichia coli* of chemically synthesized genes for human insulin. *Proceedings of the National Academy of Sciences of the United States of America, 76*(1), 106–110. DOI: 10.1073/pnas.76.1.106

Guieysse, B., Quijano Govantes, G., & Muñoz Torre, R. (2011). Airlift bioreactors—Bioreactors design. In *Comprehensive biotechnology* (2nd ed., pp. 159–170). Elsevier., DOI: 10.1016/B978-0-08-088504-9.00107-7

Hernández-Longoria, R., Hernández-Ruiz, Y., Gutiérrez-Jasso, F., & Zarazúa, A. (2021). Validation of an analytical method for the quantification of human fibrinogen in pharmaceutical products by size-exclusion liquid chromatography (SEC-HPLC). *International Journal of Hematology, 113*(4), 480–492. DOI: 10.1007/s12185-020-03045-5

Isoko, K., Cordiner, J. L., Kis, Z., & Moghadam, P. Z. (2024). Bioprocessing 4.0: A pragmatic review and future perspectives. *Digital Discovery, 3*(9), 1662–1681. DOI: 10.1039/D4DD00085B

Jagschies, G., Lindskog, E., Łącki, K., & Galliher, P. (2018). *Biopharmaceutical processing: Development, design, and implementation of manufacturing processes*. Elsevier.

Jenzsch, M., Bell, C., Buziol, S., Kepert, F., Wegele, H., & Hakemeyer, C. (2018). Trends in process analytical technology: Present state in bioprocessing. In *New bioprocessing strategies: Development and manufacturing of recombinant antibodies and proteins* (pp. 211–252). Springer., DOI: 10.1007/10_2017_48

Jia, H., Harikumar, P., Atkinson, E., Rigsby, P., & Wadhwa, M. (2021). The first WHO international standard for harmonizing the biological activity of bevacizumab. *Biomolecules, 11*(11), 1610. Advance online publication. DOI: 10.3390/biom11111610

Jiménez-González, C., & Woodley, J. M. (2010). Bioprocesses: Modeling needs for process evaluation and sustainability assessment. *Computers & Chemical Engineering, 34*(7), 1009–1017. DOI: 10.1016/j.compchemeng.2010.03.004

Khang, A., & Akhai, S. (2024). Green intelligent and sustainable manufacturing: Key advancements, benefits, challenges, and applications for transforming industry. In *Machine vision and industrial robotics in manufacturing* (pp. 405–417). CRC Press., DOI: 10.1201/9781032788487-20

Kim, H. W., Hong, S. H., & Choi, H. (2020). Effect of nitrate and perchlorate on selenate reduction in a sequencing batch reactor. *Processes (Basel, Switzerland), 8*(3), 344. Advance online publication. DOI: 10.3390/pr8030344

Kittler, S., Müller, F., Elshazly, M., Wandrey, G. B., Klein, T., Daub, A., Spadiut, O., & Kopp, J. (2025). Transferability of bioprocessing modes for recombinant protease production: From fed-batch to continuous cultivation with *Bacillus licheniformis*. *BMC Biotechnology*, *25*(1), 13. Advance online publication. DOI: 10.1186/s12896-025-00897-8

Krämer, I., & Federici, M. (2020). Implementation and microbiological stability of dose-banded ganciclovir infusion bags prepared in series by a robotic system. *European Journal of Hospital Pharmacy. Science and Practice*, *27*(4), 209–215. DOI: 10.1136/ejhpharm-2019-001925

Krause, D., Birle, S., Hussein, M. A., & Becker, T. (2011). Bioprocess monitoring and control via adaptive sensor calibration. *Engineering in Life Sciences*, *11*(4), 402–416. DOI: 10.1002/elsc.201000141

Krömer, J. O., Ferreira, R. G., Petrides, D., & Kohlheb, N. (2020). Economic process evaluation and environmental life-cycle assessment of bio-aromatics production. *Frontiers in Bioengineering and Biotechnology*, *8*, 403. Advance online publication. DOI: 10.3389/fbioe.2020.00403

Krywko-Cendrowska, A., Szweda, D., & Szweda, R. (2020). Well-defined conjugated macromolecules based on oligo(arylene ethynylene)s in sensing. *Processes (Basel, Switzerland)*, *8*(5), 539. Advance online publication. DOI: 10.3390/pr8050539

Kwon, T., Leroux, A. C., Zang, H., Pollard, D., Zehe, C., & Akbari, S. (2024). Cell-based shear stress sensor for bioprocessing. *Journal of Biotechnology*, *390*, 71–79. DOI: 10.1016/j.jbiotec.2024.05.007

Lee, S. Y. (1996). High cell-density culture of *Escherichia coli*. *Trends in Biotechnology*, *14*(3), 98–105. DOI: 10.1016/0167-7799(96)80930-9

Lisci, S., Grosso, M., & Tronci, S. (2020). A geometric observer-assisted approach to tailor state estimation in a bioreactor for ethanol production. *Processes (Basel, Switzerland)*, *8*(4), 480. Advance online publication. DOI: 10.3390/pr8040480

Madigan, M. T., Bender, K. S., Buckley, D. H., Sattley, W. M., & Stahl, D. A. (2018). Microbial growth and its control. In *Brock biology of microorganisms* (15th ed., pp. 173–208). Pearson.

Madigan, M. T., Bender, K. S., Buckley, D. H., Sattley, W. M., & Stahl, D. A. (2021). Ecological diversity of bacteria. In *Brock biology of microorganisms* (16th ed., pp. 478–518). Pearson.

Marcello, K. M. (2024). *Unraveling the genomic and adaptive strategies of Antarctic cyanobacteria: A bioinformatic analysis of survival mechanisms in extreme cold environments* [Doctoral dissertation, University of California, Davis]. ProQuest Dissertations Publishing.

McDonnell, G. E. (2020). *Antisepsis, disinfection, and sterilization: Types, action, and resistance* (2nd ed.). John Wiley & Sons.

Monod, J. (2012). The growth of bacterial cultures. In *Selected papers in molecular biology by Jacques Monod* (pp. 606–626). Academic Press. (Original work published 1949), DOI: 10.1016/B978-0-12-460482-7.50047-0

Morgado, G., Gerngross, D., Roberts, T. M., & Panke, S. (2018). Synthetic biology for cell-free biosynthesis: Fundamentals of designing novel in vitro multi-enzyme reaction networks. In *Synthetic biology—Metabolic engineering* (pp. 117–146). Springer., DOI: 10.1007/10_2016_46

Mortensen, D. N., & Williams, E. R. (2016). Surface-induced protein unfolding in submicron electrospray emitters. *Analytical Chemistry*, *88*(19), 9662–9668. DOI: 10.1021/acs.analchem.6b02512

Munro, G. (2017). ICH Q7 good manufacturing practice guide for active pharmaceutical ingredients (APIs). In *ICH quality guidelines: An implementation guide* (pp. 509–534). John Wiley & Sons. https://doi.org/DOI: 10.1002/9781118971147.ch17

Naik, S. N., Goud, V. V., Rout, P. K., & Dalai, A. K. (2010). Production of first and second generation biofuels: A comprehensive review. *Renewable & Sustainable Energy Reviews*, *14*(2), 578–597. DOI: 10.1016/j.rser.2009.10.003

Neidhardt, F. C., Ingraham, J. L., & Schaechter, M. (1990). *Physiology of the bacterial cell: A molecular approach.* Sinauer Associates.

Nielsen, J., & Keasling, J. D. (2016). Engineering cellular metabolism. *Cell*, *164*(6), 1185–1197. DOI: 10.1016/j.cell.2016.02.004

Nienow, A. W. (2006). Reactor engineering in large scale animal cell culture. *Cytotechnology*, *50*(1), 9–33. DOI: 10.1007/s10616-006-9005-0

Ögmundarson, Ó., Sukumara, S., Herrgård, M. J., & Fantke, P. (2020). Combining environmental and economic performance for bioprocess optimization. *Trends in Biotechnology*, *38*(11), 1203–1214. DOI: 10.1016/j.tibtech.2020.04.011

Ouranidis, A., Davidopoulou, C., Tashi, R. K., & Kachrimanis, K. (2021). Pharma 4.0 continuous mRNA drug products manufacturing. *Pharmaceutics*, *13*(9), 1371. Advance online publication. DOI: 10.3390/pharmaceutics13091371

Parapouli, M., Vasileiadis, A., Afendra, A. S., & Hatziloukas, E. (2020). *Saccharomyces cerevisiae* and its industrial applications. *AIMS Microbiology*, *6*(1), 1–31. DOI: 10.3934/microbiol.2020001

Pasteur, L. (1857). Mémoire sur la fermentation appelée lactique. *Annales de Chimie et de Physique*, *52*(3), 404–418.

Patel, D., Koç, J. R., & Otegbeye, F. (2025). Creating a GMP cell processing program: A focus on quality and regulation. *Best Practice & Research Clinical Haematology. Article, 101614.* Advance online publication. DOI: 10.1016/j.beha.2025.101614

Petrides, D. (2000). Bioprocess design and economics. In *Bioseparations science and engineering* (pp. 1–83). Oxford University Press.

Pirt, S. J. (1975). *Principles of microbe and cell cultivation.* Blackwell Scientific.

Qadir, A. (2023). Beyond specialization: The interconnected web of sciences and technological advancements. *SAUS-Journal of IT and Computer Sciences*, *1*(1), 15–19.

Rathore, A. S., Mishra, S., Nikita, S., & Priyanka, P. (2021). Bioprocess control: Current progress and future perspectives. *Life (Chicago, Ill.)*, *11*(6), 557. Advance online publication. DOI: 10.3390/life11060557

Rathore, A. S., & Winkle, H. (2009). Quality by design for biopharmaceuticals. *Nature Biotechnology*, *27*(1), 26–34. DOI: 10.1038/nbt0109-26

Samaras, J. J., Micheletti, M., & Ding, W. (2022). Transformation of biopharmaceutical manufacturing through single-use technologies: Current state, remaining challenges, and future development. *Annual Review of Chemical and Biomolecular Engineering*, *13*, 73–97. DOI: 10.1146/annurev-chembioeng-092220-120343

Sandle, T. (2012). Environmental monitoring: A practical approach. In *Environmental monitoring: A comprehensive handbook* (Vol. 6, pp. 29–54). Oxford University Press.

Seenivasagan, R., & Babalola, O. O. (2021). Utilization of microbial consortia as biofertilizers and biopesticides for the production of feasible agricultural product. *Biology (Basel)*, *10*(11), 1111. Advance online publication. DOI: 10.3390/biology10111111

Shintani, H. (2016). Inactivation of bacterial spore, endotoxin, lipid A, normal prion and abnormal prion by exposures to several sorts of gases plasma. *Biocontrol Science*, *21*(1), 1–12. DOI: 10.4265/bio.21.1

Shukla, A. A., & Gottschalk, U. (2013). Single-use disposable technologies for biopharmaceutical manufacturing. *Trends in Biotechnology*, *31*(3), 147–154. DOI: 10.1016/j.tibtech.2012.10.004

Shukla, A. A., & Hinckley, P. (2008). Host cell protein clearance during protein A chromatography: Development of an improved column wash step. *Biotechnology Progress*, *24*(5), 1115–1121. DOI: 10.1002/btpr.50

Shukla, A. A., & Thömmes, J. (2010). Recent advances in large-scale production of monoclonal antibodies and related proteins. *Trends in Biotechnology*, *28*(5), 253–261. DOI: 10.1016/j.tibtech.2010.02.001

Simpson, R., & Sastry, S. K. (2013). Scale-up in chemical and bioprocess engineering. In *Chemical and bioprocess engineering: Fundamental concepts for first-year students* (pp. 261–275). Springer., DOI: 10.1007/978-1-4614-9126-2_11

. Singh, R., Kumar, M., Mittal, A., & Mehta, P. K. (2016). Microbial enzymes: Industrial progress in 21st century. *3 Biotech, 6*(2), Article 174. https://doi.org/DOI: 10.1007/s13205-016-0485-8

Singh, S., Raj, D., Mathur, A., Mani, N., & Kumar, D. (2025). Current approaches in CRISPR-Cas systems for hereditary diseases. *Progress in Molecular Biology and Translational Science*, *210*, 205–229. DOI: 10.1016/bs.pmbts.2024.07.002

Tamime, A. Y. (2009). *Dairy powders and concentrated products*. Wiley-Blackwell., DOI: 10.1002/9781444322729

Tangyu, M., Muller, J., Bolten, C. J., & Wittmann, C. (2019). Fermentation of plant-based milk alternatives for improved flavour and nutritional value. *Applied Microbiology and Biotechnology, 103*(23), 9263–9275. DOI: 10.1007/s00253-019-10175-9

Tawo, O. E., & Mbamalu, M. I. (2025). Advancing waste valorization techniques for sustainable industrial operations and improved environmental safety. *International Journal of Scientific Research Archive, 14*(2), 127–149. DOI: 10.30574/ijsra.2025.14.2.0282

Trejo-Solís, C., Serrano-García, N., Castillo-Rodríguez, R. A., Robledo-Cadena, D. X., Jimenez-Farfan, D., Marín-Hernández, Á., Silva-Adaya, D., Rodríguez-Pérez, C. E., & Gallardo-Pérez, J. C. (2024). Metabolic dysregulation of tricarboxylic acid cycle and oxidative phosphorylation in glioblastoma. *Reviews in the Neurosciences, 35*(7), 813–838. DOI: 10.1515/revneuro-2024-0022

Turanli, B., Gulfidan, G., Aydogan, O. O., Kula, C., Selvaraj, G., & Arga, K. Y. (2024). Genome-scale metabolic models in translational medicine: The current status and potential of machine learning in improving the effectiveness of the models. *Molecular Omics, 20*(4), 234–247. DOI: 10.1039/D3MO00239A

Ullah, R., Ahmad, H., Rehman, F. U., & Fawad, A. (2023). Green innovation and Sustainable Development Goals in SMEs: The moderating role of government incentives. *Journal of Economic and Administrative Sciences, 39*(4), 830–846. DOI: 10.1108/JEAS-07-2022-0168

Van Dijl, J., & Hecker, M. (2013). *Bacillus subtilis*: From soil bacterium to super-secreting cell factory. *Microbial Cell Factories, 12*, 3. Advance online publication. DOI: 10.1186/1475-2859-12-3

Vegineni, G. C. (2025). Sustainable tech development: Integrating AI, XR, and CI/CD pipelines for a greener future. In *Exploring the impact of extended reality (XR) technologies on promoting environmental sustainability* (pp. 267–293). Springer., DOI: 10.1007/978-3-031-72904-1_14

Walsh, G. (2013). *Biopharmaceuticals: Biochemistry and biotechnology* (2nd ed.). John Wiley & Sons.

Wang, L., Ju, C., Han, C., Yu, Z., Bai, M. Y., & Wang, C. (2025). The interaction of nutrient uptake with biotic and abiotic stresses in plants. *Journal of Integrative Plant Biology, 67*(3), 455–487. DOI: 10.1111/jipb.13613

Yang, L., Shakeel, Q., Xu, X., Ali, L., Chen, Z., Mubeen, M., Sohail, M. A., Iftikhar, Y., Kumar, A., Solanki, M. K., & Zhou, Y. (2024). Optimized submerged batch fermentation for metabolic switching in *Streptomyces yanglinensis* 3–10 providing platform for reveromycin A and B biosynthesis, engineering, and production. *Frontiers in Microbiology, 15*, 1378834. Advance online publication. DOI: 10.3389/fmicb.2024.1378834

Zeng, A. P., & Sabra, W. (2011). Microbial production of diols as platform chemicals: Recent progresses. *Current Opinion in Biotechnology, 22*(6), 749–757. DOI: 10.1016/j.copbio.2011.05.005

Zhang, J., Bilal, M., Liu, S., Zhang, J., Lu, H., Luo, H., Luo, C., Shi, H., Iqbal, H. M., & Zhao, Y. (2020). Isolation, identification and antimicrobial evaluation of bactericides secreting *Bacillus subtilis* Natto as a biocontrol agent. *Processes (Basel, Switzerland), 8*(3), 259. Advance online publication. DOI: 10.3390/pr8030259

Zhang, J., Hou, W., & Bao, J. (2016). Reactors for high solid loading pretreatment of lignocellulosic biomass. In Bao, J., Ye, Q., & Zhong, J. J. (Eds.), *Bioreactor engineering research and industrial applications II* (pp. 75–90). Springer., DOI: 10.1007/978-3-662-48347-3_4

Zhao, X., Sun, Y., Li, Y., Jia, N., & Xu, J. (2024). Applications of machine learning in real-time control systems: A review. *Measurement Science & Technology*. Advance online publication. DOI: 10.1088/1361-6501/ad8f85

Zhu, J., Li, J., Kong, Y., Dong, M., Li, Y., & Zou, M. (2025). Study on the high-speed penetration and shear failure mechanism of beach sand. *Materials (Basel)*, *18*(9), 1922. Advance online publication. DOI: 10.3390/ma18091922

Chapter 2

Microbial and Cell Culture Systems for Bio-Manufacturing:

Cell Culture Systems in Industrial Bio-Product Formation

Ramachandra Reddy Pamuru
http://orcid.org/0000-0002-9017-974X
Yogi Vemana University, India

Tummala Chandrasekhar
Yogi Vemana University, India

Arifullah Mohammad
http://orcid.org/0000-0001-7793-8134
Koneru Lakshmaiah University, India

Mohd Tariq
Department of Academics, Sumandeep Vidyapeeth University, Vadodara, India & Department of Biotechnology, Graphic Era University, Dehradun, India

S. B. Sainath
Vikrama Simhapuri University, India

Koduru Ramesh
Yogi Vemana University, India

ABSTRACT

Bio-manufacturing is a potential area for production of biologically active products for the welfare of human beings using biological systems in the bioreactors industrially. It is well known that microbial or cell culture systems play vital role in bio-manufacturing industry. Bio-manufacturing is an interdisciplinary approach with a combination of Microbiology, Biochemistry and Chemical Engineering. Recent developments in science introduced a variety of biological systems for the production of important molecules/products. Initially, bio-manufacturing was carried out with recombinant microbial systems, later with mammalian cell cultures. This chapter emphasizes the evolution of bio-manufacturing systems, microbial and cell culture systems in producing various biological products through industrial bioreactors with special focus on wild to genetically modified cell culture systems and the challenges in quality improvement of the bio-products.

DOI: 10.4018/979-8-3373-2873-7.ch002

INTRODUCTION

The biological products have plenty of value than chemically synthesized commercial products. Pharmaceutical products that are produced biologically metabolize without difficulty in the human or other biological system. Moreover, the biological molecules have more synergic effect in the living cell than the chemically synthesized or artificially developed molecules. The use of biologically produced molecules is not new; various human civilizations are evidenced for the adaptation and usage of different biological systems or products for welfare of human beings. Direct or indirect use of bio-compounds or microbial systems is well understood from ancient days. Preparation of pickles, curdling of milk, beverages etc., is most commonly followed food preservation method through microbial fermentation. However, using fermentation modern science invaded into the production of various biologically important molecules. The process of producing biologically important molecules using microbes or biological cell lines is named as biomanufacturing. It is evolved in 1910s started producing various traditional molecules like antibiotics, ethanol and other beverages, chemicals. Modern bio-manufacturing helps in addressing critical situations such as energy crisis, food security, health issues, sustainability and climate change (Zhang et al., 2017).

Fuels, pharmaceuticals, neutraceuticals, and many other products with value addition are produced using biological systems (microbial cells or other cell cultures) in bio-manufacturing (Michels & Rosazza, 2009). The basic unit that is used in bio-manufacturing is a typical bioreactor where the fermentation process takes up in a large scale with controlled conditions. In general bioreactors with cell culture and raw materials, allows cells to grow and produce products of choice in at specified conditions. Initially batch cultures are commonly followed culturing methods of microbial cells through fermentation process in a moderate size of bioreactor. Since of its disadvantage in producing less amount of product, later fed-batch culturing of bio-manufacturing was started for the better production of bio-products like chemicals, fuels and high valued products. The production of bio-compounds has also limited the overall productivity of fed-batch culture with increased capital and operating cost of fermentation process (Xie et al., 2015). Modern technology created a way to achieve potential amount of bio-product in continuous fermentation in bioreactor with reasonable operating cost. Furthermore, modern molecular biotechnology with recombinant DNA technology has introduced genetically modified organisms to produce high amounts of valued-various bio-products through continuous fermentation process with much lowered production cost.

Continuous fermentation has great advantage in producing products of microbes and a series of studies carried out in reducing cost of bio-manufacturing with elevated product levels in the past few decades. A number of bio-products like omega-3 fatty acids (Xie et al., 2017),succinic acid(Maharaj et al., 2014; van Heerden & Nicol, 2013), ethanol, (Andersen et al., 2015; K. Liu et al., 2014; Lucio & Fermentec, 2008), organic solvents (acetone, butanol and ethanol) (Bankar et al., 2012; Vees et al., 2020), lipids (Khanal & Lenhoff, 2021; Remmers et al., 2017), lactic acid (Olszewska-Widdrat et al., 2020; Y. Wang et al., 2020), 1,3-propanediol (Menzel et al., 1997; Nakamura & Whited, 2003) and recombinant proteins (Peebo & Neubauer, 2018; Walsh, 2018) have been produced using microbial continuous fermentation process.

In the last decade, potential up gradation of continuous bio-manufacturing process has been increased with the usage of mammalian cell lines for the manufacturing of monoclonal antibodies especially in the sector of bio-pharmaceuticals (Bunnak et al., 2016; Khanal & Lenhoff, 2021).

Many products have been developed through continuous cell culture bio-manufacturing method (Ghanemi, 2015). The present chapter, emphasizes the bio-manufacturing of microbial and cell culture systems in producing a variety of bio-products with special reference to wild to genetically modified microbial and cell culture systems and the challenges in quality improvement of the bio-products.

BIO-MANUFACTURING SYSTEMS

Bio-manufacturing is a process started 9000 years ago using fruit, rice and honey mix as a substrate in the wine production (36). Since thousands of years, making and usage of fermented foods like seasonal fruit pickles (mango, lemon, tamarind, red chilli, tomato, etc.), dove for pancake (dosa) and savory cake (idly), and curdling of milk is part of Indian cultural system. Baking bread by yeast in Egypt, beer brewing practice of Babylonians and Sumerians in before 6000 BC has also been reported in the history (Y.-H. P. Zhang et al., 2017). Various fermented products are the sources for different food and other valued-products in the ancient to modern societies of various cultures all over the world. Mostly conventional methods are used to ferment the various substrates and obtained the valued-products in the ancient days, which is called pre-modern bio-manufacturing period. The commonly followed method of fermentation in this period is solid state one through anaerobic process using mixed microbes as source of fermentation inoculums. Bio-manufacturing is mentioned with 1, 2, 3, and 4 based on the advancements taken up in the fermentation process and its related aspects (**Table 1**).

Table 1. Different levels of bio-manufacturing (BM) and its advancements

S.No.	Bio-manufacturing	Salient features	References
1	Pre-Modern	Conventional fermentation products using solid state and mixed cultures with anaerobic way. Helped Louis Pasteur discovery in 1860s for the improved conventional fermentation methods.	(Fleet, 2008; McGovern et al., 2004).
2	Stage 1.0	Primary metabolites of microbes using mono-culture and liquid anaerobic fermentation. The primary products are basic components of cell which plays an important role in the control of cellular reproduction, growth and development of microbe. The findings of Chaim Weizman in 1910s and Killeffer, 1927 helped in changing the fermentation from conventional to BM 1.0.	(Demain, 2007; Lan & Liao, 2013; Sano, 2009; Vasic-Racki, 2006).
3	Stage 2.0	Secondary metabolites of microbes using mono-culture and liquid anaerobic fermentation. The secondary metabolites of a microbe play a crucial role in defense mechanism against other organisms which are used as medicine (antibiotics), fragrance and food flavoring agents used by humans. Experiments of Alexander Fleming's during 1940s, and Waksman, 1946 promoted BM 1.0 to BM 2.0. This was started during World war-II with pencillin production through fermentation. Hence, the production of microbial antibiotics is simply called BM 2.0.	(Demain, 2007; Waksman et al., 1946).

continued on following page

Table 1. Continued

S.No.	Bio-manufacturing	Salient features	References
4	Stage 3.0	Internal or external proteins and enzymes production using recombinant DNA technology produced genetically modified microbes and cell culture systems. Production of large size proteins, enzymes, polypeptides drugs has been done through recombinant microbes and human/animal cell lines. A variety of major biomolecules of different nature were produced during this period. BM 2.0 is moved to BM 3.0 with the findings of Paul Berg in 1980s.	(Afeyan & Cooney, 2006; Bornscheuer et al., 2012; Demain & Vaishnav, 2009; Liese & Hilterhaus, 2013; Michels & Rosazza, 2009; Myung et al., 2011; Siegel et al., 2015; Siegfried, 2005; Sochaj et al., 2015; Y. -H P. Zhang, 2013; Y.-H. P. Zhang, 2015).
5	Stage 4.0	Production of renewable energy and versatile foods for healthier human life using pluri potent stem cells, protein engineering, metabolic engineering and systems biology, and biotransformation with in vitro bio-synthetic systems. New revolution of bio-manufacturing for the production of new drugs and functional tissues, effective production of existing drugs and valued-products with high yield and scale-up mechanisms. A modern technology is used and upgraded from time to time after the new technology invented.	(Qin et al., 2023; Saranya et al., 2024; Tristan et al., 2021; Xu et al., 2019)

MICROBIAL AND CELL CULTURE SYSTEMS

Bio-manufacturing of valued products using microorganisms and cell culture systems is not started in the recent past. Since thousands of years, large number of groups all over the World worked on finding the right fermentation process using different substrates with multiple microorganisms. It is an interdisciplinary approach with a combination of microbial, biochemical and nano engineering systems. Technological up gradation curtailed the limitations to use any biological cell systems for bio-manufacturing of various products of biological origin through gene modifications/ manipulations including mammalian cells. Major group of microbial cell culture systems are genetically modified microorganisms or other cell culture systems that harbor specific metabolic pathways for desired product bio-synthesis. Compared to plant-based and chemical extraction methods microbial systems are often having shorter production cycles with high yields with cost effective manner.

Industrial revolution imbibed the fermentation process to produce a variety of value-added products in the last hundred years and more. A drastic change has been taken up in bio-manufacturing process with the advancement of technology. In the identification of industrially important microbes from a variety of environments has been done and was maintained in the form of pure cultures for large scale production in the industry. During this process, (J. W. Lee et al., 2016; P. C. Lee et al., 2003) isolated producers of succinic acid (*Mannheimia succiniciproducens* and *Anaerobiospirillum succiniciproducens*); (Kurosawa et al., 2015; Qiao et al., 2017) lipids and fatty acid derivatives (*Yarrowial ipolytica* and *Rhodococcus opacus*); (Eggeling & Bott, 2005) amino acids (*Corynebacterium glutamicum*); (Jansen et al., 2017; S. Yang et al., 2016) ethanol (*Zymomonas mobilis* and *Saccharomyces cerecisiae*); (Song et al., 2017) lactic acid (*Lactobacillus*); (Y.-Q. Sun et al., 2018) 1,3-propanediol (*Klebsiella pneumonia*). The most commonly used microbial host systems in bio-manufacturing industry are *Escherichia coli* (bacteria), *Sachharomyces cerevisiae* and *Pichia pastoris* (yeast species). Many constrains were swallowed with fruitful production of pure products during the development of technology, especially in the recent past. One of such examples is using the methods of biotechnology high amounts of aerobic acetic acid producing bacteria, *Acetobacter* is isolated (Yamada & Yukphan, 2008). Using the same technology microbes of producing cellulose, indole acetic acid, pigments, ascorbic acid and acetic acid were also isolated for industrial applications (Bastian et al., 1998; Fuentes-Ramírez et al., 2001; V. T. Nguyen et al., 2008). A variety of microbial strains for different products production has been evolved industrially (Jones & Woods, 1986; S. Kim et al., 2015). The role of microbes in the development of bio-manufacturing ages varies modern developments are presented in the **Table 2.**

Table 2. Products and its features of different generations of bio-manufacturing (BM) using microorganisms

BM level	Product name	Microbe	Modified features	Amount of product (g/l)	References
BM 1.0	Butanol	*Clostredium acetobutylicum*	Selection and isolation of strain	10-12	(S. Y. Lee et al., 2008)
	Pencillin	*Pencelium chrysogenum*	Selection and isolation of strain	0.06	(Demain & Elander, 1999)
	Streptomycin	*Streptomyces griseus*	Isolated strain and used peptone-meat extract medium	11.9	(Carter et al., 1945)
	Actinomycin	*Streptomyces antibioticus*	Isolation of strain and use of natural substrates	-	(Waksman et al., 1946)
BM 2.0	Pencillin	*Penceliumchrysogenum*	Mutated strain with X-rays	0.3	(Demain & Elander, 1999)
	Actinomycin	*Streptomyces antibioticus*	4(2/60) mutated strain	0.063	(Hosoya et al., 1998)
	Streptomycin	*Streptomyces griseus*	Chromatogrpahic purification	8 to 10	(Carter et al., 1945)
	Fredericamycin	*Streptomyces chattanoogensis*	46(46/100) mutated strain	0.26	(Hosoya et al., 1998)
BM 3.0	Butanol	*Clostediumaceto butylicum*	GroESL over expression	17	(S. Y. Lee et al., 2008)
	Artemisinic acid	*Saccharomyces cerevisiae*	Modification in metabolic pathways and regulatory gene expression	0.1	(Ro et al., 2006)
	1,3-Propanediol	*E. coli*	Optimized pathway design with cofactor supply	130	(Nakamura & Whited, 2003)
	L-alanine	*E. coli*	Modified alanine dehydrogenase	114	(P. Liu et al., 2022)
	Riboflavin	*Bacillus subtilis*	Mutation in zwf and gnd genes	15.7	(Z. Wang et al., 2011)
	L-valine	*Clostridium glutamicum*	Deletion of competitive pathway and balance of cofactor	150	(Hasegawa et al., 2013)
BM 4.0	2-phenyl ethanol	*Bacillus licheniformis*	Modification in phenyl pyruvate and central pathway, modulation of glucose transport and elimination of competitive pathway	6.24	(Zhan et al., 2022)

continued on following page

Table 2. Continued

BM level	Product name	Microbe	Modified features	Amount of product (g/l)	References
	1,4-butanodiol	*E. coli*	Pathway introduction, redox balance, supply of energy and cell growth	18	(Yim et al., 2011)
	Succinic acid	*Yarrowia lipolytica*	Reductive TCA rearrangement	111.9	(Cui et al., 2023)
	Polyhydroxy butyrate	*Zymomonas mobilis*	Optimization of plasmid copy number, supply of cofactors, C/N ratio, self flocculation	74%	(Li et al., 2022)
	Fatty-acid ethyl-esters	*Rhodotorula toruloides*	Elevated wax-ester synthase gene expression	9.97	(Y. Zhang et al., 2021)
	Cannabinoids	*Saccharomyces cerevisiae*	Mining of enzyme, optimization of copy number	-	(Luo et al., 2019)
	Poly-hydroxy alkanoates	*Halomonasblue phagenesis*	Morphology regulation, optimization of copy number	80	(Tan et al., 2014)

Antibodies and therapeutic proteins (insulin, growth hormone, interleukins etc.) that are used to treat various illnesses in humans are manufactured using mammalian cell culture systems. These cells are capable of performing complex post-translational modifications like glycosylation, phosphorylation, lipidation etc., crucial for their function, which lacks in prokaryotic cell systems. A number of mammalian cell culture systems are popular and most frequently used in bio-manufacturing, includes Chinese hamster ovary (CHO), human embryonic kidney (HEK), moused myeloma-derived (NS0) and mouse spleen B – lymphocytes ($SP_2/0$) (K. Byrne, 2014). On the other hand, cell lines are populations of cells derived from single cell types of different sources are engineered to produce bio-compounds industrially. Furthermore, co-cultural systems having interaction of different microbial strains are developed to produce variety of foods, compounds of high-value, treatment of wastewater for water recycling and biofuels. In these systems complex substrate molecules are simplified or simple molecules are converted into complex products. Besides cell systems, development of various types of bioreactors is developed to culture different bio-systems. The most common bio-manufacturing wide range of valuable products include biofuels, anti-biotics, various enzymes, hormones, biochemicals, food additives, pharmaceutical compounds, vitamins, organic acids, complex compounds, single cell protein, etc. The bio-manufacturing using cell culture systems has many limitations including difficulty in producing complexity molecules, higher level of contamination, variations in productivity, post-translational modifications (like glycosylated proteins) for eukaryotic proteins with microbial systems, difficulties in extraction of compounds in biologically active form, difficulty in the maintenance of bioreactor during fermentation process, control of variables, aeration etc. However, the bio-manufacturing industry at present is a potential area for production of biologically active products for the welfare of human beings using biological systems in the bioreactors industrially.

GENETIC ENGINEERING IN BIO-MANUFACTURING

Genetic engineering has emerged as a fundamental element of contemporary bio-manufacturing, facilitating the sustainable and scalable manufacture of medicines, biofuels, food additives, and industrial enzymes (Mirsalami & Mirsalami, 2025). This chapter examines the methodologies and uses of genetic engineering in bio-manufacturing, emphasising significant developments such CRISPR-Cas9, metabolic engineering, and synthetic biology (S. Zhang et al., 2020). Using modified organisms to improve industrial efficiency, lessen environmental impact, and produce new bio-based products is illustrated via case studies. Regulatory obstacles, biosafety concerns, and financial limitations are examined, along with prospective advancements in the sector (Ou & Guo, 2023).

Bio-manufacturing is the term used to describe the large-scale commercial production of goods using biological systems. With the increasing need for sustainable alternatives to petrochemicals, bio-manufacturing has become a crucial component in medicines, renewable energy, food technology, and materials science (N. Singh et al., 2022).

Genetic engineering, the direct alteration of an organism's DNA, has significantly improved bio-manufacturing capabilities, revolutionised conventional methods and facilitating the creation of innovative bioproducts. This study examines the fundamental methodologies and uses of genetic engineering in bio-manufacturing, assessing both present effects and future possibilities. One of the most impactful applications of genetic engineering is Insulin Production, Monoclonal Antibodies, Biofuels, Food and Nutrition, Bioplastics, and Polymers (Khan et al., 2016).

Microbial cells are becoming factories for the production of recombinant proteins in the bio-manufacturing field with the introduction of recombinant DNA technology. *E. coli*, a primary organism used initially as a cell factory in bio-manufacturing units. Since of less half-life (20 min.), non-pathogenic nature, grows in a simple media (Liquid Broth), easy handling made *E. coli* as one of the model organisms for any kind of microbial experimentations. In recent past, E. coli is replaced with other bacterial host as cell factories for bio-manufacturing due to the variation in the potentiality of biosynthetic pathways, cellular growth at diversified conditions and having diversity in metabolic pathways. Major group of these organisms are potential cell factories for the production of recombinant cell biomanufacturars (Ferrer-Miralles & Villaverde, 2013; Rasala & Mayfield, 2015). Best example comes under this category is Lactic acid bacteria and used conventionally for the microbial food industry (Arendt et al., 2011; de Vos, 2011; Rhee et al., 2011; Teusink et al., 2011). Research has been upgraded and made lactic acid bacteria via r-DNA technology as to produce protein especially protein delivery and drug display (Bermúdez-Humarán et al., 2011; Daniel et al., 2011; García-Fruitós, 2012; Hu et al., 2011; Morello et al., 2008; Peterbauer et al., 2011; Pontes et al., 2011; Scavone et al., 2007). Moreover, the genetic modification through r-DNA technology is a safe one to continue further. **Table 3** shows various bacterial cell factories used for the production of different recombinant proteins.

Techniques in Genetic Engineering for Bio-Manufacturing

Recombinant DNA Technology

Recombinant DNA technology, one of the earliest and most fundamental genetic engineering techniques, is the insertion of genes from one organism into another to bestow new functionalities, such as enzyme synthesis or the expansion of metabolic pathways.

Bioprocessing procedures are employed to manufacture biopharmaceuticals, such as monoclonal antibodies, vaccines, hormones, and enzymes. These biopharmaceuticals are crucial for the treatment of several ailments, including cancer, diabetes, and infectious disorders. The use of recombinant DNA technology in insulin synthesis transformed diabetes therapy, becoming insulin broadly accessible and economical (Gottschalk et al., 2012).

Metabolic Engineering

Metabolic engineering is a field that modifies cellular biosynthetic pathways for new product creation or enhanced production of desired compounds. This method emphasises the reprogramming of cellular metabolism to enhance the production of desired chemicals. It frequently entails many gene knockouts and insertions to enhance precursor availability, enzyme expression, and pathway flow. A number of engineered pathways are introduced into the microbial and cell culture systems for enhanced productivity (Bikram et al., 2014). Using metabolic engineering developed *Lactobacillus* and *Enterococcus* strains with enhanced production of lactic acid with lower maintenance and reduced pollution (Christopher et al., 2014; Subramanian et al., 2015). In microbes, metabolic engineering helps for *in vitro* and *in vivo* synthetic metabolic pathway construction (Lindberg et al., 2010; Steen et al., 2010; Zhao et al., 2013; Alonso-Gutierrez et al., 2013), enzyme engineering (Siegel et al., 2010; Tobias et al., 2017), product enhancement (Lian et al., 2014; Whitaker et al., 2017), and optimal pathway prediction through *in silico* methods (McShan et al., 2003; Cho et al., 2010; Moriya et al., 2010).

Metabolic engineering has not stopped modifying the pathways in eukaryotic cell systems. *Yarrowia lipolytica* a yeast species served as superior host for metabolic pathway engineering. Products like biodiesel, carotenoids and functional fatty acid pathways are engineered in the *Yerrowia lipolytica* (Zhu and Jackson, 2015). It is well known that metabolic engineering can be operated in both plants and animals to produce various secondary metabolites of pharmacological importance. Moreover, this process is very efficient one with less investment for discovering and producing effective drugs (Harvey et al., 2015; Dhakal et al., 2017).

CRISPR-Cas9 and Genome Editing

CRISPR-Cas9 facilitates accurate, targeted alterations to the genome. In addition to increasing yields and decreasing strain optimisation costs, it has expedited the creation of novel microbial strains. CRISPR-Cas9 technology facilitates the editing of industrially important microbial or eukaryotic cell genome precisely and efficiently. It also helps in simultaneous editing of multiple genes in cells (Hsu et al., 2013). CRISPR-Cas9 technology became inevitable in the engineering of industrial microbes. Liang et al., 2025), presented the role of gene editing in the industrially important microorganisms. Using this technology, developed microbial strains with elevated levels of desired products with stress sustainable capacities. In Cyanobacteria using *FnCas12a* deleted *nblA* single gene with 100% selective media (Baldanta et al., 2022). Deletion of *avtA, ilvE* and *ilvA* genes are reported with efficacy of 88, 67 and 58% in *Corynebacterium glutamicum* using *FnCas 12a* (Su et al., 2023). There is genome manipulation in eukaryotic cells using CRISPR-based technologies. However, need further attention to improve the strains of important microbes and cell culture of bio-manufacturing systems using CRISPR-Cas9 technology for enhanced productivity of products with stress sustainable organisms.

Table 3. Different bacterial groups as recombinant protein cell factories in the bio-manufacturing industry

S.No.	Bacterial Species	Character(s) of the gene	Host bacteria	Recombinant protein	References
1	*Halomonas elongate*	Enhanced Solubility	*Halophilic bacteria*	Beta-lactamase	(Tokunaga et al., 2010)
2	*Pseudomonas fluorescens*	High secretions	*Pseudomonads*	Granulocyte stimulating-factor of humans	(Jin et al., 2011)
3	*Caulobacter crescentus*	RSaA fusion protein elevated secretion	*Caulobacteria*	Capsid protein of hematopoietic necrosis virus	(Simon et al., 2001)
4	*Pseudoalteromonas haloplanktis*	High levels of protein folding	*Bacteria adopted to cold conditions*	Human nerve-growth factor	(Vigentini et al., 2006)
5	*Bacillus subtilis*	Elevated protein synthesis and secretion	*Bacillus*	Beta-galactosidase	(M. Yang et al., 2013)
6	*Streptomyces lividans*	Elevated protein secretion	*Streptomycetes*	Antigens for *Mycobacterium tuberculosis*	(Ayala et al., 2013)
7	*Labtobacillus plantarum*	GRAS and protein secretion	*Lactic acid producing bacteria*	Beta-galactosidase	(T.-T. Nguyen et al., 2012)
8	*Bacillus amyloliquefaciens*	Elevated protein secretion	*Bacillus*	Amylase enzyme	(Deb et al., 2013)
9	*Brevibaterium lactofermentum*	GRAS and elevated protein synthesis and secretion	*Coryneforms*	Enzymes cellulases	(Paradis et al., 1987)
10	*Bacillus megaterium*	Elevated protein secretion	*Bacillus*	Antibodies	(David et al., 2011)
11	*Mycobacterium smegmatis*	Change in post-translational modifications	*Mycobateria*	Fusion protein (Hsp65-hIL-2) and proteins of *Mycobaterium*	(Guo et al., 2012; Noens et al., 2011)

Synthetic Biology

Synthetic biology integrates engineering ideas with biological sciences to develop novel biological components, technologies, or systems. It is utilised to engineer "chassis organisms" or synthetic pathways absent in nature (Pandey et al., 2024).

Microbial fermentation is employed to generate bioethanol, biodiesel, and biogas from renewable biomass sources. The advancement of sophisticated biofuels, like cellulosic ethanol, has enhanced the sustainability and economic feasibility of biofuel production. Cellulosic ethanol is derived from non-food biomass, including agricultural leftovers and lignocellulosic plants, hence diminishing competition with food resources.

Genetic engineering has revolutionised bio-manufacturing, rendering it more sustainable, efficient, and inventive. As methodologies and technologies advance, bio-manufacturing will be crucial in tackling worldwide issues related to health, energy, and materials. Ongoing investment in research, infrastructure, and public education is crucial to realise its whole potential (Samoraj et al., 2024).

Fermentation technology has long been a cornerstone of microbial manufacturing for meeting the growing demand for industrially important biomolecules. However, industries continue to face significant challenges in developing novel methods to boost biomolecule productivity while keeping costs low (Nehal et al., 2022). Nanodrug delivery systems have gained attention for their ability to enhance solubility and bioavailability, enabling targeted therapies. Likewise, nanomaterials with exceptional physicochemical properties and antimicrobial activity are applied in areas such as crop protection, bioremediation, and food processing. Despite these advantages, producing biocompatible and non-toxic nanodelivery systems through cost-effective processes remains a major hurdle. In recent years, integrating microbial fermentation with nanotechnology has emerged as a promising approach for creating safe, biocompatible nanostructures. This chapter highlights the role of microbial fermentation in generating valuable biomolecules and explores how coupling this technology with nanotechnology can enhance the productivity of industrially significant biomolecules. Enhanced microbial efficiency can be achieved with many processes. They are immobilization of enzymes and cells real-time monitoring, improved mass transfer, product recovery, and purification (Lv et al., 2024).

IMPACTS OF NANOTECHNOLOGY ON BIOMANUFACTURING

Nanotechnology has become essential in enhancing microbial and mammalian cell culture systems for biomanufacturing. The incorporation of nanomaterials, nanosensors, and nano-encapsulation methods improves productivity, stability, real-time monitoring, and bioprocess control. Particular uses in single-cell encapsulation, nano-scaffold formation, enzyme immobilisation, and purification based on nanoparticles are thoroughly investigated (Shahcheraghi et al., 2022). Biomanufacturing utilises living cells, particularly microbial and mammalian systems, to generate valuable products including therapeutic proteins, vaccines, and enzymes. Conventional culture techniques encounter limitations concerning scalability, contamination, process inefficiency, and product consistency (Tang et al., 2023). Nanotechnology, by manipulating matter at the 1–100 nm scale, provides innovative solutions to address these challenges. Nanotechnology enhances cell viability, facilitates dynamic monitoring, improves delivery systems, and optimises downstream processing in microbial and cell culture systems (Zhu et al., 2021).

Nano-Encapsulation of Microbial and Mammalian Cells

Nanoencapsulation represents a novel approach in biomanufacturing, characterised by the application of nano-meter thick, semi-permeable coatings on individual microbial or mammalian cells. This method enhances cell viability, stress tolerance, immune evasion, and process control. This technology shows considerable potential for improving fermentation processes, facilitating therapeutic cell delivery, and advancing tissue engineering applications (Arratia-Quijada et al., 2024). A method that encapsulates cells in nanoscale coatings usually composed of polymers, silica, or hybrid materials to safeguard them while facilitating selective exchange of nutrients and metabolites. Microbial systems utilise processes such as fermentation enhancement, stress resistance, and synthetic consortia, whereas mammalian systems employ cell therapy and controlled differentiation. It provides advantages Enhances cellular robustness and productivity, facilitates intelligent regulation of cellular behaviour, and minimises variability in therapeutic applications (Zheng et al., 2024).

Nanoencapsulation serves as an effective method for enhancing the performance of microbial and mammalian cells in biomanufacturing. Ongoing advancements in materials and regulatory frameworks are poised to significantly influence the future of industrial biotechnology and cell-based therapies (A. K. Singh et al., 2023).

Nanostructured Scaffolds and Surfaces

Nanostructured scaffolds and surfaces represent significant advancements in contemporary biomanufacturing. By replicating the nanoscale structure of natural extracellular matrices, they improve cell adhesion, proliferation, differentiation, and metabolic activity (Sindhi et al., 2025). This technique examines the design, materials, applications, and future prospects of nanostructured platforms in microbial and mammalian cell culture systems, focussing on their significance in tissue engineering, therapeutic protein production, and lab-grown biomaterials. Traditional two-dimensional culture systems frequently do not accurately mimic the intricate microenvironment necessary for optimal cellular function (S. Liu et al., 2023). Nanostructured surfaces, designed at the 1–100 nm scale, enhance cell-substrate interactions and more effectively direct cellular behaviour. In microbial and mammalian cell culture systems, these structures enhance productivity, mitigate cellular stress, and facilitate scalable biomanufacturing processes. The materials utilised include natural substances such as collagen, gelatin, chitosan, and silk fibroin; synthetic materials including polycaprolactone (PCL), polylactic acid (PLA), and polydimethylsiloxane (PDMS); and hybrid materials comprising functionalised nanocomposites with graphene, hydroxyapatite, or carbon nanotubes.

Nanostructured surfaces and scaffolds offer a potent foundation for biomanufacturing advancement. In both microbial and mammalian systems, they improve cellular function and scalability via nanoscale replication of the original microenvironment. These technologies have the potential to completely transform the cell-based synthesis of biologics, biofuels, and tailored tissues as manufacturing becomes more accessible and repeatable (Yi et al., 2025).

Nanoparticle-Assisted Gene and Protein Delivery

Because they allow for the precise, effective, and low-toxicity transfer of biomolecules into cells, nanoparticles have completely changed gene and protein delivery methods. Delivery via nanoparticles is essential for metabolic engineering, synthetic biology, and the synthesis of biopharmaceuticals in microbial and mammalian cell systems (Yusuf et al., 2023). A key component of biotechnology is the transfer of genes and proteins into cells. Conventional techniques, such as viral vectors or electroporation, frequently have poor immunogenicity, cytotoxicity, or efficiency. Because of their surface chemistry, biocompatibility, and adjustable size, nanoparticles (NPs) provide a potent non-viral substitute for delivering therapeutic proteins, enzymes, and nucleic acids into cells (Yusuf et al., 2023). This has significant ramifications for the development of vaccines, gene editing, synthetic biology, and recombinant protein synthesis. Different types of nanoparticles are used in gene and protein delivery: lipid nanoparticles (which are widely used for mRNA and plasmid delivery, such as in CHO cells); polymeric nanoparticles (which are biodegradable and have a controlled release); gold/magnetic nanoparticles (which allow for targeted and visible delivery); and dendrimers (which have a high payload capacity for proteins and nucleic acids) (Jung et al., 2022).

Gene and protein transport aided by nanoparticles has become a game-changing technique in mammalian and microbial cell engineering. By facilitating the targeted, scalable, and highly efficient delivery of biomolecules, it gets beyond the drawbacks of conventional techniques. Future biomanufacturing and therapeutic applications will heavily rely on nanoparticle systems as material science and bioengineering continue to progress (Zhu et al., 2024).

Enzyme Immobilization on Nanocarriers

An innovative method for enhancing enzyme performance in commercial biocatalysis is enzyme immobilisation on nanocarriers. Enzymes are biological catalysts that speed up chemical reactions by lowering activation energy without altering reaction equilibrium. Their stability like resistance to denaturation from factors like extreme pH, solvents, salts, and heat is essential for both basic and applied enzymology. Stabilization helps understand how enzymes loses its function and links structural integrity to activity, with the goal of producing durable, commercially viable enzymes. Denaturation, triggered by stressors such as strong acids, bases, salts, or organic solvents, disrupts the quaternary, tertiary, and secondary structures of enzymes, altering their active sites and overall shape, and thus impairing their function (Ding et al., 2015). Enzyme immobilization: a breakthrough solution for challenges in microbial manufacturing.

The enzyme immobilization focuses on two primary strategies for improving the stability and industrial applicability of microbial enzymes immobilization and chemical modification using polysaccharides. Enzymes are crucial biocatalysts used extensively in medicine, food processing, environmental remediation, and renewable energy production, but their practical use is often limited by instability under harsh conditions such as extreme pH, solvents, temperature, or mechanical stress. Enhancing their stability not only improves performance but also enables repeated use, lowering operational costs (Wahab, 2025).

Immobilization is highlighted as one of the most widely applied and cost-effective stabilization approaches. Also discusses traditional techniques such as adsorption, covalent bonding, cross-linking, encapsulation, and entrapment with detailing their mechanisms, advantages, and drawbacks. While adsorption is simple and reversible, it suffers from enzyme leakage; covalent bonding offers strong stability but may reduce activity; cross-linking improves rigidity but involves harsh reagents; and encapsulation or entrapment protects enzymes within membranes or gels but can cause diffusion limitations. Advances in support materials, such as biocompatible polymers, eco-friendly carriers, nanomaterials (graphene, MOFs, magnetic nanoparticles), and nanoporous gold, have further enhanced immobilization efficiency. Novel approaches like microwave-assisted immobilization, photo-immobilization, carrier-free systems such as cross-linked enzyme aggregates (CLEAs) and crystals (CLECs), and protein-coated microcrystals (PCMC) are also explored for their ability to improve activity, reusability, and process scalability (Khafaga et al., 2024).

The second major stabilization method examined is chemical modification via conjugation with chemically altered polysaccharides, such as acetylated, phosphorylated, sulfated, or carboxymethylated derivatives. These modifications can improve enzyme heat stability, solubility, and resistance to denaturation, while sometimes imparting additional bioactivities, including anticancer, antibacterial, and immune-stimulating properties. Polysaccharide conjugation also facilitates the creation of more intra- and intermolecular bonds within enzyme structures, thereby increasing durability (Wahab, 2025).

In medicine, immobilized enzymes are used in biosensors for rapid disease detection, in the production of antibiotics, and in targeted cancer therapy through enzyme-prodrug systems. In environmental biotechnology, they enable efficient bioremediation of pollutants such as dyes and phenolic compounds. In the energy sector, immobilized lipases serve as catalysts for biodiesel production, offering cleaner and more sustainable alternatives to chemical catalysts. In the food industry, they are used to produce lactose-free milk, high-fructose syrup, and nutraceuticals, with improved operational stability over free enzymes (Khafaga et al., 2024). Schematic representation showing applications in the field of bio-manufacturing is presented in **Figure 1.**

Figure 1. The scope of nano-materials in the field ofbio-manufacturing

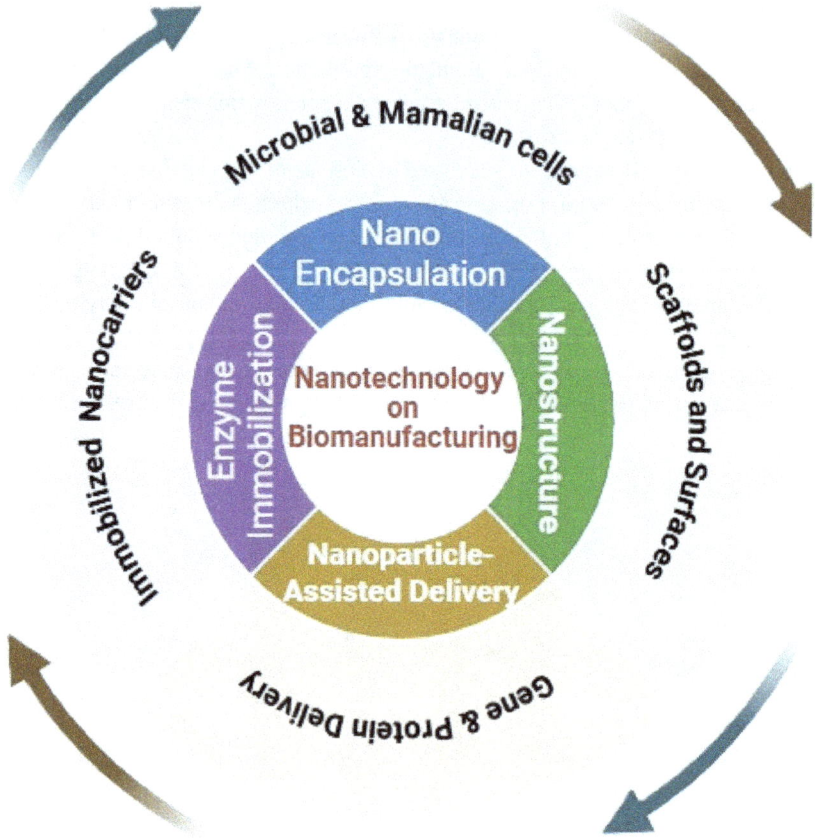

CHALLENGES IN BIO-MANUFACTURING SYSTEMS

The role of *E. coli* in the recombinant technology is well understood in the microbial production of valued-products industrially. However, host burden in producing recombinant proteins is one of the major constrains in industrial production of proteins. A number of strategies have been developed to alleviate the host burden with increased recombinant protein production (Zhang et al., 2021) have reported the strategies required for the high quality and quantity production of recombinant proteins in *E. coli*. They found the following strategies for high quality recombinant protein production with reduced stress of introducing foreign DNA in *E. coli*. They are: 1) regulating T7 RNA polymerase for high amounts of protein and its activity (Jeong et al., 2009; Kim et al., 2017; Z. Sun et al., 2021) 2) high amounts of mRNA synthesis by induction of RNA polymerase levels in the cell (Graumann & Premstaller, 2006; Z. Li & Rinas, 2020; Mittal et al., 2018; S.-I. Tan & Ng, 2020) 3) inducing recombinant protein expression at the level of pET-plasmid (Anilionyte et al., 2018; Chaudhary & Lee, 2015; Mirzadeh et al., 2015, 2020; Nie et al., 2020) 4) maintaining recombinant protein expression and bacterial cell growth (Cheng et al., 2017; Fuentes et al., 2013; Kumar et al., 2020; Minton, 1984; Yari et al., 2012) 5) balancing of growth and production with optimization and decoupling the process (Ceroni et al., 2015; Segall-Shapiro et al., 2014; Yari et al., 2012) 6) production decoupling between bacterial cell growth and recombinant protein (Galindo Casas et al., 2020; Kasari et al., 2022; Kolber et al., 2021; Menacho-Melgar et al., 2020; Ye et al., 2021) 7) recombinant protein activity optimization (Gawin et al., 2020; McElwain et al., 2022; Tripathi & Shrivastava, 2019; Yadwad et al., 1994; Ytterberg et al., 2019) 8) Inclusion bodies elimination (Huang et al., 2018; T. Kim et al., 2023; Ko et al., 2021). General production process and optimization of recombinant protein is depicted in **Figure 2**.

Figure 2. General recombinant protein (r-protein) optimization procedure in the microbial cells for industrial production of protein

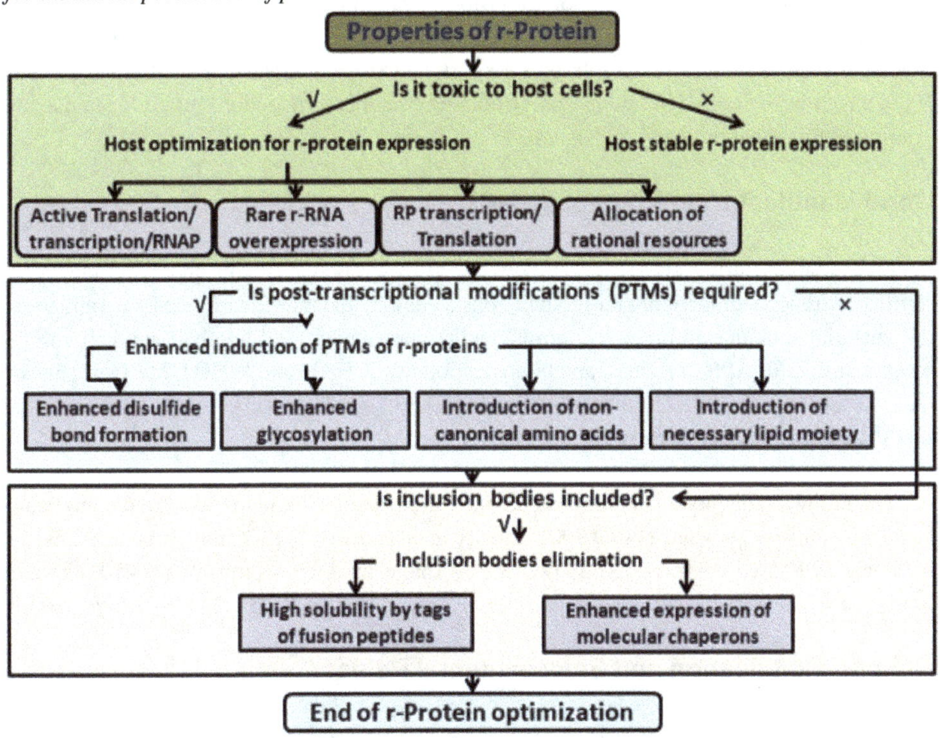

Where RNAP: RNA Polymerase; RP: recombinant protein; √: Yes; ×: No

BIOMANUFACTURING RULES FOR MICROBIAL AND CELL CULTURE SYSTEMS

Among all it is important that biomanufacturing industry strictly follow the rules and regulations framed and released by the Governments from time to time. Regulations governing microbial and cell culture systems in biomanufacturing aim to ensure the safety, quality, and consistency of products, particularly when utilized in pharmaceuticals, food, agriculture, or environmental applications. These frameworks generally encompass biosafety, quality management, and adherence to Good Manufacturing Practices (GMP).

Biosafety Regulations

The following biosafety regulations are to be followed in biomanufacturing industry. 1) Biosafety Levels (BSL-1 to BSL-4) delineate containment practices for the management of microorganisms based on their associated risk categories 2) Safe handling and containment procedures are outlined in the WHO Laboratory Biosafety Manual as well as the National Institutes of Health Guidelines for Research Involving Recombinant or Synthetic Nucleic Acid Molecules 3) Rules for the Manufacture, Use, Import, Export, and Storage of Hazardous Microorganisms, 1989, which were enacted in India as part of the Environment Protection Act, for example, are examples of national biosafety legislation.

Good Manufacturing Practice (GMP)

Basic manufacturing practices to follow are 1) Controls manufacturing environments for sterility, cross-contamination, and product consistency 2) Includes facility design, validation, raw material sourcing, in-process controls, and documentation 3) Microbial and cell culture manufacturing for APIs, vaccines, and biologics follows ICH Q7 and WHO GMP Guidelines.

Quality and Product Safety

The following quality and product safety measurements are to be followed in the biomanufacturing industry. They are 1) ISO 9001 (quality management) 2) ISO 13485 (medical devices involving cell-based components) 3) ISO 20387 (biotechnology – biobanking) 4) Endotoxin limits (USP <85> Bacterial Endotoxins Test) 5) Sterility testing (USP <71> Sterility Tests).

Genetic Modification and Environmental Release

The Cartagena Protocol on Biosafety regulates the transboundary movement of genetically modified organisms. National guidelines for GMOs encompass the approval, containment, and monitoring of recombinant microbial strains.

Specific Product Regulations

The specific product regulations to be followed are: 1) Biopharmaceuticals: The EMA and US FDA have released product-specific guidelines pertaining to cell-based therapies, vaccines, and recombinant proteins 2) Food and Feed: The European Food Safety Authority (EFSA) and the Food and Drug Administration (FDA) oversee the regulation of probiotics, fermented products, and microbial-derived food additives 3) Industrial enzymes and biochemicals are subject to REACH regulations in the EU and TSCA requirements in the US for chemical safety during export and import activities.

CONCLUSION

Bio-manufacturing systems are the bacterial systems in earlier days. At present permitting variety of biological cell as cell culture systems for bio-product production through technological advancements. To meet the demand of various products of industrially important are producing by following r-DNA technology in a variety of cell culture systems, including human cells. The present chapter emphasized the evolution of various types of cell systems using advanced technologies like gene manipulations and nanotechnology from the conventional biomanufacturing. The role of advanced modern science like r-DNA technology, metabolic engineering, CRSPR-Cas9 and genome editing, nano-encapsulation, nano-assisted gene and protein delivery, and nano-carrier mediated enzyme immobilization in enhancing the high valued compounds production using microbial and cell culture systems in biomanufacturing are also outlined. This chapter also projected various challenges facing by the bio-manufacturing industry in the present scenario along with rules and regulations to follow in bio-product synthesis. However, the researchers working for the development of microbial and cell culture systems for biomanufacturing are need to focus on more effective computational models with the support of artificial intelligence, integrating metabolic pathways, cell signaling, gene regulatory mechanisms and protein-protein interaction networks along with production kinetics of bioreactor industrially to gather with detailed system knowledge including proper regulatory guidelines for the production of new desired drugs and products.

ACKNOWLEDGEMENT

Authors are grateful to RUSA 2.0 (file No. RUSA-ANU/YVU/Research project-01/Sanction order/2024 Dated: 01.06.2024), Government of India, New Delhi and Government of Andhra Pradesh, A.P. for financial support sanctioned to Prof. P. Ramachandra Reddy, PI, Department of Biochemistry, Yogi Vemana University, Vemanapuram, Kadapa. Authors are thankful to authorities of Yogi Vemana University, Kadapa for providing facilities to writing this book chapter.

REFERENCES

Afeyan, N. B., & Cooney, C. L. (2006). Professor Daniel I.C. Wang: A legacy of education, innovation, publication, and leadership. *Biotechnology and Bioengineering*, *95*(2), 206–217. DOI: 10.1002/bit.21078

Alonso-Gutierrez, J., Chan, R., Batth, T. S., Adams, P. D., Keasling, J. D., Petzold, C. J., & Lee, T. S. (2-13). Metabolic engineering of *Escherichia coli* for limonene and perillyl alcohol production. *Metabolic Engineering*, *19*, 33–41.

Andersen, R. L., Jensen, K. M., & Mikkelsen, M. J. (2015). Continuous Ethanol Fermentation of Pretreated Lignocellulosic Biomasses, Waste Biomasses, Molasses and Syrup Using the Anaerobic, Thermophilic Bacterium Thermoanaerobacter italicus Pentocrobe 411. *PLoS One*, *10*(8), e0136060. DOI: 10.1371/journal.pone.0136060

Anilionyte, O., Liang, H., Ma, X., Yang, L., & Zhou, K. (2018). Short, auto-inducible promoters for well-controlled protein expression in Escherichia coli. *Applied Microbiology and Biotechnology*, *102*(16), 7007–7015. DOI: 10.1007/s00253-018-9141-z

Arendt, E. K., Moroni, A., & Zannini, E. (2011). Medical nutrition therapy: use of sourdough lactic acid bacteria as a cell factory for delivering functional biomolecules and food ingredients in gluten free bread. *Microbial Cell Factories, 10 Suppl 1*(Suppl 1), S15. https://doi.org/DOI: 10.1186/1475-2859-10-S1-S15

Arratia-Quijada, J., Nuño, K., Ruíz-Santoyo, V., & Andrade-Espinoza, B. A. (2024). Nano-encapsulation of probiotics: Need and critical considerations to design new non-dairy probiotic products. *Journal of Functional Foods*, *116*, 106192. DOI: 10.1016/j.jff.2024.106192

Ayala, J. C., Pimienta, E., Rodríguez, C., Anné, J., Vallín, C., Milanés, M. T., King-Batsios, E., Huygen, K., & Van Mellaert, L. (2013). Use of Strep-tag II for rapid detection and purification of Mycobacterium tuberculosis recombinant antigens secreted by Streptomyces lividans. *Journal of Microbiological Methods*, *94*(3), 192–198. DOI: 10.1016/j.mimet.2013.06.004

Baldanta, S., Guevara, G., & Navarro-Llorens, J. M. (2022). SEVA-Cpf1, a CRISPR-Cas12a vector for genome editing in cyanobacteria. *Microbial Cell Factories*, *21*(1), 103. DOI: 10.1186/s12934-022-01830-4

Bankar, S. B., Survase, S. A., Singhal, R. S., & Granström, T. (2012). Continuous two stage acetone–butanol–ethanol fermentation with integrated solvent removal using Clostridium acetobutylicum B 5313. *Bioresource Technology, 106*, 110–116. DOI: 10.1016/j.biortech.2011.12.005

Bastian, F., Bernard, C., Lyon, U., Cohen, A., Piccoli, P., Luna, M. V., Bastián, F., Luna, V., Baraldi, R., & Bottini, R. (1998). Production of indole-3-acetic acid and gibberellins A_1 and A_3 by Acetobacter diazotrophicus and Herbaspirillum seropedicae in chemically-defined culture media Production of indole-3-acetic acid and gibberellins A 1 and A 3 by Acetobacter diazotrophicus and Herbaspirillum seropedicae in chemically-defined culture media. In *Plant Growth Regulation* (Vol. 24, Issue 7). https://www.researchgate.net/publication/263453138

Bermúdez-Humarán, L. G., Kharrat, P., Chatel, J.-M., & Langella, P. (2011). Lactococci and lactobacilli as mucosal delivery vectors for therapeutic proteins and DNA vaccines. *Microbial Cell Factories, 10*(S1), S4. DOI: 10.1186/1475-2859-10-S1-S4

Bikram, P. U., Linda, C. D., & Lew, P. C. (2014). Metabolic engineering as a tool for enhanced lactic acid production. *Trends in Biotechnology, 32*(12), 637–644. DOI: 10.1016/j.tibtech.2014.10.005

Bornscheuer, U. T., Huisman, G. W., Kazlauskas, R. J., Lutz, S., Moore, J. C., & Robins, K. (2012). Engineering the third wave of biocatalysis. *Nature, 485*(7397), 185–194. DOI: 10.1038/nature11117

Bunnak, P., Allmendinger, R., Ramasamy, S. V., Lettieri, P., & Titchener-Hooker, N. J. (2016). Life-cycle and cost of goods assessment of fed-batch and perfusion-based manufacturing processes for mAbs. *Biotechnology Progress, 32*(5), 1324–1335. DOI: 10.1002/btpr.2323

Byrne, K. (2014). High density CHO cell cultures: Improved productivity and product quality. A thesis submitted to Dublin City University, Dublin, Ireland.

Carter, H. E., Clark, R. K., Dickman, S. R., Loo, Y. H., Skell, I. S., & Strong, W. A. (1945). *ISOLATION AND PURIFICATION OF STREPTOMYCIN*.*

Ceroni, F., Algar, R., Stan, G.-B., & Ellis, T. (2015). Quantifying cellular capacity identifies gene expression designs with reduced burden. *Nature Methods, 12*(5), 415–418. DOI: 10.1038/nmeth.3339

Chaudhary, A. K., & Lee, E. Y. (2015). Tightly regulated and high level expression vector construction for Escherichia coli BL21 (DE3). *Journal of Industrial and Engineering Chemistry, 31*, 367–373. DOI: 10.1016/j.jiec.2015.07.011

Cheng, L., Yang, X., Li, S., Fu, Q., Fu, S., Wang, J., Li, F., Lei, L., & Shen, Z. (2017). Impact of gene modification of phosphotransferase system on expression of glutamate dehydrogenase protein of *Streptococcus suis* in *Escherichia coli. Biotechnology, Biotechnological Equipment, 31*(3), 612–618. DOI: 10.1080/13102818.2017.1304179

Cho, A., Yun, H., Park, J. H., Lee, S. Y., & Park, S. (2010). Prediction of novel synthetic pathways for the production of desired chemicals. *BMC Systamatic Biology, 4*(1), 35.

Christopher, L. P., Kapatral, V., Vaisvil, B., Emel, G., & DeVeaux, L. C. (2014). Draft Genome Sequence of a New Homofermentative, Lactic Acid-Producing *Enterococcus faecalis* Isolate, CBRD01. *Genome Announcements*, *2*(2), e00147–e14. DOI: 10.1128/genomea.00147-14

Cui, Z., Zhong, Y., Sun, Z., Jiang, Z., Deng, J., Wang, Q., Nielsen, J., Hou, J., & Qi, Q. (2023). Reconfiguration of the reductive TCA cycle enables high-level succinic acid production by Yarrowia lipolytica. *Nature Communications*, *14*(1), 8480. DOI: 10.1038/s41467-023-44245-4

Daniel, C., Roussel, Y., Kleerebezem, M., & Pot, B. (2011). Recombinant lactic acid bacteria as mucosal biotherapeutic agents. *Trends in Biotechnology*, *29*(10), 499–508. DOI: 10.1016/j.tibtech.2011.05.002

David, F., Steinwand, M., Hust, M., Bohle, K., Ross, A., Dübel, S., & Franco-Lara, E. (2011). Antibody production in *Bacillus megaterium*: Strategies and physiological implications of scaling from microtiter plates to industrial bioreactors. *Biotechnology Journal*, *6*(12), 1516–1531. DOI: 10.1002/biot.201000417

de Vos, W. M. (2011). Systems solutions by lactic acid bacteria: From paradigms to practice. *Microbial Cell Factories*, *10*(Suppl 1), S2. DOI: 10.1186/1475-2859-10-S1-S2

Deb, P., Talukdar, S. A., Mohsina, K., Sarker, P. K., & Sayem, S. A. (2013). Production and partial characterization of extracellular amylase enzyme from *Bacillus amyloliquefaciens* P-001. *SpringerPlus*, *2*(1), 154. DOI: 10.1186/2193-1801-2-154

Demain, A. L. (2007). REVIEWS: The business of biotechnology. *Industrial Biotechnology (New Rochelle, N.Y.)*, *3*(3), 269–283. DOI: 10.1089/ind.2007.3.269

Demain, A. L., & Elander, R. P. (1999). The β-lactam antibiotics: Past, present, and future. *Antonie van Leeuwenhoek*, *75*(1–2), 5–19. DOI: 10.1023/A:1001738823146

Demain, A. L., & Vaishnav, P. (2009). Production of recombinant proteins by microbes and higher organisms. *Biotechnology Advances*, *27*(3), 297–306. DOI: 10.1016/j.biotechadv.2009.01.008

Dhakal, D., Dhakal, Y., & Sohng, J. K. (2017). Book review: antibody-drug conjugates: fun- damentals, drug development, and clinical outcomes to target cancer. *Frontiers in Pharmacology*, *8*, 771.

Ding, S., Cargill, A. A., Medintz, I. L., & Claussen, J. C. (2015). Increasing the activity of immobilized enzymes with nanoparticle conjugation. *Current Opinion in Biotechnology*, *34*, 242–250. DOI: 10.1016/j.copbio.2015.04.005

Eggeling, L., & Bott, M. (Eds.). (2005). *Handbook of Corynebacterium glutamicum*. CRC Press., DOI: 10.1201/9781420039696

Ferrer-Miralles, N., & Villaverde, A. (2013). Bacterial cell factories for recombinant protein production; expanding the catalogue. *Microbial Cell Factories*, *12*(1), 113. DOI: 10.1186/1475-2859-12-113

Fleet, G. H. (2008). Wine yeasts for the future. *FEMS Yeast Research*, *8*(7), 979–995. DOI: 10.1111/j.1567-1364.2008.00427.x

Fuentes, L. G., Lara, A. R., Martínez, L. M., Ramírez, O. T., Martínez, A., Bolívar, F., & Gosset, G. (2013). Modification of glucose import capacity in Escherichia coli: Physiologic consequences and utility for improving DNA vaccine production. *Microbial Cell Factories, 12*(1), 42. DOI: 10.1186/1475-2859-12-42

Fuentes-Ramírez, L. E., Bustillos-Cristales, R., Tapia-Hernández, A., Jiménez-Salgado, T., Wang, E. T., Martínez-Romero, E., & Caballero-Mellado, J. (2001). Novel nitrogen-fixing acetic acid bacteria, Gluconacetobacter johannae sp. nov. and Gluconacetobacter azotocaptans sp. nov., associated with coffee plants. *International Journal of Systematic and Evolutionary Microbiology, 51*(4), 1305–1314. DOI: 10.1099/00207713-51-4-1305

Galindo Casas, M., Stargardt, P., Mairhofer, J., & Wiltschi, B. (2020). Decoupling Protein Production from Cell Growth Enhances the Site-Specific Incorporation of Noncanonical Amino Acids in *E. coli. ACS Synthetic Biology, 9*(11), 3052–3066. DOI: 10.1021/acssynbio.0c00298

García-Fruitós, E. (2012). Lactic acid bacteria: A promising alternative for recombinant protein production. *Microbial Cell Factories, 11*(1), 157. DOI: 10.1186/1475-2859-11-157

Gawin, A., Ertesvåg, H., Hansen, S. A. H., Malmo, J., & Brautaset, T. (2020). Translational regulation of periplasmic folding assistants and proteases as a valuable strategy to improve production of translocated recombinant proteins in Escherichia coli. *BMC Biotechnology, 20*(1), 24. DOI: 10.1186/s12896-020-00615-0

Ghanemi, A. (2015). Cell cultures in drug development: Applications, challenges and limitations. *Saudi Pharmaceutical Journal : SPJ : the Official Publication of the Saudi Pharmaceutical Society, 23*(4), 453–454. DOI: 10.1016/j.jsps.2014.04.002

Gottschalk, U., Brorson, K., & Shukla, A. A. (2012). The need for innovation in biomanufacturing. *Nature Biotechnology, 30*(6), 489–492. DOI: 10.1038/nbt.2263

Graumann, K., & Premstaller, A. (2006). Manufacturing of recombinant therapeutic proteins in microbial systems. *Biotechnology Journal, 1*(2), 164–186. DOI: 10.1002/biot.200500051

Guo, X.-Q., Wei, Y.-M., & Yu, B. (2012). Recombinant Mycobacterium smegmatis expressing Hsp65–hIL–2 fusion protein and its influence on lymphocyte function in mice. *Asian Pacific Journal of Tropical Medicine, 5*(5), 347–351. DOI: 10.1016/S1995-7645(12)60056-X

Harvey, A. L., Edrada-Ebel, R., & Quinn, R. J. (2015). The re-emergence of natural products for drug discovery in the genomics era. *Nature Reviews. Drug Discovery, 14*(2), 111.

Hasegawa, S., Suda, M., Uematsu, K., Natsuma, Y., Hiraga, K., Jojima, T., Inui, M., & Yukawa, H. (2013). Engineering of Corynebacterium glutamicum for High-Yield <scp>l</scp> -Valine Production under Oxygen Deprivation Conditions. *Applied and Environmental Microbiology, 79*(4), 1250–1257. DOI: 10.1128/AEM.02806-12

Hosoya, Y., Okamoto, S., Muramatsu, H., & Ochi, K. (1998). Acquisition of Certain Streptomycin-Resistant (*str*) Mutations Enhances Antibiotic Production in Bacteria. *Antimicrobial Agents and Chemotherapy, 42*(8), 2041–2047. DOI: 10.1128/AAC.42.8.2041

Hsu, P. D., Scott, D. A., & Weinstein, J. A. (2013). DNA targeting specificity of RNA-guided Cas9 nucleases. *Nature Biotechnology, 31*(9), 827–832. DOI: 10.1038/nbt.2647

Hu, S., Kong, J., Sun, Z., Han, L., Kong, W., & Yang, P. (2011). Heterologous protein display on the cell surface of lactic acid bacteria mediated by the s-layer protein. *Microbial Cell Factories, 10*(1), 86. DOI: 10.1186/1475-2859-10-86

Huang, M. nan, Lu, X. yao, Zong, H., Zhuge, B., & Shen, W. (2018). Bioproduction of trans-10,cis-12-Conjugated Linoleic Acid by a Highly Soluble and Conveniently Extracted Linoleic Acid Isomerase and an Extracellularly Expressed Lipase from Recombinant Escherichia coli Strains. *Journal of Microbiology and Biotechnology, 28*(5), 739–747. DOI: 10.4014/jmb.1802.02007

Jansen, M. L. A., Bracher, J. M., Papapetridis, I., Verhoeven, M. D., de Bruijn, H., de Waal, P. P., van Maris, A. J. A., Klaassen, P., & Pronk, J. T. (2017). Saccharomyces cerevisiae strains for second-generation ethanol production: From academic exploration to industrial implementation. *FEMS Yeast Research, 17*(5). Advance online publication. DOI: 10.1093/femsyr/fox044

Jeong, H., Barbe, V., Lee, C. H., Vallenet, D., Yu, D. S., Choi, S.-H., Couloux, A., Lee, S.-W., Yoon, S. H., Cattolico, L., Hur, C.-G., Park, H.-S., Ségurens, B., Kim, S. C., Oh, T. K., Lenski, R. E., Studier, F. W., Daegelen, P., & Kim, J. F. (2009). Genome Sequences of Escherichia coli B strains REL606 and BL21(DE3). *Journal of Molecular Biology, 394*(4), 644–652. DOI: 10.1016/j.jmb.2009.09.052

Jin, H., Cantin, G. T., Maki, S., Chew, L. C., Resnick, S. M., Ngai, J., & Retallack, D. M. (2011). Soluble periplasmic production of human granulocyte colony-stimulating factor (G-CSF) in Pseudomonas fluorescens. *Protein Expression and Purification, 78*(1), 69–77. DOI: 10.1016/j.pep.2011.03.002

Jones, D. T., & Woods, D. R. (1986). Acetone-butanol fermentation revisited. *Microbiological Reviews, 50*(4), 484–524. DOI: 10.1128/mr.50.4.484-524.1986

Jung, H. N., Lee, S.-Y., Lee, S., Youn, H., & Im, H.-J. (2022). Lipid nanoparticles for delivery of RNA therapeutics: Current status and the role of *in vivo* imaging. *Theranostics, 12*(17), 7509–7531. DOI: 10.7150/thno.77259

Kasari, M., Kasari, V., Kärmas, M., & Jõers, A. (2022). Decoupling Growth and Production by Removing the Origin of Replication from a Bacterial Chromosome. *ACS Synthetic Biology, 11*(8), 2610–2622. DOI: 10.1021/acssynbio.1c00618

Khafaga, D. S. R., Muteeb, G., Elgarawany, A., Aatif, M., Farhan, M., Allam, S., Almatar, B. A., & Radwan, M. G. (2024). Green nanobiocatalysts: Enhancing enzyme immobilization for industrial and biomedical applications. *PeerJ, 12*, e17589. DOI: 10.7717/peerj.17589

Khan, S., Ullah, M. W., Siddique, R., Nabi, G., Manan, S., Yousaf, M., & Hou, H. (2016). Role of Recombinant DNA Technology to Improve Life. *International Journal of Genomics, 2016*, 1–14. DOI: 10.1155/2016/2405954

Khanal, O., & Lenhoff, A. M. (2021). Developments and opportunities in continuous biopharmaceutical manufacturing. *mAbs, 13*(1). Advance online publication. DOI: 10.1080/19420862.2021.1903664

Kim, S., Jang, Y.-S., Ha, S.-C., Ahn, J.-W., Kim, E.-J., Hong Lim, J., Cho, C., Shin Ryu, Y., Kuk Lee, S., Lee, S. Y., & Kim, K.-J. (2015). Redox-switch regulatory mechanism of thiolase from Clostridium acetobutylicum. *Nature Communications*, *6*(1), 8410. DOI: 10.1038/ncomms9410

Kim, S. K., Lee, D.-H., Kim, O. C., Kim, J. F., & Yoon, S. H. (2017). Tunable Control of an *Escherichia coli* Expression System for the Overproduction of Membrane Proteins by Titrated Expression of a Mutant *lac* Repressor. *ACS Synthetic Biology*, *6*(9), 1766–1773. DOI: 10.1021/acssynbio.7b00102

Kim, T., Chung, H. S., Lee, H.-S., Uthaman, S., Park, I.-K., & Park, K. (2023). Effects of retinoid-loaded hyaluronic acid nanomicelles on vaginal epithelium in a murine menopause model. *Investigative and Clinical Urology*, *64*(2), 182. DOI: 10.4111/icu.20220366

Ko, H., Kang, M., Kim, M.-J., Yi, J., Kang, J., Bae, J.-H., Sohn, J.-H., & Sung, B. H. (2021). A novel protein fusion partner, carbohydrate-binding module family 66, to enhance heterologous protein expression in Escherichia coli. *Microbial Cell Factories*, *20*(1), 232. DOI: 10.1186/s12934-021-01725-w

Kolber, N. S., Fattal, R., Bratulic, S., Carver, G. D., & Badran, A. H. (2021). Orthogonal translation enables heterologous ribosome engineering in E. coli. *Nature Communications*, *12*(1), 599. DOI: 10.1038/s41467-020-20759-z

Kumar, J., Chauhan, A. S., Shah, R. L., Gupta, J. A., & Rathore, A. S. (2020). Amino acid supplementation for enhancing recombinant protein production in *E. coli*. *Biotechnology and Bioengineering*, *117*(8), 2420–2433. DOI: 10.1002/bit.27371

Kurosawa, K., Plassmeier, J., Kalinowski, J., Rückert, C., & Sinskey, A. J. (2015). Engineering l-arabinose metabolism in triacylglycerol-producing Rhodococcus opacus for lignocellulosic fuel production. *Metabolic Engineering*, *30*, 89–95. DOI: 10.1016/j.ymben.2015.04.006

Lan, E. I., & Liao, J. C. (2013). Microbial synthesis of n-butanol, isobutanol, and other higher alcohols from diverse resources. *Bioresource Technology*, *135*, 339–349. DOI: 10.1016/j.biortech.2012.09.104

Lee, J. W., Yi, J., Kim, T. Y., Choi, S., Ahn, J. H., Song, H., Lee, M.-H., & Lee, S. Y. (2016). Homo-succinic acid production by metabolically engineered Mannheimia succiniciproducens. *Metabolic Engineering*, *38*, 409–417. DOI: 10.1016/j.ymben.2016.10.004

Lee, P. C., Lee, S. Y., Hong, S. H., Chang, H. N., & Park, S. C. (2003). Biological conversion of wood hydrolysate to succinic acid by Anaerobiospirillum succiniciproducens. *Biotechnology Letters*, *25*(2), 111–114. DOI: 10.1023/A:1021907116361

Lee, S. Y., Park, J. H., Jang, S. H., Nielsen, L. K., Kim, J., & Jung, K. S. (2008). Fermentative butanol production by clostridia. *Biotechnology and Bioengineering*, *101*(2), 209–228. DOI: 10.1002/bit.22003

Li, Y., Wang, Y., Wang, R., Yan, X., Wang, J., Wang, X., Chen, S., Bai, F., He, Q., & Yang, S. (2022). Metabolic engineering of *Zymomonas mobilis* for continuous co-production of bioethanol and poly-3-hydroxybutyrate (PHB). *Green Chemistry*, *24*(6), 2588–2601. DOI: 10.1039/D1GC04522A

Li, Z., & Rinas, U. (2020). Recombinant protein production associated growth inhibition results mainly from transcription and not from translation. *Microbial Cell Factories*, *19*(1), 83. DOI: 10.1186/s12934-020-01343-y

Lian, J., Chao, R., & Zhao, H. (2014). Metabolic engineering of a Saccharomyces cere- visiae strain capable of simultaneously utilizing glucose and galactose to pro- duce enantiopure (2r, 3r)-butanediol. *Metabolic Engineering*, *23*, 92–99.

Liang, L., Tan, H., & Liu, R. (2025). Emerging gene editing in industrial microbiology beyond CRISPR-Cas9. *Trends in Biotechnology*, *43*(4), 742–744. DOI: 10.1016/j.tibtech.2024.09.012

Liese, A., & Hilterhaus, L. (2013). Evaluation of immobilized enzymes for industrial applications. *Chemical Society Reviews*, *42*(15), 6236. DOI: 10.1039/c3cs35511j

Lindberg, P., Park, S., & Melis, A. (2010). Engineering a platform for photosynthetic iso- prene production in cyanobacteria, using Synechocystis as the model organism. *Metabolic Engineering*, *12*(1), 70–79.

Liu, K., Atiyeh, H. K., Stevenson, B. S., Tanner, R. S., Wilkins, M. R., & Huhnke, R. L. (2014). Continuous syngas fermentation for the production of ethanol, n-propanol and n-butanol. *Bioresource Technology*, *151*, 69–77. DOI: 10.1016/j.biortech.2013.10.059

Liu, P., Xu, H., & Zhang, X. (2022). Metabolic engineering of microorganisms for L-alanine production. *Journal of Industrial Microbiology & Biotechnology*, *49*(2). Advance online publication. DOI: 10.1093/jimb/kuab057

Liu, S., Yu, J.-M., Gan, Y.-C., Qiu, X.-Z., Gao, Z.-C., Wang, H., Chen, S.-X., Xiong, Y., Liu, G.-H., Lin, S.-E., McCarthy, A., John, J. V., Wei, D.-X., & Hou, H.-H. (2023). Biomimetic natural biomaterials for tissue engineering and regenerative medicine: New biosynthesis methods, recent advances, and emerging applications. *Military Medical Research*, *10*(1), 16. DOI: 10.1186/s40779-023-00448-w

Lucio, M., & Fermentec, L. (2008). Continuous and batch fermentation processes: Advantages and disadvantages of these processes in the Brazilian ethanol production. In *Article in International Sugar Journal*. https://www.researchgate.net/publication/289874380

Luo, X., Reiter, M. A., d'Espaux, L., Wong, J., Denby, C. M., Lechner, A., Zhang, Y., Grzybowski, A. T., Harth, S., Lin, W., Lee, H., Yu, C., Shin, J., Deng, K., Benites, V. T., Wang, G., Baidoo, E. E. K., Chen, Y., Dev, I., & Keasling, J. D. (2019). Complete biosynthesis of cannabinoids and their unnatural analogues in yeast. *Nature*, *567*(7746), 123–126. DOI: 10.1038/s41586-019-0978-9

Lv, Y., Li, W., Liao, W., Jiang, H., Liu, Y., Cao, J., Lu, W., & Feng, Y. (2024). Nano-Drug Delivery Systems Based on Natural Products. *International Journal of Nanomedicine*, *19*, 541–569. DOI: 10.2147/IJN.S443692

Maharaj, K., Bradfield, M. F. A., & Nicol, W. (2014). Succinic acid-producing biofilms of Actinobacillus succinogenes: Reproducibility, stability and productivity. *Applied Microbiology and Biotechnology*, *98*(17), 7379–7386. DOI: 10.1007/s00253-014-5779-3

McElwain, L., Phair, K., Kealey, C., & Brady, D. (2022). Current trends in biopharmaceuticals production in Escherichia coli. *Biotechnology Letters*, *44*(8), 917–931. DOI: 10.1007/s10529-022-03276-5

McGovern, P. E., Zhang, J., Tang, J., Zhang, Z., Hall, G. R., Moreau, R. A., Nuñez, A., Butrym, E. D., Richards, M. P., Wang, C., Cheng, G., Zhao, Z., & Wang, C. (2004). Fermented beverages of pre- and proto-historic China. *Proceedings of the National Academy of Sciences of the United States of America*, *101*(51), 17593–17598. DOI: 10.1073/pnas.0407921102

McShan, D. C., Rao, S., & Shah, I. (2003). Pathminer: Predicting metabolic pathways by heuristic search. *Bioinformatics (Oxford, England)*, *19*(13), 1692–1698.

Menacho-Melgar, R., Moreb, E. A., Efromson, J. P., Yang, T., Hennigan, J. N., Wang, R., & Lynch, M. D. (2020). Improved two-stage protein expression and purification via autoinduction of both autolysis and auto DNA/RNA hydrolysis conferred by phage lysozyme and DNA/RNA endonuclease. *Biotechnology and Bioengineering*, *117*(9), 2852–2860. DOI: 10.1002/bit.27444

Menzel, K., Zeng, A.-P., & Deckwer, W.-D. (1997). High concentration and productivity of 1,3-propanediol from continuous fermentation of glycerol by Klebsiella pneumoniae. *Enzyme and Microbial Technology*, *20*(2), 82–86. DOI: 10.1016/S0141-0229(96)00087-7

Michels, P., & Rosazza, J. (2009). The evolution of microbial transformations for industrial applications. *SIM News*, 36–59.

Minton, N. P. (1984). Improved plasmid vectors for the isolation of translational lac gene fusions. *Gene*, *31*(1–3), 269–273. DOI: 10.1016/0378-1119(84)90220-8

Mirsalami, S. M., & Mirsalami, M. (2025). Advances in genetically engineered microorganisms: Transforming food production through precision fermentation and synthetic biology. *Future Foods : a Dedicated Journal for Sustainability in Food Science*, *11*, 100601. DOI: 10.1016/j.fufo.2025.100601

Mirzadeh, K., Martínez, V., Toddo, S., Guntur, S., Herrgård, M. J., Elofsson, A., Nørholm, M. H. H., & Daley, D. O. (2015). Enhanced Protein Production in *Escherichia coli* by Optimization of Cloning Scars at the Vector–Coding Sequence Junction. *ACS Synthetic Biology*, *4*(9), 959–965. DOI: 10.1021/acssynbio.5b00033

Mirzadeh, K., Shilling, P. J., Elfageih, R., Cumming, A. J., Cui, H. L., Rennig, M., Nørholm, M. H. H., & Daley, D. O. (2020). Increased production of periplasmic proteins in Escherichia coli by directed evolution of the translation initiation region. *Microbial Cell Factories*, *19*(1), 85. DOI: 10.1186/s12934-020-01339-8

Mittal, P., Brindle, J., Stephen, J., Plotkin, J. B., & Kudla, G. (2018). Codon usage influences fitness through RNA toxicity. *Proceedings of the National Academy of Sciences of the United States of America*, *115*(34), 8639–8644. DOI: 10.1073/pnas.1810022115

Morello, E., Bermúdez-Humarán, L. G., Llull, D., Solé, V., Miraglio, N., Langella, P., & Poquet, I. (2008). <i>Lactococcus lactis,</i> an Efficient Cell Factory for Recombinant Protein Production and Secretion. *Microbial Physiology, 14*(1–3), 48–58. https://doi.org/DOI: 10.1159/000106082

Moriya, Y., Shigemizu, D., Hattori, M., Tokimatsu, T., Kotera, M., Goto, S., & Kanehisa, M. (2010). Pathpred: An enzyme-catalyzed metabolic pathway prediction server. *Nucleic Acids Research, 38*(2), W138–W143.

Myung, S., Zhang, X., & Percival Zhang, Y.-H. (2011). Ultra-stable phosphoglucose isomerase through immobilization of cellulose-binding module-tagged thermophilic enzyme on low-cost high-capacity cellulosic adsorbent. *Biotechnology Progress, 27*(4), 969–975. DOI: 10.1002/btpr.606

Nakamura, C. E., & Whited, G. M. (2003). Metabolic engineering for the microbial production of 1,3-propanediol. *Current Opinion in Biotechnology, 14*(5), 454–459. DOI: 10.1016/j.copbio.2003.08.005

Nehal, N., Mathur, A., Ganguli, M., & Singh, P. (2022). Fermentation Process Versus Nanotechnology. In *Nanomaterials in Clinical Therapeutics* (pp. 115–175). Wiley., DOI: 10.1002/9781119857747.ch4

Nguyen, T.-T., Nguyen, H. A., Arreola, S. L., Mlynek, G., Djinović-Carugo, K., Mathiesen, G., Nguyen, T.-H., & Haltrich, D. (2012). Homodimeric β-Galactosidase from Lactobacillus delbrueckii subsp. *bulgaricus* DSM 20081: Expression in Lactobacillus plantarum and Biochemical Characterization. *Journal of Agricultural and Food Chemistry, 60*(7), 1713–1721. DOI: 10.1021/jf203909e

Nguyen, V. T., Flanagan, B., Gidley, M. J., & Dykes, G. A. (2008). Characterization of Cellulose Production by a Gluconacetobacter xylinus Strain from Kombucha. *Current Microbiology, 57*(5), 449–453. DOI: 10.1007/s00284-008-9228-3

Nie, Z., Luo, H., Li, J., Sun, H., Xiao, Y., Jia, R., Liu, T., Chang, Y., Yu, H., & Shen, Z. (2020). High-Throughput Screening of T7 Promoter Mutants for Soluble Expression of Cephalosporin C Acylase in E. coli. *Applied Biochemistry and Biotechnology, 190*(1), 293–304. DOI: 10.1007/s12010-019-03113-y

Noens, E. E., Williams, C., Anandhakrishnan, M., Poulsen, C., Ehebauer, M. T., & Wilmanns, M. (2011). Improved mycobacterial protein production using a Mycobacterium smegmatis groEL1ΔCexpression strain. *BMC Biotechnology, 11*(1), 27. DOI: 10.1186/1472-6750-11-27

Olszewska-Widdrat, A., Alexandri, M., López-Gómez, J. P., Schneider, R., & Venus, J. (2020). Batch and Continuous Lactic Acid Fermentation Based on A Multi-Substrate Approach. *Microorganisms, 8*(7), 1084. DOI: 10.3390/microorganisms8071084

Ou, Y., & Guo, S. (2023). Safety risks and ethical governance of biomedical applications of synthetic biology. *Frontiers in Bioengineering and Biotechnology, 11*. Advance online publication. DOI: 10.3389/fbioe.2023.1292029

Pandey, K., Pandey, M., Kumar, V., Aggarwal, U., & Singhal, B. (2024). Bioprocessing 4.0 in biomanufacturing: Paving the way for sustainable bioeconomy. *Systems Microbiology and Biomanufacturing, 4*(2), 407–424. DOI: 10.1007/s43393-023-00206-y

Paradis, F. W., Warren, R. A. J., Kilburn, D. G., & Miller, R. C. (1987). The expression of Cellulomonas fimi cellulase genes in Brevibacterium lactofermentum. *Gene, 61*(2), 199–206. DOI: 10.1016/0378-1119(87)90114-4

Peebo, K., & Neubauer, P. (2018). Application of Continuous Culture Methods to Recombinant Protein Production in Microorganisms. *Microorganisms, 6*(3), 56. DOI: 10.3390/microorganisms6030056

Peterbauer, C., Maischberger, T., & Haltrich, D. (2011). Food-grade gene expression in lactic acid bacteria. *Biotechnology Journal, 6*(9), 1147–1161. DOI: 10.1002/biot.201100034

Pontes, D. S., de Azevedo, M. S. P., Chatel, J.-M., Langella, P., Azevedo, V., & Miyoshi, A. (2011). Lactococcus lactis as a live vector: Heterologous protein production and DNA delivery systems. *Protein Expression and Purification, 79*(2), 165–175. DOI: 10.1016/j.pep.2011.06.005

Qiao, K., Wasylenko, T. M., Zhou, K., Xu, P., & Stephanopoulos, G. (2017). Lipid production in Yarrowia lipolytica is maximized by engineering cytosolic redox metabolism. *Nature Biotechnology, 35*(2), 173–177. DOI: 10.1038/nbt.3763

Qin, Y., Li, Q., Fan, L., Ning, X., Wei, X., & You, C. (2023). *Biomanufacturing by In Vitro Biotransformation (ivBT).* Using Purified Cascade Multi-enzymes., DOI: 10.1007/10_2023_231

Rasala, B. A., & Mayfield, S. P. (2015). Photosynthetic biomanufacturing in green algae; production of recombinant proteins for industrial, nutritional, and medical uses. *Photosynthesis Research, 123*(3), 227–239. DOI: 10.1007/s11120-014-9994-7

Remmers, I. M., Hidalgo-Ulloa, A., Brandt, B. P., Evers, W. A. C., Wijffels, R. H., & Lamers, P. P. (2017). Continuous versus batch production of lipids in the microalgae Acutodesmus obliquus. *Bioresource Technology, 244*, 1384–1392. DOI: 10.1016/j.biortech.2017.04.093

Rhee, S., Lee, J.-E., & Lee, C.-H. (2011). Importance of lactic acid bacteria in Asian fermented foods. *Microbial Cell Factories, 10*(Suppl 1), S5. DOI: 10.1186/1475-2859-10-S1-S5

Ro, D.-K., Paradise, E. M., Ouellet, M., Fisher, K. J., Newman, K. L., Ndungu, J. M., Ho, K. A., Eachus, R. A., Ham, T. S., Kirby, J., Chang, M. C. Y., Withers, S. T., Shiba, Y., Sarpong, R., & Keasling, J. D. (2006). Production of the antimalarial drug precursor artemisinic acid in engineered yeast. *Nature, 440*(7086), 940–943. DOI: 10.1038/nature04640

Samoraj, M., Çalış, D., Trzaska, K., Mironiuk, M., & Chojnacka, K. (2024). Advancements in algal biorefineries for sustainable agriculture: Biofuels, high-value products, and environmental solutions. *Biocatalysis and Agricultural Biotechnology, 58*, 103224. DOI: 10.1016/j.bcab.2024.103224

Sano, C. (2009). History of glutamate production. *The American Journal of Clinical Nutrition, 90*(3), 728S–732S. DOI: 10.3945/ajcn.2009.27462F

Saranya, S., Thamanna, L., & Chellapandi, P. (2024). Unveiling the potential of systems biology in biotechnology and biomedical research. *Systems Microbiology and Biomanufacturing, 4*(4), 1217–1238. DOI: 10.1007/s43393-024-00286-4

Scavone, P., Miyoshi, A., Rial, A., Chabalgoity, A., Langella, P., Azevedo, V., & Zunino, P. (2007). Intranasal immunisation with recombinant Lactococcus lactis displaying either anchored or secreted forms of Proteus mirabilis MrpA fimbrial protein confers specific immune response and induces a significant reduction of kidney bacterial colonisation in mice. *Microbes and Infection, 9*(7), 821–828. DOI: 10.1016/j.micinf.2007.02.023

Segall-Shapiro, T. H., Meyer, A. J., Ellington, A. D., Sontag, E. D., & Voigt, C. A. (2014). A 'resource allocator' for transcription based on a highly fragmented T7 <scp>RNA</scp> polymerase. *Molecular Systems Biology*, *10*(7). Advance online publication. DOI: 10.15252/msb.20145299

Shahcheraghi, N., Golchin, H., Sadri, Z., Tabari, Y., Borhanifar, F., & Makani, S. (2022). Nanobiotechnology, an applicable approach for sustainable future. *3 Biotech, 12*(3), 65. https://doi.org/DOI: 10.1007/s13205-021-03108-9

Siegel, J. B., Smith, A. L., Poust, S., Wargacki, A. J., Bar-Even, A., Louw, C., Shen, B. W., Eiben, C. B., Tran, H. M., Noor, E., Gallaher, J. L., Bale, J., Yoshikuni, Y., Gelb, M. H., Keasling, J. D., Stoddard, B. L., Lidstrom, M. E., & Baker, D. (2015). Computational protein design enables a novel one-carbon assimilation pathway. *Proceedings of the National Academy of Sciences of the United States of America, 112*(12), 3704–3709. DOI: 10.1073/pnas.1500545112

Siegel, J. B., Zanghellini, A., Lovick, H. M., Kiss, G., Lambert, A. R., St.Clair, J. L., Gallaher, J. L., Hilvert, D., Gelb, M. H., Stoddard, B. L., Houk, K. N., Michael, F. E., & Baker, D. (2010). Computational Design of an Enzyme Catalyst for a Stereoselective Bimolecular Diels-Alder Reaction. *Science, 329*(5986), 309–313. 1190239

Siegfried, T. (2005). In Praise of Hard Questions. *Science*, *309*(5731), 76–77. DOI: 10.1126/science.309.5731.76

Simon, B., Nomellini, J., Chiou, P., Bingle, W., Thornton, J., Smit, J., & Leong, J. (2001). Recombinant vaccines against infectious hematopoietic necrosis virus: Production by the Caulobacter crescentus S-layer protein secretion system and evaluation in laboratory trials. *Diseases of Aquatic Organisms*, *44*, 17–27. DOI: 10.3354/dao044017

Sindhi, K., Pingili, R. B., Beldar, V., Bhattacharya, S., Rahaman, J., & Mukherjee, D. (2025). The role of biomaterials-based scaffolds in advancing skin tissue construct. *Journal of Tissue Viability*, *34*(2), 100858. DOI: 10.1016/j.jtv.2025.100858

Singh, A. K., Pal, P., Pandey, B., Goksen, G., Sahoo, U. K., Lorenzo, J. M., & Sarangi, P. K. (2023). Development of "Smart Foods" for health by nanoencapsulation: Novel technologies and challenges. *Food Chemistry: X*, *20*, 100910. DOI: 10.1016/j.fochx.2023.100910

Singh, N., Ogunseitan, O. A., Wong, M. H., & Tang, Y. (2022). Sustainable materials alternative to petrochemical plastics pollution: A review analysis. *Sustainable Horizons*, *2*, 100016. DOI: 10.1016/j.horiz.2022.100016

Sochaj, A. M., Świderska, K. W., & Otlewski, J. (2015). Current methods for the synthesis of homogeneous antibody–drug conjugates. *Biotechnology Advances*, *33*(6), 775–784. DOI: 10.1016/j.biotechadv.2015.05.001

Song, A. A.-L., In, L. L. A., Lim, S. H. E., & Rahim, R. A. (2017). A review on Lactococcus lactis: From food to factory. *Microbial Cell Factories*, *16*(1), 55. DOI: 10.1186/s12934-017-0669-x

Steen, E. J., Kang, Y., Bokinsky, G., Hu, Z., Schirmer, A., McClure, A., Del Cardayre, S. B., & Keasling, J. D. (2010). Microbial production of fatty-acid-derived fuels and chemicals from plant biomass. *Nature*, *463*(7280), 559–562.

Su, R., Ting, W., Taidong, B., Ningyun, C., Meng, Y., Chen, W., & Hao, J., Huadong, & P., Ning, C. (2023). Enhanced production of d-pantothenic acid in *Corynebacterium glutamicum* using an efficient CRISPR–Cpf1 genome editing method. *Microbial Cell Factories*, *22*, 3. DOI: 10.1186/s12934-023-02017-1

Subramanian, M. R., Suvarna, T., & Christopher, L. P. (2015). Production of lactic acid using a new homofermentative *Enterococcus faecalis* isolate. *Microbial Biotechnology*, *8*(2), 221–229. DOI: 10.1111/1751-7915.12133

Sun, Y.-Q., Shen, J.-T., Yan, L., Zhou, J.-J., Jiang, L.-L., Chen, Y., Yuan, J.-L., Feng, E., & Xiu, Z.-L. (2018). Advances in bioconversion of glycerol to 1,3-propanediol: Prospects and challenges. *Process Biochemistry*, *71*, 134–146. DOI: 10.1016/j.procbio.2018.05.009

Sun, Z., Wu, B., Ren, Y., Wang, Z., Zhao, C., Hai, M., Weitz, D. A., & Chen, D. (2021). Diverse Particle Carriers Prepared by Co-Precipitation and Phase Separation: Formation and Applications. *ChemPlusChem*, *86*(1), 49–58. DOI: 10.1002/cplu.202000497

Tan, D., Wu, Q., Chen, J.-C., & Chen, G.-Q. (2014). Engineering Halomonas TD01 for the low-cost production of polyhydroxyalkanoates. *Metabolic Engineering*, *26*, 34–47. DOI: 10.1016/j.ymben.2014.09.001

Tan, S.-I., & Ng, I.-S. (2020). New Insight into Plasmid-Driven T7 RNA Polymerase in *Escherichia coli* and Use as a Genetic Amplifier for a Biosensor. *ACS Synthetic Biology*, *9*(3), 613–622. DOI: 10.1021/acssynbio.9b00466

Tang, C., Wang, L., Zang, L., Wang, Q., Qi, D., & Dai, Z. (2023). On-demand biomanufacturing through synthetic biology approach. *Materials Today. Bio*, *18*, 100518. DOI: 10.1016/j.mtbio.2022.100518

Teusink, B., Bachmann, H., & Molenaar, D. (2011). Systems biology of lactic acid bacteria: A critical review. *Microbial Cell Factories*, *10*(Suppl 1), S11. DOI: 10.1186/1475-2859-10-S1-S11

Tobias, J. Erb., Patrik, Jones, R., & Bar-Even, A. (2017). Synthetic metabolism: Metabolic engineering meets enzyme design. *Current Opinion in Chemical Biology*, *37*, 56–62. DOI: 10.1016/j.cbpa.2016.12.023

Tokunaga, H., Arakawa, T., & Tokunaga, M. (2010). Novel soluble expression technologies derived from unique properties of halophilic proteins. *Applied Microbiology and Biotechnology*, *88*(6), 1223–1231. DOI: 10.1007/s00253-010-2832-8

Tripathi, N. K., & Shrivastava, A. (2019). Recent Developments in Bioprocessing of Recombinant Proteins: Expression Hosts and Process Development. *Frontiers in Bioengineering and Biotechnology*, *7*. Advance online publication. DOI: 10.3389/fbioe.2019.00420

Tristan, C. A., Ormanoglu, P., Slamecka, J., Malley, C., Chu, P.-H., Jovanovic, V. M., Gedik, Y., Jethmalani, Y., Bonney, C., Barnaeva, E., Braisted, J., Mallanna, S. K., Dorjsuren, D., Iannotti, M. J., Voss, T. C., Michael, S., Simeonov, A., & Singeç, I. (2021). Robotic high-throughput biomanufacturing and functional differentiation of human pluripotent stem cells. *Stem Cell Reports*, *16*(12), 3076–3092. DOI: 10.1016/j.stemcr.2021.11.004

van Heerden, C. D., & Nicol, W. (2013). Continuous and batch cultures of Escherichia coli KJ134 for succinic acid fermentation: Metabolic flux distributions and production characteristics. *Microbial Cell Factories*, *12*(1), 80. DOI: 10.1186/1475-2859-12-80

Vasic-Racki, D. (2006). *History of Industrial Biotransformations-Dreams and Realities.*

Vees, C. A., Neuendorf, C. S., & Pflügl, S. (2020). Towards continuous industrial bioprocessing with solventogenic and acetogenic clostridia: Challenges, progress and perspectives. *Journal of Industrial Microbiology & Biotechnology*, *47*(9–10), 753–787. DOI: 10.1007/s10295-020-02296-2

Vigentini, I., Merico, A., Tutino, M. L., Compagno, C., & Marino, G. (2006). Optimization of recombinant human nerve growth factor production in the psychrophilic Pseudoalteromonas haloplanktis. *Journal of Biotechnology*, *127*(1), 141–150. DOI: 10.1016/j.jbiotec.2006.05.019

Wahab, W. A. A. (2025). Review of research progress in immobilization and chemical modification of microbial enzymes and their application. *Microbial Cell Factories*, *24*(1), 167. DOI: 10.1186/s12934-025-02791-0

Waksman, S. A., Reilly, H. C., & Johnstone, D. B. (1946). Isolation of Streptomycin-producing Strains of Streptomyces griseus. *Journal of Bacteriology*, *52*(3), 393–397.

Walsh, G. (2018). Biopharmaceutical benchmarks 2018. *Nature Biotechnology*, *36*(12), 1136–1145. DOI: 10.1038/nbt.4305

Wang, Y., Chan, K.-L., Abdel-Rahman, M. A., Sonomoto, K., & Leu, S.-Y. (2020). Dynamic simulation of continuous mixed sugar fermentation with increasing cell retention time for lactic acid production using Enterococcus mundtii QU 25. *Biotechnology for Biofuels*, *13*(1), 112. DOI: 10.1186/s13068-020-01752-6

Wang, Z., Chen, T., Ma, X., Shen, Z., & Zhao, X. (2011). Enhancement of riboflavin production with Bacillus subtilis by expression and site-directed mutagenesis of zwf and gnd gene from Corynebacterium glutamicum. *Bioresource Technology*, *102*(4), 3934–3940. DOI: 10.1016/j.biortech.2010.11.120

Whitaker, W. B., Jones, J. A., Bennett, R. K., Gonzalez, J. E., Vernacchio, V. R., Collins, S. M., Palmer, M. A., Schmidt, S., Antoniewicz, M. R., & Koffas, M. A.. (2017). Engineering the biological conversion of methanol to specialty chemicals in Escherichia coli. *Metabolic Engineering*, *39*, 49–59.

Xie, D., Jackson, E. N., & Zhu, Q. (2015). Sustainable source of omega-3 eicosapentaenoic acid from metabolically engineered Yarrowia lipolytica: From fundamental research to commercial production. *Applied Microbiology and Biotechnology*, *99*(4), 1599–1610. DOI: 10.1007/s00253-014-6318-y

Xie, D., Miller, E., Sharpe, P., Jackson, E., & Zhu, Q. (2017). Omega-3 production by fermentation of *Yarrowia lipolytica* : From fed-batch to continuous. *Biotechnology and Bioengineering*, *114*(4), 798–812. DOI: 10.1002/bit.26216

Xu, Y., Chen, C., Hellwarth, P. B., & Bao, X. (2019). Biomaterials for stem cell engineering and biomanufacturing. *Bioactive Materials*, *4*, 366–379. DOI: 10.1016/j.bioactmat.2019.11.002

Yadwad, V. B., Wilson, S., & Ward, O. P. (1994). Production of human epidermal growth factor by an ampicillin resistant recombinant Escherichia coli strain. *Biotechnology Letters*, *16*(9), 885–890. DOI: 10.1007/BF00128619

Yamada, Y., & Yukphan, P. (2008). Genera and species in acetic acid bacteria. *International Journal of Food Microbiology*, *125*(1), 15–24. DOI: 10.1016/j.ijfoodmicro.2007.11.077

Yang, M., Zhang, W., Ji, S., Cao, P., Chen, Y., & Zhao, X. (2013). Generation of an Artificial Double Promoter for Protein Expression in Bacillus subtilis through a Promoter Trap System. *PLoS One*, *8*(2), e56321. DOI: 10.1371/journal.pone.0056321

Yang, S., Fei, Q., Zhang, Y., Contreras, L. M., Utturkar, S. M., Brown, S. D., Himmel, M. E., & Zhang, M. (2016). *Zymomonas mobilis* as a model system for production of biofuels and biochemicals. *Microbial Biotechnology*, *9*(6), 699–717. DOI: 10.1111/1751-7915.12408

Yari, K., Fatemi, S. S.-A., & Tavallaei, M. (2012). High level expression of recombinant BoNT/A-Hc by high cell density cultivation of Escherichia coli. *Bioprocess and Biosystems Engineering*, *35*(3), 407–414. DOI: 10.1007/s00449-011-0579-y

Ye, Z., Li, S., Hennigan, J. N., Lebeau, J., Moreb, E. A., Wolf, J., & Lynch, M. D. (2021). Two-stage dynamic deregulation of metabolism improves process robustness & scalability in engineered E. coli. *Metabolic Engineering*, *68*, 106–118. DOI: 10.1016/j.ymben.2021.09.009

Yi, W., Hu, S., Qian, X., Yan, W., & Li, Y. (2025). Synthetic Biology-Based Engineering Cells for Drug Delivery. *Exploration*, *5*(2). Advance online publication. DOI: 10.1002/EXP.20240095

Yim, H., Haselbeck, R., Niu, W., Pujol-Baxley, C., Burgard, A., Boldt, J., Khandurina, J., Trawick, J. D., Osterhout, R. E., Stephen, R., Estadilla, J., Teisan, S., Schreyer, H. B., Andrae, S., Yang, T. H., Lee, S. Y., Burk, M. J., & Van Dien, S. (2011). Metabolic engineering of Escherichia coli for direct production of 1,4-butanediol. *Nature Chemical Biology*, *7*(7), 445–452. DOI: 10.1038/nchembio.580

Ytterberg, A. J., Zubarev, R. A., & Baumgarten, T. (2019). Posttranslational Targeting of a Recombinant Protein Promotes Its Efficient Secretion into the Escherichia coli Periplasm. *Applied and Environmental Microbiology*, *85*(13). Advance online publication. DOI: 10.1128/AEM.00671-19

Yusuf, A., Almotairy, A. R. Z., Henidi, H., Alshehri, O. Y., & Aldughaim, M. S. (2023). Nanoparticles as Drug Delivery Systems: A Review of the Implication of Nanoparticles' Physicochemical Properties on Responses in Biological Systems. *Polymers*, *15*(7), 1596. DOI: 10.3390/polym15071596

Zhan, Y., Shi, J., Xiao, Y., Zhou, F., Wang, H., Xu, H., Li, Z., Yang, S., Cai, D., & Chen, S. (2022). Multilevel metabolic engineering of Bacillus licheniformis for de novo biosynthesis of 2-phenylethanol. *Metabolic Engineering*, *70*, 43–54. DOI: 10.1016/j.ymben.2022.01.007

Zhang, S., Guo, F., Yan, W., Dai, Z., Dong, W., Zhou, J., Zhang, W., Xin, F., & Jiang, M. (2020). Recent Advances of CRISPR/Cas9-Based Genetic Engineering and Transcriptional Regulation in Industrial Biology. *Frontiers in Bioengineering and Biotechnology*, *7*. Advance online publication. DOI: 10.3389/fbioe.2019.00459

Zhang, Y., Peng, J., Zhao, H., & Shi, S. (2021). Engineering oleaginous yeast Rhodotorula toruloides for overproduction of fatty acid ethyl esters. *Biotechnology for Biofuels*, *14*(1), 115. DOI: 10.1186/s13068-021-01965-3

Zhang, Y.-H. P. (2013). Next generation biorefineries will solve the food, biofuels, and environmental trilemma in the energy–food–water nexus. *Energy Science & Engineering*, *1*(1), 27–41. DOI: 10.1002/ese3.2

Zhang, Y.-H. P. (2015). Production of biofuels and biochemicals by in vitro synthetic biosystems: Opportunities and challenges. *Biotechnology Advances*, *33*(7), 1467–1483. DOI: 10.1016/j.biotechadv.2014.10.009

Zhang, Y.-H. P., Sun, J., & Ma, Y. (2017). Biomanufacturing: History and perspective. *Journal of Industrial Microbiology & Biotechnology*, *44*(4–5), 773–784. DOI: 10.1007/s10295-016-1863-2

Zhao, J., Li, Q., Sun, T., Zhu, X., Xu, H., Tang, J., Zhang, X., & Ma, Y. (2013). Engineering central metabolic modules of Escherichia coli for improving β-carotene production. *Metabolic Engineering*, *17*, 42–50.

Zheng, C., Gao, L., Sun, H., Zhao, X.-Y., Gao, Z., Liu, J., & Guo, W. (2024). Advancements in enzymatic reaction-mediated microbial transformation. *Heliyon*, *10*(19), e38187. DOI: 10.1016/j.heliyon.2024.e38187

Zhu, C., Ji, Z., Ma, J., Ding, Z., Shen, J., & Wang, Q. (2021). Recent Advances of Nanotechnology-Facilitated Bacteria-Based Drug and Gene Delivery Systems for Cancer Treatment. *Pharmaceutics*, *13*(7), 940. DOI: 10.3390/pharmaceutics13070940

Zhu, C., Mu, J., & Liang, L. (2024). Nanocarriers for intracellular delivery of proteins in biomedical applications: Strategies and recent advances. *Journal of Nanobiotechnology*, *22*(1), 688. DOI: 10.1186/s12951-024-02969-5

Zhu, Q., & Jackson, E. N. (2015). Metabolic engineering of *Yarrowia lipolytica* for industrial applications. *Current Opinion in Biotechnology*, *36*, 65–72. DOI: 10.1016/j.copbio.2015.08.010

Chapter 3
Metabolic Engineering and Synthetic Biology:
Pioneering Innovations for Optimized Biomanufacturing

Preeti Mehta Kakkar
https://orcid.org/0000-0002-0997-7796
Amity University, Noida, India

Ajay Yadav
https://orcid.org/0009-0005-4189-6565
Amity Institute of Biotechnology, Amity University, Noida, India

Mayuk Majumder
Amity Institute of Biotechnology, Amity University, Noida, India

Sumit Sharma
Independent Researcher, USA

Tanu Allen
Amity Institute of Biotechnology, Amity University, Noida, India

Ruchi Jakhmola Mani
Amity Institute of Biotechnology, Amity University, Noida, India

ABSTRACT

Metabolic engineering and synthetic biology are enhancing the design and production of microbial cells with scaled capabilities for producing high-demand bio-based products, such as biofuels, enzymes, nutraceuticals, and food industry products. Metabolic engineering provides cellular metabolism to maximize product yields and minimize wastages. Synthetic biology further modifies and enables the production of complex molecules that are difficult to synthesize through other methods. This chapter provides an in-depth exploration and study of the latest innovations and developments, highlighting their transformative impact on optimized biomanufacturing processes. It also highlights the advanced genetic tools, genome-scale modelling, etc. Additionally, it discusses prospects, challenges, and potential solutions for next-generation biomanufacturing, emphasizing the role of Artificial Intelligence (AI) and Machine Learning (ML) in system metabolic engineering.

DOI: 10.4018/979-8-3373-2873-7.ch003

INTRODUCTION

Scientists have produced a comprehensive collection of tools and frameworks that have moved both metabolic engineering and synthetic biology forward considerably. These two fields have not evolved in a vacuum; they are becoming increasingly codependent, and each is strengthening the other's capabilities. Synthetic biology aims to design and build genetic parts (e.g., modular devices, regulatory genetic circuits) that allow for predictable biological behavior [Buecherl & Myers, 2022; Schladt et al., 2021; Nikolados et al., 2019]. Progress in synthetic biology, much like the progress in metabolic engineering, depends heavily on quantitative analysis and models that enable accurate predictions of biological systems' dynamics and models/ biological engineering. Metabolic engineering is concerned with optimizing cellular pathways for the conversion of cheap substrates into valuable products of commercial value. The predominant method of performing metabolic engineering is through manipulating the metabolic fluxes - using many of the elaborated databases and environmental conditions - to generate the desired target product as quickly as possible [Kuroda, et al. 2017; Matsuda et al., 2017]. Synthetic biology and metabolic engineering are complementary fields, and together they provide a coherent conceptual grounding for efficient and sustainable design of biological systems catering to health, education, pharmaceuticals, biofuels, and industrial biotechnology.

Metabolic engineering, historically centered on the alteration of endogenous biochemical pathways to increase metabolite yields, has become a data-driven discipline. The metabolic pathway can be constructed either in the natural host by repeating the addition and elimination of new genes or in an appropriate heterologous host by combinatorial biosynthetic pathway assembly. When a native host organism is a slow-growing strain or difficult to manipulate genetically, biosynthetic pathways are generally first constructed or optimized in a heterologous host. Although *E. coli* is most commonly utilized for that purpose, other hosts like *Bacillus subtilis* [Liu, et al. 2016], *Pichia pastoris* [Sun, et al. 2019], *Saccharomyces cerevisiae* [Zhao, *et al. 2024],* and *Trichoderma reesei* [Luu, et al. 2023] have been utilized as well, with each providing advantages for expression of sophisticated biosynthetic gene clusters. The successful microbial production of insulin that are using recently have focused on optimizing expression systems, particularly in yeast species like *Saccharomyces cerevisiae* [Kjeldsen, et al. 2023] and artemisinin, a vital antimalarial compound, Notably, *Saccharomyces cerevisiae* has been engineered to produce artemisinin acid, a precursor to artemisinin, through the integration of a multi-enzyme biosynthetic pathway[Guo, et al. 2025] Constituted major milestones in metabolic engineering, as they established the viably of reconditioning biology by introducing designed pathways into heterologous hosts. These successes have opened up avenues for the development of microbial cell factories for the production of a vast set of valuable compounds.

The metabolic engineering innovations are supported by synthetic biology for higher industrial output. For instance, the engineering of *Pichia pastoris* to produce soy leghemoglobin has revolutionized the plant-based food market by replicating the taste and experience of traditional meat products. Pharmaceutical biotechnology, with the help of Synthetic biology, has enabled the production of bioactive compounds. Recent applications include the biosynthesis of therapeutic molecules such as semaglutide, the active ingredient in diabetes treatments, and the development of antibody-drug conjugates for targeted cancer therapy. Also, the synthetic biology has allowed for monoclonal antibodies [Goulet & Atkins, 2020], vaccines [Pfeifer *et al, 2023],* and rare plant chemicals such as Taxol [Xie et al, 2024]to be biosynthesized. In the bio energy sector, synthetic *cyanobacteria* and algae transform the sun into biodiesel without incurring the carbon footprint of conventional fossil fuels [Majhi, 2025]

Biomanufacturing is an advanced type of industrial production that uses biological systems like engineered microorganisms or cell cultures to create pharmaceuticals, biofuels, food ingredients, and even biodegradable materials. Its value is in providing scalable and ecologically sound solutions to chemical manufacturing that uses toxic byproducts and fossil fuels. Biomanufacturing furthers the transition to a bio-based economy by decreasing greenhouse gas emissions and conserving resources through circular production systems. With the help of synthetic biology, which allows for the precise redesign of biological systems to optimize production pathways, enhance yield, and add new functions, biomanufacturing has even greater efficiency and versatility. Synthetic biology helps biomanufacturing expand into other sectors and tackle the sophisticated challenge of developing high-value, complex products. Together, they serve as the pillars of industrial biotechnology, advancing health, energy, agriculture, and materials science, but also advancing global sustainability challenges, economic stability, and public health readiness.

HISTORICAL CONTEXT AND EVOLUTION

Figure 1. Evolution of metabolic engineering and synthetic biology (1960 to 2016)

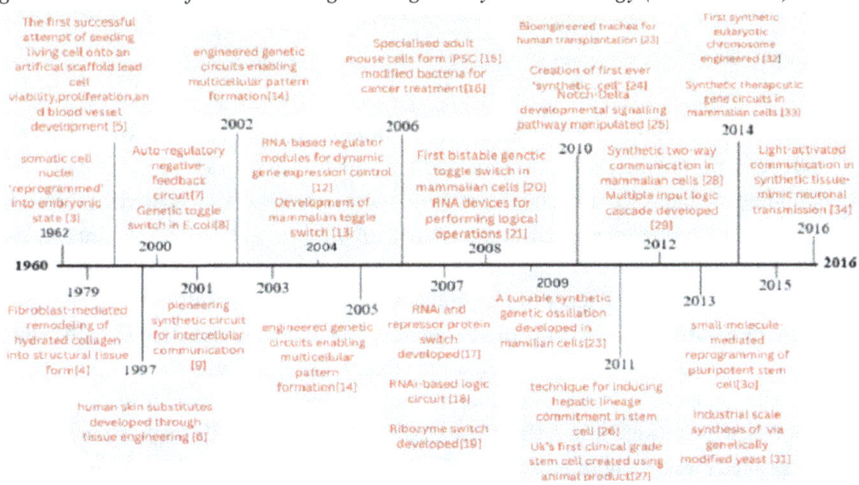

Origins of Metabolic Engineering

Metabolic engineering, formally recognized as an independent discipline in the late 1980s and early 1990s, is the rational and systematic redirection of cellular metabolism to optimize the production of target compounds. This approach analyzes the metabolic engineering pathways of the microbes to determine the limitations and the consequent effect on the targeted products. It then uses genetic engineering to overcome these limitations in an attempt to maximize the yield of the target products, which undergo genetic modifications by using chemically induced mutation, and only those desired metabolites are selected that have a mutant strain. Some successful metabolic engineering examples from the beginning of metabolic engineering and synthetic biology [Figure 1], this innovation with the timeframe. Some points are: (i) genetic modification of *Corynebacterium glutamicum* to maximize and improve the production of lysin, (ii) using reverse beta oxidation pathway for the efficient production of fatty acids and alcohols and synthesis of chemicals and biofuels using catalytic conversion, (iii) enhancement in the production of 3-Deoxy-D-arabino-heptulosonate 7-phosphate (DAHP) a aromatic compound synthesized by *E-coli* as a intermediate. [Buchner, 1897; Fischer et, al, 1894]

Biochemical Revolution: foundation for metabolic engineering:

Concurrently, the beginning of the 20th century witnessed pioneering developments in the science of biochemistry that established the scientific foundation for metabolic engineering. Isolation and definition of enzymes – the protein catalysts that control each step in a metabolic pathway – were revolutionary. Eduard Buchner's demonstration of cell-free fermentation (1897) fixed metabolic activity in soluble fractions, as opposed to cells. The "lock-and-key" model of enzyme specificity theory (Emil Fischer) and the realization that enzymes catalyze step-by-step chemical conversions started illuminating the intricate network of metabolic pathways. [Embden et al. 1934]

Key Milestones

Glycolysis Explanation: The painstaking work of Gustav Embden, Otto Meyerhof, Jacob Parnas, and others during the 1920s-30s followed the stepwise conversion of glucose into pyruvate, determining the intermediates and the enzymes. The earlier work on coenzymes by Arthur Harden and William Young suggested the involvement of other factors. [Krebs & Johnson, 1937]

Discovery of the TCA Cycle: The discovery of the citric acid cycle by Hans Krebs (1937) provided the basis for aerobic energy production and precursor availability.

Biosynthetic Routes: The discovery of how microbes made complex molecules such as amino acids, vitamins, and nucleotides uncovered interlinked networks extending from core metabolism.

This growing adoption of metabolic blueprints was the necessary "groundwork" in the initial statement. Scientists were aware that the carbon and energy flow through these connected pathways regulated the amount of any desired final product. If one knew the enzymes and their regulation – how activity was regulated by substrates, products, or other molecules (allosteric control, feedback inhibition) – one could, in principle, step in to "unclog" bottlenecks or redirect flux. For example, the observation that the end-product of an amino acid pathway inhibited the first enzyme in the pathway (feedback inhibition) explained natural constraints on production. This knowledge immediately suggested that bypassing this inhibition, by mutation or later by genetic engineering, could raise yields, a fundamental principle of metabolic engineering. The main motive of metabolic engineering and synthetic biology is to use microorganisms and their genetic modification for the large-scale production of valuable products using industrial innovation and technology to make them economically efficient. For example, the use of yeast in the production of alcohols (wine, beer), cheese, and biopharmaceuticals. These advancements are also employed in the development of oil crops and enhance the crops and genetically modified crops (e.g, BT Cotton, golden rice variety, etc.). The main strategies employed by metabolic engineering and synthetic biology are as follows: (i) expression of rate-limiting and gene-coding enzymes for the biosynthesis pathways, (ii) blocking the biosynthesis pathways' competitors, (iii) expression of heterologous genes, and (iii) bioenzyme engineering development. At the industrial scale, metabolic engineering is becoming more convenient and cost-effective. The metabolic engineering and synthetic biology also show high-end effectiveness in competing with global climate and environmental problems, like the production of biofuels from renewable biomass, which helps in reducing greenhouse gas (GHG) emissions. Biofuels such as short-chain alcohols, alkanes, which replace gasoline, the combination of fatty acid and methyl ester and fatty alcohol (replacing diesel), and fatty acid and isoprenoid-based biofuels use replace diesel [Stephanopoulos et, al, 2012; Nielsen & Keasling. 2016].

Emergence of Synthetic Biology

French biologist Stéphane Leduc first used the phrase "synthetic biology" in his 1910 book Théorie physico-chimique de la vie et générations spontanées. Leduc aimed to create "life-like" systems from self-organizing inorganic chemistry, experimenting with diffusion gradients in salts and gels in an attempt to construct complex mineral structures in the form of biological organisms like algae or fungi. His "osmotic growths" were intended to demonstrate that morphology could be the product of physical laws and not depend on vital forces, disproving vitalism by suggesting life was a physicochemical process of some sophistication. Philosophically ambitious, Leduc's approach had no molecular biological basis and was mostly discredited as imitative. British biologist John Burdon Sanderson Haldane condemned it in 1912 as "pseudo-synthetic biology," attacking it for overlooking the genetic nature of life—a shortcoming that would persist for decades. The idea slumbered until the advent of molecular biology. Mid-20th century advances—Watson and Crick's identification of DNA structure (1953), Jacob and Monod's operon theory (1961), and the development of recombinant DNA technology (1970s)—gave scientists the means to engineer biology rather than just watch it happen. The 1970s-80s witnessed researchers such as Wacław Szybalski envision "synthetic biology" as designing working genomes de novo. The first synthetic gene, a yeast tRNA, was constructed by Arminius and Polke in 1978, and the 1980 construction of a working peptide-coding gene by Khorana's laboratory foreshadowed the large-scale assembly. However, the discipline was still patchy, with no unifying engineering principles. [Khorana, et al. 1980; Smith, et al. 2003].

The emergence of the modern paradigm around 2000 came from scaled advances that converged:

1. **Sequencing of a genome** (e.g., *Haemophilus influenzae*, 1995) produces biological "parts lists."
2. **Rapidly declining costs of DNA synthesis** (from \$10+/base in 2000 to < \$0.05/base by 2020), there emerged a realization that genes could be assembled
3. **Movement toward standardization** (e.g, MIT's Tom Knight pioneered the development of BioBricks in 2003, and made standardized DNA parts that had interchangeable ends).
4. **The Foundational Projects** (e.g, the synthesis of a functional bacteriophage, phiX174 in 2003 and the minimal genome of *Mycoplasma genitalium* in 2008) demonstrated that an intricate biological system could be designed from scratch.

Institutions formalized the discipline: the first International Meeting on Synthetic Biology (2004) and the iGEM competition at MIT (2004) spurred a generation of engineers to think of biology as a programmable thing. Fundamental principles followed: design can be decoupled from natural evolution, abstraction hierarchies exist (DNA → devices → systems), and standardization provides predictability. Major advances in metabolic engineering improved existing biological pathways for yield, while the goal of synthetic biology was new biological functions, ranging from genetic circuits that oscillate like electronic timers, to microbes that produced artemisinin (2013), the first drug derived from a synthetic biology organism. Alongside technical progress, ethical discussions escalated. The synthesis of the horsepox virus (2017) raised concerns about dual-use risks. The precision of CRISPR forced the reckoning with heritable genome edits. Today, synthetic biology has a new meaning that conjoined Leduc's visionary term with an engineering style and established a form of biotechnology as a design science across medicine, agriculture, and sustainable manufacturing. [Keasling, 2010; Khalil & Collins, 2010].

Convergence of Disciplines

The Engineered Cell Factory Paradigm

Bringing together the design-oriented perspective of synthetic biology and the optimization-centered view of metabolic engineering has transformed industrial biotechnology. Microbial hosts (e.g., *E. coli, S. cerevisiae*) can be engineered as "chassis" to build de novo pathways using:

- Standardized genetic parts (promoters, RBSs, terminators) enabling more predictable expression.
- CRISPR-based genome editing technologies allow multiplexed gene knockouts/inserts.
- Computational models (FBA, kinetic modeling) to predict flux bottlenecks.

The confluence of these products provides a means of specifically re-routing carbon/nitrogen fluxes to make the product of interest while imposing minimal metabolic burden.

Synthetic Pathways

Creatively combined multiple genes from Artemisia annua (ADS, CYP71AV1)+ ADH1 from C. cinerea into *S. cerevisiae*. Developed an engineered synthetic amorphadiene pathway using an inducible GAL promoter system

Metabolic Optimization: Upregulated mevalonate pathway genes (tHMG1, ERG12, ERG8) to increase the supply of precursor (FPP). Deleted ERG9 (squalene synthase) to disable the competitive sterol pathway. Deleted ERG9 (squalene synthase) to disable the competitive sterol pathway. Added an engineered synthetic electron transport system (cytochrome P450 reductase) to enhance the activity of CYP71AV1

Systems-Level Tuning: Utilized quantitative PCR (qPCR) and metabolomics to balance the quantities of enzymes expressed. Titered up from <1 mg/L to >25 g/L using fed-batch fermentation, [Casini, et al. 2015].

Impact

Cost Savings will reduce costs for artemisinin synthesis by>80%, facilitating semi-synthesis. Supply Chain Stability can reduce dependence on seasonal harvests of Artemisia, assuring up to 150 million patients annually from malaria. Proof of Concept that Established a validated microbial factory for complex plant-derived pharmaceuticals, [Esvelt & Wang, 2013].

METABOLIC FLUXES AND THEIR ANALYSIS

Metabolic flux is the flow of metabolite compounds through metabolic pathways within a cell. The metabolic flux analysis (MFA) stands out as a powerful and systematic approach for quantifying the rates of metabolic engineering reactions. Within a living cell. Leveraging a stoichiometric model that accounts for key intracellular biochemical reactions and the mass balancing of metabolites. These Metabolic fluxes are fundamental to cellular bio-physiology; they help in dictating the allocation of resources among competing biological processes and determine cell functions. Accurate flux estimation and quantification are very critical, particularly in metabolic engineering and synthetic biology, where the main objective is often to maximize the conversion of substrates into useful and valuable products. MFA provides an understanding of cellular metabolism, offering insights on (i) identification of major branching points in cellular metabolic pathways, (ii) estimation of non-measured extracellular fluxes, (iii) identification of alternative pathways, and (iv) calculation of maximum theoretical product yields. The systematic analysis of metabolic fluxes takes place in three stages: (i) methods are developed for monitoring metabolic pathways and estimation of metabolic fluxes through the use of radiolabeled isotopic tracing, (ii) introduction of targeted perturbations to the metabolic network, such as altering enzyme activities, to asses the flexibility of metabolic nodes, (iii) the effect of these perturbations are analyzed to reveal the biochemical reactions that determines the metabolic flux distributions/network.

The notable advancement in MFA's ability to accurately model cellular metabolic pathways using known biochemical pathway knowledge, without the help of detailed enzymatic parameters. This enables genetic scientists to predict the effect of genetic modifications, such as enzyme deletion or biosynthetic pathway insertions, on the metabolic network. Furthermore, MFAs can infer fluxes through pathways that are experimentally inaccessible and guide metabolic engineering efforts by identifying the promising interventions for improved product yields. [Singh, 2021]

Recent advancements and developments in Metabolic Flux Analysis (MFA) have expanded its capabilities through the integration and use of stable isotopes (e.g., 13C), which can be detected by mass spectrometry (MS) and nuclear magnetic resonance (NMR) spectroscopy. In 13C-MFA, cells are supplied with 13C-labeled substrates [e.g., 1,2-13C Glucose]; [1,6-13C Glucose], allowing bioengineering researchers to trace the incorporation of labeled carbon atoms source for cell growth and throughout the metabolic pathway network. This approach believes in achieving both the metabolic pathway and the isotopic steady states, ensuring that measured flux distributions are representative of the system under steady state. However, one limitation is that certain cell types, such as mammalian cells, may require more time (4 hours or even a day) to achieve this isotopic steady state. This [13C] isotope technique for analysis of metabolic flux is an essential tool in systems biotechnology, providing an active role in medicine, biochemistry, metabolic engineering, and synthetic biology fields. [Figure 2], [Sinreih, et al. 2015].

Figure 2. The standard carbon labelling experiment workflow

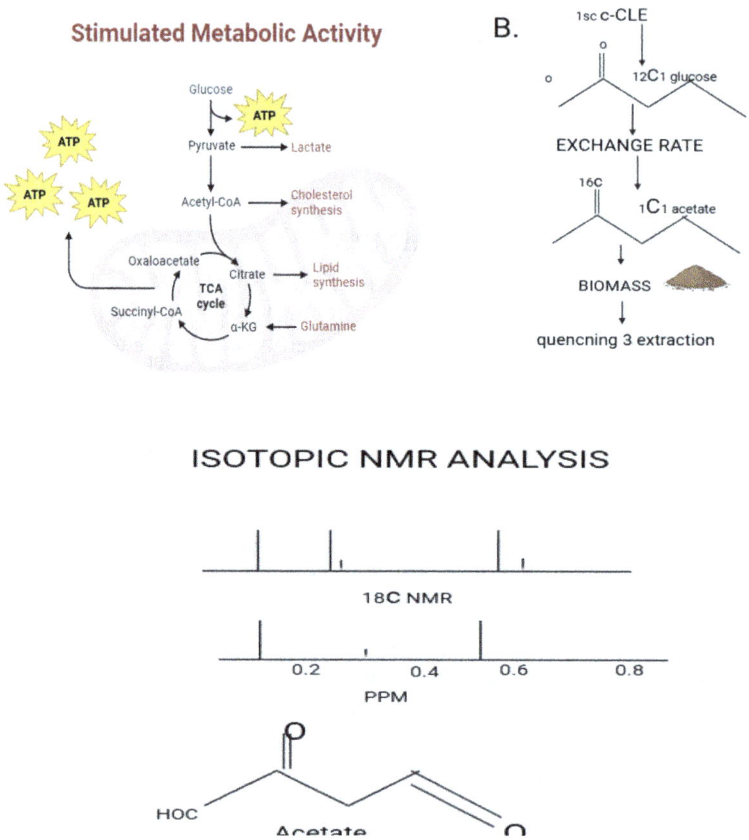

(A) Initially, a metabolic model of cellular metabolism is constructed. (B) Cells are cultivated with 13C-labeled isotopes. (C) The extracted samples are analyzed using MS and NMR spectroscopy. (D) Determination of intracellular fluxes through internal and external rate measurement and flux analysis using a metabolic network

Synthetic Metabolic Pathway Construction and Flux Analysis

Synthetic biology has fundamentally transformed the way bioengineering researchers approach metabolic engineering and synthetic biology. Instead of waiting for a long time for nature to evolve new pathways, biotechnologists have designed and developed synthetic biological pathways using genetic modification from various organisms (e.g., promoters and coding sequences). For instance, to produce n-butanol by the conversion of acetyl-CoA, using *Ralstonia eutropus*, *Clostridium acetobutylicum*, and *Streptomyces collinus*. However, these synthetic pathways are not inherently optimized. Unlike naturally evolved pathways, which undergo selection to minimize toxic intermediates and flux balancing. The synthetic biological routes lead to the accumulation of metabolically harmful products/intermediates, which directly impact negatively on cell growth and productivity. To overcome this, a biotechnologist employs advanced regulatory strategies and techniques, such as synthetic and dynamic regulatory networks, for example, CRISPRi, TALE-based transcription factors, and synthetic sRNAs, to modulate gene expression and enzyme activity [Figure 3.]. Further advancement includes the spatial organization of enzyme-mediated pathways through protein, DNA, or RNA scaffolds are used to enhance metabolic flux by co-localizing relevant enzymes in a physically bound manner.

Figure 3. Metabolic pathway engineering

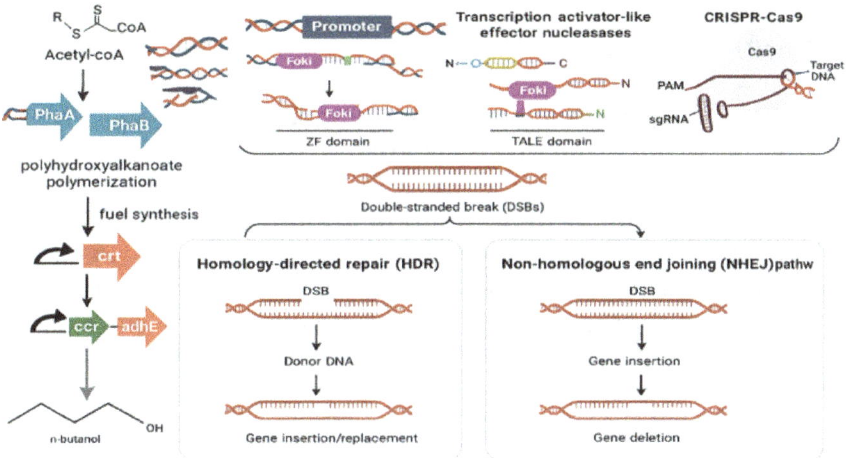

Due to the inherent complexity of gene expression and enzyme kinetics, these systems, computational and mathematical models, integrated with Artificial Intelligence (AI) and machine learning (ML) algorithms, are increasingly incorporated to predict metabolic engineering and synthetic biology pathway behaviour and optimization, ensuring robust and predictable early production outcomes.

There are several notable examples of successful and advanced microbial cell factories engineered for enhanced biosynthesis. High-titer n-butanol production in *E. coli* has been achieved using a chimeric pathway comprising enzymes from three organisms. The major and notable challenge in metabolic engineering pathways is reversibility. The well-known biotechnologist Bond–Watta discovered and constructed a biosynthetic pathway for n-butanol production by extracting enzymes from different microbial (bacteria) sources; the phaA (acetoacetyl-CoA synthase) and phaB (3-Hydroxybutyral-CoA dehydrogenase) from bacteria *R. eutrophus*, *C. acetobutylicum* produce crotonase (crt), adhE2, and crotonyl-CoA reductase (crr) obtained from *S. collinus*. This pathway includes the incorporation of heterologous enzymes and the deletion of competing metabolic functions, for example, ldhA deletion to prevent lactic acid formation under low oxygen availability, resulting in improved product titer. [Ellis, et al. 2011; Matsumoto, et al. 2017]

Beyond n-butanol, engineered microbes (bacteria, yeast, fungi, etc.) have been developed for the biological synthesis of various compounds like succinic acid, 2,4-dihydroxybutyric acid, and maleate. Some have reached commercial application, particularly in food industries as preservatives and as enhancers.

Despite these advancements, the synthetic biology pathways remain labour-intensive, often requiring multiple rounds of cloning and assembly. To minimize these, the Randomized BioBrick Assembly (RBBA) has been introduced, enabling rapid combination and screening of gene constituents. Promoters, ribosomes, binding sites, and terminators have achieved a significant milestone in product titering (30% in E. coli), as demonstrated in the lycopene biosynthesis pathway. [Figure 4], [Jones, et al. 2015; Erb, et al. 2017]

TOOLS AND TECHNIQUES

CRISPR (Clustered Regularly Interspaced Short Palindromic Repeats) -Cas System and Precision Editing

Plasmid-based systems, despite their widespread use, lead to limitations which including significant consumption of cellular energy due to high-end metabolic pathway demand, and the recent challenges of maintenance of plasmid maintenance. As a result, there has been a need to shift towards chromosomal integration of genes for more stable and enhanced enzyme expression. The recent advanced biotechnologies in genomic editing, particularly those involving CRISPR-Cas, have facilitated the integration of entire metabolic engineering pathways into host genomes. [Noda, et al. 2017; Weber, Engler, et al. 2011]. The noteworthy example is the delta integration CRISPR-Cas platform, which enhances homologous recombination efficiency by employing guided RNA sequences that specifically target multiple delta sites within the bacterium *S. cerevisiae* genome. [Shi, et al. 2016]. In this approach, a plasmid expressing the Cas9 protein and delta-targeting guide RNA is introduced alongside large donor DNA fragments (typically ranging from 8 to 24 kb) flanked by delta homology arms. This method has successfully enabled integration of synthetic biology and metabolic engineering pathways for (R, R)-2,3-butanediol production, incorporating genes such as acetolactate synthase and (R, R)-butanediol dehydrogenase from bacteria *B. subtilis*, as well as acetolactate decarboxylase from *Enterobacter aerogenes*. Beyond these examples, numerous other studies have noted the use of the CRISPR-Cas system for the chromosomal integration of heterologous pathways. The most recent one that which CRISPR-Cas has been used to regulate gene expression more efficiently than conventional techniques. More recently, clustered, regularly interspaced, short palindromic repeat (CRISPR)-Cas9 systems have been used to regulate gene expression more efficiently than conventional methods. Therefore, these synthetic transcription factors could be the key to synthetic biology and metabolic engineering.

The CRISPR-Cas9 has rapidly gained an enormous achievement to become the tool for genome editing across diverse microorganisms, enabling precise and efficient editing and modification by altering the target DNA sequence. This system utilizes a combination of sRNAs (crRNAs and tracrRNA), the Cas9 nuclease, and the host RNase III, together guiding Cas9 to a specific DNA locus adjacent to a protospacer-adjacent motif (PAM), where Cas9 introduces a targeted double-strand break. [Jiang et al. 2013; Keasling, 2010; Sander & Joung, 2014].

The recent research has demonstrated the efficiency and effectiveness of CRISPR-Cas9 for introducing point mutation and codon modification in the *E. coli* genomic sequence, facilitating metabolic engineering and synthetic biology optimized strategies. Biotechnologists have also systematically optimized and analyzed the metabolic pathways, such as beta-carotene biosynthetic and methylerythritol-phosphate pathways, through genome editing cycles, achieving beta-carotene production levels as highest i.e., 2.0 g/L in fed-batch fermentation.

Beyond this genome editing, the CRISPR interference approach employs a catalytically inactive Cas9 (dCas9) for modulation of gene expression without introduction of DNA lysis. dCase9 causes mutations in both RuvC (D10A) and HNH (H840A) domains, can bind target DNA, and function as a transcriptional repressor by blocking RNA polymerase binding. The CRISPRi has been applied to mitigate leaky expressions of toxic proteins and activate transcription by fusing with dCas9 with transcriptional activators, such as the RNA polymerase omega subunit.

The CRISPR-Cas9 system has enabled rapid, highly efficient, with accurate multi-locus editing and metabolic engineering. Table 1 highlights numerous applications of CRISPR in different bacterial species, which include *E. coli, Streptococcus, Clostridium, Cyanobacteria, Bacillus*, lactic acid bacteria, and various pathogenic bacteria.

Application of CRISPR-Cas9 in Microbes

CRISPR-Cas9 emerged as a highly influential technological advancement in microbial gene editing. Its precision and accuracy have enabled researchers and biotechnologists to manipulate a wide array of bacterial species, for example, E. coli, LAB, and various others. These microbes function as efficient biological production units, capable of utilizing inexpensive and economically renewable materials, even generating valuable products from waste. By harnessing CRISPR-Cas9, biotechnologists can engineer microbial genomes to optimize the production of specific metabolites or byproducts.

Cyanobacteria

They are unique among microorganism classifications due to their ability to perform photosynthesis, reducing carbon dioxide and harnessing solar energy as the primary source of food. They can synthesize a variety of bioproducts such as biofuels, pharmaceuticals, and essential nutrients. Despite their potential, genetic modification of cyanobacteria provides emerging challenges. These are often polyploid, possessing numerous chromosomal copies (ranging from 3 to 218 per cell), which complicates the homogenous genomic edits.

To remove these challenges, the advanced gene editing tool CRISPR-Cas9 and Cas12 have been incorporated. Recent research reports have successfully shown the application of these tools in species like *Synechococcus elongatus* UTEX2973 and *S. elongatus* P7942. While Cas9 can exhibit cytotoxic effects, transient expression strategies have enabled effective Knock-IN and Knock-OUT experiments, leading to the production of targeted compounds such as succinate. [Genomics & its impact on med.,2001; Plant science vol.1, 2001; Agbiotech omics, 2003; Chen et al. 2021; Ou et al. 2020].

Lactic Acid Bacteria (LAB)

LAB represents a diverse group of gram-positive low-GC-content bacteria that play an essential role in fermentation and probiotics in humans, it also maintains the gut health of humans. These bacteria have small genomic sequences, robust sugar metabolism, acid tolerance, and the capacity to thrive in harsh environmental conditions. Such traits make scientists attracted to them in the production of secondary metabolites, including enzymes.

CRISPR-Cas9 has become the principal tool for genome editing of LAB. It enabled gene insertion and deletion with efficiencies ranging from 25% to 62%. [Painter et al. 2013; Blazej, et al. 2006; Kohlstedt, & Wittman, 2019].

Table 1. Metabolically engineered microbes with their potential application

Species name	Strategies	Applications
S. elongatus	CRISPR-Cas9	Biological studies
Synechococcus	Cas12a	Biological studies
Anabaena	Cas12a	Biological researches
Synecocystis	Cas12a	Biological experiments
L. casei	CRISPR-Cas9	Biological studies
L. reuteri	CRISPR-Cas9	Biological studies
C. beijerinckii	CRISPR-Cas9	Biological studies
C. saccharoperbutylacetonicum	CRISPR-Cas9	Butanol synthesis
C. ljungdahlii	CRISPR-Cas9	Biofuels synthesis from artificial gas
C. tyrobutyricum	CRISPR-Cas9	Butanol synthesis
C. pasteurianum	CRISPR-Cas9	Butanol synthesis from waste glycerol
S. aureus	CRISPR-Cas9	Biological studies

Omics Technologies (Genomics, Proteomics, Metabolomics)

"OMICS" technologies have fundamentally transformed the way of thinking of biotechnological researchers in studying biological systems. Rather than focusing solely on individual components, these large-scale data-driven methods enable comprehensive analysis of the entire biological system at multiple levels. This shift, combining traditional " bottom-up" experiments with holistic "top-down" approaches it has yielded a deeper understanding of biological complexities, [Ayoglu, et al. 2011].

Figure 4. Omics field, including genomics, transcriptomics, proteomics, metabolomics, and fluxomics. Each provides a distinct examination of biological processes

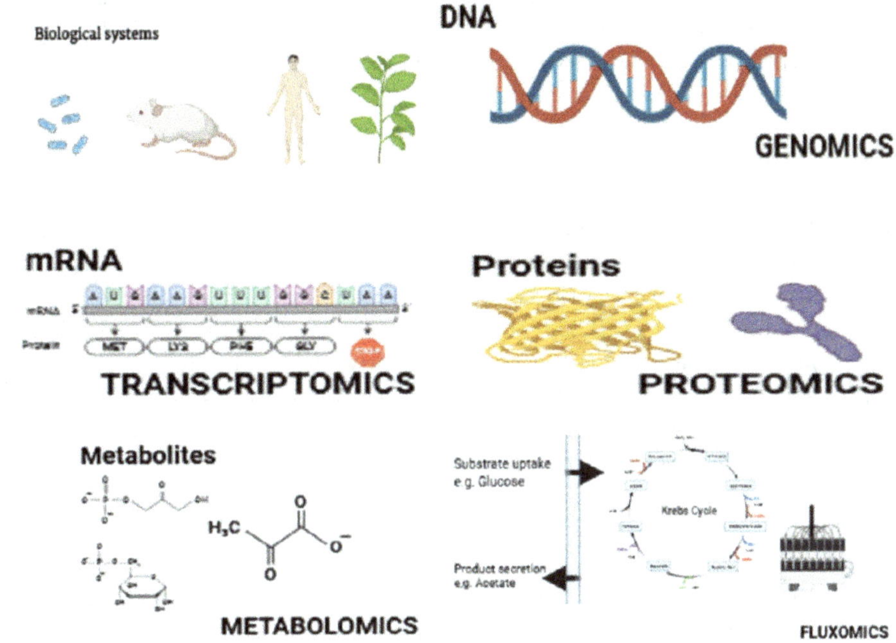

Genomics

Genomics, as a field, is concerned with the identification and alteration of the genetic sequence of a microbe or eukaryote. It also investigates gene function, comparing genomes across species, and determining the 3-D structures of proteins. In agricultural science, genomics is more valuable because it helps in mapping the entire genetically modified crop plants, such as *BT* Cotton, golden rice, etc. This facilitates crops to be pathogen-resistant, increases productivity with high nutrient content, and makes them environmentally sustainable. The flow of genetic information follows the Central Dogma from DNA replication to protein synthesis.DNA is transformed into mRNA, producing the transcriptome. The resulting mRNA molecules carry genetic instructions to the ribosomal units, where proteins are synthesized, [Bailey, et al. 2007].

Proteomics

The study of proteins in the cell is a dynamic field that aims to understand the structure, functions, and interactions of proteins. The proteome is highly responsive to environmental conditions, changing over time and responding to various stimuli.

Example: The proteomics research conducted at Iowa State University, USA includes:

For example, proteomics research at Iowa State University, USA includes:

- an examination of changes in protein in the corn proteome during low temperatures, which is a major problem for young corn seedlings;
- analysis of the differences that occur in the genome expression in developing soybean stressed by high temperatures; and
- identification of protein expressed sequences in response to diseased crops, e.g., soybean cyst nematodes, [Fagerberg et al. 2011].

Metabolomics

It is a relatively recent advancement in "omics". The metabolome incorporates the full array of low molecular weight compounds present within the biological samples. These molecules function as both substrates and byproducts in enzyme reactions, and play a direct and crucial role in shaping the phenotype of a cell. Metabolomics enables agricultural scientists to distinguish differences in the abundance of thousands of molecules between healthy and diseased crop specimens. However, the advancement in technologies and the instruments in evaluating nutritional differences between conventional and genetically modified crops help in the identification of specialized metabolites involved in plant defense mechanisms, [Drexler et al. 2011].

Fluxomics

It is a contemporary application that arises from metabolomics, and it focuses on the actual rates of flow within metabolic networks. Measuring the metabolic fluxes directly is not feasible due to the dynamic and complex nature of the metabolic pathway. The "omics" fields are the holistic scope, the fluxome, which represents the complete set of metabolic fluxes within a cell arising from the omes, most notably the proteome and the metablome, [Aon & Cortassa, 2015].

Computational Tools and Artificial Intelligence

Metabolic engineering and synthetic biology mainly focus on the modification of biosynthetic pathways to enhance the production of bio-compounds in highly efficient and cost-effective ways. Yet, many key active ingredients in traditional medicine the artemisinin acid, glycyrrhizic acid, and similar molecules, tend to have intricate chemical structures that pose significant challenges for conventional metabolic engineering approaches in the development/production of desired products. Hence, this led to the development and integration of the emerging field of computational knowledge, i.e., Artificial Intelligence (AI), into metabolic engineering technologies. Machine learning (ML) Algorithms are increasingly being utilized to optimize gene expression and regulation of metabolic pathways, significantly boosting the yield of required products in medicinal plants. AI-driven models can efficiently predict and analyze the enzyme activity and metabolic flux, allowing for more precise adjustments and improvement, as shown in Figure 2, [Zhang, et al. 2024].

Additionally, deep learning enables researchers to identify and modification of critical nodes within the metabolic networks framework, further increasing the production of bioactive compounds. By incorporating metabolomics data, AI can analyse and provide comprehensive metabolite dynamics, supporting more informed optimization strategies. This approach not only accelerates the production capacity but also reduces the experimental and production time by enabling rapid screening through simulation and predictive modeling.

Figure 5. The application of ML in the analysis of plant-based traditional therapeutics. This computational paradigm enables detailed elucidation of natural products through an advanced analysis system (AI)

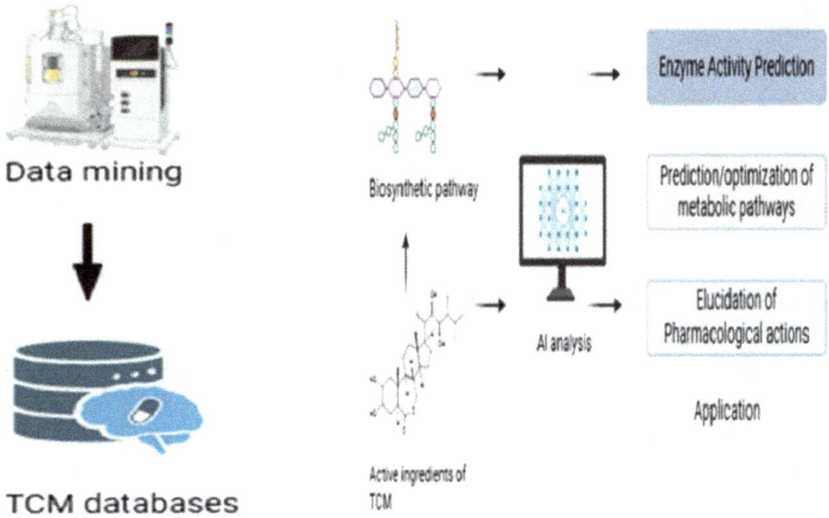

The continued advancement of computational biology and artificial intelligence has enhanced their fusion. For example, machine learning algorithms are used to predict: (1) whether the engineered and modulated pathways are behaving as anticipated, (2) to optimize heterologous and recombinant gene expression, and (3) to find potential bottlenecks to flow through the metabolic super-network putative targets. This computational assistance improves the efficiency and specificity of designing multi-genomic systems. Some of the recent AI-powered outcomes are Artemisinin Scale-Up: Keasling team engaged optKnock algorithms to identify ERG9 knockout targets, increasing the titer levels of amorphadiene product by 40% and reducing experimental screening time by 90%. Biofuels: LanzaTech AI platform engineered bacterial strains of Clostridium capable of producing acetone or isopropanol from CO_2 to produce 150% higher yields due to bootstrapping co-factors from the enhanced redox recycling process. Pharmaceuticals: Bactabolize (2023) used available data to predict edits to an *E. coli* genome for morphine synthesis de novo, repressing other metabolites by 78% through pathway compartmentalization.

APPLICATIONS IN BIOMANUFACTURING

Biomanufacturing, at its highest point, refers to the use of biological systems such as enzymes, microbes, or engineered genetically modified organisms to produce biofuels, nutraceuticals, pharmaceuticals, and other useful and valuable products from renewable resources. The history given in [section 2]. The latest biomanufacturing phase, known as phase 4.0, is characterized by its main focus on addressing urgent needs for global challenges, such as energy crises, health concerns, food security, climate change, and overall sustainability.

Central to most biomanufacturing processes is fermentation within a bioreactor, where raw materials are converted into target products by biological catalysts. Since the 1950s, batch and fed-batch fermentation methods have dominated commercial practice. These approaches are favored for their relatively straightforward reactor design, scalability, and adaptability to different products. Despite these advantages, batch and fed-batch processes suffer from inherent inefficiencies—namely, significant downtime between batches and suboptimal production rates—which ultimately limit overall productivity and drive up both capital and operating costs. Over the past several decades, scientific advances in synthetic biology, metabolic engineering, and protein biochemistry have outpaced the capabilities of conventional batch processes. Modern, engineered cells have the potential for much greater productivity, but existing manufacturing paradigms often fail to fully realize this potential. Consequently, there is a pressing need to transition toward fully controlled, continuous biomanufacturing processes, which promise to deliver biofuels, commodity chemicals, and high-value products more efficiently and at lower cost. Continuous fermentation has been the focus of considerable research aiming to increase productivities and reduce manufacturing expenses. This approach has been explored for a variety of products, including biofuels (such as ethanol for gasoline and lipids for biodiesel), commodity chemicals (e.g., acetone–butanol–ethanol solvents, lactic acid, succinic acid, 1,3-propanediol), and specialty molecules (such as omega-3 fatty acids and recombinant proteins). Recently, the biopharmaceutical sector has also started to adopt continuous manufacturing, particularly for the production of monoclonal antibodies with mammalian cells. Despite these developments, the bulk of commercial biomanufacturing still relies on batch or fed-batch methods. Widespread adoption of continuous processing will require technological breakthroughs in both strain development and process engineering to overcome significant technical hurdles, [Genomics & med. 2001; Atsumi et al. 2007; Nielsen, et al. 2009; Steen, et al. 1997; Park, et al. 2003; Chen & Blascheck, 1999].

Synthetic Biology in Biofuels Production

Synthetic biology is an especially promising field that supports these advances. This discipline focuses on the rational design and construction of biological systems from standardized components, enabling the creation of programmable cells tailored for specific functions. In the context of biofuels, synthetic biology facilitates the integration of new genes and pathways into host cell metabolism and the fine-tuning of these systems for maximum productivity and yield—a critical consideration given the economic sensitivity of biofuel production to costs such as raw materials and downstream processing.

The synthetic biology toolkit includes DNA, RNA, and protein-level elements that allow precise regulation of gene expression and metabolic pathways. Examples range from engineered promoters for controlled gene expression to complex regulatory systems involving tunable intergenic regions, riboregulators, ribozymes, and chromosomal amplification strategies. These innovations are vital for constructing robust, industrial strains. Computational models have also been developed to optimize ribosome binding sites, achieving wide-ranging control over protein expression levels. Together, these tools and approaches position synthetic biology as a key driver in the ongoing transformation of biomanufacturing, offering the potential for significant improvements in efficiency, scalability, and sustainability. Synthetic biology is able to provide tools and design principles to guide the development of such biomanufacturing processes ref. [Figure 6], [Connor & Liao, 2008; Smith, et al. 2010].

Figure 6. DNA level, RNA level, and Protein level, showing metabolies synthesis pathways

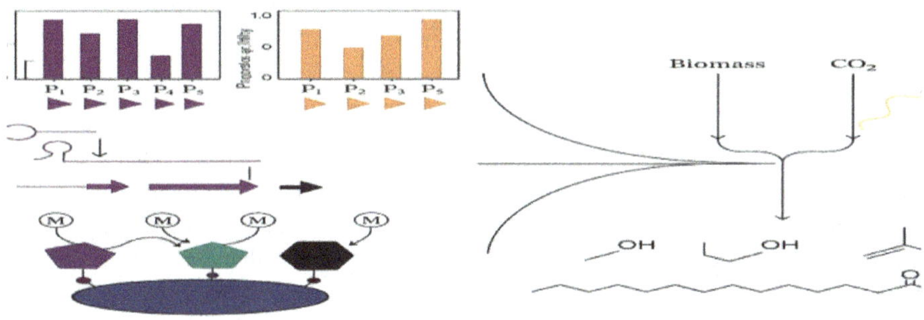

CASE STUDIES

Microbial Cell Factories for Drug Synthesis

The area of drug development and manufacturing is in the midst of a profound change perpetuated by synthetic biology and metabolic engineering. Microbial Cell Factories (MCFs) - living microorganisms (mostly bacteria and yeast) that have been genetically programmed to act as energy-efficient replicating bio-catalysts that enable sustainable production of complex pharmaceuticals - are going to be the vehicles of change. MCFs can offer a compelling alternative to classic chemical synthesis and natural product extraction - thus having the potential to offer enhanced sustainability, more cost-effective product manufacturing, and eventually access to drug molecules that in the past would have been thought to be too expensive and complex productions.

The advantages of MCFs are able to function under mild conditions (aqueous, room temperature and pressure), resulting in far less energy usage, fewer hazardous solvents, and much less toxic waste than multi-step chemical syntheses. MCFs also use renewable carbon sources that fit within the circular bioeconomy principles. Cost-Effective & Scalable: Fermentation processes are fundamentally scalable, and already utilize industrial infrastructure. After a successful strain is developed, production can be scaled-up in huge bioreactors, and the origin of the complexity also lowers expensive production costs - especially for complex molecules. Access to Complexity: Most pharmaceuticals, like all natural products (i.e., alkaloids, polyketides, and terpenes), have complex chemical structures with multiple chiral centers. To chemically synthesize most natural products, numerous steps are required, typically with low yields. MCFs allow complex scaffolds to be built in an affordable manner using the exquisite stereo- and regio-selectivity of enzyme catalysis. Security of Supply Chain & Independence: Production can be separated from the geographical limits, seasonal changes, political instability, or ecological stresses on plants or animals sourcing the starting materials. This leads to a more reliable and consistent delivery of important medicines. Novelty & Biosynthesis: New analogs ("unnatural natural products") can be produced via biosynthesis using combinatorial biosynthesis or engineered biosynthetic pathways, which may lead to drugs with better efficacy, fewer side effects, or activity against resistant pathogens. [Wijffels, et al. 2016; Hansen, et al. 2009; Liew, et al. 2022]

The Case of Artemisinin

The semi-synthetic production of artemisinin was a remarkable success story and serves to demonstrate the malaria control framework for global health. [**Ro,** et al. 2006]. The Challenge: Artemisinin (isolated only from sweet wormwood [Artemisia annua]) is the active pharmaceutical ingredient (API) at the core of artemisinin-based combination therapies (ACTs), which has been designated by the World Health Organization (WHO) as the first-line treatment for malaria.

Extending the MCF Pharmaceutical Pipeline

The success of artemisinin has opened the doors for MCFs to develop a range of pharmaceuticals:

Therapeutic Proteins & Peptides

Insulin: The introduction of recombinant human insulin expressed in *E. coli* or *S. cerevisiae* has transformed the therapeutic option for diabetes, allowing for the termination of animal-sourced insulin while producing the product with more purity and consistency than was previously possible. Researchers are working continuously to lower costs in insulin production, providing improvements in strain and process [Li& Neubauer, 2020].

Monoclonal Antibodies (mAbs)

The majority of complex mAbs are produced in mammalian cells in high volume, however, microbial systems (particularly with yeasts such as *Pichia pastoris*) are replacing mammalian cells for antibody fragments (scFvs, Fabs), bispecific antibodies, and simpler mAbs, offering rapid fermentation and potentially lower costs.

Hormones & Growth Factors: Human growth hormone (hGH), erythropoietin (EPO), interferons, and granulocyte colony-stimulating factor (G-CSF) can all be produced routinely in *E. coli* or mammalian cells, but viral systems are employed for the production of non-glycosylated versions.

Vaccine Antigens

Vaccine subunits (Hepatitis B surface antigen in yeast) and virus-like particles (VLPs) can be produced in situ for MCF large-scale hosting.

Complex Small Molecule APIs (Active Pharmaceutical Ingredients)

Opioid Analgesics

Yeast strains can now produce thebaine (a precursor to opioid production), derived from sugar, which may allow for a more consistent and traceable supply chain than current poppy farmed sources. Ongoing work is in progress for hydrocodone and oxycodone. Anticancer Agents: The production of complex chemotherapeutics, including the production of taxol (paclitaxel) precursors in either yeast or E. coli for production is actively being researched to improve upon the slow growth and agricultural yield of the yew tree. There are also a few ongoing projects with vinca alkaloids (e.g., vinblastine, & vincristine).

Alkaloids

Taking one step further beyond opioid production, the microbial production of bioactive alkaloids beyond opioids, for example, noscapine (as a cough suppressant/anticancer), berberine (as an antimicrobial), and macrolides originating from plants (e.g., Erythromycin precursors) is being developed in the lab. [Frick, et al. 2007]

Vitamins & Nutraceuticals

Microbial fermentation represents the main method of industrial synthesis of vitamin B2 (riboflavin), vitamin B12 (cobalamin), vitamin C (ascorbic acid using a two-step fermentation process), beta-carotene, and astaxanthin. [Shiio & Nakamori, 1969]

Engineered Yeast for Flavor Compounds

Over $30 billion in sales globally, the flavor and fragrance industries depend on the supply of more complex molecules from different starting points, often plants, synthetic, or traditional fermentation routes. All of these supplies have constraints: the plants are often not abundant, seasonal or take considerable energy and land; the synthetic versions of flavor molecules may be viewed as having less authenticity and it may lead producers to label them as "artificial;" and traditional fermentation approaches have difficulty showcasing varieties. Through engineered *Saccharomyces cerevisiae* (baker's yeast), we can develop yeast into small factories for the sustainability, high-purity, "natural" flavor and fragrance molecules they desire. These methods enable researchers to integrate plant, microbial, or potentially, synthetic new pathways directly into yeast, allowing us to utilize yeast's rapid growth cycle, its well-characterized genetics, and ease of scaling with industrial fermentation to make important molecules like vanillin, nootkatone, valencene, raspberry ketone, and other complex terpenes. This process takes advantage of metabolic engineering in the yeast - yeast often survive on sugars, however metabolic engineering will utilize that resource and redirect carbon flux in the metabolic network to the creation of desired flavor molecules [Hirst & Richter, 2016]. Metabolic engineering will produce the desired flavors in a variety of ways, which include optimizing the expression of the fermentative and flavor biosynthetic enzymes of the yeast in the metabolic network, increasing the availability of precursors necessary for flavor synthesis, and limiting or suppressing the toxicity of the product to yeast. The case for metabolic engineering yeast - sustainability (limited land and water use, lower carbon footprint, etc.) uses renewable resources, the potential for lower cost strategies and risk to eventual scale-up, and an increased range and varieties to flavor compounds. [Peter, et al. 2018]

Engineering yeast towards flavor production is a complex process of pathway reconstruction and optimization. Heterologous Pathway Introduction: Genes encoding enzymes from plants (vanillin biosynthesizing enzymes from Vanilla planifolia), bacteria or fungi are codon optimized and placed into yeast. For example, to produce the citrus flavor nootkatone, the pathway would require valencene synthase (from orange), a cytochrome P450 enzyme (like CYP71AV8 from chamomile or engineered related versions) plus its reductase partner, and also required optimization of the mevalonate pathway to provide a precursor FPP. Host Engineering: Competing native yeast pathways consuming precursors (particularly sterol biosynthesis using FPP) are down regulated. Pathways for precursors (such as shikimate pathway for vanillin precursors or the mevalonate pathway for terpenes) are needed to be amplified with an overexpressed first enzyme. Transporters may be engineered to secrete the products, thus reducing the intracellular toxic levels.[Gellissen, et al. 2005]

Enzyme Engineering

Natural enzymes can have low activity, be unstable, or have poor specificity in yeast. Directed evolution or rational design can generate enzyme variants that have improved catalytic efficiencies, solubility, substrate specificity, and cofactor recycling (e.g., regaining NADPH).

Commercial Outcomes and Notable Compounds

Vanillin made by the leading company Evolva (with IFF) was able to successfully commercialize fermented vanillin ("Vanillin Natural"), produced using an engineered yeast. This venture circumvents the long wait of cultivating vanilla beans, the complexities of extracting vanillin by using a consistent, sustainable, and "natural" approach to replace synthetic vanillin. It competes for the most considerable slice of the most valuable natural vanillin market. Nootkatone: Proposed natural insect repellent with grapefruit aroma. Nootkatone is a highly valued compound made by companies like Allylix (Evolva, then IFF), or Conagen. Each company is developing a commercial yeast platform, wherein engineered yeast produces valencene and more efficiently oxidizes it to nootkatone based on overcoming low natural P450 activity from yeast via enzyme engineering. [Cankar, et al., 2015]. Valencene is the key precursor to orange flavor and is easily produced in yeast. [Peralta-Yahya et al., 2011]., as at example, by Conagen- as part of its end product or as feed stock for nootkatone. Raspberry Ketone: The compound that gives raspberries their "raspberry" characteristic aroma. This is an example when numpy created a pathway in engineered yeast that could be a more sustainable approach than the experimentation of extraction from scarce raspberries. High-Value Terpenes: Terra Incognita: Beyond citrus, engineered yeast can produce other terpenes: Linalool (Florals), santalols (sandalwood), patchoulol (earthy), bisabolol (soothing, cosmetic ingredient). These compounds are produced for perfumery and cosmetics.

Table 2. Comparison of flavor compound production methods

Features	Plant Extraction	Chemical Synthesis	Engineered Yeast Fermentation
Source	Crops e.g. vanilla orchids	Petrochemical feedstocks	Sugar e.g. Glucose, Sucrose
Sustainability	High land/water use, seasonal weather-dependent	High energy, hazardous waste, fossil carbon	Low land footprint, renewable carbon, lower carbon dioxide
Scalability	Limited by crop yield and geography	Highly scalable	High Scalable (industrial fermentation)
Cost	Very high e.g. natural vanillin	Low-Medium	Medium (decreasing with optimization)
Purity/Consistency	Variable (pesticides, contaminants, possible)	High (but may contain isomers/ byproducts)	High and Consistent
Natural label	Yes	No	Yes (US/EU compliant processes)

CHALLENGES AND LIMITATIONS

Metabolic Burden and Cellular Trade-offs

Metabolic burden is a major hurdle when engineering surfaces, be it inserting foreign genetic elements or over-expressing native pathways, in both synthetic biology and metabolic engineering. Metabolic burden describes the drain on a host's limited repertoire (energy, precursors, macromolecular machinery, etc.) that is introduced by the operation of a heterologous or amplified genetic construct. This burden pressures the cell into cellular trade-offs that are allocations of resources away from growth and maintenance and towards maintaining the engineered functions, often resulting in performance that is below par or the engineered system failing altogether. Metabolic burden arises from a "web" of factors that have interrelated demands:

Resource Consumption for Expression

The processes of transcription and translation are not a free lunch, and the energy costs is considerable. The expression of foreign genes requires the consumption of ATP, GTP, nucleotides, and amino acids. This consumption is particularly pronounced when the gene is being high-level expressed under strong constitutive promoters [Ceroni, et al. 2015]. The process of high-level expression can ultimately cause a "strain" on the transcriptional apparatus (i.e., RNA polymerase) and the translational machinery (i.e., ribosomes, tRNAs, aminoacyl-tRNA synthetases). Protein Synthesis and Folding: The synthesis of large and/or complex heterologous proteins consumes amino acid stocks, and the folding of proteins requires co-factors and at times chaperones which further depletes energy (ATP) that is available to the organism. In turn, misfolded proteins then stress the organism through proteolytic systems to dispose of them. Enzymatic Activity and Flux of Pathways: The operation of heterologous metabolic pathway proceeds by "consuming" central metabolites such as acetyl-CoA, pyruvate, phosphoenolpyruvate, NADPH, ATP, etc. [Glick, 1995]. to either react, act as co-factors, or provide energy. Thus, if the host and heterologous metabolic pathway are competing for these employed, or vital, intermediates in a given pathway. Genetic Element Maintenance: Maintaining, replicating, and keeping plasmid DNA (a preferentially high-copy number plasmid) consumes nucleotides, and requires DNA polymerase activity, which takes away resources from chromosomal DNA, which is replicating and is subjected to repairs. Toxicity and Stress: Lastly, there are instances of toxic heterologous proteins and stress from intermediates within pathways that have competing metabolism or are detrimental to cell homeostasis (i.e., membrane proteins about membrane integrity or reactive oxygen species about in induction of oxidative stress) that will trigger stress responses, which then use additional resources.

Mitigation Strategies

Understanding metabolic burden is essential for successfully implementing engineering strategies for Promoter Engineering. tune is using tunable (inducible) or weaker promoters; it avoids unnecessarily high constitutive expression and genomic Integration. Replacing high-copy plasmids with single or low-copy genomic integrations reduces the replication burden, leading to enhanced genetic stability. Pathway Balancing has fine-tuned expression levels of individual enzymes within a heterologous pathway to mitigate bottlenecks and toxically accumulated intermediates without overexpressing non-rate-limiting enzymes. Dynamic Regulation builds genetic circuits that enable pathway expression only after significant biomass build-up or under specific conditions (e.g. nutrient starvation). Host Engineering: The host strain is to be more robust. for example, increase precursor/cofactor supply (for example, overexpress NADPH generating enzymes), increase protein folding capacity, delete competing pathways or use evolved strains to tolerate specific burdens it will reduces Genetic Load to minimize size of inserted DNA, use codon-optimized genes to avoid unnecessary translational costs, use genes without unnecessary genetic elements.

Table 3. Key aspects of metabolic burden and cellular trades-offs

Feature	Description	Primary Consequence (Trade-off)	Example of Mitigation Strategy
Resource Consumptions (Expression)	Energy (ATP/GTP), nucleotides, amino acids, ribosomes, RNAP used for transcription/translation	Reduced native protein synthesis; slower growth	Weaker/tunable promoters, codon optimization
Protein synthesis/ folding	Demand for amino acids, ATP, and cofactors for folding complex proteins	Energy depletion, proteotoxic stress	Fusion tags/ solubility enhancers, chaperone co-expression
Enzymatic activity/ pathway flux	Drain on central metabolites (acetyl-CoA, PEP), energy carriers (ATP, NADPH), cofactors	Flux imbalance, reduced precursor for biomass/ native metabolism.	Pathway balancing cofactor engineering
Genetic element maintenance	Nucleotides, polymerases for plasmid replication, occupied the regulatory sites	Competition with chromosome replication/ repair, genetic instability	Genomic integration, minimized plasmid backbones

continued on following page

Table 3. Continued

Feature	Description	Primary Consequence (Trade-off)	Example of Mitigation Strategy
Toxicity/stress	Disruption of membranes, pH, redox balance, generation of reactive species by intermediates/products	Activation of stress responses, cell lysis	Toxicity screening, pathway compartmentalization, and efflux pumps
Genetic instability	Selection pressure favors cells that lose or mutate the burden-imposing construct	Loss of productivity over time, culture heterogeneity	Strong selection markers, genomic integration, and dynamic control

Metabolic burden and the resulting cellular compromises represent a fundamental constraint in synthetic biology and metabolic engineering due to the competition for finite cellular resources between designed functions and the host's intrinsic needs for growth and survival. It dictates whether a designed biological system ultimately succeeds or fails. It is essential to conceptualize all of the sources and manifestations of burden. Future progress depends on better engineering practices – including smarter dynamic regulatory practices, better host chassis engineering, and computationally derived burden predictions – that reduce trade-offs and explore the full capacity of engineered biological systems for sustainable bioproduction and novel biological applications.

Scalability and Industrial Translation

Moving synthetic biology and metabolic engineering achievements from the safety of the laboratory flask to the challenging environment of the industrial bioreactor is a significant challenge of scale, and we call this scale-up. Just because something works in a shake flask of a few milliliters does not guarantee its success in a fermenter of thousands of liters. Industrial translation of laboratory innovation (besides physical scale) is a uniquely complex effort that aims to develop and optimize the whole bioprocess (upstream and downstream) for economic feasibility, operational robustness, compliance with regulatory requirements, and manufacturability within current manufacturing infrastructure. This challenge is often considered the biggest hurdle to realizing the commercial potential of modified biological systems.

The key hurdle in successful transitions of engineered biological systems to industrial bioreactors is the translational step of **scalability,** or practical limitations beyond small laboratory-scale experiments. In laboratory-scale experiments, conditions are controlled, homogeneous, and consistent across small scales (nutrients levels, oxygen levels, pH, temperature, etc.), but are lost in large-scale fermentation. Scale can change key physical and biological parameters non-linearly, for example, mass transfer limitations, will make oxygen limitation a severe bottleneck due to surface-to-volume ratios, mixing heterogeneity will create spatial gradients of nutrients, pH, dissolved oxygen, and temperature and shear stress from the limited physical agitation/aeration needed to mitigate these issues. These factors will expose cells to fluctuating, often, non-optimal microenvironments, creating population heterogeneity in toxicity, physiological and metabolic parameters, so cells will grow slower, as well as exhibit varied performance of the engineered strain optimized under ideal lab conditions. Additionally, engineered strains are more sensitive to these stresses, and will worsen, for instance, with genetic instability, or lower productivity on a small scale. Therefore, obtaining similar titers, yields, and productivities at industrial is not as straightforward, giving a significant process development risk (Delvigne & Goffin, 2014).

Industrial translation is more than just a large-scale "scale-up", it is an optimization of the entire bioprocess to be economically viable, robust, and compliant with regulations. Navigating the complexities of large-scale process control (dealing with delays, spatial variations), the much higher costs and technical challenges of downstream processes (DSP) for purifying product from large volumes, and the relentless economic pressure of needing high space-time yields and cheapest feedstocks, all become considerable challenges. Moreover, regulatory standards (e.g., FDA GMP for therapeutics) necessitate that product quality and safety are reproducibly achieved, which requires considerable validation through scale-downs and pilot plants. Some strategies around overcoming these challenges include using scale-down approaches (replicating some, if not all, of the industrial heterogeneities within lab systems); predictive strain and process optimization with scale downs; engineered hosts for sophistication (robustness and tolerance to stress, genetic stability, efficient substrate utilization); advanced bioprocess control (PAT, model-predictive feeding) and initiating integrated bioprocess design ("Design for Purification") early in the development journey to lessen DSP bottlenecks. In the end, successful industrial translation must treat biological performance, engineering restraints, and commercial realities holistically from the start (Junker, 2021; Liew et al., 2022).

Table 4. Key challenges in scaling-up engineered biological systems

Challenge category	**Laboratory scale reality**	**Industrial scale challenges**	**Primary impact**	**Mitigation strategy examples**
Mass transfer (oxygen/ substrates)	Easily achieved (high S/V ratio)	Severely limited, major bottleneck	Reduced growth/ productivity, anaerobic zones	High sparge/agitation, reactor design, oxygen vectors
Mixing/homogeneity	Near perfect mixing	Significant gradients (nutrients, pH, dO2, temperature)	Cell heterogeneity, stress, reduced yield	Impeller design, baffling, CFD modeling control
Process control	Precise, responsive	Delays, overshoots, spatial variation	Instability, suboptimal conditions	PAT sensors, model-predictive control, robust strains
Downstream processing	Relatively simple low volume	Major cost driver, complexity increases	High CoGs, product loss, purification failures	Early design for purification, secretion engineering
Economics/ regulation	Focus on proof-of-concept	Paramount, high Cogs, Strict	Commercial viability, market barriers	Robust processes, high-yield strains, low cost feeds

Scalability and industrial translation continue to be significant bottlenecks in synthetic biology and metabolic engineering. The very large differences between lab-level and industrial-level contexts mean that moving a discovery further along the translation pathway needs to occur more systematically, combining new strain engineering that has been integrated into robustness and performance during stress, to advance bioprocess design and control approaches that accommodate mass constraints, and early thought toward downstream processing and economic reality. Delivering on this transition will be critical if the underlying potential of engineered biology is to have the potential for real, sustainable, and economically viable processes that provide societal value.

CONCLUSION AND FUTURE RESEARCH IN METABOLIC ENGINEERING AND SYNTHETIC BIOLOGY APPROACH

The convergence of the disciplines of metabolic engineering and synthetic biology has transformed the biomanufacturing industry with unprecedented access to directing cellular systems for sustainable and viable production of high-value bio-products. In the last few decades, the convergence of the two disciplines has revolutionized our capability to design, engineer, and optimize metabolic pathways, not only to mimic nature but also to improve it by designing novel biological systems with tailored functionalities. Metabolic engineering targets the redesign of endogenous and exogenous biochemical networks to enhance metabolite yield and efficiency of production. Synthetic biology targets the same through the introduction of standardized genetic building blocks, programming of artificial regulatory circuits, and enabling de novo assembly of full pathways. Collectively, these technologies have enabled successful microbial production of biofuels, medicines such as artemisinin and semiglutide, food products such as soy leghemoglobin, and industrial chemicals through microbial cell factories engineered.

The discovery and use of highly effective technologies like CRISPR-Cas systems, omics technologies (genomics, transcriptomics, proteomics, metabolomics), and metabolic flux analysis have greatly enhanced our precision to engineer biological systems. The introduction of AI and machine learning in this arsenal is revolutionizing the face of biological engineering. AI facilitates the prediction of enzyme activity, metabolic flux distribution, pathway optimization, and strain performance. AI also facilitates data-driven decisions, speeds up the Design-Build-Test-Learn (DBTL) cycle, and saves time and cost significantly in pathway engineering and strain development. Despite such advancements, there are several challenges that still exist. Metabolic burden, competition for resources within the cell, pathway instability, and the problem of scaling from laboratory to industrial scale are some of the major issues. Further, coupling of non-natural synthetic routes tends to pose toxicity or flux imbalance, thereby decreasing overall productivity. Research Directions: AI-Driven Pathway Design: Future studies will rely more and more on AI algorithms for de novo pathway prediction, multi-objective optimization, and automation of strain design, enabling more iteration cycles and more stable production systems. Genome Editing Tools: Tools besides CRISPR, such as base editors and prime editing, will offer greater control over genetic elements and regulatory mechanisms. Adaptive Laboratory Evolution (ALE) in combination with Machine Learning: Such technologies will facilitate dynamic optimization of microbes in varying environmental conditions, with AI tracking evolution trajectories and predicting beneficial mutations. Whole-Cell Modeling and Digital Twins: Computational models will model whole cell systems ("digital twins") to predict outcomes before the actual biological experimentation, with much higher accuracy and efficiency. Expanded Chassis and Non-Model Organisms: In addition to the use of model organisms like E. coli and S. cerevisiae, more emphasis will be placed on the engineering of stable non-model hosts like cyanobacteria, Pichia pastoris, and extremophiles for specific applications. Sustainable Bioprocessing: Metabolic engineering and renewable feedstocks combined with green chemistry will enable the creation of environmentally friendly, circular bioeconomy systems. Synthetic Ecologies and Co-Culture Engineering: Designing microbial consortia capable of co-operating in sophisticated bioconversions provides solutions to issues not possible by single strains. Automation and Biofoundries: Automated biofoundries, supported by AI-driven decision-making and quality control, will facilitate high-throughput screening and design of engineered organisms. Regulatory and Ethical Frameworks: With the development of synthetic biology technologies, ethical, safety, and regulatory concerns will become increasingly more salient. It will be interested in risk assessment, policies for containment, and responsible innovation. Global Health and Climate Solutions: In the end, microbes will unlock answers to global problems, including the development of low-cost therapeutics, biodegradable plastics, carbon sequestration technologies, and renewable energy solutions.

REFERENCES

Aon, M. A., & Cortassa, S. (2015). Systems biology of the fluxome. *Processes (Basel, Switzerland), 3*(3), 607–618. DOI: 10.3390/pr3030607

Atsumi, S., Cann, A. F., Connor, M. R., Shen, C. R., Smith, K. M., Brynildsen, M. P., Chou, K. J. Y., Hanai, T., & Liao, J. C. (2007). Metabolic engineering of *Escherichia coli* for 1-butanol production. *Metabolic Engineering, 10*(6), 305–311. DOI: 10.1016/j.ymben.2007.08.003 PMID: 17942358

Ayoglu, B., Häggmark, A., Neiman, M., Igel, U., Uhlén, M., Schwenk, J. M., & Nilsson, P. (2011). Systematic antibody and antigen-based proteomic profiling with microarrays. *Expert Review of Molecular Diagnostics, 11*(2), 219–234. DOI: 10.1586/erm.10.110 PMID: 21405972

Bailey, R. C., Kwong, G. A., Radu, C. G., Witte, O. N., & Heath, J. R. (2007). DNA-encoded antibody libraries: A unified platform for multiplexed cell sorting and detection of genes and proteins. *Journal of the American Chemical Society, 129*(7), 1959–1967. DOI: 10.1021/ja065930i PMID: 17260987

Blazej, R. G., Kumaresan, P., & Mathies, R. A. (2006). Microfabricated bioprocessor for integrated nanoliter-scale Sanger DNA sequencing. *Proceedings of the National Academy of Sciences of the United States of America, 103*(19), 7240–7245. DOI: 10.1073/pnas.0602476103 PMID: 16648246

Buchner, E. (1897). Alkoholische Gärung ohne Hefezellen. *Berichte der Deutschen Chemischen Gesellschaft, 30*(1), 117–124. DOI: 10.1002/cber.18970300121

Buecherl, L., & Myers, C. J. (2022). Engineering genetic circuits: Advancements in genetic design automation tools and standards for synthetic biology. *Current Opinion in Microbiology, 68*, 102155. DOI: 10.1016/j.mib.2022.102155 PMID: 35588683

Cankar, K., van Houwelingen, A., Bosch, D., Sonke, T., Bouwmeester, H., & Beekwilder, J. (2015). A chicory cytochrome P450 mono-oxygenase CYP71AV8 for the oxidation of (+)-valencene. *FEBS Letters, 589*(1), 9–16. DOI: 10.1016/j.febslet.2014.11.020 PMID: 21115006

Casini, A., Storch, M., Baldwin, G. S., & Ellis, T. (2015). Bricks and blueprints: Methods and standards for DNA assembly. *Nature Reviews. Molecular Cell Biology, 16*(9), 568–576. DOI: 10.1038/nrm4014 PMID: 26081612

Ceroni, F., Algar, R., Stan, G. B., & Ellis, T. (2015). Quantifying cellular capacity identifies gene expression designs with reduced burden. *Nature Methods, 12*(5), 415–418. DOI: 10.1038/nmeth.3339 PMID: 25849635

Chen, C. K., & Blaschek, H. P. (1999). Acetate enhances solvent production and prevents degeneration in *Clostridium beijerinckii* BA101. *Applied Microbiology and Biotechnology, 52*(2), 170–173. DOI: 10.1007/s002530051504 PMID: 10499256

Chen, X., Dong, Y., Huang, Y., Fan, J., Yang, M., & Zhang, J. (2021). Whole-genome resequencing using next-generation and Nanopore sequencing for molecular characterization of T-DNA integration in transgenic poplar 741. *BMC Genomics*, *22*, 329. DOI: 10.1186/s12864-021-07625-y PMID: 33957867

Connor, M. R., & Liao, J. C. (2008). Engineering of an *Escherichia coli* strain for the production of 3-methyl-1-butanol. *Applied and Environmental Microbiology*, *74*(18), 5769–5775. DOI: 10.1128/AEM.00468-08 PMID: 18676713

Delvigne, F., & Goffin, P. (2014). Microbial heterogeneity affects bioprocess robustness: Dynamic single-cell analysis contributes to understanding of microbial populations. *Biotechnology Journal*, *9*(1), 61–72. DOI: 10.1002/biot.201300119 PMID: 24408611

Drexler, D. M., Reily, M. D., & Shipkova, P. A. (2011). Advances in mass spectrometry applied to pharmaceutical metabolomics. *Analytical and Bioanalytical Chemistry*, *399*(8), 2645–2653. DOI: 10.1007/s00216-010-4370-8 PMID: 21107980

Ellis, T., Adie, T., & Baldwin, G. S. (2011). DNA assembly for synthetic biology: From parts to pathways and beyond. *Integrative Biology*, *3*(2), 109–118. DOI: 10.1039/C0IB00070A PMID: 21246151

Embden, G., Meyerhof, O., & Parnas, J. (1934). Glycolysis and the Embden-Meyerhof pathway. *Biochemische Zeitschrift*, *273*, 416–429.

Erb, T. J., Jones, P. R., & Bar-Even, A. (2017). Synthetic metabolism: Metabolic engineering meets enzyme design. *Current Opinion in Chemical Biology*, *37*, 56–62. DOI: 10.1016/j.cbpa.2016.12.023 PMID: 28152442

Esvelt, K. M., & Wang, H. H. (2013). Genome-scale engineering for systems and synthetic biology. *Molecular Systems Biology*, *9*(1), 641. DOI: 10.1038/msb.2012.66 PMID: 23340847

Fagerberg, L., Strömberg, S., El-Obeid, A., Gry, M., Nilsson, K., Uhlén, M., Pontén, F., & Asplund, A. (2011). Large-scale protein profiling in human cell lines using antibody-based proteomics. *Journal of Proteome Research*, *10*(9), 4066–4075. DOI: 10.1021/pr200263f PMID: 21726073

Fischer, E. (1894). Einfluss der Configuration auf die Wirkung der Enzyme. *Berichte der Deutschen Chemischen Gesellschaft*, *27*(3), 2985–2993. DOI: 10.1002/cber.18940270364

Frick, S., Kramell, R., & Kutchan, T. M. (2007). Metabolic engineering with a morphine biosynthetic P450 in opium poppy surpasses breeding. *Metabolic Engineering*, *9*(2), 169–176. DOI: 10.1016/j.ymben.2006.10.004 PMID: 17189709

Gellissen, G., Kunze, G., Gaillardin, C., Cregg, J. M., Berardi, E., Veenhuis, M., & van der Klei, I. (2005). New yeast expression platforms based on methylotrophic *Hansenula polymorpha* and *Pichia pastoris* and on dimorphic *Arxula adeninivorans* and *Yarrowia lipolytica*—A comparison. *FEMS Yeast Research*, *5*(11), 1079–1096. DOI: 10.1016/j.femsyr.2005.06.004 PMID: 16144775

Glick, B. R. (1995). Metabolic load and heterologous gene expression. *Biotechnology Advances*, *13*(2), 247–261. DOI: 10.1016/0734-9750(95)00004-A PMID: 14537822

Goulet, D. R., & Atkins, W. M. (2020). Considerations for the design of antibody-based therapeutics. *Journal of Pharmaceutical Sciences, 109*(1), 74–103. DOI: 10.1016/j.xphs.2019.05.031 PMID: 31173761

Guo, Z., Zhou, Y., Li, J., Liu, D., Huang, Y., Zhang, Y., Yu, R., & Zhu, J. (2025). Dihydroartemisinic acid dehydrogenase-mediated alternative route for artemisinin biosynthesis. *Nature Communications, 16*(1), 3888. DOI: 10.1038/s41467-025-59312-1 PMID: 40274872

Hansen, E. H., Møller, B. L., Kock, G. R., Bünner, C. M., Kristensen, C., Jensen, O. R., Okkels, F. T., Olsen, C. E., Motawia, M. S., & Hansen, J. (2009). De novo biosynthesis of vanillin in fission yeast (*Schizosaccharomyces pombe*) and baker's yeast (*Saccharomyces cerevisiae*). *Applied and Environmental Microbiology, 75*(9), 2765–2774. DOI: 10.1128/AEM.02681-08 PMID: 19286778

Hirst, M. B., & Richter, C. L. (2016). Review of aroma formation through metabolic pathways of *Saccharomyces cerevisiae* in beverage fermentations. *American Journal of Enology and Viticulture, 67*(4), 361–370. DOI: 10.5344/ajev.2016.15098

Iowa State University. (2001). *Plant Sciences Institute update. Iowa State University Plant Sciences Institute Newsletter, 2*(1).

Jiang, W., Bikard, D., Cox, D., Zhang, F., & Marraffini, L. A. (2013). RNA-guided editing of bacterial genomes using CRISPR-Cas systems. *Nature Biotechnology, 31*(3), 233–239. DOI: 10.1038/nbt.2508 PMID: 23360965

Jones, J. A., Toparlak, Ö. D., & Koffas, M. A. (2015). Metabolic pathway balancing and its role in the production of biofuels and chemicals. *Current Opinion in Biotechnology, 33*, 52–59. DOI: 10.1016/j.copbio.2014.11.013 PMID: 25445548

Junker, B. H. (2021). Scale-up methodologies for *Escherichia coli* and yeast fermentation processes. *Journal of Bioscience and Bioengineering, 131*(3), 245–256. DOI: 10.1016/j.jbiosc.2020.11.011 PMID: 16233642

Keasling, J. D. (2010). Manufacturing molecules through metabolic engineering. *Science, 330*(6009), 1355–1358. DOI: 10.1126/science.1193990 PMID: 21127247

Keasling, J. D. (2010). Advanced biofuel production in microbes. *Biotechnology Journal, 5*(2), 147–162. DOI: 10.1002/biot.200900233 PMID: 20084640

Khalil, A. S., & Collins, J. J. (2010). Synthetic biology: Applications come of age. *Nature Reviews. Genetics, 11*(5), 367–379. DOI: 10.1038/nrg2775 PMID: 20395970

Khorana, H. G., Buchi, H., Ghosh, H., Gupta, N., Jacob, T. M., Kossel, H., Morgan, R., Narang, S. A., Ohtsuka, E., & Wells, R. D. (1980). Total synthesis of a gene for an alanine transfer RNA from yeast. *Nature, 283*(5743), 273–278. DOI: 10.1038/283273a0

Kjeldsen, T., Andersen, A. S., Hubálek, F., Johansson, E., Kreiner, F. F., Schluckebier, G., & Kurtzhals, P. (2023). Molecular engineering of insulin for recombinant expression in yeast. *Trends in Biotechnology, 42*(4), 464–478. DOI: 10.1016/j.tibtech.2023.09.012 PMID: 37880066

Kohlstedt, M., & Wittmann, C. (2019). GC-MS-based 13C metabolic flux analysis resolves the parallel and cyclic glucose metabolism of *Pseudomonas putida* KT2440 and *Pseudomonas aeruginosa* PAO1. *Metabolic Engineering*, *54*, 35–53. DOI: 10.1016/j.ymben.2019.01.008 PMID: 30831266

Krebs, H. A., & Johnson, W. A. (1937). The role of citric acid in intermediate metabolism in animal tissues. *Enzymologia*, *4*, 148–156.

Li, J., & Neubauer, P. (2020). *Escherichia coli* as a cell factory for heterologous production of nonribosomal peptides and polyketides. *New Biotechnology*, *59*, 1–11. DOI: 10.1016/j.nbt.2020.06.003 PMID: 24704144

Liew, F. E., Nogle, R., Abdalla, T., Rasor, B. J., Canter, C., Jensen, R. O., Wang, L., Strutz, J., Chirania, P., De Tissera, S., Mueller-Cajar, O., & Köpke, M. (2022). Carbon-negative production of acetone and isopropanol by gas fermentation at industrial pilot scale. *Nature Biotechnology*, *40*(3), 335–344. DOI: 10.1038/s41587-021-01195-w PMID: 35190685

Liu, Q., Liu, Y., & Qi, Q. (2016). Microbial production of natural and non-natural flavors: Pathways, engineering, and challenges. *Current Opinion in Biotechnology*, *70*, 1–9. DOI: 10.1016/j.copbio.2020.10.010

Liu, Q., Shen, Q., Bian, X., Chen, H., Fu, J., Wang, H., Lei, P., Guo, Z., Chen, W., Li, D., & Zhang, Y. (2016). Simple and rapid direct cloning and heterologous expression of natural product biosynthetic gene cluster in *Bacillus subtilis* via Red/ET recombineering. *Scientific Reports*, *6*, 34623. DOI: 10.1038/srep34623 PMID: 27687863

Luu, X. C., Shida, Y., Suzuki, Y., Kuwahara, D., Fujimoto, T., Takahashi, Y., Sato, N., Nakamura, A., & Ogasawara, W. (2023). Ultrahigh-throughput screening of *Trichoderma reesei* strains capable of carbon catabolite repression release and cellulase hyperproduction using a microfluidic droplet platform. *Bioscience, Biotechnology, and Biochemistry*, *87*(11), 1393–1406. DOI: 10.1093/bbb/zbad108 PMID: 37550222

Majhi, B. K. (2025). Cyanobacteria: Photosynthetic cell factories for biofuel production. *Journal of Bioresources and Bioproducts*, *10*(2), 128–144. DOI: 10.1016/j.jobab.2024.10.001

Matsuda, F., Toya, Y., & Shimizu, H. (2017). Learning from quantitative data to understand central carbon metabolism. *Biotechnology Advances*, *35*(8), 971–980. DOI: 10.1016/j.biotechadv.2017.09.006 PMID: 28928003

Matsumoto, T., Tanaka, T., & Kondo, A. (2017). Engineering metabolic pathways in *Escherichia coli* for constructing a "microbial chassis" for biochemical production. *Bioresource Technology*, *245*(Pt B), 1362–1368. https://doi.org/DOI: 10.1016/j.biortech.2017.05.171

Monod, J., Changeux, J. P., & Jacob, F. (1961). Allosteric proteins and cellular control systems. *Journal of Molecular Biology*, *6*(4), 306–329. DOI: 10.1016/S0022-2836(63)80091-1 PMID: 13936070

Nielsen, D. R., Leonard, E., Yoon, S. H., Tseng, H. C., Yuan, C., & Prather, K. L. J. (2009). Engineering alternative butanol production platforms in heterologous bacteria. *Metabolic Engineering*, *11*(4–5), 262–273. DOI: 10.1016/j.ymben.2009.05.003 PMID: 19464384

Nielsen, J., & Keasling, J. D. (2016). Engineering cellular metabolism. *Cell, 164*(6), 1185–1197. DOI: 10.1016/j.cell.2016.02.004 PMID: 26967285

Nikolados, E. M., Weiße, A. Y., Ceroni, F., & Oyarzún, D. A. (2019). Growth defects and loss-of-function in synthetic gene circuits. *ACS Synthetic Biology*, *8*(6), 1231–1240. DOI: 10.1021/acssynbio.8b00531 PMID: 31181895

Noda, S., Shirai, T., Mori, Y., Oyama, S., & Kondo, A. (2017). Engineering a synthetic pathway for maleate in *Escherichia coli. Nature Communications*, *8*, 1153. DOI: 10.1038/s41467-017-01253-9 PMID: 29074856

Ou, Y. J., Ren, Q. Q., Fang, S. T., Wu, J. G., Jiang, Y. X., Chen, Y. R., Zhang, Y., & Song, J. (2020). Complete genome insights into *Lactococcus petauri* CF11 isolated from a healthy human gut using second- and third-generation sequencing. *Frontiers in Genetics*, *11*, 119. DOI: 10.3389/fgene.2020.00119 PMID: 32174973

Painter, H. J., Altenhofen, L. M., Kafsack, B. F., & Llinás, M. (2013). Whole-genome analysis of *Plasmodium* spp. utilizing a new Agilent Technologies DNA microarray platform. *Methods in Molecular Biology (Clifton, N.J.)*, *923*, 213–219. DOI: 10.1007/978-1-62703-026-7_14 PMID: 22990780

Park, S. H., Zarrinpar, A., & Lim, W. A. (2003). Rewiring MAP kinase pathways using alternative scaffold assembly mechanisms. *Science*, *299*(5609), 1061–1064. DOI: 10.1126/science.1076979 PMID: 12511654

Peralta-Yahya, P. P., Ouellet, M., Chan, R., Mukhopadhyay, A., Keasling, J. D., & Lee, T. S. (2011). Identification and microbial production of a terpene-based advanced biofuel. *Nature Communications*, *2*, 483. DOI: 10.1038/ncomms1494 PMID: 21952217

Peter, J., Chiara, M. D., Friedrich, A., Yue, J., Pflieger, D., Bergström, A., Sigwalt, A., Barre, B., Freel, K., & Llored, A.. (2018). Genome evolution across 1,011 *Saccharomyces cerevisiae* isolates. *Nature*, *556*(7701), 339–344. DOI: 10.1038/s41586-018-0030-5 PMID: 29643504

Pfeifer, B. A., Beitelshees, M., Hill, A., & Jones, C. H. (2023). Harnessing synthetic biology for advancing RNA therapeutics and vaccine design. *npj Systems Biology and Applications, 9*, 60. https://doi.org/DOI: 10.1038/s41540-023-00323-3

Ro, D. K., Paradise, E. M., Ouellet, M., Fisher, K. J., Newman, K. L., Ndungu, J. M., Ho, K. A., Eachus, R. A., Ham, T. S., Kirby, J., Chang, M. C. Y., Withers, S. T., Shiba, Y., Sarpong, R., & Keasling, J. D. (2006). Production of the antimalarial drug precursor artemisinic acid in engineered yeast. *Nature*, *440*(7086), 940–943. DOI: 10.1038/nature04640 PMID: 16612385

Sander, J. D., & Joung, J. K. (2014). CRISPR-Cas systems for editing, regulating and targeting genomes. *Nature Biotechnology*, *32*(4), 347–355. DOI: 10.1038/nbt.2842 PMID: 24584096

Schladt, T., Engelmann, N., Kubaczka, E., Hochberger, C., & Koeppl, H. (2021). Automated design of robust genetic circuits: Structural variants and parameter uncertainty. *ACS Synthetic Biology*, *10*(6), 1393–1405. DOI: 10.1021/acssynbio.0c00608 PMID: 34807573

Shi, S., Liang, Y., Zhang, M. M., Ang, E. L., & Zhao, H. (2016). A highly efficient single-step, markerless strategy for multi-copy chromosomal integration of large biochemical pathways in *Saccharomyces cerevisiae*. *Metabolic Engineering*, *33*, 19–27. DOI: 10.1016/j.ymben.2015.10.011 PMID: 26546089

Shiio, I., & Nakamori, S. (1969). Microbial production of L-threonine part I. Production by *Escherichia coli* mutant resistant to α-amino-β-hydroxyvaleric acid. *Agricultural and Biological Chemistry*, *33*(8), 1152–1160. DOI: 10.1080/00021369.1969.10859439

Singh, V. (Ed.). (2021). *Microbial cell factories engineering for production of biomolecules*. Academic Press.

Sinreih, M., Zukunft, S., Sosič, I., Cesar, J., Gobec, S., Adamski, J., & Lanišnik Rižner, T. (2015). Combined application of *in silico* and *in vitro* screening for AKR1B10 inhibitors. *PLoS One*, *10*(2), e0117984. DOI: 10.1371/journal.pone.0117984 PMID: 25680188

Smith, H. O., Hutchison, C. A., Pfannkoch, C., & Venter, J. C. (2003). Generating a synthetic genome by whole genome assembly: PhiX174 bacteriophage from synthetic oligonucleotides. *Proceedings of the National Academy of Sciences of the United States of America*, *100*(26), 15440–15445. DOI: 10.1073/pnas.2237126100 PMID: 14657399

Smith, K. M., Cho, K. M., & Liao, J. C. (2010). Engineering *Corynebacterium glutamicum* for isobutanol production. *Applied Microbiology and Biotechnology*, *87*(3), 1045–1055. DOI: 10.1007/s00253-010-2522-6 PMID: 20376637

Steen, E. J., Chan, R., Prasad, N., Myers, S., Petzold, C. J., Redding, A., Ouellet, M., & Keasling, J. D. (2008). Metabolic engineering of *Saccharomyces cerevisiae* for the production of n-butanol. *Microbial Cell Factories*, *7*, 36. DOI: 10.1186/1475-2859-7-36 PMID: 19055772

Stephanopoulos, G. (2012). Synthetic biology and metabolic engineering. *ACS Synthetic Biology*, *1*(11), 514–525. DOI: 10.1021/sb300094q PMID: 23656228

Sun, X., Liu, H., Wang, P., Wang, Y., & Lu, L. (2019). Construction of a novel MK-4 biosynthetic pathway in *Pichia pastoris* through heterologous expression of HsUBIAD1. *Microbial Cell Factories*, *18*, 169. DOI: 10.1186/s12934-019-1215-9 PMID: 31601211

Weber, E., Engler, C., Gruetzner, R., Werner, S., & Marillonnet, S. (2011). A modular cloning system for standardized assembly of multigene constructs. *PLoS One*, *6*(2), e16765. DOI: 10.1371/journal.pone.0016765 PMID: 21364738

Wijffels, R. H., Barbosa, M. J., & Eppink, M. H. M. (2016). Microalgae for the production of bulk chemicals and biofuels. *Biofuels, Bioproducts & Biorefining*, *4*(3), 287–295. DOI: 10.1002/bbb.215

Xie, L., Gao, J., & Zhou, Y. J. (2024). Synthetic biology for Taxol biosynthesis and sustainable production. *Trends in Biotechnology*, *42*(6), 674–676. DOI: 10.1016/j.tibtech.2024.04.001 PMID: 38609783

Zhang, P., Zhang, D. F., Zhou, W., Wang, Q., Zhang, Y., & Li, Y. (2024). Network pharmacology: Towards the artificial intelligence-based precision traditional Chinese medicine. *Briefings in Bioinformatics*, *25*(1), bbad518. Advance online publication. DOI: 10.1093/bib/bbad518 PMID: 38197310

Zhao, M., Ma, J., Zhang, L., Huang, Y., Zhang, Y., & Yu, R. (2024). Engineering strategies for enhanced heterologous protein production by *Saccharomyces cerevisiae*. *Microbial Cell Factories*, *23*, 32. DOI: 10.1186/s12934-024-02299-z PMID: 38247006

Chapter 4
Advanced Bioreactor Systems and Design Principles for Scalable Bio-Manufacturing

Rishabh Garg
https://orcid.org/0000-0001-9813-9630
Birla Institute of Technology, India

Ayush Madan
https://orcid.org/0000-0001-5089-1794
People's University, India

ABSTRACT

A bioreactor is a specialized vessel designed to facilitate biological reactions, harnessing the capabilities of microorganisms, mammalian cells, or other biological systems to convert raw materials into valuable products. Bioreactor systems serve as the central hub of bioprocessing, from laboratory-scale experiments to pilot and industrial-scale manufacturing, bridging upstream and downstream operations. Their design and optimization are critical for achieving high productivity, maintaining process efficiency, and ensuring cost-effectiveness. This chapter provides a comprehensive overview of advanced bioreactor systems, including stirred-tank, airlift, perfusion, and single-use bioreactors, highlighting their advantages, limitations, and applications. It explores key design principles such as oxygen transfer, mixing dynamics, shear stress minimization, and real-time process monitoring.

INTRODUCTION

Biomanufacturing is the process of using biological systems, such as cells, enzymes, or organisms, to produce commercially valuable products on an industrial scale. This approach integrates biotechnology with manufacturing principles to produce a wide array of products, including biopharmaceuticals (like vaccines, monoclonal antibodies, and therapeutic proteins),

DOI: 10.4018/979-8-3373-2873-7.ch004

biofuels, industrial enzymes, and food additives (Zhang et al., 2017). Biomanufacturing typically involves the cultivation of living cells either microbial, plant, or animal in controlled environments where they express the target molecule or product. The process is often divided into upstream processing (which includes cell line development, media preparation, and cultivation in bioreactors) and downstream processing (which includes product recovery, purification, and formulation). One of the key advantages of biomanufacturing is the ability to produce complex molecules that are difficult or impossible to synthesize chemically, making it indispensable in modern medicine and biotechnology.

Biomanufacturing is a critical component of the biotechnology and pharmaceutical industries, involving the production of biological products such as vaccines, therapeutic proteins, enzymes, and biofuels using living cells. As the demand for bioproducts increases, the development of advanced bioreactor systems and scalable design principles becomes essential to ensure consistent, efficient, and high-yield production (Averesch et al., 2023). Modern bioreactor technologies are evolving to accommodate the needs of scalability, automation, process control, and regulatory compliance.

Fermentation is a biochemical process that involves the conversion of substrates (usually carbohydrates) into desired products through the metabolic activity of microorganisms such as bacteria, yeast, or fungi. It is one of the oldest forms of biotechnology and remains a cornerstone of industrial microbiology (Wang et al., 2024). While traditional fermentation was primarily used in food and beverage production (e.g., bread, alcohol, yogurt), modern industrial fermentation plays a crucial role in the production of antibiotics, amino acids, organic acids, vitamins, bioethanol, and recombinant proteins. Fermentation can be aerobic (requiring oxygen) or anaerobic (occurring in the absence of oxygen), depending on the type of microorganism and the end product desired Ross et al., 2002; Ezemba et al., 2022). Controlled fermentation processes occur in specialized equipment called fermenters, where conditions such as temperature, pH, oxygen levels, and nutrient supply are tightly regulated to maximize product yield and quality. For this the devices which are used are bioreactors or fermenters.

Importance of Bioreactors in Biomanufacturing

Bioreactor

A bioreactor is a sophisticated vessel or system designed to support biologically active environments for the cultivation of cells or microorganisms. It provides a controlled setting for various biochemical processes, such as cell growth, protein expression, and product synthesis. Bioreactors are an essential component of both biomanufacturing and fermentation industries (Liden, 2002). They are designed to regulate key process parameters such as temperature, pH, dissolved oxygen, agitation speed, and nutrient feed rate to maintain optimal growth conditions for the biological system in use. There are various types of bioreactors based on operation mode (batch, fed-batch, or continuous), design (stirred-tank, airlift, packed-bed, fluidized-bed), and usage (laboratory, pilot-scale, or production-scale). Advanced bioreactors may incorporate automated monitoring systems, sensors, and control algorithms to ensure reproducibility and scalability. In mammalian cell culture processes, bioreactors are vital for producing therapeutic proteins and vaccines, while microbial bioreactors are used in the production of antibiotics, enzymes, and other biomolecules. The versatility and precise control offered by bioreactors make them indispensable in modern biotechnology (Nguyen et al., 2024).

Fermenter

A fermenter is a specific type of bioreactor that is primarily used for microbial fermentation processes. It is a closed system designed to cultivate microorganisms under optimal conditions for the production of biochemical products. The fermenter provides the necessary environment for microbial cells to grow, metabolize, and convert substrates into desired products such as ethanol, antibiotics, organic acids, or enzymes. Typical features of a fermenter include a vessel made of stainless steel or glass, an aeration system for oxygen transfer (in aerobic fermentation), an agitation system for uniform mixing, and various ports for inoculation, sampling, nutrient addition, and waste removal. Fermenters are equipped with sensors to monitor and control critical parameters such as temperature, pH, and dissolved oxygen (Chettri et al., 2024). They are available in a range of sizes, from a few millilitres in laboratory-scale systems to thousands of litres in industrial-scale operations. Unlike bioreactors that are used for both microbial and mammalian cell cultures, fermenters are predominantly associated with microbial cultures and are optimized to meet the specific physiological needs of these organisms. The design and operation of fermenters are crucial for achieving high productivity and product consistency in industrial fermentation processes (Sheikh et al., 2024).

Evolution of Bioreactor Technology

The development of bioreactor technology has undergone significant evolution over the past century, driven by the growing need for efficient, scalable, and controlled systems for the production of biologically-derived products. From rudimentary fermentation vessels used in traditional food production to highly sophisticated, computer-controlled systems used in modern biotechnology, the progression of bioreactor technology reflects advancements in engineering, microbiology, and process control (Thon et al., 2017).

The earliest forms of bioreactors were simple containers used for fermentation in ancient civilizations. Traditional fermentation practices, such as brewing beer, fermenting wine, and producing yogurt or vinegar, relied on natural microbial activity in open or closed vessels like clay pots, wooden barrels, or ceramic jars. These processes lacked control over environmental parameters and were prone to contamination, resulting in inconsistent product quality (Hemmerich et al., 2018). Although primitive, these systems laid the foundation for understanding microbial growth and metabolism. A comparative trends analysis is shown in the Figure 1, where the development of bioreactors design has taken place between 2003 and 2023.

Figure 1. Evolution of the number of publications involving the keywords "bioreactors" and "bioreactor design" between 2003 and 2023

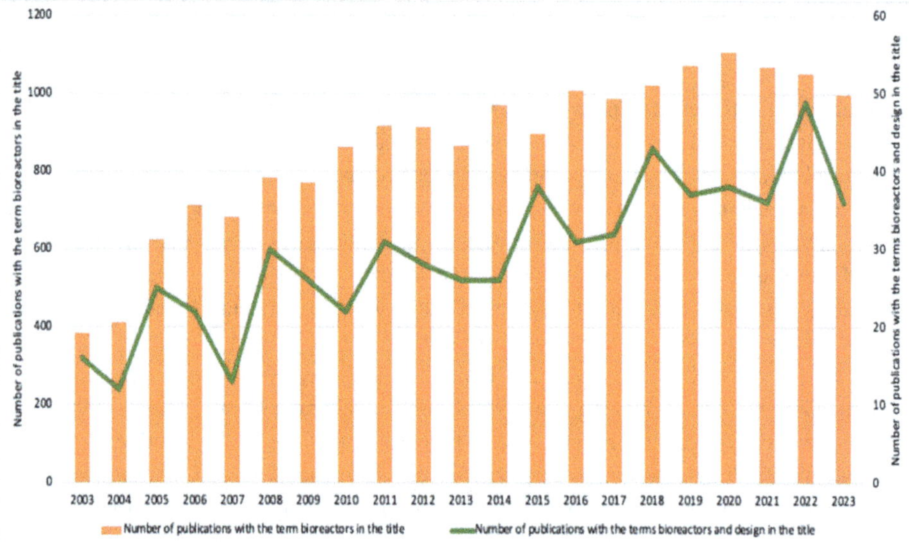

(Palladino et al., 2024)

Industrial Fermentation: The First Controlled Systems

With the advent of the Industrial Revolution in the 19th and early 20th centuries, bioreactor technology began to take on a more scientific and engineered form. The discovery of microorganisms and their role in fermentation by scientists such as Louis Pasteur led to more controlled and efficient fermentation processes (Chisti and Moo-Young, 2006). The production of ethanol, acetic acid, and butanol through microbial fermentation marked the beginning of industrial bioprocessing (Kendall, 2022; Pörtner et al., 2022).

During World War I and II, the need for large-scale production of solvents and antibiotics (like penicillin) drove the development of the first **stirred-tank fermenters**, which allowed for mechanical agitation and better aeration (Sevda and Kumar, 2024). These early stainless-steel bioreactors featured spargers, impellers, and basic monitoring tools, enabling improved control over oxygen transfer and mixing. This era represented the transition from artisanal fermentation to scientifically optimized industrial-scale bioproduction.

Post-War Advancements: Scaling and Diversification

In the decades following World War II, bioreactor design and operation saw rapid advancements. The pharmaceutical and chemical industries expanded the use of fermentation for producing antibiotics, vitamins, amino acids, and enzymes. Key developments during this period included Better sterilization methods (autoclaving, steam-in-place systems), Improved impeller designs for enhanced mixing, development of sensors and control systems for pH, temperature, and dissolved oxygen, Introduction of fed-batch and continuous operation modes, improving yields and productivity (Raj and Karanth, 2005). This period also saw the diversification of bioreactor types, such as airlift, bubble column, and packed-bed reactors, to accommodate different biological systems, including immobilized cells and anaerobic microorganisms (Ashok et al., 2017).

Biotechnological Revolution: Cell Culture and Genetic Engineering

The 1970s and 1980s marked a significant milestone in the evolution of bioreactors with the rise of recombinant DNA technology and mammalian cell culture (Pörtner et al., 2022).. The ability to genetically modify cells to produce therapeutic proteins, hormones, and monoclonal antibodies led to new demands on bioreactor technology. Mammalian cells are more fragile than microbes and require precise environmental control, low shear conditions, and specialized media. This era also saw the emergence of hollow-fiber and wave bioreactors, particularly for cell therapy and vaccine production (Altman, 2003; Lazim and Nazir, 2025). Bioreactors were adapted to accommodate these needs, with features such as:

a. Low-shear impellers (e.g., marine impellers).
b. Advanced temperature and gas control systems (CO_2 and O_2 supplementation).
c. Nutrient feed strategies tailored to cell growth and productivity.
d. Aseptic and closed-system designs to meet regulatory standards for biologics.

Single-Use Bioreactors and Disposable Technology

In the early 2000s, the introduction of single-use bioreactors (SUBs) marked a paradigm shift in bioreactor technology. These systems, made from polymeric materials and designed for one-time use, offered several advantages reduced cleaning and sterilization requirements, Faster turnaround between batches, Lower risk of cross-contamination and Scalability from bench to pilot and production scale (Oosterhuis and Junne, 2016). SUBs became particularly popular in biologics and vaccine production, where flexibility and sterility are paramount. Companies developed scalable platforms, such as wave-mixed, rocking-motion, and stirred-substitute systems that emulate traditional stainless-steel reactors (Jossen et al., 2019).

Smart Bioreactors and Digital Integration

Recent years have seen the emergence of smart bioreactors equipped with advanced process analytical technologies (PAT), automation, and integration with Industry. These include Real-time monitoring and control of multiple parameters using sensors and software, Automated feeding and harvesting systems, integration with machine learning and artificial intelligence for predictive control and optimization and modular, flexible bioreactor platforms suitable for multi-product facilities (Wang et al., 2020; Lee et al., 2024; Palladino et al., 2024). Digital twins, cloud-based analytics, and remote process monitoring are now being incorporated to increase productivity and ensure regulatory compliance in real-time.

CLASSIFICATION OF BIOREACTOR SYSTEMS

Bioreactors can be categorized based on the type of cells they cultivate (microbial, animal, or plant), their physical design (stirred tank, bubble column, airlift, or fluidized bed), and their mode of operation (batch, fed-batch, or continuous) (Geada et al., 2024). Additionally, they are classified according to their particular function (e.g., photobioreactors for algae) and the substrate (submerged or solid-state).

Stirred-Tank Bioreactors

Stirred tank bioreactors (STRs) are among the most commonly used and versatile types of bioreactors employed in both research and industrial-scale bioprocesses. These bioreactors consist of a cylindrical vessel, typically made from stainless steel or borosilicate glass, equipped with one or more mechanical agitators (impellers) mounted on a central shaft (Figure 2). The primary function of the impellers is to ensure thorough mixing of the culture medium, facilitating uniform distribution of nutrients, maintaining homogeneity, and enhancing gas-liquid mass transfer. Stirred tank bioreactors are often fitted with spargers that introduce air or oxygen into the liquid medium, making them highly effective for aerobic microbial and mammalian cell cultures (Julien & Whitford, 2024). They are also equipped with baffles to prevent vortex formation and to improve mixing efficiency. STRs allow precise control over critical process parameters such as pH, temperature, dissolved oxygen, agitation speed, and foam formation, often monitored and regulated via integrated sensors and feedback systems. The design can accommodate various operational modes batch, fed-batch, or continuous depending on the production strategy. Due to their robust design, scalability, and compatibility with a wide range of biological systems, STRs are extensively used in the production of pharmaceuticals, enzymes, biofuels, and vaccines. Moreover, their adaptability to both microbial and mammalian systems, combined with ease of operation and maintenance, makes stirred tank bioreactors a foundational tool in modern biomanufacturing (Candia-Sanchez et al., 2017).

A continuous stirred tank bioreactor consists of a cylindrical vessel with motor driven central shaft that supports one or more agitators (impellers). The shaft is fitted at the bottom of the bioreactor. The number of impellers is variable and depends on the size of the bioreactor i.e., height to diameter ratio, referred to as aspect ratio. Several types of impellers (Rustom disc, concave bladed, marine propeller etc.) are in use. The air is added to the culture medium under pressure through a device called sparger (Brindhadevi et al., 2021; Lin and Gu, 2021). The sparger may be a ring with many holes or a tube with a single orifice. The sparger along with impellers (agitators) enables better gas distribution system throughout the vessel. The bubbles generated by sparger are broken down to smaller ones by impellers and dispersed throughout the medium. This enables the creation of a uniform and homogeneous environment throughout the bioreactor (Nienow, 2014). There are many advantages of STRs like the efficient gas transfer to growing cells. Good mixing of the contents and flexible operating conditions, besides the commercial availability of the bioreactors.

Figure 2. Classical composition of a stirred tank bioreactor (4) equipped with a motor (1), mechanical seal (2), air inlet (3), shaft (5), baffles (6), impellers (7), double jacket for heat transfer (8), sparger (9) and bottom drain (10). H, vessel height; D, vessel diameter

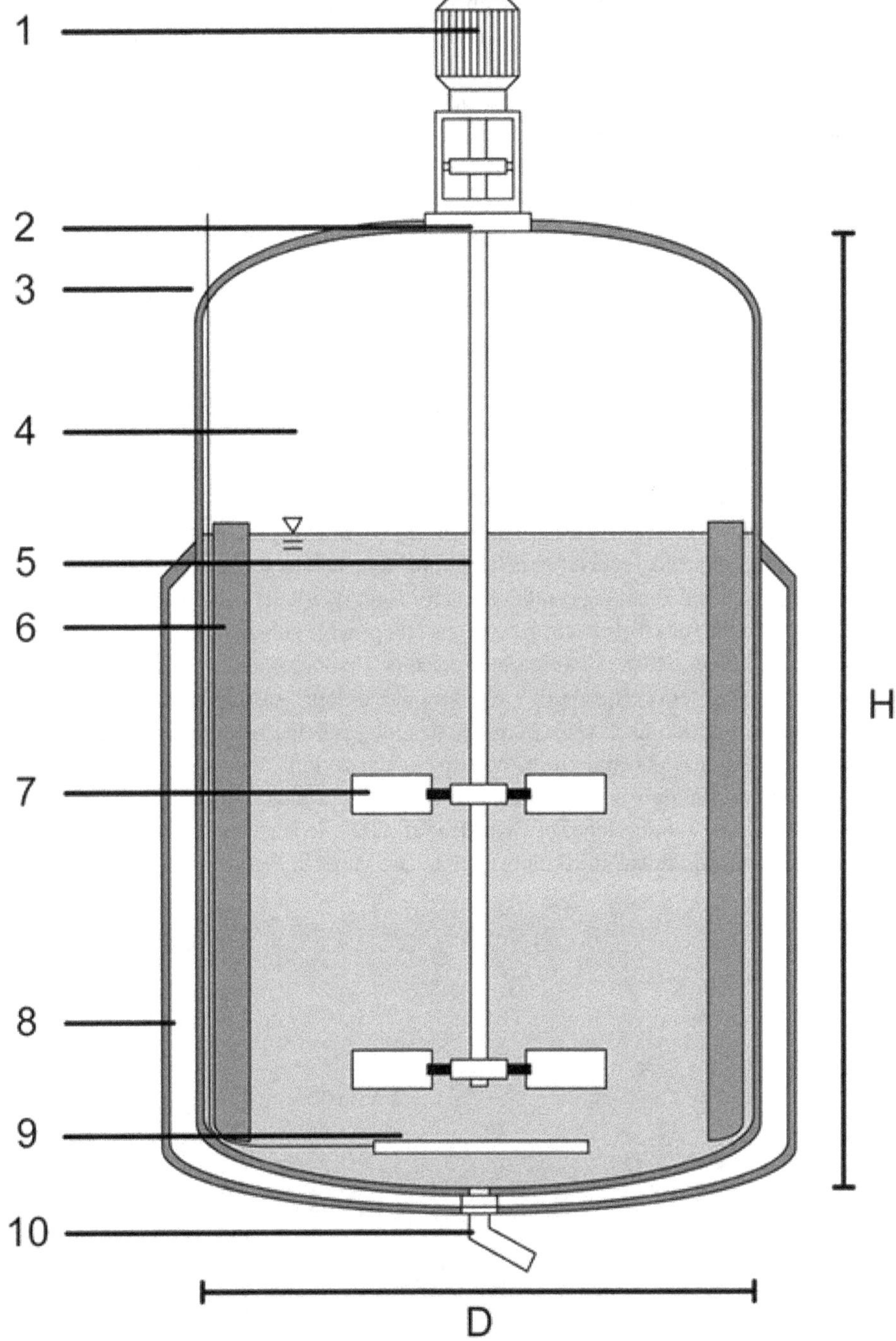

(Schirmer et al., 2021)

Airlift and Bubble Column Bioreactors

In airlift fermenter the liquid culture volume of the vessel is divided into two interconnected zones by means of a baffle or draft tube. Only one of the two zones is sparged with air or other gas and this sparged zone is known as the riser. The other zone that receives no gas is called down-comer (Cerrone and O'Connor, 2025). The bulk density of the gas-liquid dispersion in the gas-sparged riser tends to be lower than the bulk density in the down-comer. Consequently the dispersion flows up in the riser zone and down-flow occurs in the down-comer. Airlift fermenters are highly energy-efficient. They are often used in large-scale manufacture of biopharmaceutical proteins obtained from fragile animal cells. Heat and mass transfer capabilities of airlift reactors are at least as good as those of other systems. Airlift reactors are more effective in suspending solids than are bubble column fermenters. All performance characteristics of airlift -fermenter are related ultimately to the gas injection rate and the resulting rate of liquid circulation (Bokelmann et al., 2025).

The rate of liquid circulation increases with the square root of the height of the airlift device. Because the liquid circulation is driven by the gas hold-up difference between the riser and the down-comer. Circulation is enhanced if there is little or no gas in the down-comer. All the gas in the down-comer comes from being entrained in with the liquid as it flows into the down-comer from the riser near the top of the reactor (Lee et al., 2014; Pino et al., 2018).

Rectangular airlift bioreactors have demonstrated better mixing and mass transfer capabilities compared to their cylindrical counterparts. This improvement is largely attributed to the influence of geometric design and operating conditions on the fluid flow and mass transfer behaviour. Research has shown that rectangular airlift loop reactors provide enhanced gas holdup and higher mass transfer coefficients than cylindrical loop reactors (Drandev et al., 2016). In fact, the average volumetric mass transfer coefficient (k_a) in rectangular designs was reported to be around 40% higher. Preliminary experiments also confirmed that the gas holdup and mass transfer efficiency in rectangular airlift reactors outperform those in circular designs, aligning well with previously published findings. Building on these advantages, a new rectangular dynamic membrane airlift bioreactor (RDMAB) was developed by Ganlu Li et al., 2022. Schematic diagrams of the RDMAB and a conventional cylindrical airlift bioreactor are presented in Figure 3.

Figure 3. (a) Schematic diagram of the rectangular dynamic membrane airlift bioreactor, (b) the dynamic membrane, (c) the rectangular cover, and (d) the conventional cylinder airlift bioreactor. (1: Bioreactor tank; 2: draft tube; 3: steam inlet or cooling water outlet; 4: sampling outlet; 5: air inlet; 6: continuous fermentation inlet; 7: continuous fermentation outlet; 8: thermometer, pH meter, and dissolved oxygen meter (DO) in downcomer; 9: condensate water outlet or cooling water inlet; 10: dynamic membrane blade; 11: inoculation inlet; 12: tail gas outlet; 13: feeding inlet, and 14: DO meter in riser)

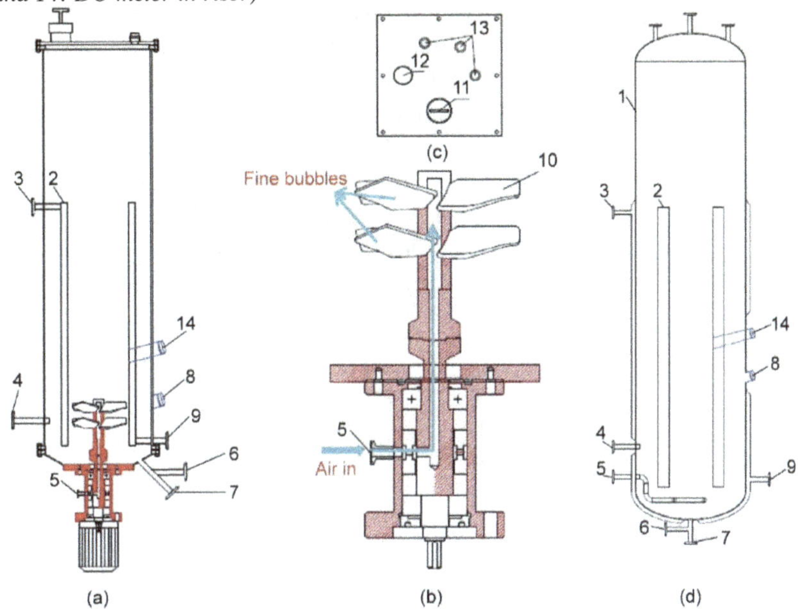

(Reprinted from Li et al., 2022)

Packed Bed and Fixed Bed Bioreactors

Packed bed bioreactors (PBRs), also known as fixed bed bioreactors, are specialized systems designed primarily for the cultivation of immobilized cells or microorganisms. In these reactors, the cells are either physically entrapped or chemically bound to solid support materials such as glass beads, porous ceramics, polymer matrices, or sponge-like carriers, which are packed tightly into a column or cylindrical vessel (Warnock et al., 2005). The liquid nutrient medium is continuously or intermittently passed through this packed bed, allowing substrates to diffuse into the immobilized cells while metabolic products are carried away. These systems are particularly suited for processes requiring long-term, stable operation and are widely used in applications such as enzyme production, wastewater treatment, and the manufacturing of secondary metabolites (Mitchell et al., 2023). One of the main advantages of packed bed bioreactors is the high cell density that can be maintained, which often results in increased productivity and reduced reactor volume. Additionally, because the biomass remains immobilized, the reactor can operate continuously for extended periods without the need for cell separation. However, challenges such as mass transfer limitations, channelling (non-uniform flow through the bed), and clogging can arise, especially when the biomass grows excessively or forms aggregates. Despite these limitations, packed/fixed bed bioreactors offer a highly efficient and stable environment for specific bioprocesses where cell retention and long residence times are desirable, making them particularly valuable in both industrial and environmental biotechnology (Gomes et al., 2023).

A bed of solid particles, with biocatalysts on or within the matrix of solids, packed in a column constitutes a packed bed bioreactor. The solids used may be porous or non-porous gels, and they may be compressible or rigid in nature. A nutrient broth flows continuously over the immobilized biocatalyst. The products obtained in the packed bed bioreactor are released into the fluid and removed (Mitchell et al., 2023). While the flow of the fluid can be upward or downward, down flow under gravity is preferred. The concentration of the nutrients (and therefore the products formed) can be increased by increasing the flow rate of the nutrient broth. Because of poor mixing, it is rather difficult to control the pH of packed bed bioreactors by the addition of acid or alkali (Eibl et al., 2009; Gomes et al., 2023)). However, these bioreactors are preferred for bioprocessing technology involving product-inhibited reactions. The packed bed bioreactors do not allow accumulation of the products to any significant extent. Figure 4 shows diagram of a typical laboratory based packed bed bioreactor.

Figure 4. Simplified diagram of a laboratory based packed bed bioreactor

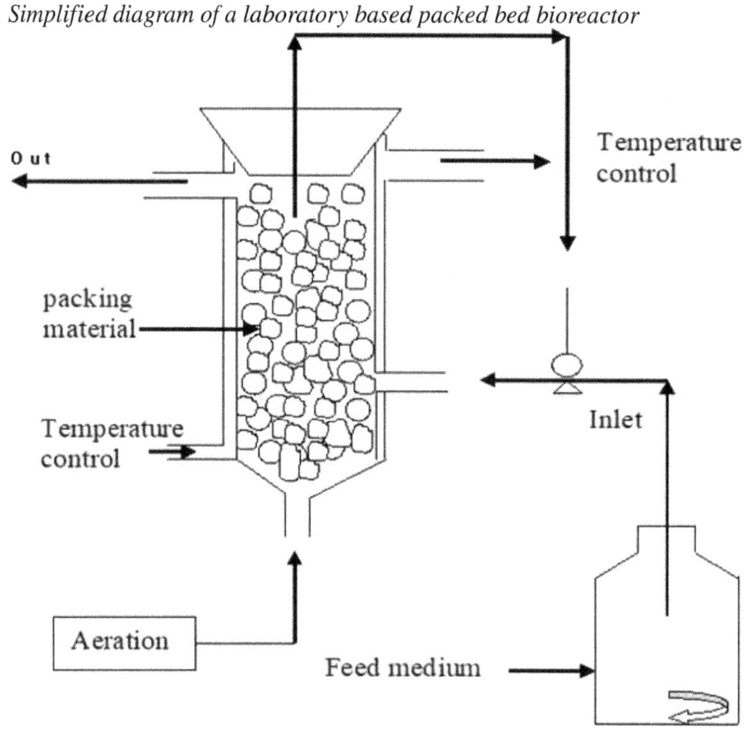

(Reprinted from Tekere, 2019)

Single-Use Bioreactors

Single-use bioreactors (SUBs) represent a transformative innovation in modern bioprocessing, offering flexibility, efficiency, and cost-effectiveness compared to traditional stainless-steel systems. These bioreactors are designed with disposable plastic bags or chambers typically made from multilayer polymer films that replace the need for cleaning and sterilization between production runs (Jossen et al., 2019). SUBs have gained widespread acceptance, particularly in the biopharmaceutical industry, for processes involving cell culture, vaccine production, monoclonal antibody synthesis, and personalized therapies. Their popularity has grown significantly due to the increasing demand for agile manufacturing systems that can quickly adapt to new products, scale-out strategies, and rapid development timelines (Junne and Neubauer, 2018).

The main advantage of single-use bioreactors lies in their operational simplicity. By eliminating the need for cleaning, sterilization, and validation associated with reusable systems, SUBs significantly reduce turnaround time between batches. This feature not only improves production efficiency but also minimizes the risk of cross-contamination, a critical concern in the manufacture of biologics. In addition, the lower capital investment and smaller facility footprint make SUBs an attractive option for small and medium-sized enterprises as well as large-scale biomanufacturing facilities adopting multi-product lines (Löffelholz et al., 2013). Technologically, SUBs come in various designs including wave-mixed, stirred tank, rocking motion, and pneumatic mixing systems. These designs are engineered to provide adequate mixing, gas transfer, and temperature control, often incorporating disposable sensors for pH, dissolved oxygen, and temperature monitoring. Modern SUBs also support a wide range of working volumes from a few milliliters in development stages to over 2,000 liters in commercial production allowing seamless scalability. However, challenges such as limited mechanical strength, lower oxygen transfer rates compared to stainless steel systems, and material compatibility issues with certain cell lines or products do exist (Oosterhuis and Junne, 2016). Environmental concerns related to plastic waste have also prompted discussions on sustainable disposal and recycling methods for single-use components.

Despite these limitations, the flexibility and performance of single-use bioreactors have made them a key enabler of innovations in cell and gene therapy, personalized medicine, and modular biomanufacturing. They are especially beneficial in clinical development and multi-product manufacturing settings, where speed and adaptability are crucial. As automation, sensor technology, and material science continue to evolve, the next generation of SUBs is expected to overcome current limitations and further integrate into advanced biomanufacturing platforms (Junne and Neubauer, 2018). Overall, single-use bioreactors have revolutionized bioprocessing by simplifying operations, reducing costs, and enabling faster, more flexible production cycles in the rapidly growing biopharmaceutical sector.

DESIGN PRINCIPLES OF BIOREACTORS

The design and construction of a typical and successful bioreactor or fermenter consists of a closed container, large-scale industrial fermenters are almost always constructed of stainless steel. A fermenter is a large cylinder closed at the top and the bottom and various pipes and valves are fitted into it. Since most industrial fermentation process is aerobic, the construction of a typical aerobic fermenter is the following:

Fluid Dynamics and Mixing

The fermenter is fitted externally with a cooling jacket through which steam (for sterilization) or cooling water (for cooling) is run. Cooling jacket is necessary because sterilization of the nutrient medium and removal of the heat generated are obligatory for successful completion of the fermentation in the fermenter (Nadal-Rey et al., 2021).

A typical biofermentor, even in its basic form, except in special cases, is equipped with a set of baffles and an agitation system. Agitation refers to the proper mixing of the liquid contents, including nutrients, within the fermenter (Garcıa-Ochoa et al., 2000). It helps prevent the coagulation of the medium and ensures the uniform distribution of the input medium, the formed product, and waste materials, thereby facilitating maximum productivity. The motion generated by agitation, in combination with the baffles and the regulated inflow and outflow of contents, is studied under the principles of fluid dynamics. This fluid behaviour is influenced by the type of microorganism used and must be compatible with the selected microbe, culture medium, and the desired product (Nadal-Rey et al., 2022).

Oxygen Transfer and Aeration

Oxygen transfer and aeration are critical parameters in aerobic fermentation and bioprocessing, directly influencing cell growth, metabolism, and product formation. In bioreactors, especially those cultivating aerobic microorganisms or mammalian cells, oxygen must be supplied efficiently to meet the biological demand of the cells (Kirk and Szita, 2013). However, oxygen has low solubility in aqueous solutions, which makes its effective delivery to the cells a complex challenge that requires careful engineering. Aeration refers to the process of introducing air or pure oxygen into the liquid culture medium within a bioreactor. This is typically achieved through spargers, devices that disperse air as fine bubbles at the bottom of the reactor. These bubbles rise through the liquid and provide a large surface area for gas exchange, allowing oxygen to dissolve into the medium while carbon dioxide is simultaneously removed. The efficiency of aeration depends on the size and distribution of bubbles, the gas flow rate, and the total surface area for mass transfer (Germain and Stephenson, 2005).

Oxygen transfer is quantitatively described by the oxygen transfer rate (OTR) and the volumetric mass transfer coefficient, which together determine how quickly oxygen can move from the gas phase into the liquid and become available for cellular uptake. The rate of oxygen transfer must match or exceed the oxygen uptake rate (OUR) of the growing cells; otherwise, oxygen limitation may occur, leading to reduced growth, altered metabolism, and lower yields (Garcia-Ochoa and Gomez, 2009). The value depends on several factors including agitation speed, type of impeller, aeration rate, temperature, viscosity of the medium, and the reactor design itself.

Agitation plays a vital role in enhancing oxygen transfer by breaking up large bubbles into smaller ones, maintaining uniform mixing, and reducing the boundary layer around gas bubbles, which promotes faster diffusion. In stirred-tank bioreactors, the combination of spargers and mechanical agitation is commonly used to optimize oxygen availability. In systems with shear-sensitive cells, such as mammalian or insect cells, low-shear mixing strategies and oxygen-enriched air are used to maintain adequate oxygen levels without damaging the cells (Kirk and Szita, 2013).

In large-scale bioreactors, maintaining efficient oxygen transfer becomes more challenging due to increased culture volume and reduced surface area-to-volume ratios. Strategies to overcome these limitations include using pure oxygen instead of air, employing multiple spargers, optimizing impeller configurations, and implementing dynamic control of gas flow rates based on real-time dissolved oxygen monitoring. Ultimately, oxygen transfer and aeration are essential to sustaining optimal cell physiology and productivity in aerobic bioprocesses (Ma et al., 2005; Löffelholz et al., 2014). A well-designed oxygenation system not only ensures adequate cell respiration but also supports the overall stability and scalability of the bioreactor operation.

Shear Stress and Cell Viability

Shear stress is a mechanical force generated by fluid movement within bioreactors, primarily due to agitation and aeration, and it plays a crucial role in influencing cell viability and productivity. While efficient mixing and oxygen transfer are essential for maintaining a homogeneous environment and supporting cell metabolism, excessive shear forces can be detrimental particularly to shear-sensitive cells such as mammalian, insect, or hybridoma cells (Fadlallah et al., 2016; Chabanon et al., 2019). These cells typically lack a rigid cell wall and are therefore more susceptible to mechanical damage caused by high-speed impellers, turbulent flow, or bursting gas bubbles. Shear stress can lead to membrane disruption, cell lysis, reduced viability, and altered metabolic behavior, ultimately impacting the yield and quality of the desired bioproducts. To mitigate these effects, bioreactor designs and operating parameters are carefully optimized. Strategies include the use of low-shear impellers (e.g., marine or pitched-blade impellers), lower agitation speeds, bubble-free aeration systems, and protective agents such as Pluronic F-68 that enhance cell membrane stability (Jung et al., 2011; Wyma et al., 2018). Additionally, single-use bioreactors and wave-mixed systems are often preferred for culturing shear-sensitive cells due to their gentler mixing profiles. Balancing adequate mixing and oxygen transfer with minimal shear damage is essential for maintaining high cell viability, especially in large-scale bioprocesses where the mechanical forces are significantly amplified. Hence, understanding and controlling shear stress is fundamental to the successful cultivation of fragile cell lines and the consistent production of high-quality biologics.

Nutrient and Waste Management in Bioreactors

Effective nutrient and waste management is essential for maintaining optimal growth conditions and ensuring high productivity in bioreactor-based bioprocesses. Microorganisms and cultured cells require a continuous and balanced supply of nutrients such as carbon sources, nitrogen, vitamins, minerals, and growth factors to sustain metabolism, proliferation, and product formation (Bajić et al., 2022). In parallel, metabolic activities generate various byproducts, including organic acids, ammonia, carbon dioxide, and other inhibitory compounds that can accumulate over time and negatively affect cell viability and process efficiency. If not properly managed, nutrient depletion or waste accumulation can lead to reduced growth rates, stress responses, altered metabolic pathways, and a decline in product yield and quality (Sablayrolles and Mouret, 2022).

To address these challenges, different feeding strategies and process modes are employed, including batch, fed-batch, and continuous culture systems. In fed-batch systems, nutrients are added in a controlled manner during cultivation to avoid both depletion and excess, which helps maintain cells in their exponential growth phase for a longer duration (Warnock et al., 2005). In continuous cultures, fresh medium is continuously supplied while spent medium containing waste products is simultaneously removed, maintaining a steady-state environment. Additionally, real-time monitoring of nutrient concentrations and metabolic byproducts using biosensors and control systems allows for precise adjustment of feeding and aeration strategies (Chandrashekhar and Rao, 2010).

Advanced bioreactors also integrate feedback-controlled perfusion systems, especially in mammalian cell cultures, which allow continuous removal of waste products and replenishment of essential nutrients without disturbing the cells. This enhances cell density, viability, and productivity over extended periods (Schirmer et al., 2021). Moreover, the use of high-efficiency filtration systems and membrane bioreactors further aids in selective removal of toxic metabolites while retaining valuable cells or proteins (Sahu and Panda, 2018). Overall, proper nutrient supply and effective waste removal are fundamental to achieving consistent bioprocess performance and high-quality bioproducts, making nutrient and waste management a critical component of modern bioreactor operation.

SCALE-UP STRATEGIES AND CHALLENGES

Achieving good volumetric productivity in a batch system depends on the amount of product produced per unit volume of production bioprocessor per unit time (or, in crude terms "how fast does the process go"). High Volumetric Productivity minimises the contribution of fixed costs to the cost of the product. Fixed costs are business expenses that are not dependent on the level of product produced. They tend to be time-related, such as salaries plant, power, etc (Garcia-Ochoa et al., 2010). Maximising the proportion of time spent at the fastest production rate. Minimising the lag before maximum production starts by practices like inoculum development and avoiding subsequent phases of slower/zero production. Extending the length of time spent in active production which in turn can be achieved by fed batch (Junker, 2004; Xie, 2022). Finally the things which ensure that the production is rapid are choice of medium and organism, high concentration of active organisms and most importantly the type of fermentation bioreactor used accordingly (Figure 5).

Figure 5. Graphical representation of the fermentation process, product vs time with factors involved to enhance the production inside the bioreactor: (A) fastest production ideal graph; (B) Lag phase; (C) stationary or concentration phase; (D) exponential phase achieved again by process advancements; (E) process advancement achieved by fermenter type selection for optimum production

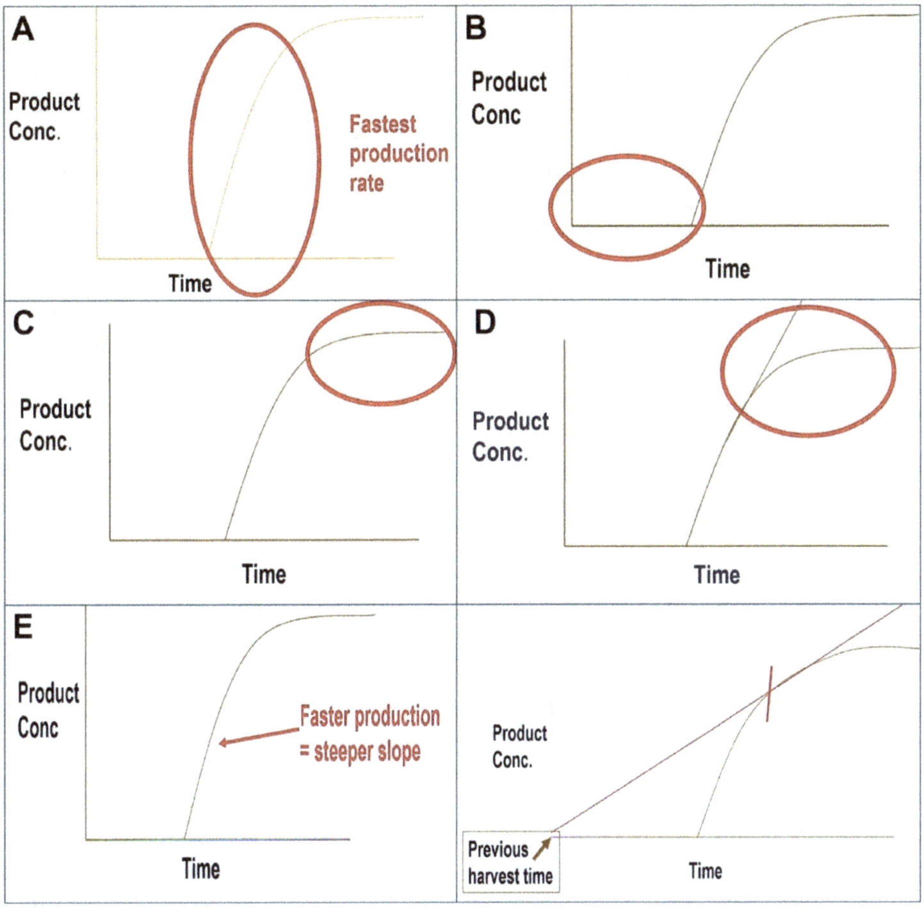

EMERGING TRENDS IN BIOREACTOR TECHNOLOGY

As biomanufacturing becomes more complex with the production of cell and gene therapies, personalized medicine, and synthetic biology products, bioreactor technology continues to evolve. The convergence of engineering, biology, and data science is expected to revolutionize bioreactor design and operation, making them more adaptive, efficient, and intelligent (Estevez and Navarro, 2017; Abdallah and Estévez, 2023).

Future trends include:

a. 3D-printed and customizable bioreactor components.
b. Microbioreactors for rapid process development and high-throughput screening.
c. Perfusion and continuous bioreactors for higher productivity and lower footprint.
d. Integration of omics data (genomics, proteomics, and metabolomics) into bioreactor control systems.

Modern bioreactors incorporate sophisticated features to enhance performance and scalability. The following are some of the most prominent types of advanced bioreactor systems: Single-use bioreactors are pre-sterilized, disposable systems that eliminate the need for cleaning and sterilization between batches. They are typically made from polymer films and are widely used in the production of monoclonal antibodies and vaccines. Their advantages include reduced cross-contamination risk, faster turnaround time, and lower capital costs. SUBs are scalable from millilitre to several thousand litres. Perfusion systems continuously remove waste and replenish nutrients while retaining cells within the reactor (Mitra and Murthy, 2022). This enables prolonged cell culture and higher product yields. These systems are particularly useful for producing labile or toxic products and are used extensively in stem cell and cell therapy manufacturing.

Continuous bioreactors maintain cells in a steady-state condition, offering enhanced productivity and consistent product quality. Advances in control strategies and online monitoring have made continuous processing more viable for industrial-scale applications (Chaachouay and Zidane, 2024). These miniaturized systems are designed for high-throughput screening and process development. They allow simultaneous testing of multiple conditions at a small scale, accelerating process optimization before scaling up. Modular bioreactors allow for flexible and scalable production setups. Automation facilitates real-time monitoring, reduces human error, and supports GMP (Good Manufacturing Practice) compliance. Integration with PAT (Process Analytical Technology) ensures tight control over critical process parameters (Xie, 2022).

Scalability is a fundamental requirement for translating laboratory-scale processes to industrial production. The following principles guide the design of bioreactors suitable for scalable biomanufacturing: Scaling up a bioreactor must preserve key physical parameters such as mixing time, shear stress, oxygen transfer rate, and power input per volume (Connelly et al., 2017; Junne and Neubauer, 2018). Geometric similarity ensures that the shape and proportion of the reactor are consistent across scales, while hydrodynamic similarity maintains the fluid dynamics critical to cell viability and productivity. Adequate oxygen and nutrient supply is essential for high-density cultures. Design elements such as sparger types, impeller configuration, and agitation speed must be optimized to maximize oxygen transfer rate and volumetric mass transfer coefficient (kLa) without damaging cells (Achar et al., 2025).

Advanced sensors and control systems are integrated into bioreactor designs to monitor parameters like pH, dissolved oxygen, temperature, and metabolite concentrations. The application of feedback and feedforward control algorithms enables dynamic adjustments to maintain optimal conditions. Designs must comply with aseptic operation requirements, including the use of clean-in-place and sterilize-in-place systems for reusable bioreactors (O'Mara et al., 2018). For single-use systems, sterile connectors and filters are employed to maintain sterility. Bioreactor materials must be biocompatible, non-toxic, and resistant to degradation under operating conditions. Stainless steel is commonly used in traditional systems, while high-grade polymers are employed in disposable bioreactors (Busse et al., 2017).

Scalable designs must accommodate changes in production volume with minimal alterations to the process. Modular systems and platform technologies offer the flexibility needed to adjust scale while maintaining consistent product quality. Despite significant progress, challenges remain in scaling up bioprocesses, especially for complex biologics like cell and gene therapies. Some of the key issues include: Maintaining cell viability and productivity during scale-up; Ensuring uniform mixing and nutrient distribution in large volumes; Adapting to the diverse requirements of different cell types and products; Addressing regulatory concerns regarding new materials and automation systems.

Future trends in bioreactor development include the integration of artificial intelligence and machine learning for predictive process control, the use of 3D-printed components for customized designs, and the development of hybrid systems that combine the benefits of different bioreactor types.

CONCLUSION

Advanced bioreactor systems and scalable design principles are crucial for the success of modern biomanufacturing. Innovations in reactor technology, process control, and automation have significantly enhanced the ability to produce high-quality biological products efficiently and reliably. As biotechnology continues to evolve, the role of sophisticated bioreactor systems will become even more pivotal in meeting the growing global demand for biopharmaceuticals and other biologics. The evolution of bioreactor technology reflects the progress of biotechnology as a whole, transitioning from basic fermentation vessels to highly specialized systems capable of producing life-saving therapeutics and sustainable bio-based products. Each phase of development has been shaped by the needs of science and industry, with continuous innovation ensuring that bioreactors remain at the heart of scalable and efficient biomanufacturing processes.

REFERENCES

Abdallah, Y. K., & Estévez, A. T. (2023). 3D-printed bioreceptive tiles of reaction–diffusion (Gierer–Meinhardt model) for multi-scale algal strains' passive immobilization. *Buildings (Basel, Switzerland), 13*(8), 1972. DOI: 10.3390/buildings13081972

Achar, S. S., Mohanty, S. K., Indu, B. K., Suhasa, G., & Shilpa, P. (2025). Bioreactors. In *In Vitro Production of Plant Secondary Metabolites: Theory and Practice* (pp. 205–226). Springer Nature Singapore.

Altman, A. (2003). From plant tissue culture to biotechnology: Scientific revolutions, abiotic stress tolerance, and forestry. *In Vitro Cellular & Developmental Biology. Plant, 39*, 75–84. DOI: 10.1079/IVP2002379

Ashok, A., Doriya, K., Rao, D. R. M., & Kumar, D. S. (2017). Design of solid state bioreactor for industrial applications: An overview to conventional bioreactors. *Biocatalysis and Agricultural Biotechnology, 9*, 11–18. DOI: 10.1016/j.bcab.2016.10.014

Averesch, N. J., Berliner, A. J., Nangle, S. N., Zezulka, S., Vengerova, G. L., Ho, D., & Arkin, A. P. (2023). Microbial biomanufacturing for space-exploration—What to take and when to make. *Nature Communications, 14*(1), 2311. DOI: 10.1038/s41467-023-37910-1 PMID: 37085475

Bajić, B., Vučurović, D., Vasić, Đ., Jevtić-Mučibabić, R., & Dodić, S. (2022). Biotechnological production of sustainable microbial proteins from agro-industrial residues and by-products. *Foods, 12*(1), 107. DOI: 10.3390/foods12010107 PMID: 36613323

Bokelmann, C., Bromley, J., & Takors, R. (2025). Pros and cons of airlift and bubble column bioreactors: How internals improve performance. *Biochemical Engineering Journal, 213*, 109539. DOI: 10.1016/j.bej.2024.109539

Brindhadevi, K., Shanmuganathan, R., Pugazhendhi, A., Gunasekar, P., & Manigandan, S. (2021). Biohydrogen production using horizontal and vertical continuous stirred tank reactor-a numerical optimization. *International Journal of Hydrogen Energy, 46*(20), 11305–11312. DOI: 10.1016/j.ijhydene.2020.06.155

Busse, C., Biechele, P., de Vries, I., Reardon, K. F., Solle, D., & Scheper, T. (2017). Sensors for disposable bioreactors. *Engineering in Life Sciences, 17*(8), 940–952. DOI: 10.1002/elsc.201700049 PMID: 32624843

Candia-Sanchez, L. F., Álvarez-Cervantes, J., Díaz, R., & Díaz-Godínez, G. (2017). Uso potencial de biorreactores para la producción de lacasas de hongos basidiomicetos. *Mexican Journal of Biotechnology, 2*(1), 15–36. DOI: 10.29267/mxjb.2017.2.1.15

Cerrone, F., & O'Connor, K. E. (2025). Cultivation of filamentous fungi in airlift bioreactors: Advantages and disadvantages. *Applied Microbiology and Biotechnology, 109*(1), 41. DOI: 10.1007/s00253-025-13422-4 PMID: 39928147

Chaachouay, N., & Zidane, L. (2024). Plant-derived natural products: A source for drug discovery and development. *Drugs and Drug Candidates, 3*(1), 184–207. DOI: 10.3390/ddc3010011

Chabanon, M., Duval, H., Grenier, J., Beauchesne, C., Goyeau, B., & David, B. (2019). Histological method to study the effect of shear stress on cell proliferation and tissue morphology in a bioreactor. *Tissue Engineering and Regenerative Medicine, 16*, 225–235. DOI: 10.1007/s13770-019-00181-3 PMID: 31205852

Chandrashekhar, H., & Rao, J. V. (2010). An overview of fermenter and the design considerations to enhance its productivity. *Pharmacologyonline, 1*, 261–301.

Chettri, D., Verma, A. K., Chirania, M., & Verma, A. K. (2024). Optimization Strategies for Enhanced Production of Microbial Products. In *Industrial Microbiology and Biotechnology: A New Horizon of the Microbial World* (pp. 465–487). Springer Nature Singapore., DOI: 10.1007/978-981-97-6270-5_15

Chisti, Y., & Moo-Young, M. (2006). Bioreactor design. *Basic biotechnology, 3*, 181-200. ISBN 978-0-521-54958-5

Connelly, S., Shin, S. G., Dillon, R. J., Ijaz, U. Z., Quince, C., Sloan, W. T., & Collins, G. (2017). Bioreactor scalability: Laboratory-scale bioreactor design influences performance, ecology, and community physiology in expanded granular sludge bed bioreactors. *Frontiers in Microbiology, 8*, 664. DOI: 10.3389/fmicb.2017.00664 PMID: 28507535

Drandev, S., Penev, K. I., & Karamanev, D. (2016). Study of the hydrodynamics and mass transfer in a rectangular air-lift bioreactor. *Chemical Engineering Science, 146*, 180–188. DOI: 10.1016/j.ces.2016.02.041

Eibl, R., Eibl, D., Pörtner, R., Catapano, G., Czermak, P., Catapano, G., & Pörtner, R. (2009). Bioreactor design and scale-up. *Cell and Tissue Reaction Engineering: With a Contribution by Martin Fussenegger and Wilfried Weber*, 173-259. https://doi.org/DOI: 10.1007/978-3-540-68182-3_5

Estevez, A. T., & Navarro, D. (2017). Biomanufacturing the future: Biodigital architecture & genetics. *Procedia Manufacturing, 12*, 7–16. DOI: 10.1016/j.promfg.2017.08.002

Ezemba, C., Ekwegbalu, E. A., & Ezemba, A. S. (2022). Fermentation, types of fermenters, design & uses of fermenters and optimization of the fermentation process. *Department of Microbiology, Chukwuemeka Odumegwu Ojukwu UniversityPress.* https://www.researchgate.net/publication/358265321_FERMENTATION_TYPES OF_FERMENTERS_DESIGN_USES_OF_FERMENTERS_AND_OPTIMZATI ON_OF_FERMENTATION_PROCESS. ISBN: 978-620-2-05649-6

Fadlallah, H., Jarrahi, M., Herbert, E., Ferrari, R., Mejean, A., & Peerhossaini, H. (2016). Effects of shear stress on the growth rate of micro-organisms in agitated reactors. In *Fluids Engineering Division Summer Meeting* (Vol. 50282, p. V01AT13A006). American Society of Mechanical Engineers. https://doi.org/DOI: 10.1115/FEDSM2016-7590

Garcia-Ochoa, F., & Gomez, E. (2009). Bioreactor scale-up and oxygen transfer rate in microbial processes: An overview. *Biotechnology Advances, 27*(2), 153–176. DOI: 10.1016/j.biotechadv.2008.10.006 PMID: 19041387

Garcia-Ochoa, F., Gomez, E., Santos, V. E., & Merchuk, J. C. (2010). Oxygen uptake rate in microbial processes: An overview. *Biochemical Engineering Journal, 49*(3), 289–307. DOI: 10.1016/j.bej.2010.01.011

Garcıa-Ochoa, F., Santos, V. E., Casas, J. A., & Gómez, E. (2000). Xanthan gum: Production, recovery, and properties. *Biotechnology Advances, 18*(7), 549–579. DOI: 10.1016/S0734-9750(00)00050-1 PMID: 14538095

Geada, P., Vicente, A. A., & Teixeira, J. A. (2024) Bioreactor: General Configuration, Classification, and Bioreactor Types. In *Bioreactor Technology in Food Processing* (pp. 36-58). CRC Press. https://doi.org/DOI: 10.1201/9780429424236

Germain, E., & Stephenson, T. (2005). Biomass characteristics, aeration and oxygen transfer in membrane bioreactors: Their interrelations explained by a review of aerobic biological processes. *Reviews in Environmental Science and Biotechnology, 4*, 223–233. DOI: 10.1007/s11157-005-2097-3

Gomes, D. G., Coelho, E., Silva, R., Domingues, L., & Teixeira, J. A. (2023). Bioreactors and engineering of filamentous fungi cultivation. In *Current developments in biotechnology and bioengineering* (pp. 219–250). Elsevier., DOI: 10.1016/B978-0-323-91872-5.00018-1

Hemmerich, J., Noack, S., Wiechert, W., & Oldiges, M. (2018). Microbioreactor systems for accelerated bioprocess development. *Biotechnology Journal, 13*(4), 1700141. DOI: 10.1002/biot.201700141 PMID: 29283217

Jossen, V., Eibl, R., & Eibl, D. (2019). Single-use bioreactors–an overview. *Single-use technology in biopharmaceutical manufacture*, 37-52. https://doi.org/DOI: 10.1002/9781119477891.ch4

Jossen, V., Eibl, R., & Eibl, D. (2019). Single-use bioreactors–an overview. *Single-use technology in biopharmaceutical manufacture*, 37-52. https://doi.org/DOI: 10.1002/9781119477891.ch4

Julien, C., & Whitford, W. (2007). Bioreactor monitoring, modeling, and simulation. *BioProcess International, 5*(01), S10–S17.

Jung, I. S., Oh, M. K., Cho, Y. C., & Kong, I. S. (2011). The viability to a wall shear stress and propagation of Bifidobacterium longum in the intensive membrane bioreactor. *Applied Microbiology and Biotechnology, 92*, 939–949. DOI: 10.1007/s00253-011-3387-z PMID: 21681403

Junker, B. H. (2004). Scale-up methodologies for Escherichia coli and yeast fermentation processes. *Journal of Bioscience and Bioengineering, 97*(6), 347–364. DOI: 10.1016/S1389-1723(04)70218-2 PMID: 16233642

Junne, S., & Neubauer, P. (2018). How scalable and suitable are single-use bioreactors? *Current Opinion in Biotechnology, 53*, 240–247. DOI: 10.1016/j.copbio.2018.04.003 PMID: 29753977

Kendall, E. C. (2022). *Bioreactors: Design, background, and applications* (No. LA-UR-22-29370). Los Alamos National Laboratory (LANL), Los Alamos, NM (United States). https://doi.org/DOI: 10.2172/1887112

Kirk, T. V., & Szita, N. (2013). Oxygen transfer characteristics of miniaturized bioreactor systems. *Biotechnology and Bioengineering*, *110*(4), 1005–1019. DOI: 10.1002/bit.24824 PMID: 23280578

Lazim, N. A. M., & Nazir, N. M. (2025). Biotechnology and Genetic Engineering: Unlocking New Possibilities. In *Evolving Landscapes of Research and Development: Trends, Challenges, and Opportunities* (pp. 109-122). IGI Global Scientific Publishing. https://doi.org/DOI: 10.4018/979-8-3693-7101-5.ch005

Lee, J., Kim, H., Lim, H. R., Kim, Y. S., Hoang, T. T. T., Choi, J., & Yeo, W. H. (2024). Large-scale smart bioreactor with fully integrated wireless multivariate sensors and electronics for long-term in situ monitoring of stem cell culture. *Science Advances*, *10*(7), eadk6714. Advance online publication. DOI: 10.1126/sciadv.adk6714 PMID: 38354246

Lee, K. Y., Buldum, G., Mantalaris, A., & Bismarck, A. (2014). More than meets the eye in bacterial cellulose: Biosynthesis, bioprocessing, and applications in advanced fiber composites. *Macromolecular Bioscience*, *14*(1), 10–32. DOI: 10.1002/mabi.201300298 PMID: 23897676

Li, G., Chen, K., Wei, Y., Zeng, J., Yang, Y., He, F., & Ouyang, P. (2022). Mass transfer, gas holdup, and kinetic models of batch and continuous fermentation in a novel rectangular dynamic membrane airlift bioreactor. *Engineering*, *13*, 153–163. DOI: 10.1016/j.eng.2021.07.025

Lidén, G. (2002). Understanding the bioreactor. *Bioprocess and Biosystems Engineering*, *24*, 273–279. DOI: 10.1007/s004490100263

Lin, Y. H., & Gu, Y. J. (2021). Biodegradation kinetic studies of phenol and P-cresol in a batch and continuous stirred-tank bioreactor with Pseudomonas putida ATCC 17484 cells. *Processes (Basel, Switzerland)*, *9*(1), 133. DOI: 10.3390/pr9010133

Löffelholz, C., Husemann, U., Greller, G., Meusel, W., Kauling, J., Ay, P., & Eibl, D. (2013). Bioengineering parameters for single-use bioreactors: Overview and evaluation of suitable methods. *Chemieingenieurtechnik (Weinheim)*, *85*(1-2), 40–56. DOI: 10.1002/cite.201200125

Löffelholz, C., Kaiser, S. C., Kraume, M., Eibl, R., & Eibl, D. (2014). Dynamic single-use bioreactors used in modern liter-and m 3-scale biotechnological processes: engineering characteristics and scaling up. *Disposable bioreactors II*, 1-44. https://doi.org/DOI: 10.1007/10_2013_187

Ma, N., Mollet, M., & Chalmers, J. J. (2005). Aeration, mixing and hydrodynamics in bioreactors. In *Cell culture technology for pharmaceutical and cell-based therapies* (pp. 243–266). CRC Press., DOI: 10.1201/9780849351068

Mitchell, D. A., Ruiz, H. A., & Krieger, N. (2023). A critical evaluation of recent studies on packed-bed bioreactors for solid-state fermentation. *Processes (Basel, Switzerland)*, *11*(3), 872. DOI: 10.3390/pr11030872

Mitra, S., & Murthy, G. S. (2022). Bioreactor control systems in the biopharmaceutical industry: A critical perspective. *Systems Microbiology and Biomanufacturing*, , 1–22. DOI: 10.1007/s43393-021-00048-6 PMID: 38624976

Nadal-Rey, G., McClure, D. D., Kavanagh, J. M., Cassells, B., Cornelissen, S., Fletcher, D. F., & Gernaey, K. V. (2022). Computational fluid dynamics modelling of hydrodynamics, mixing and oxygen transfer in industrial bioreactors with Newtonian broths. *Biochemical Engineering Journal, 177,* 108265. DOI: 10.1016/j.bej.2021.108265

Nadal-Rey, G., McClure, D. D., Kavanagh, J. M., Cornelissen, S., Fletcher, D. F., & Gernaey, K. V. (2021). Understanding gradients in industrial bioreactors. *Biotechnology Advances, 46,* 107660. DOI: 10.1016/j.biotechadv.2020.107660 PMID: 33221379

Nguyen, N. T., Vo, T. S., Tran-Nguyen, P. L., Nguyen, M. N., Pham, V. H., Matsuhashi, R., & Vo, T. T. B. C. (2024). A comprehensive review of aeration and wastewater treatment. *Aquaculture (Amsterdam, Netherlands), 741113.* Advance online publication. DOI: 10.1016/j.aquaculture.2024.741113

Nienow, A. W. (2014). Stirring and stirred-tank reactors. *Chemieingenieurtechnik (Weinheim), 86*(12), 2063–2074. DOI: 10.1002/cite.201400087

O'Mara, P., Farrell, A., Bones, J., & Twomey, K. (2018). Staying alive! Sensors used for monitoring cell health in bioreactors. *Talanta, 176*, 130–139. DOI: 10.1007/978-981-97-8808-8_16 PMID: 28917732

Oosterhuis, N. M., & Junne, S. (2016). Design, Applications, and Development of Single-Use Bioreactors. *Bioreactors: Design, Operation and Novel Applications*, 261-294. https://doi.org/ DOI: 10.1002/9783527683369.ch9

Oosterhuis, N. M., & Junne, S. (2016). Design, Applications, and Development of Single-Use Bioreactors. *Bioreactors: Design, Operation and Novel Applications*, 261-294. https://doi.org/ DOI: 10.1002/9783527683369.ch9

Palladino, F., Marcelino, P. R. F., Schlogl, A. E., José, Á. H. M., Rodrigues, R. D. C. L. B., Fabrino, D. L., & Rosa, C. A. (2024). Bioreactors: Applications and Innovations for a sustainable and healthy future-a critical review. *Applied Sciences (Basel, Switzerland), 14*(20), 9346. DOI: 10.3390/app14209346

Pino, M. S., Rodríguez-Jasso, R. M., Michelin, M., Flores-Gallegos, A. C., Morales-Rodriguez, R., Teixeira, J. A., & Ruiz, H. A. (2018). Bioreactor design for enzymatic hydrolysis of biomass under the biorefinery concept. *Chemical Engineering Journal, 347*, 119–136. DOI: 10.1016/j.cej.2018.04.057

Pörtner, R., Nagel-Heyer, S., Goepfert, C., Adamietz, P., & Meenen, N. M. (2005). Bioreactor design for tissue engineering. *Journal of Bioscience and Bioengineering, 100*(3), 235–245. DOI: 10.1263/jbb.100.235 PMID: 16243271

Raj, A. E., & Karanth, N. G. (2005). 03 Fermentation Technology and Bioreactor Design. In *Food Biotechnology* (pp. 60–113). CRC Press.

Ross, R. P., Morgan, S., & Hill, C. (2002). Preservation and fermentation: Past, present and future. *International Journal of Food Microbiology, 79*(1-2), 3–16. DOI: 10.1016/S0168-1605(02)00174-5 PMID: 12382680

Sablayrolles, J. M., & Mouret, J. R. (2022). Nitrogen management during fermentation. In *White Wine Technology* (pp. 143–154). Academic Press., DOI: 10.1016/B978-0-12-823497-6.00027-2

Sahu, L., & Panda, S. K. (2018). Innovative technologies and implications in fermented food and beverage industries: an overview. *Innovations in technologies for fermented food and beverage industries*, 1-23. https://doi.org/DOI: 10.1007/978-3-319-74820-7_1

Schirmer, C., Maschke, R. W., Pörtner, R., & Eibl, D. (2021). An overview of drive systems and sealing types in stirred bioreactors used in biotechnological processes. *Applied Microbiology and Biotechnology, 105*, 2225–2242. DOI: 10.1007/s00253-021-11180-7 PMID: 33649923
Schirmer, C., Maschke, R. W., Pörtner, R., & Eibl, D. (2021). An overview of drive systems and sealing types in stirred bioreactors used in biotechnological processes. *Applied Microbiology and Biotechnology, 105*, 2225–2242. DOI: 10.1007/s00253-021-11180-7 PMID: 33649923
Sevda, S., & Kumar, S. (2024). Introduction of bioreactor. In *Bioreactor design concepts for viral vaccine production* (pp. 1–34). Academic Press., DOI: 10.1016/B978-0-443-15378-5.00001-2

Sheikh, H., Anand, G. G., & Shivanna, G. B. (2024). Fermentation: A Potential Strategy for Microbial Metabolite Production. https://doi.org/DOI: 10.5772/intechopen.114814

Tekere, M. (2019). Microbial bioremediation and different bioreactors designs applied. In *Biotechnology and bioengineering*. IntechOpen., DOI: 10.5772/intechopen.83661

Thon, J. N., Dykstra, B. J., & Beaulieu, L. M. (2017). Platelet bioreactor: Accelerated evolution of design and manufacture. *Platelets, 28*(5), 472–477. DOI: 10.1080/09537104.2016.1265922 PMID: 28112988

Wang, B., Wang, Z., Chen, T., & Zhao, X. (2020). Development of novel bioreactor control systems based on smart sensors and actuators. *Frontiers in Bioengineering and Biotechnology, 8*, 7. DOI: 10.3389/fbioe.2020.00007 PMID: 32117906

Wang, G., Xie, L., Huang, Z., & Xie, J. (2024). Recent advances in polysaccharide biomodification by microbial fermentation: Production, properties, bioactivities, and mechanisms. *Critical Reviews in Food Science and Nutrition, 64*(33), 12999–13023. DOI: 10.1080/10408398.2023.2259461 PMID: 37740706

Warnock, J. N., Bratch, K., & Al-Rubeai, M. (2005). Packed bed bioreactors. In *Bioreactors for Tissue Engineering: Principles, Design and Operation* (pp. 87–113). Springer Netherlands., DOI: 10.1007/1-4020-3741-4

Wyma, A., Martin-Alarcon, L., Walsh, T., Schmidt, T. A., Gates, I. D., & Kallos, M. S. (2018). Non-Newtonian rheology in suspension cell cultures significantly impacts bioreactor shear stress quantification. *Biotechnology and Bioengineering, 115*(8), 2101–2113. DOI: 10.1002/bit.26723 PMID: 29704461

Xie, D. (2022). Continuous biomanufacturing with microbes—Upstream progresses and challenges. *Current Opinion in Biotechnology, 78*, 102793. DOI: 10.1016/j.copbio.2022.102793 PMID: 36088736

Zhang, Y. H. P., Sun, J., & Ma, Y. (2017). Biomanufacturing: History and perspective. *Journal of Industrial Microbiology & Biotechnology*, *44*(4-5), 773–784. DOI: 10.1007/s10295-016-1863-2 PMID: 27837351

Chapter 5
Advances in Bioprocess Monitoring and Control Systems

Rahul Kumar
https://orcid.org/0009-0000-1323-2220
Graphic Era University, India

Sourav Chattaraj
Siksha 'O' Anusandhan, India

Gökhan Boyno
University of Van Yuzuncu Yil, Turkey

Wiem Alloun
University Mentouri Constantine, Algeria

Snežana Andjelković
https://orcid.org/0000-0003-0436-3530
Institute for Forage Crops, Kruševac, Serbia

Sanja Živković
University of Niš, Serbia

Guerra Sierra B. E.
Facultad de Ciencias, Universidad de Santander, Colombia

Debasis Mitra
https://orcid.org/0000-0003-0525-8812
Graphic Era University, India

ABSTRACT

The bioprocess monitoring market, valued at $12.3 billion in 2023, is expected to grow at a CAGR of 9.1% to reach $20.5 billion by 2030. This growth is driven by biosensors, machine learning, and Industry 4.0. Innovations like Raman spectroscopy and NMR have improved metabolite profiling accuracy, leading to enhanced process control. Artificial intelligence-driven models have reduced batch variability by 20%, while digital twin technologies have reduced process development time by 25%. Automated fed-batch strategies have increased recombinant protein yields by 15-25%, while microfluidic bioreactors enable high-throughput screening with a 5-fold reduction in reagent costs. Soft-sensor technologies have adjusted metabolic flux projections by 35%, reducing process variation. IoT-enabled bioprocessing has reduced manual interventions by 40%, improving operational effectiveness.

DOI: 10.4018/979-8-3373-2873-7.ch005

INTRODUCTION

The complexity of biomanufacturing activities the demand for biopharmaceuticals and the development of Industry 4.0 expertise has all influenced to meaningful enhancements in bioprocess monitoring and management systems (Pandey et al., 2024). With a cumulative annual growth rate (CAGR) of 8.3%, the global market for bioprocess technology will reach USD 37.3 billion by 2030 (Issaoui et al., 2022). This is driven by the emergence of cell and gene therapy, biosimilars, biologics, and individualized or personalized medicine, all of which require precision at a high level in real time, with the sort of reliability associated with well-crafted control schemes. As over 70% of biopharmaceutical companies currently employ at least one process analytical technology (PAT) device in their manufacturing process, the adoption of high-tech monitoring systems has gained momentum because of PAT implementation (Rantanen and Khinast, 2015). Real-time bioprocess understanding has been significantly enhanced by the development of compact, non-invasive sensors, including optical sensors for pH and DO, Raman and near-infrared spectroscopy for measuring metabolites, and dielectric spectroscopy for cell viability (Reyes et al., 2022). To control the nonlinear and multivariate nature of modern bioprocesses, sophisticated control techniques, such as model predictive control (MPC), fuzzy logic, neural networks, and reinforcement learning algorithms, have been integrated into bioprocess control. Group of data from compound production sites improved process visualization and isolated method monitoring have all been supported by a grouping of cloud computing and Internet of Things (IoT) technology (Kumar et al., 2023). Digital twins in bioprocessing have developed in nearly 20% cost reserves in manufacturing and a 25–40% reduction in development time (Chen et al., 2020). Industry tendencies point toward a robust direction for more participated, automated, and smart bioprocess operations, even though challenges in the implementation of keen adaptive bioprocess control organisms (Rathore et al., 2021). To close the gap between laboratory-scale development and industrial-scale application academic institutions, biotechnology startups, and major pharmaceutical partnerships are working together to build next-generation bioprocessing proposals.

BIOPROCESS MONITORING AND CONTROL

In advanced biotechnology and biomanufacturing the control and supervising of bioprocesses are searching for ensuring the efficacy, security, and quality of products taken from biological sources. In these activities live cells or their components are employed to manufacture imports such as food additives, pharmaceuticals, vaccines, enzymes, and biofuels (Goshtasbi et al., 2023). They are involved and sensitive to numerous equipped and environmental parameters such as cell density, temperature, pH, dissolved oxygen (DO), disturbance speed, and nutrient composition. Good monitoring and control approaches are required to maintain optimal situation throughout life (Frangopol and Liu, 2019). Traditionally, offline sampling and laboratory tests have been used in bioprocess observing which often result in stays and raised chances of contamination. However, the alteration towards in-line and real-time monitoring notably improves the product consistency and manage productivity (Bowler et al., 2020). To enable real-time decision-making and greater control over vital process parameters and quality characteristics advanced sensors and analytical equipment such as optical sensors for DO and pH dielectric spectroscopy for cell viability, and spectroscopic methods such as near-infrared (NIR) and Raman spectroscopy enable continuous and non-invasive data acquisition (Rösner et al., 2022). Through the integration of advanced monitoring technology, regulatory authorities, such as the U.S. FDA, have driven Process Analytical Technology (PAT) strategies, enhanced process reliability, and reduced the need for end-product testing (Känsäkoski et al., 2006). Modern control methods, such as model predictive control (MPC), fuzzy logic, and machine learning, allow for dynamic and adaptive responses to changes in processes, raising yields, and reducing variability, although standard proportional-integral-derivative (PID) controllers remain the tools of choice for simple regulation (Tang and Ahmad, 2024). With Internet-of-things (IoT) connectivity, cloud-based software, and digital twins facilitating deep monitoring and optimization, digital bioprocessing has completely transformed the landscape (Isoko et al., 2024).

IMPORTANCE IN BIOTECHNOLOGY, PHARMACEUTICALS, AND INDUSTRIAL APPLICATIONS

In most industries, including biotechnology, pharmaceuticals, and industrial use, the control and monitoring of bioprocesses is very important (Rathore et al., 2021). In biotechnology, precise control over variables, such as temperature, pH, and dissolved oxygen, is critical for optimal microbial growth and metabolite production (Kumar et al., 2024). Rigorous control in the pharmaceutical industry ensures product safety, quality, and compliance with regulations (Wang et al., 2023). Deviations from critical process parameters can lead to noncompliance, product loss, or batch failure. Strong control systems in industrial biotechnology support resource optimization, process scaling, and environmental sustainability (Straathof et al., 2019). Environmental biotechnology and food technology monitoring systems assist in pollution management in wastewater treatment management (Gupta et al., 2025) and bioremediation and ensure product safety and consistency in fermentation processes (Kumar et al., 2025a). Advanced monitoring and control systems are key instruments in modern bioprocessing as they enhance sustainability, productivity, and quality assurance (Table 1).

Table 1. Importance of bioprocesses in control and monitoring

Applications	Sector	Control and monitoring importance	References
Enzyme production, microbial fermentation	Biotechnology	Minimizes contamination risk, ensures optimal microbial growth, maximizes yield	(Patel et al., 2023)
Monoclonal antibodies, vaccines	Pharmaceuticals	Ensures regulatory compliance (GMP, QbD, PAT),	(Covarrubias et al., 2022)
Organic acids, biofuels, bioplastics	Industrial Biotech	Supports large scale continuous, Enhances productivity and process sustainability	(Vasilakis et al., 2023)
Enzyme based processing, fermented foods, probiotics	Food and Beverages	Controls flavor, texture, safety and shelf life of products	(Dai et al., 2024)
Bioremediation, wastewater treatment	Environmental Biotech	Monitors microbial activity and nutrient levels effective pollution control	(Saeed et al., 2022; Kumar et al., 2025c)

FUNDAMENTALS OF BIOPROCESS MONITORING

Process Parameters

In bioprocessing, critical process parameters (CPPs) are key to confirming the value and effectiveness of a produce. These involve temperature, pH, dissolved oxygen (DO), biomass value, and glucose concentration (Liao et al., 2011). A simple and susceptible parameter, pH, impacts metabolite formation, nutrient uptake, cell membrane absorptivity and enzyme action. Cell stress and lowered production or even cell death could be a consequence of these variations. It is essential to measure the pH continually and exactly often using in-line optical or electrochemical sensors (Steinegger et al., 2020). Automated control routines with the adding of base or acid ensure constant environmental conditions throughout the culture process (Reyes et al., 2022). The dose is another necessary parameter specifically in cell cultures or aerobic fermentation methods. Lower growth rates and unwanted results could be the result of replaces in cellular metabolism from aerobic to anaerobic setting because of inadequate DO levels (Müller et al., 2012). Cascade control schemes are employed in modern bioreactors to modulate oxygen enhancement, gas movement rate, and agitation rate as per real-time DO sensor performances (Tamborini et al., 2018). Temperature control is also paramount as it influences cell viability, protein expression, and enzymatic reaction rates. Every microbe or cell line has an optimum temperature range, and deviations result in the thermal inactivation of biological elements, protein folding errors, or stress responses of the cells (Somero, 2020). To provide stable thermal conditions throughout the process, advanced bioprocess systems utilize highly accurate temperature-control equipment, often in combination with heating/cooling jackets. Because glucose is the primary source of carbon and energy in most bioprocesses, it must be carefully monitored and regulated (Mulukutla et al., 2016; Karmakar et al., 2025). Real-time glucose monitoring using biosensors or spectroscopic techniques allows dynamic feed regimens to achieve optimal metabolic balance and enhance the yield. In certain protocols, automated glycemic control has been shown to enhance therapeutic protein yield by up to 30% (Perkins et al., 2021).

Real-Time vs. Offline Monitoring Methods

The accurate monitoring of critical process parameters (CPPs) is mandatory for consistent bioprocessing product quality, yield, and compliance with regulations. Real-time (online or offline) and offline analysis methods are two common techniques (Wasalathanthri et al., 2020). Through complex sensors and analysis equipment, real-time monitoring involves the frequent or ongoing measurement of process variables within the bioreactor or through an associated loop system (Reyes et al., 2022). In adding to more sophisticated machineries such as near-infrared (NIR) spectroscopy, Raman spectroscopy, dielectric spectroscopy, and capacitance probes, these devices can monitor variable quantity such as pH, temperature, dissolved oxygen, agitation frequency, and exposure to air rate (Zainurin et al., 2022). The benefits of real-time monitoring contain improved control accuracy, process automation, and permanent data grouping. It reduces the probability of batch breakdown by identifying deviations and acknowledging for sudden remedial action. However, because real-time systems require exclusive sensors, processor units, and calibration methods, they can come at an expensive price. Some parameters must be delivered via offline procedures, particularly those including complex molecular reviews (Trabucco et al., 2022). The samples were yourself removed from the bioreactor and considered in the laboratory as part of offline observing. This method is regularly applied to measurements such as cell feasibility, metabolite profiling, substrate/product titres, and specific activeness tests. Offline analysis often develops equipment, such as spectrophotometers, flow cytometers, GC-MS, and HPLC (Chen et al., 2020). Although offline examining is time-consuming and labour-intensive it is still imperative for verifying the accuracy of real-time measuring device validating projecting models, and conducting comprehensive excellence tests (Xu et al., 2025). Offline and real-time monitoring practices are indispensable in bioprocessing. Although offline methods influence to depth and accuracy for confirmation in analysis real-time systems play an important role in dynamic control and ongoing advancement (Zhao et al., 2024). Both approaches are often merged in a consolidated approach to ensure a complete process understanding and healthy product quality.

Manage Analytical Technology Methods

Process Analytical Technology (PAT) and Quality by Design (QbD) have reformed biopharmaceutical and biological improvement, supervising, and control. PAT, firstly working by the FDA generates massive amounts of data to understand development behavior and notice abnormalities by engaging sensors and analytical instrumentation to continuously monitor dangerous quality and performance qualities (Kim et al., 2021). It gathers speed time-to-market with real-time product supply, reduces offline testing support, and accepts constant process verification (CPV). To confirm dependability and conformance with laws implementation wants robust data supervision, calibration models, and justification protocols (Mustapää et al., 2022). The systematically detecting and understanding the connections between formulation factors, process variables, and product quality, QbD highlights bringing quality into the product at the lead of development. The identification of Critical Quality Attributes (CQAs), development of a Design Area, risk reviews, and a Quality Target Product Profile (QTPP) are all dangerous elements of QbD (Namjoshi et al., 2020). Producers can design more forceful and variable processes using QbD principles which will lead to smaller amount deviations, fewer batch failures, and more streamlined regulatory sanctions.

ADVANCED SENSOR TECHNOLOGIES IN BIOPROCESSING

Biosensors

Biosensors are necessary for online checking and management of bioprocesses because they offer rapid and precise revealing of biological and chemical parameters. They consist of a transducer that transfers the biological answer into an electrical or optical signal that can be measured and a built-in biological recollection component (Kozitsina et al., 2018). Biosensors are required for monitoring basic analysis, such as glucose, lactate, oxygen, ammonia, and biomass through bioprocessing. Electrochemical biosensors detect variations in electrical belongings, including current, possible, or impedance, induced by metabolic methods (Brett, 2022). Their low cost, fast reaction time, high sensitivity, and ease of reduction make them in high want. However, fouling, signal drift, and intervening chemicals in complex bioprocess fluids can destroy the electrochemical sensors necessitating routine calibration and conservation (Xu et al., 2024).

Optical biosensors which use light to identify metabolic variations are highly limited and non-invasive. Advanced optical techniques such as Raman and near-infrared (NIR) spectroscopy can simultaneously monitor various analysis (Hang et al., 2022). Real-time analysis, minimal sample usage, and low electromagnetic noise restriction are some of the advantages of visual biosensors. Acoustic wave properties improved by contact of analysis with the sensor surface are measured using acoustic biosensors, incorporating surface acoustic wave (SAW) devices and quartz crystal microbalance (QCM) tools (Länge, 2019). Biomolecules at low concentrations can be discovered because of their sympathy to mass variations at the sensor apparent.

Spectroscopy-Based Monitoring

Spectroscopy-based observing has become an impressive tool for precise real-time bioprocess observes. Complex chemical fingerprints of biological arrangements are gained using techniques such as nuclear magnetic resonance (NMR), Fourier-transform infrared (FTIR), and Raman spectroscopy (Balan et al., 2019). These fingerprints enabled precise metabolite reporting, nutritional monitoring, and quality monitor. These methodologies increase the precision and efficiency of metabolite reporting by 30–40% associated to traditional methods (Aretz and Meierhofer, 2016). Raman spectroscopy is a vibrational technique that measures the inelastic scattering of monochromatic light and requires thorough molecular information about the chemical constituents of cells and their products. Owing to its sophisticated chemometric models, low sample planning time, and non-destructive characteristics, it is ideal for in-line fermentation and cell culture method examining (Chen et al., 2020). Through a study of the chemical bonds in a samples capacity to recognize infrared light FTIR spectroscopy can finance insight into the dynamics of functional groups and the overall composition of molecules (Koczoń et al., 2023). It permits for the rapid identification of transfers in metabolism and is employed both in line for bioprocesses. Nuclear magnetic resonance (NMR) spectroscopy is an informative technique for the non-destructive gaining of structural and dynamic information observing molecules is nuclear magnetic resonance (NMR) spectroscopy (Burns et al., 2020). It is ideal for complete metabolic profiling because it can simultaneously identify and measure a broad limit of metabolites. It is now more reasonable for online bioprocess applications, owing to improves in flow-cell integration and benchtop NMR (Mehendale et al., 2020). These methods offer complementary benefits for bioprocess monitoring, progression understanding, decrease of the development timeline, and regulatory agreement. Through their combination into Process Analysis Tool (PAT) templates metabolite profiling is augmented by 30–40%, and the shift regarding automated intelligent biomanufacturing structures is assisted (Williams et al., 2023).

Microfluidic Sensors

Microfluidic sensors have reformed bioprocess supervising particularly high-throughput screening (HTS). Microfluidic sensors function in microfluidic approaches which employ controlled avenues to deal with small quantities of fluid. Microfluidic sensors provide accurate, rapid, and cost-effective multiplexed measurements of biochemical and cellular factors in real-time by incorporating biosensing elements (Luka et al., 2015). By reducing reagent and sample utilization by as much as five-fold, microfluidic devices can make HTS more cost-effective and sustainable. High amounts of chemicals and medium and biological samples are wanted for high throughput examining via traditional methods. This control is addressed by microfluidic sensors which decrease the reaction levels while maintaining or attractive the analytical sensitivity (Salim and Lim, 2018). Because of its small size HTS is cost-effective and balanced. For bioprocess use numerous microfluidic devices have been developed, comprising optical sensors based on fluorescence or absorbance to display cell viability and protein expression, electrochemical sensors to monitor metabolites, and impedance-based sensors to monitor cell growth and their morphology (Goker et al., 2020). In pharmaceutical biotechnology sophisticated microfluidic systems integrating lab-on-a-chip designs are valuable for cell-line development media optimization. The single-cell analysis is increasingly important in accuracy medicine and synthetic biology and is consistent with microfluidic sensors (Taha et al., 2024). Microfluidic droplets can confine specific cells to individual microenvironments during the choice of strains or the design of bioprocesses allowing enhanced decision-making (Alexandre-Franco et al., 2024). Real-time feedback control because nonstop streams of data permit vigorous regulation of factors such as oxygen, pH, and provision of nutrients. The capability of microfluidics in intelligent biomanufacturing has been improved by the addition of AI and machine learning (Galan et al., 2020). High-throughput microfluidic information can be engaged to train forecast models that can precisely model process deviations or identify the optimum development conditions (Table 2).

Table 2. Benefits and features of microfluidic sensors

Feature	Description	Benefits in HTS	References
Miniaturization	Operates with micro to nano liter volumes of reagents and samples	5-fold reduction in reagent cost, reduced waste	(Puumala et al., 2022)
Multiplexing	Allow simultaneous testing of multiple analysis or conditions	Speeds up parallel screening increase throughput	(Anfossi et al., 2018)
Sensor	Impedance based sensors, electrochemical and optical	Enables real time monitoring of glucose, lactate, pH, etc	(Holzer et al., 2020)
Single cell analysis	Droplet based microfluidics isolate and monitor individual cells	Supports precision screening of strain variants	(Gérard et al., 2020)
Integration with automation	Compatible with robotic liquid handlers and automated platforms	Enhances reproducibility, reduces labour requirements	(Holland and Davies, 2020)
Real time feedback control	Continuous data streams for dynamic parameter adjustments	Improves process stability and product yield	(Diehl et al., 2002)
Data analytics compatibility	Interfaces with AI/ML for pattern recognition and process optimization	Enables predictive modelling and digital twin development	(Karkaria et al., 2025)
Lab chip format	Combines mixing, reaction, separation and detection on a single chip	Efficient, compact, and cost-effective design	(Dkhar et al., 2023)
Applications	Strain screening, media optimization, drug testing, enzyme activity assay	Versatile tool for biotech, pharma, and synthetic biology	(Sarnaik et al., 2020)

ARTIFICIAL INTELLIGENCE AND MACHINE LEARNING IN BIOPROCESS CONTROL

One significant move concerning smarter, more flexible, and dynamic manufacturing systems in pharmaceuticals and biotechnology is the relevance of artificial intelligence (AI) and machine learning (ML) in bioprocess control. The complication of bioprocesses which are often data rich makes it challenging for accepted control systems to realize maximum performance (Gargalo et al., 2020). To improve process robustness, product quality, and overall effectiveness. AI and ML offer advanced data-driven processes that can learn from historical and surviving process information, identify shapes, predict results, and permit for dynamic decision-making (Machireddy et al., 2021). Among AI and ML, the most valuable influence on bioprocess and biocontrol control is predictive modelling (Kumar et al., 2025d). To predict key outputs such as biomass concentration product titre and metabolite concentrations, machine learning (ML) methods like provision vector machines (SVM), artificial neural networks (ANN), decision trees, and casual forests can be cultured from historical progression data (Imamoglu, 2024). These predictive models are often more precise and stretcher than traditional mechanistic models mostly in cases where the original biology is not well-understood. A second essential application of AI-based control techniques is the real-time monitoring processes control. AI-based control systems can combine information from multiple sensors and examine it in real time to detect aberrations, optimize feeding regimens, and environmental situation (Rath et al., 2024). Through trial-and-error interactions with the method environment and learning action which is a subset of machine learning has shown promise in the automation of the control of bioprocesses. AI and ML are critical for anomaly finding and fault diagnosis because they support quick helpful action, reduce downtime, improve product quality, and regulatory defiance (Chukwunweike et al., 2024).

EMERGING TRENDS IN BIOPROCESS CONTROL SYSTEMS

Real-Time Metabolic Flux Analysis

One impressive method for understanding and overseeing cellular metabolism through bioprocessing is real-time metabolic flow analysis (rMFA). It provides vigorous real-time information on intracellular instabilities allowing a 35% improvement in flux prediction accuracy. This enhances the regularity, productivity, and optimization of bioprocesses (Isoko et al., 2024). Process technologists can monitor how variations in culture situations affect metabolic action using rMFA, which contains the integration of computational models and real-time data streams from sensors, spectroscopy, and biosensors to expect intracellular metabolic conditions in real time (Chu et al., 2022). Technological improvements such as high-frequency data acquisition schemes the integration of Process Analytical Technology (PAT) equipment, FTIR or Raman spectroscopy, and the use of Machine Learning (ML) algorithms to interpret nonlinear biological replies are all liable for enhancing flux prediction (Rolinger et al., 2020). Assessed with static models ML-augmented FBA provides more accurate reconstructions of the cells metabolic state by collaborative internal flux displays to live real-time outer metabolite absorptions. Another breakthrough is 13C-MFA, which agrees the exact resolution of carbon fluxes concluded key metabolic pathways. This is critical for strain engineering and reasonable metabolic create (Guo et al., 2015). In biomanufacturing real-time MFA is also arising as fundamental part of digital twins in which virtual duplications simulate real-time bioprocesses using real-time data to predict system behaviours, optimize operations, and prevent mistakes. The approach adheres to continuous production and Quality by Design (QbD) paradigms that demand precise and stable product quality, and it enables adaptive control plans (Ganesh et al., 2020). With a 35% improvement in prediction accuracy rMFA represents a substantial advance in system-level bioprocess management and genetic improvement (Mahakur et al., 2025) that will permit researchers and industry professionals to make improved choices maximize microbial or mammalian cell speed up development schedules.

Soft Sensors and Adaptive Control Mechanisms

Soft sensors and adaptive control systems are vital tools in bioprocessing that enhance system operation, decision-making, and process monitoring. Intelligent systems provide new ways of dealing with complex, dynamic, and nonlinear biological processes where it is often impractical or too costly to measure crucial variables directly (Rojas et al., 2025). Soft sensors, also called software or virtual sensors, utilize measurable inputs such as dissolved oxygen, substrate concentration, pH, or off-gas composition to approximate unmeasurable or hard-to-measure process parameters in real time. They are particularly useful in bioprocesses where accurate, direct, and continuous measurement is not possible due to sensor limitations, cost, or sampling constraints because they apply mathematical, statistical, or machine learning models to draw inferences about hidden variables (Zhu et al., 2020). Soft sensors can estimate biomass growth with inputs from easily available Internet instruments because they are flexible and affordable. Kalman filtering, partial least squares regression (PLSR), and advanced machine learning methods, such as artificial neural networks (ANN) and support vector regression (SVR), may all be utilized to tailor them for specific bioprocesses (Imamoglu, 2024). Adaptive control tools permit dynamic process parameter adjustments to sustain optimal conditions, facilitating smarter, more responsive, and efficient bioprocess operations. These tools are particularly valuable for Quality by Design (QbD) and Process Analytical Technology (PAT) philosophies, where real-time adjustment is vital for sustaining critical quality attributes (CQAs) (Nishal et al., 2024). With biomanufacturing embracing Industry 4.0, these tools will prove critical to highly automated, predictive, and quality-focused production systems. The models can be retrained or refreshed with new data as the process evolves while maintaining accuracy (Figure 1).

Figure 1. Soft sensors adaptation

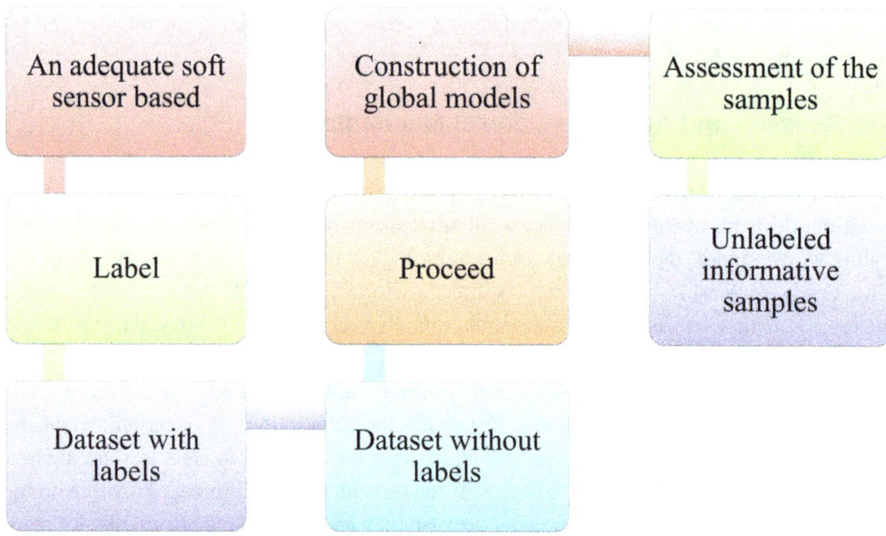

DIGITAL TRANSFORMATION IN BIOMANUFACTURING (INDUSTRY 4.0 APPLICATIONS)

Through the integration of cyber-physical systems, cloud computing, big data analytics, the Internet of Things (IoT), and artificial intelligence (AI) into production environments, Industry 4.0 is revolutionizing biomanufacturing (Gurawalia et al., 2024). The biopharmaceutical and industrial biotechnology sectors are moving into a new age of precision, productivity, and versatility due to this revolution in the production, manufacturing, and supply of biological products. Perhaps the most significant of all the technologies that have facilitated this shift is the Industrial Internet of Things (IIoT), which continuously generates high-resolution sensor and device data in the bioprocess setup (Vrchota et al., 2020). These data make predictive and prescriptive bioprocess control feasible and allow for automatic adjustment and remote monitoring. Another critical technology that facilitates advanced process optimization, scenario analysis, and failure forecasting is digital twins, which are virtual replicas of real bioprocesses. Through simplification of storing, sharing, and analyzing large sets of data in different departments and locations, cloud computing and unified data lakes enable data integrity and cooperation across functions (Nambiar and Mundra, 2022). Real-time control of processes, predictive maintenance, and root-cause analysis driven by automation are additional uses of AI and big-data analytics. Artificial intelligence systems, for example, can predict mechanical failures prior to their occurrence, keeping unscheduled downtime to a minimum, and extending the lifespan of machinery (Rojek et al., 2023). To enhance safety, eliminate the new-hire learning curve, and support troubleshooting in highly regulated applications without shutting down in-process production, alternate reality (AR) and virtual reality (VR) technologies have been utilized for operator training, remote maintenance, and visualization of plant layouts (Yazdi, 2024). Industry 4.0-fostered digital transformation in biomanufacturing is making the industry more agile, scalable, and quality oriented. Biomanufacturers can meet the growing global need for biologics and personalized drugs, enhance process resilience, reduce costs, and accelerate innovation by leveraging digital technologies (Mirakhori and Niazi, 2025). An era of truly intelligent biotechnology manufacturing will begin as digital infrastructure evolves and will play an increasingly significant role in shaping the trajectory of bioproduction (Figure 2).

Figure 2. Digital transformation keys

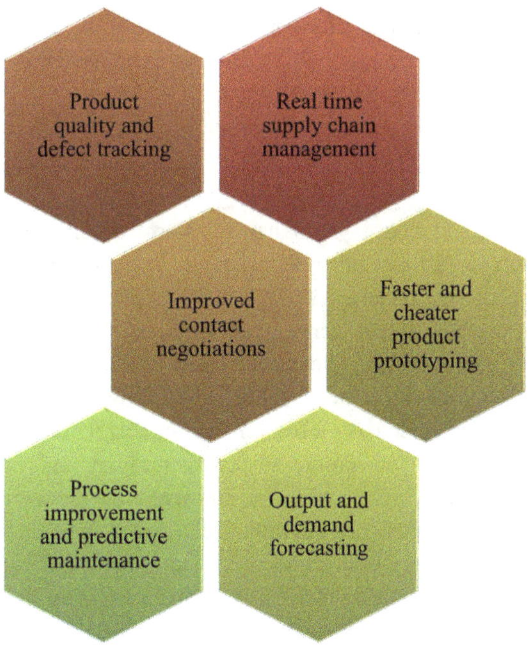
Product quality and defect tracking
Real time supply chain management
Improved contact negotiations
Faster and cheater product prototyping
Process improvement and predictive maintenance
Output and demand forecasting

CHALLENGES AND FUTURE PERSPECTIVES

The scalability, consistency, and efficiency of biomanufacturing can be revolutionized entirely by bioprocess monitoring and control systems. However, these technologies suffer from management problems, data integration, sensor limitations, machine learning (ML) models, corporate culture, and employee readiness (Sun and Jung, 2024). The extremely high amounts of data generated by multiple sources, such as sensors, spectrometers, bioreactors, and control systems, pose a challenge for data integration. The lack of established data protocols and hardware and software system compatibility (Aminizadeh et al., 2024). Poor generalizability and robustness are other major issues with machine-learning models applied to process prediction and control. The validation, traceability, and interpretability of AI and ML algorithms are significant concerns in highly regulated industries, such as pharmaceuticals (Suri et al., 2024). AI-based process control is still being integrated into regulatory guidelines, and additional guidance is needed to facilitate its safe and legal application in Good Manufacturing Practice (GMP) settings. Another limitation of real-time bioprocess monitoring is sensor limitations. However, spectroscopy-based methods and biosensors have improved, robust, non-invasive, and scalable sensors that can accurately monitor intracellular metabolites, protein folding states, or other important quality attributes (CQAs) are still lacking (Fisher et al., 2019). Other issues include the company culture and employee readiness. Despite these challenges, there are some promising features for bioprocess monitoring and control. Process precision will be significantly enhanced through the development of next-generation bioreactors with smart sensors, edge-computing hardware, and real-time feedback systems. Quantum computing and further development of digital twins have the potential to radically change multivariate data processing and biological modeling.

CONCLUSION

Bioprocess monitoring and control systems have transformed the manufacturing sector through real-time data collection, sophisticated analysis techniques, and computational intelligence. These systems control critical process parameters (CPPs), such as pH, dissolved oxygen, temperature, glucose concentration, and biomass, influencing cell or microbial culture performance, metabolic activity, and quality of the product. Predictive and adaptive bioprocessing is made possible by Process Analytical Technology (PAT), and Quality by Design principles, maintaining consistent product quality and regulatory compliance for recycling technology (Kumar et al., 2025b). Dynamic process optimization is aided by soft sensors, adaptive controllers, and real-time metabolic flux analysis to minimize waste, maximize production, and accelerate innovation. The integration of Artificial Intelligence (AI) and Machine Learning (ML) results in predictive deviations in processes, remediation steps, and detection of underlying trends in complicated datasets. Advanced process simulation and AI-driven digital twins create a virtual world for stress testing, stimulating innovation and decision-making. Challenges remain, including data integration, model validation, regulation approval, and the harmonization of technologies. With emerging technologies, such as wearable bioreactors, autonomous control algorithms, and quantum computing-enabled process analytics driving biomanufacturing, bioprocess monitoring and control will continue to advance.

REFERENCES

Alexandre-Franco, M. F., Kouider, R., Kassir Al-Karany, R., Cuerda-Correa, E. M., & Al-Kassir, A. (2024). Recent Advances in Polymer Science and Fabrication Processes for Enhanced Microfluidic Applications: An Overview. *Micromachines, 15*(9), 1137. PMID: 39337797

Aminizadeh, S., Heidari, A., Dehghan, M., Toumaj, S., Rezaei, M., Navimipour, N. J., & Unal, M. (2024). Opportunities and challenges of artificial intelligence and distributed systems to improve the quality of healthcare service. *Artificial Intelligence in Medicine, 149*, 102779. PMID: 38462281

Anfossi, L., Di Nardo, F., Cavalera, S., Giovannoli, C., & Baggiani, C. (2018). Multiplex lateral flow immunoassay: An overview of strategies towards high-throughput point-of-need testing. *Biosensors (Basel), 9*(1), 2. PMID: 30587769

Aretz, I., & Meierhofer, D. (2016). Advantages and pitfalls of mass spectrometry based metabolome profiling in systems biology. *International Journal of Molecular Sciences, 17*(5), 632. PMID: 27128910

Balan, V., Mihai, C. T., Cojocaru, F. D., Uritu, C. M., Dodi, G., Botezat, D., & Gardikiotis, I. (2019). Vibrational spectroscopy fingerprinting in medicine: From molecular to clinical practice. *Materials (Basel), 12*(18), 2884. PMID: 31489927

Bowler, A. L., Bakalis, S., & Watson, N. J. (2020). A review of in-line and on-line measurement techniques to monitor industrial mixing processes. *Chemical Engineering Research & Design, 153*, 463–495.

Brett, C. M. (2022). Electrochemical impedance spectroscopy in the characterisation and application of modified electrodes for electrochemical sensors and biosensors. *Molecules (Basel, Switzerland), 27*(5), 1497. PMID: 35268599

Burns, N. K., Theakstone, A. G., Zhu, H., O'Dell, L. A., Pearson, J. R., Ashton, T. D., & Conlan, X. A. (2020). The identification of synthetic cannabinoids surface coated on herbal substrates using solid-state nuclear magnetic resonance spectroscopy. *Analytica Chimica Acta, 1104*, 105–109. PMID: 32106940

Chen, X., Hu, R., Hu, L., Huang, Y., Shi, W., Wei, Q., & Li, Z. (2020). Portable analytical techniques for monitoring volatile organic chemicals in biomanufacturing processes: Recent advances and limitations. *Frontiers in Chemistry, 8*, 837. PMID: 33024746

Chen, Y., Yang, O., Sampat, C., Bhalode, P., Ramachandran, R., & Ierapetritou, M. (2020). Digital twins in pharmaceutical and biopharmaceutical manufacturing: A literature review. *Processes (Basel, Switzerland), 8*(9), 1088.

Chu, S. S., Nguyen, H. A., Zhang, J., Tabassum, S., & Cao, H. (2022). Towards multiplexed and multimodal biosensor platforms in real-time monitoring of metabolic disorders. *Sensors (Basel), 22*(14), 5200. PMID: 35890880

Chukwunweike, J., Anang, A. N., Adeniran, A. A., & Dike, J. (2024). Enhancing manufacturing efficiency and quality through automation and deep learning: addressing redundancy, defects, vibration analysis, and material strength optimization Vol. 23. *World Journal of Advanced Research and Reviews. GSC Online Press.*

Covarrubias, C. E., Rivera, T. A., Soto, C. A., Deeks, T., & Kalergis, A. M. (2022). Current GMP standards for the production of vaccines and antibodies: An overview. *Frontiers in Public Health, 10*, 1021905. PMID: 36743162

Dai, Y., Chen, Y., Lin, X., & Zhang, S. (2024). Recent Applications and Prospects of Enzymes in Quality and Safety Control of Fermented Foods. *Foods, 13*(23), 3804. PMID: 39682876

Diehl, M., Bock, H. G., Schlöder, J. P., Findeisen, R., Nagy, Z., & Allgöwer, F. (2002). Real-time optimization and nonlinear model predictive control of processes governed by differential-algebraic equations. *Journal of Process Control, 12*(4), 577–585.

Dkhar, D. S., Kumari, R., Malode, S. J., Shetti, N. P., & Chandra, P. (2023). Integrated lab-on-a-chip devices: Fabrication methodologies, transduction system for sensing purposes. *Journal of Pharmaceutical and Biomedical Analysis, 223*, 115120. PMID: 36343538

Fisher, A. C., Kamga, M. H., Agarabi, C., Brorson, K., Lee, S. L., & Yoon, S. (2019). The current scientific and regulatory landscape in advancing integrated continuous biopharmaceutical manufacturing. *Trends in Biotechnology, 37*(3), 253–267. PMID: 30241924

Frangopol, D. M., & Liu, M. (2019). Maintenance and management of civil infrastructure based on condition, safety, optimization, and life-cycle cost. *Structures and infrastructure systems*, 96-108.

Galan, E. A., Zhao, H., Wang, X., Dai, Q., Huck, W. T., & Ma, S. (2020). Intelligent microfluidics: The convergence of machine learning and microfluidics in materials science and biomedicine. *Matter, 3*(6), 1893–1922.

Ganesh, S., Su, Q., Nagy, Z., & Reklaitis, G. (2020). Advancing smart manufacturing in the pharmaceutical industry. In *Smart manufacturing* (pp. 21–57). Elsevier.

Gargalo, C. L., Udugama, I., Pontius, K., Lopez, P. C., Nielsen, R. F., Hasanzadeh, A., & Gernaey, K. V. (2020). Towards smart biomanufacturing: A perspective on recent developments in industrial measurement and monitoring technologies for bio-based production processes. *Journal of Industrial Microbiology & Biotechnology: Official Journal of the Society for Industrial Microbiology and Biotechnology, 47*(11), 947–964. PMID: 32895764

Gérard, A., Woolfe, A., Mottet, G., Reichen, M., Castrillon, C., Menrath, V., & Brenan, C. (2020). High-throughput single-cell activity-based screening and sequencing of antibodies using droplet microfluidics. *Nature Biotechnology, 38*(6), 715–721. PMID: 32231335

Goker, M., Kurbanoglu, S., Huri, P. Y., Sezgintürk, M. K., & Ozkan, S. A. (2020). Bioprocess monitoring by biosensor-based technologies. In *Commercial Biosensors and Their Applications* (pp. 259–285). Elsevier.

Goshtasbi, H., Okolodkov, Y. B., Movafeghi, A., Awale, S., Safary, A., Barar, J., & Omidi, Y. (2023). Harnessing microalgae as sustainable cellular factories for biopharmaceutical production. *Algal Research*, *74*, 103237.

Guo, W., Sheng, J., & Feng, X. (2015). 13C-metabolic flux analysis: An accurate approach to demystify microbial metabolism for biochemical production. *Bioengineering (Basel, Switzerland)*, *3*(1), 3. PMID: 28952565

Gupta, N., Wijenayake, W. P. T., Roy, D., Kumar, R., Rangot, M., Chugh, P., Santoyo, G., Chattaraj, S., Bhaskar, S. S., Andjelković, S., & Guerra-Sierra, B. E. (2025). Smart Recycling and Sustainable Lignocellulosic Waste Management. In *Value Addition and Utilization of Lignocellulosic Biomass: Through Novel Technological Interventions* (pp. 221–250). Springer Nature Singapore.

Gurawalia, H., Shinde, P. B., & Sharma, K. K. (2024). Embracing Industry 4.0 Ingredients in Synthetic Biology for the Development of Carbon–Neutral Economy. In *Biorefinery and Industry 4.0: Empowering Sustainability* (pp. 215–252). Springer Nature Switzerland.

Hang, Y., Boryczka, J., & Wu, N. (2022). Visible-light and near-infrared fluorescence and surface-enhanced Raman scattering point-of-care sensing and bio-imaging: A review. *Chemical Society Reviews*, *51*(1), 329–375. PMID: 34897302

Holland, I., & Davies, J. A. (2020). Automation in the life science research laboratory. *Frontiers in Bioengineering and Biotechnology*, *8*, 571777. PMID: 33282848

Holzer, R., Bloch, W., & Brinkmann, C. (2020). Minimally invasive electrochemical patch-based sensor system for monitoring glucose and lactate in the human body—A survey-based analysis of the end-user's perspective. *Sensors (Basel)*, *20*(20), 5761. PMID: 33050656

Imamoglu, E. (2024). Artificial Intelligence and/or Machine Learning Algorithms in Microalgae Bioprocesses. *Bioengineering (Basel, Switzerland)*, *11*(11), 1143. PMID: 39593803

Imamoglu, E. (2024). Artificial Intelligence and/or Machine Learning Algorithms in Microalgae Bioprocesses. *Bioengineering (Basel, Switzerland)*, *11*(11), 1143. PMID: 39593803

Isoko, K., Cordiner, J. L., Kis, Z., & Moghadam, P. Z. (2024). Bioprocessing 4.0: A pragmatic review and future perspectives. *Digital Discovery*, *3*(9), 1662–1681.

Isoko, K., Cordiner, J. L., Kis, Z., & Moghadam, P. Z. (2024). Bioprocessing 4.0: A pragmatic review and future perspectives. *Digital Discovery*, *3*(9), 1662–1681.

Issaoui, M., Jellali, S., Zorpas, A. A., & Dutournie, P. (2022). Membrane technology for sustainable water resources management: Challenges and future projections. *Sustainable Chemistry and Pharmacy*, *25*, 100590.

Känsäkoski, M., Kurkinen, M., von Weymarn, N., Niemelä, P., Neubauer, P., Juuso, E., & Suhonen, P. (2006). Process analytical technology (PAT) needs and applications in the bioprocess industry. *VTT Technical Research Centre of Finland*, *60*, 99.

Karkaria, V., Tsai, Y. K., Chen, Y. P., & Chen, W. (2025). An optimization-centric review on integrating artificial intelligence and digital twin technologies in manufacturing. *Engineering Optimization*, *57*(1), 161–207.

Karmakar, R., Behera, N. R., Mandal, A., Sharma, P. K., Toomey, J. B., Kundu, K., & Kumar, R. (2025). State-of-the-Art in algal biofuel research: Waste-algae as a sustainable energy solution. *Journal of Solid Waste Technology Management*, *51*(3), 385–404.

Kim, E. J., Kim, J. H., Kim, M. S., Jeong, S. H., & Choi, D. H. (2021). Process analytical technology tools for monitoring pharmaceutical unit operations: A control strategy for continuous process verification. *Pharmaceutics*, *13*(6), 919. PMID: 34205797

Koczoń, P., Hołaj-Krzak, J. T., Palani, B. K., Bolewski, T., Dąbrowski, J., Bartyzel, B. J., & Gruczyńska-Sękowska, E. (2023). The analytical possibilities of FT-IR spectroscopy powered by vibrating molecules. *International Journal of Molecular Sciences*, *24*(2), 1013. PMID: 36674526

Kozitsina, A. N., Svalova, T. S., Malysheva, N. N., Okhokhonin, A. V., Vidrevich, M. B., & Brainina, K. Z. (2018). Sensors based on bio and biomimetic receptors in medical diagnostic, environment, and food analysis. *Biosensors (Basel)*, *8*(2), 35. PMID: 29614784

Kumar, R., Gupta, G., Hussain, A., Rani, A., Thapliyal, A., Gunsola, D., & Mitra, D. (2025a). Pioneering zero-waste technologies utilization and its framework on sustainable management: International, national and state level. *Discover Applied Sciences*, *7*(3), 224.

Kumar, R., Kamboj, N., & Mitra, D. (2024). Microbial innovations in agriculture: Interdisciplinary approaches to leveraging microbes for food sustainability and security. *Indian Journal of Microbiology Research*, *11*(3), 129–139.

Kumar, R., Kamboj, N., Mitra, D., & Ray, A. (2025b). Strengthening Local Communities Through Advanced Recycling Technology for Sustainable Growth. In Mitra, D., Choudhury, T., Madan, A., Chattaraj, S., & Pellegrini, M. (Eds.), *AI Technologies for Enhancing Recycling Processes* (pp. 393–420). IGI Global Scientific Publishing.

Kumar, R., Kamboj, N., Mitra, D., Verma, D., & Choudhury, T. (2025c). Bacterial Strategies: Novel Pathways for Sustainable Development Through Wastewater. In Mitra, D., Choudhury, T., Madan, A., Chattaraj, S., & Pellegrini, M. (Eds.), *AI Technologies for Enhancing Recycling Processes* (pp. 421–440). IGI Global Scientific Publishing.

Kumar, R., Lakhera, A., Gulati, M., Rani, A., Thapliyal, A., Gunsola, D., & Mitra, D. (2025d). Genome Mining of Biocontrol Agents for Bioprospecting Action Modes. In Mitra, D., de los Santos Villalobos, S., Rani, A., Elena Guerra Sierra, B., & Andjelković, S. (Eds.), *Bio-control Agents for Sustainable Agriculture*. Springer.

Kumar, R., Sangwan, K. S., Herrmann, C., & Thakur, S. (2023). A cyber physical production system framework for online monitoring, visualization and control by using cloud, fog, and edge computing technologies. *International Journal of Computer Integrated Manufacturing*, *36*(10), 1507–1525.

Länge, K. (2019). Bulk and surface acoustic wave sensor arrays for multi-analyte detection: A review. *Sensors (Basel)*, *19*(24), 5382. PMID: 31817599

Liao, B. Q., Lin, H. J., Langevin, S. P., Gao, W. J., & Leppard, G. G. (2011). Effects of temperature and dissolved oxygen on sludge properties and their role in bioflocculation and settling. *Water Research*, *45*(2), 509–520. PMID: 20875910

Luka, G., Ahmadi, A., Najjaran, H., Alocilja, E., DeRosa, M., Wolthers, K., & Hoorfar, M. (2015). Microfluidics integrated biosensors: A leading technology towards lab-on-a-chip and sensing applications. *Sensors (Basel)*, *15*(12), 30011–30031. PMID: 26633409

Machireddy, J. R., Rachakatla, S. K., & Ravichandran, P. (2021). Leveraging AI and machine learning for data-driven business strategy: A comprehensive framework for analytics integration. *African Journal of Artificial Intelligence and Sustainable Development*, *1*(2), 12–150.

Mahakur, B., Bedaprabha, A., Barik, D. P., Gupta, S., Kumar, R., Mitra, D., & Verma, D. (2025). Hairy Root Culture: An Effective Method for Production of Plant Bioactive Compounds. Genetic Improvement and Conservation Practices of Medicinal Plants. First Edition (2025) | CRC Press, Pages: 9 | eBook ISBN: 9781003482659

Mehendale, N., Jenne, F., Joshi, C., Sharma, S., Masakapalli, S. K., & MacKinnon, N. (2020). A nuclear magnetic resonance (NMR) platform for real-time metabolic monitoring of bioprocesses. *Molecules (Basel, Switzerland)*, *25*(20), 4675. PMID: 33066296

Mirakhori, F., & Niazi, S. K. (2025). Harnessing the AI/ML in Drug and Biological Products Discovery and Development: The Regulatory Perspective. *Pharmaceuticals*, *18*(1), 47. PMID: 39861110

Müller, M., Mentel, M., van Hellemond, J. J., Henze, K., Woehle, C., Gould, S. B., & Martin, W. F. (2012). Biochemistry and evolution of anaerobic energy metabolism in eukaryotes. *Microbiology and Molecular Biology Reviews : MMBR*, *76*(2), 444–495. PMID: 22688819

Mulukutla, B. C., Yongky, A., Le, T., Mashek, D. G., & Hu, W. S. (2016). Regulation of glucose metabolism–a perspective from cell bioprocessing. *Trends in Biotechnology*, *34*(8), 638–651. PMID: 27265890

Mustapää, T., Nummiluikki, J., & Viitala, R. (2022). Digitalization of calibration data management in pharmaceutical industry using a multitenant platform. *Applied Sciences (Basel, Switzerland)*, *12*(15), 7531.

Nambiar, A., & Mundra, D. (2022). An overview of data warehouse and data lake in modern enterprise data management. *Big Data and Cognitive Computing*, *6*(4), 132.

Namjoshi, S., Dabbaghi, M., Roberts, M. S., Grice, J. E., & Mohammed, Y. (2020). Quality by design: Development of the quality target product profile (QTPP) for semisolid topical products. *Pharmaceutics*, *12*(3), 287. PMID: 32210126

Nishal, S., Kumar, V., Phogat, P., Garg, V., & Dureja, H. (2024). Selection of Design of PAT. In *Introduction to Quality by Design (QbD) From Theory to Practice* (pp. 59–89). Springer Nature Singapore.

Pandey, K., Pandey, M., Kumar, V., Aggarwal, U., & Singhal, B. (2024). Bioprocessing 4.0 in biomanufacturing: Paving the way for sustainable bioeconomy. *Systems Microbiology and Biomanufacturing*, *4*(2), 407–424.

Patel, A. K., Dong, C. D., Chen, C. W., Pandey, A., & Singhania, R. R. (2023). Production, purification, and application of microbial enzymes. In *Biotechnology of microbial enzymes* (pp. 25–57). Academic Press.

Perkins, B. A., Sherr, J. L., & Mathieu, C. (2021). Type 1 diabetes glycemic management: Insulin therapy, glucose monitoring, and automation. *Science*, *373*(6554), 522–527. PMID: 34326234

Puumala, L. S., Grist, S. M., Morales, J. M., Bickford, J. R., Chrostowski, L., Shekhar, S., & Cheung, K. C. (2022). Biofunctionalization of multiplexed silicon photonic biosensors. *Biosensors (Basel)*, *13*(1), 53. PMID: 36671887

Rantanen, J., & Khinast, J. (2015). The future of pharmaceutical manufacturing sciences. *Journal of Pharmaceutical Sciences*, *104*(11), 3612–3638. PMID: 26280993

Rath, K. C., Khang, A., Rath, S. K., Satapathy, N., Satapathy, S. K., & Kar, S. (2024). Artificial intelligence (AI)-enabled technology in medicine-advancing holistic healthcare monitoring and control systems. In *Computer Vision and AI-Integrated IoT Technologies in the Medical Ecosystem* (pp. 87–108). CRC Press.

Rathore, A. S., Mishra, S., Nikita, S., & Priyanka, P. (2021). Bioprocess control: Current progress and future perspectives. *Life (Chicago, Ill.)*, *11*(6), 557. PMID: 34199245

Rathore, A. S., Mishra, S., Nikita, S., & Priyanka, P. (2021). Bioprocess control: Current progress and future perspectives. *Life (Chicago, Ill.)*, *11*(6), 557. PMID: 34199245

Reyes, S. J., Durocher, Y., Pham, P. L., & Henry, O. (2022). Modern sensor tools and techniques for monitoring, controlling, and improving cell culture processes. *Processes (Basel, Switzerland)*, *10*(2), 189.

Rojas, L., Yepes, V., & Garcia, J. (2025). Complex Dynamics and Intelligent Control: Advances, Challenges, and Applications in Mining and Industrial Processes. *Mathematics*, *13*(6), 961.

Rojek, I., Jasiulewicz-Kaczmarek, M., Piechowski, M., & Mikołajewski, D. (2023). An artificial intelligence approach for improving maintenance to supervise machine failures and support their repair. *Applied Sciences (Basel, Switzerland)*, *13*(8), 4971.

Rolinger, L., Rüdt, M., & Hubbuch, J. (2020). A critical review of recent trends, and a future perspective of optical spectroscopy as PAT in biopharmaceutical downstream processing. *Analytical and Bioanalytical Chemistry*, *412*, 2047–2064. PMID: 32146498

Rösner, L. S., Walter, F., Ude, C., John, G. T., & Beutel, S. (2022). Sensors and techniques for on-line determination of cell viability in bioprocess monitoring. *Bioengineering (Basel, Switzerland)*, *9*(12), 762. PMID: 36550968

Saeed, M. U., Hussain, N., Sumrin, A., Shahbaz, A., Noor, S., Bilal, M., & Iqbal, H. M. (2022). Microbial bioremediation strategies with wastewater treatment potentialities–A review. *The Science of the Total Environment*, *818*, 151754. PMID: 34800451

Salim, A., & Lim, S. (2018). Review of recent metamaterial microfluidic sensors. *Sensors (Basel)*, *18*(1), 232. PMID: 29342953

Sarnaik, A., Liu, A., Nielsen, D., & Varman, A. M. (2020). High-throughput screening for efficient microbial biotechnology. *Current Opinion in Biotechnology*, *64*, 141–150. PMID: 32302926

Somero, G. N. (2020). The cellular stress response and temperature: Function, regulation, and evolution. *Journal of Experimental Zoology. Part A, Ecological and Integrative Physiology*, *333*(6), 379–397. PMID: 31944627

Steinegger, A., Wolfbeis, O. S., & Borisov, S. M. (2020). Optical sensing and imaging of pH values: Spectroscopies, materials, and applications. *Chemical Reviews*, *120*(22), 12357–12489. PMID: 33147405

Straathof, A. J., Wahl, S. A., Benjamin, K. R., Takors, R., Wierckx, N., & Noorman, H. J. (2019). Grand research challenges for sustainable industrial biotechnology. *Trends in Biotechnology*, *37*(10), 1042–1050. PMID: 31054854

Sun, Y., & Jung, H. (2024). Machine Learning (ML) Modeling, IoT, and Optimizing Organizational Operations through Integrated Strategies: The Role of Technology and Human Resource Management. *Sustainability*, *16*(16), 6751.

Suri, G. S., Kaur, G., & Shinde, D. (2024). Beyond boundaries: Exploring the transformative power of AI in pharmaceuticals. *Discover Artificial Intelligence*, *4*(1), 82.

Taha, B. A., Abbas, E. M., Kadhim, A. C., Azzahrani, A. S., Haider, A. J., Chaudhary, V., & Arsad, N. (2024). Needle scattered light guided chiplets-interfaced with AI for advanced biomedical application. *Microelectronic Engineering*, *292*, 112228.

Tamborini, L., Fernandes, P., Paradisi, F., & Molinari, F. (2018). Flow bioreactors as complementary tools for biocatalytic process intensification. *Trends in Biotechnology*, *36*(1), 73–88. PMID: 29054312

Tang, H. H., & Ahmad, N. S. (2024). Fuzzy logic approach for controlling uncertain and nonlinear systems: A comprehensive review of applications and advances. *Systems Science & Control Engineering*, *12*(1), 2394429.

Trabucco, B., Geng, X., Kumar, A., & Levine, S. (2022, June). Design-bench: Benchmarks for data-driven offline model-based optimization. In *International Conference on Machine Learning* (pp. 21658-21676). PMLR.

Vasilakis, P., Pyrgakis, K., Psycha, M., Biundo, A., & Kokossis, A. (2023). A novel industrial biotechnology approach to valorize fatty acids to bioplastics: Scope for scale-up and process efficiency using an integrated approach. [). Elsevier.]. *Computer-Aided Chemical Engineering*, *52*, 2563–2568.

Vrchota, J., Pech, M., Rolinek, L., & Bednář, J. (2020). Sustainability outcomes of green processes in relation to industry 4.0 in manufacturing: Systematic review. *Sustainability, 12*(15), 5968.

Wang, H., Chen, Y., Wang, L., Liu, Q., Yang, S., & Wang, C. (2023). Advancing herbal medicine: Enhancing product quality and safety through robust quality control practices. *Frontiers in Pharmacology, 14*, 1265178. PMID: 37818188

Wasalathanthri, D. P., Feroz, H., Puri, N., Hung, J., Lane, G., Holstein, M., & Li, Z. J. (2020). Real-time monitoring of quality attributes by in-line Fourier transform infrared spectroscopic sensors at ultrafiltration and diafiltration of bioprocess. *Biotechnology and Bioengineering, 117*(12), 3766–3774. PMID: 32776504

Williams, T., Kalinka, K., Sanches, R., Blanchard-Emmerson, G., Watts, S., Davies, L., & Dikicioglu, D. (2023). Machine learning and metabolic modelling assisted implementation of a novel process analytical technology in cell and gene therapy manufacturing. *Scientific Reports, 13*(1), 834. PMID: 36646795

Xu, F., Su, L., Gao, H., Wang, Y., Ben, R., Hu, K., & Tian, X. (2025). Harnessing near-infrared and Raman spectral sensing and artificial intelligence for real-time monitoring and precision control of bioprocess. *Bioresource Technology*, •••, 132204. PMID: 39923859

Xu, X., Zuo, Y., Chen, S., Hatami, A., & Gu, H. (2024). Advancements in brain research: The in vivo/in vitro electrochemical detection of neurochemicals. *Biosensors (Basel), 14*(3), 125. PMID: 38534232

Yazdi, M. (2024). Augmented reality (AR) and virtual reality (VR) in maintenance training. In *Advances in Computational Mathematics for Industrial System Reliability and Maintainability* (pp. 169–183). Springer Nature Switzerland.

Zainurin, S. N., Wan Ismail, W. Z., Mahamud, S. N. I., Ismail, I., Jamaludin, J., Ariffin, K. N. Z., & Wan Ahmad Kamil, W. M. (2022). Advancements in monitoring water quality based on various sensing methods: A systematic review. *International Journal of Environmental Research and Public Health, 19*(21), 14080. PMID: 36360992

Zhao, X., Sun, Y., Li, Y., Jia, N., & Xu, J. (2024). Applications of machine learning in real-time control systems: A review. *Measurement Science & Technology.*

Zhu, X., Rehman, K. U., Wang, B., & Shahzad, M. (2020). Modern soft-sensing modeling methods for fermentation processes. *Sensors (Basel), 20*(6), 1771. PMID: 32210053

Chapter 6
Automation and Advanced Control Systems in Bio-Manufacturing:
Ensuring Precision and Consistency

Vinay Jain
https://orcid.org/0000-0003-2186-3801
ShriRam College of Pharmacy, India

Aditya Yadav
https://orcid.org/0009-0005-2793-6276
Shri Ram College of Pharmacy, India

ABSTRACT

Effective monitoring and control of bioprocesses in the biotechnology and pharmaceutical sectors helps to maximize both biopharmaceutical manufacture and enzyme production of bio-based chemical outputs. Real-time tracking of significant elements including regulatory controls of temperature and pH and nutritional parameters with biomass concentration follows through regulatory controls. Modern technologies combining sensors, data analytics, automaton, ion, and data analysis improve yield, process efficiency, and product quality and maintenance. Through these techniques, nutraceuticals, food and beverage sectors as well as pharmaceuticals items have industrial-scale bioprocessing. Different sectors have developed to demand sophisticated process monitoring and control systems; so, enhanced process control becomes indispensable for maximizing yields and improving processes. Innovations in healthcare engineering such as automated living materials and stem cell production open new opportunities but also demand solutions to technological challenges and operational constraints.

DOI: 10.4018/979-8-3373-2873-7.ch006

INTRODUCTION

Background and Importance

Biomanufacturing, which is vital to the biotechnology and pharmaceutical industries, is evolving due to increased product quality, improved process efficiency, and stringent regulatory compliance. The production of complex biologics, such as monoclonal antibodies, vaccines, and gene therapies, may be hampered by the variability, scalability issues, and inefficiencies of traditional manufacturing processes, which are frequently manual and batch-based. To address these growing challenges, biomanufacturing environments are gradually incorporating automation and advanced control systems. Automation reduces human error, ensures repeatability, and boosts throughput, (Rathore & Winkle, 2009), while contemporary control systems enable real-time monitoring and dynamic adjustments to maintain critical quality attributes (CQAs) within acceptable bounds. These technologies, such as Process Analytical Technology (PAT) systems and Quality by Design (QbD) frameworks, are not only essential for ensuring product consistency, but they also aid in meeting regulatory requirements, (Kroll et al., 2017). The importance of automation and control is further highlighted by the rise of customized medicine and the increasing complexity of therapeutic products, which call for adaptable, scalable, and intelligent production systems, (Lee et al., 2020).

Objectives of the Chapter

This chapter's main goal is to look at how advanced control systems and automation could change modern biomanufacturing. The chapter's main goal is to stress how important it is to monitor and control important bioprocess parameters like temperature, pH, nutrient concentration, and biomass levels in real time, (FDA, 2004; Gronemeyer, Ditz, & Strube, 2014).

- Talk about how data analytics, sensor technologies, and automation make the processes of making biopharmaceuticals and enzymes more efficient, productive, and high-quality.
- See how advanced control measures help to make sure that regulatory standards are met by lowering the risk of contamination and lowering production costs, (FDA, 2004).
- Talk about new ideas in healthcare engineering that are being worked on right now, such as making stem cells and automated living materials, as well as the technical and operational problems they face.
- This chapter's goals are to give you a full understanding of the technological advances that are taking biomanufacturing to a new level of accuracy, consistency, and creativity.

Scope and Structure

Automation and advanced control systems are changing the biomanufacturing business in the pharmaceutical, nutraceutical, food, and beverage industries. This chapter goes into great detail about these changes. It deals with integrating real-time monitoring, smart data processing, and advanced feedback control systems into both upstream and downstream processes, (Gronemeyer, Ditz, & Strube, 2014).

The chapter is set up in the following divisions:

- Section 1: Key Technologies in Automation and Control talks about basic technologies like sensors, SCADA (Supervisor Control and Data Acquisition), DCS (Distributed Control Systems), robotics, and AI-driven analytics.
- Section 2: Implementation in Biomanufacturing-looks at how these technologies can be used in real-world bioprocessing, with case studies from a number of different industries.
- Section 3: Regulatory Compliance and Quality Assurance—Looks at models like Process Analytical Technology (PAT) and Quality by Design (QbD) to see how well they work with automated systems.
- Section 4: Challenges and Future Directions—Lists the problems that automation faces right now and talks about possible future developments, such as decision support based on artificial intelligence and automated stem cell production.
- Section 5: Conclusion-summarizes the main points and gives strategic advice to people looking for advanced biomanufacturing solutions. The chapter's goal is to help researchers, business leaders, and students fully understand how automation will affect the future of bioprocessing through this framework.

OVERVIEW OF THE BIOTECHNOLOGY AND PHARMACEUTICAL INDUSTRY

Growth and Trends in Biomanufacturing

Over the past 20 years, biomanufacturing, which is making therapeutic biological products using living systems, has grown a lot. The global biopharmaceutical market, which includes vaccines, monoclonal antibodies, and recombinant proteins, is expected to reach over USD 600 billion by 2030. This is because chronic diseases are becoming more common, people want personalized medicine, and molecular biology is making progress.

Key Trends Include:

- The rise of biosimilars was caused by the expiration of patents on popular biologics.
- More and more cost-effective and flexible single-use technology applications.
- Move toward constant manufacturing to make process control and scalability better.
- Using digital and AI-based tools to make decisions and improve processes These changes show that things are moving toward agile, data- driven, more efficient production systems that can meet both global demand and strict regulatory requirements, (Rathore & Winkle, 2009; Kroll et al., 2017; Lee et al., 2020; FDA, 2004; Walsh, 2018).

Challenges in Conventional Bioprocessing

Conventional bioprocessing is mostly done in batches and by hand, which makes it less efficient and harder to scale up:

- A lot of variation in the process: It's hard to keep things consistent from batch to batch because of the complexity of biology and the need for human intervention.

- Takes a lot of time and money: Old ways of doing things are slow, require a lot of human work, and cost a lot of money to run, especially when it comes to quality testing and compliance.
- Limited control in real time: Batch systems often put off fixing problems based on offline sampling, which makes deviations more likely.
- Problems with scaling up: Optimized processes that work well on a small scale usually can't keep up with performance on a commercial scale without a lot of reengineering, (Gronemeyer, Ditz, & Strube, 2014). These issues show that we need more modern ways of making things as products get more complicated and regulators stress Quality by Design (QbD).

Need for Automation and Advanced Control

In biomanufacturing, automation and better process control are becoming more and more important to meet the needs of the industry as they change and go beyond the limits of current methods.

Automation makes it possible to:

- Lower human error through consistent procedures;
- Improve operational efficiency and throughput.
- Data capture and electronic records have made it easier to track things and follow the rules, (EMA, 2020).
- Advanced control systems like Process Analytical Technology (PAT) and Model Predictive Control (MPC) let you watch important process parameters (CPRs) and quality characteristics (CQAs) in real time.
- Dynamic control of bioprocess parameters ensures the highest product quality and yields.
- Predictive insights allow for proactive decision-making through the use of artificial intelligence and machine learning ., (Rathore & Winkle, 2009).
- Automation and better control are not just new ideas; they are also necessary for modern, compliant, and competitive biomanufacturing. This is because regulatory agencies encourage the use of these technologies through programs like the FDA's PAT and Emerging Technology Programs.

Table 1. Comparison of conventional and automated biomanufacturing approaches

Feature	Conventional Manufacturing	Automated Biomanufacturing
Process Control	Manual/Semi-automated	Fully automated with real-time feedback
Data Management	Paper-based	Digitalized (e.g., SCADA, MES)
Error Rate	High	Low (due to minimal human intervention)
Scalability	Moderate	High (modular and flexible systems)
Regulatory Compliance	Manual documentation	Integrated electronic batch records

The contrast between conventional and automated approaches is summarized in this Table highlighting improvements in process control, scalability, and compliance, (Walsh, 2018).

Basic Ideas Behind Biomanufacturing Processes

Biomanufacturing is the foundation of modern biotechnology. It uses living cells and biological systems to make medicines, vaccines, diagnostics, and other useful biomolecules. The process is made up of a series of carefully planned steps that ensure that the final products are all the same, safe, and efficient. This chapter talks about the basics of biomanufacturing, such as upstream and downstream operations, Critical Quality Attributes (CQAs), process parameters, and the rules that govern the industry.

Processes that go Up and Down

There are usually two main steps in biomanufacturing: upstream processing and downstream processing. These steps are the most important parts of any biologics manufacturing system, and they must be perfectly tuned to make a high-quality product.

Processing Upstream

This phase includes all the steps needed to create and keep biological production systems, like cells from microbes, mammals, or insects. The main goal is to get the most out of the desired biomolecule while keeping the cells alive and reducing contamination.

Some of the most important parts are:

- Cell Line Development: Choosing and improving cell lines to make the target protein. For steady production, stable lines are better. This means using clonal selection and genetic engineering to add the gene you want.
- Media Optimization: The health and productivity of cells are greatly affected by the growth media. They have important nutrients, growth factors, amino acids, trace elements, and they can be based on serum or not. Optimizing media increases yield and lowers costs, (European Commission, 2015).
- Bioreactor Design and Operation: Bioreactors create controlled spaces for cells to grow. In real time, things like pH, temperature, oxygen, agitation, and feeding strategies are changed. People often use fed-batch and perfusion systems.
- Scale-Up: After optimizing on a small scale (like in shake flasks or bioreactors),
- The process is scaled up for industrial production, keeping the same quality and consistency from pilot to commercial volumes (hundreds to thousands of liters).
- Control of contamination: It is very important to keep viruses, bacteria, and fungi from getting into things. This includes keeping an eye on things, using filtered air, sterile parts, and cleanroom conditions.

Processing Downstream

This step is all about recovering, cleaning up, and making the product. Downstream processes are usually more complicated and expensive than upstream ones because they need to be very pure and get rid of all pollutants.

Key Steps Include:

- Harvesting: Centrifugation, depth filtration, or microfilament separation of biomass or cells from the culture media Harvesting for intracellular products disturbs cells.
- Cell Lysis (if required): Usually by mechanical (e.g., homogenization), chemical, or enzymatic techniques, breaking open the cells releases the intended product
- Initial Clarification: Eliminating insoluble components and cellular trash helps to ready the solution for more purification.
- **Purification**: This step involves multiple chromatographic techniques:
  - o Affinity Chromatography: Highly specific purification using ligand-resin systems, particularly effective for monoclonal antibodies.
  - o Ion Exchange Chromatography (IEX): Separates molecules based on charge differences.
  - o Size Exclusion Chromatography (SEC): Separates proteins based on size.
  - o Hydrophobic Interaction Chromatography (HIC): Useful for proteins with exposed hydrophobic regions.
- Polishing: Final purification techniques eliminate trace contaminants including DNA, endotoxins, host cell proteins (HCPs), or aggregates.
- Formulation and Filling: Before being aseptically filled into vials, syringes, or other administration forms, (Walsh, 2018, European Commission, 2015), the pure product is stabilized with appropriate excipients and adjusted for isotonicity, pH, and shelf-life.
- Reducing manufacturing costs, improving scalability, and guaranteeing regulatory compliance depend on effective integration of upstream and downstream operations, (Ghosh et al., 2020).

Critical Quality Attributes (CQAs) and Process Parameters

In biomanufacturing, maintaining product quality throughout the manufacturing process rather than only a last testing stage. Understanding and regulating the elements influencing Critical Quality Attributes (CQAs) helps one to emphasis developing quality into the process by Design (QbD), (Rathore & Winkle, 2009; Lang, Meyer, & Smith, 2020).

Critical Quality Attributes (CQAs)

To guarantee the intended product quality, CQAs—physical, chemical, biological, or microbiological traits—must be within set limits.

Common CQAs include:

- Purity: absence of other process-related pollutants, DNA, or host cell proteins.
- Potency: a metric of therapeutic product biological activity and efficacy.

- Identity: Verification of the product's intended biologic nature by molecular or analytical methods assures us of this.
- Sterility and Endotoxin Levels: Particularly important for parenteral formulations, when contamination can cause death, (Ghasemi & Behzadnia, 2018).
- Stability: The capacity of the product to keep safe and efficient over its shelf life.
- Aggregation and Glycosylation: Immunogenicity results from protein aggregation. Especially for monoclonal antibodies, glycosylation patterns influence bioavailability and effectiveness.
- Usually combining preclinical data, process knowledge, and risk analysis methodologies like Failure Mode and Effects Analysis (FMEA), CQA identification calls.
- Critical Process Parameters (CPPs)
- Variables like CPPs can influence CQAs, hence they need to be under control during manufacture. These consist among:
- Temperature: influences cell metabolism and enzyme activity. Protein expression and folding can be impacted by even minute changes.
- pH: kept under control by buffers or regulated additions. It influences enzymatic interactions, solubility, and product degradation.
- Dissolved Oxygen (DO): Crucially important for aerobic cell cultures. Gas mixes enriched in oxygen, sparging, and agitation help to control DO levels.
- Agitation Speed: Impacts shear tension, gas exchange, and mixing. While poor mixing might produce nutritional gradients, too strong shear can injure cells.
- Feeding Strategy: Nutrient feeds are tuned to avoid accumulation of harmful byproducts (such as lactate, ammonia) or depletion. QbD calls for defining a design space, a reasonable range for CPPs inside which product quality is guaranteed. Real-time monitoring of these factors made possible by advanced instruments like Process Analytical Technology (PAT) enables adaptive contro, (Ghosh et al., 2020; Lang, Meyer, & Smith, 2020).

Regulatory Framework and Compliance

Biomanufacturing is under strict rules considering the complexity and the hazards connected with biologics. Making sure all items are safe, efficient, and of great quality comes first, (Ghasemi & Behzadnia, 2018; Shukla & Thömmes, 2010).

Global Regulatory Bodies

- U.S. Food and Drug Administration (FDA): supervises both investigational and marketed biologics and enforces the Food, Drug, and Cosmetic Act.
- European Medicines Agency (EMA): coordinates EU medical product evaluation and monitoring of standards.
- World Health Organization (WHO): issues worldwide standards and rules, particularly for vaccinations and goods used in international health projects.
- International Council for Harmonisation (ICH): offers standardized rules based on ICH Q-series accepted in the USA, Japan, and Europe.

Key Regulatory Guidelines

- **Good Manufacturing Practices (GMP)**: Provides uniform guidelines grounded on ICH Q-series approved in Europe, Japan, and the USA.
- **ICH Guidelines**:
  - o **ICH Q8**: Encourages understanding product and process development.
  - o **ICH Q9**: Offers tools for quality risk management.
  - o **ICH Q10**: Describes a pharmaceutical quality system encompassing product lifecycle.

- **Good Manufacturing Practices (GMP)**: Provides uniform guidelines grounded on ICH Q-series approved in Europe, Japan, and the USA.
- **ICH Guidelines**:
  - o **ICH Q8**: Encourages understanding product and process development.
  - o **ICH Q9**: Offers tools for quality risk management.
  - o **ICH Q10**: Describes a pharmaceutical quality system encompassing product lifecycle.

- Biosafety Regulations: Include NIH Guidelines and local laws governing the containment and handling of biological agents.
- **Compliance Strategies**
- Process Validation: Comprises three stages—process design, process qualification, and continued process verification. It ensures that manufacturing processes consistently produce quality products.
- Analytical Method Validation: Demonstrates that testing methods are accurate, specific, precise, and robust.
- Documentation and Record-Keeping: Comprehensive documentation supports traceability and is often a focus of inspections. This includes batch production records, deviations, investigations, and corrective actions.
- Audits and Inspections: Regulatory authorities conduct pre-approval inspections and periodic audits. Internal audits are also critical for ongoing compliance and identifying potential issues.
- Change Control: Formal system for managing changes in manufacturing processes, equipment, or raw materials. Recent advances also include digital transformation through electronic batch records, automation, and real-time data monitoring, which support better regulatory compliance and facilitate continuous improvement, (Ghosh et al., 2020; Lang, Meer, & Smith, 2020; Ghasemi & Behzadnia, 2018; Shukla & Thömmes, 2010; Langer, 2015).

AUTOMATION IN BIOMANUFACTURING

Definition and Scope

In biomanufacturing, automation is the application of technology systems and machines to minimally humanly involved manufacturing operations. From upstream (e.g., cell culture and fermentation) to downstream (e.g., purification and formulation) procedures in the manufacturing of biological products including vaccines, monoclonal antibodies, and cell treatments, these processes cover all. Improvements in control systems, robotics, and digitalization have fundamentally changed the extent of automation used in biomanufacturing. Automation today not only improves production speed and uniformity but also supports real-time monitoring, lowers the danger of contamination, guarantees compliance with strict regulatory criteria, and enables scalable manufacturing, (European Commission, 2015). Among the several systems and tools automation covers are sensors, programmable logic controllers (PLCs), supervisory systems, and robotics. These components help data acquisition, process management, and analytics to be seamlessly integrated across biomanufacturing sites. Modern environments call for automation as a key enabler of smart biomanufacturing or "Biomanufacturing 4.0," a phrase consistent with Industry 4.0 ideas, therefore fostering real-time decision-making and adaptive production systems.

Key Automation Technologies

Figure 1. Hierarchical structure showing the integration of SCADA, DCS, PAT, and AI systems within biomanufacturing processes. The layered design demonstrates the transition from sensor-level data acquisition to enterprise-level decision-making platforms

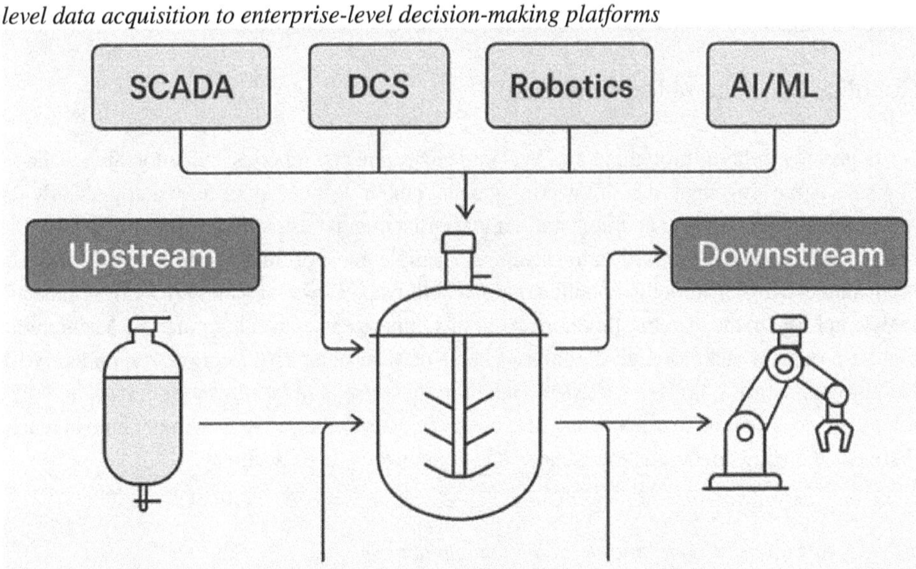

(Rathore & Saxena, 2023)

Supervisory Control and Data Acquisition (SCADA)

Monitoring and regulating biomanufacturing processes depend critically on SCADA systems. These systems gather real-time data from sensors and equipment spread around the facility, therefore offering centralized control. All of which are vital for preserving ideal conditions in bioprocessing, SCADA systems let operators monitor key parameters including temperature, pH, dissolved oxygen, and agitation speed. Users of SCADA interfaces may create reports, raise alarms for out-of-spec circumstances, and see process trends. Modern SCADA systems also provide data historizing, cloud integration, and remote access, thereby supporting predictive maintenance and quality assurance. In mammalian cell culture systems, for example, SCADA systems can dynamically change aeration and nutrient delivery depending on sensor feedback, therefore guaranteeing a stable environment fit for high cell viability and productivity.

Distributed Control Systems (DCS)

With control elements spread over several subsystems, distributed control systems offer a more dispersed method of automation. Large-scale biomanufacturing plants, where several bioreactors, purification skids, and support utilities run concurrently, benefit greatly from DCS designs. Managing particular facets of the production process, each DCS node or controller interacts with a central supervisory system. This flexibility lets unit operations be independently scaled and increases fault tolerance. Often combined with Manufacturing Execution Systems (MES) and Enterprise Resource Planning (ERP) systems, DCS systems help to create a seamless information flow from the shop floor to corporate level decision-making. DCS can guarantee strict control over parameters over several unit processes in continuous biomanufacturing systems, hence minimizing batch-to- batch variability, (Rathore & Saxena, 2023).

Robotics and Automated Equipment

Especially in high-throughput and hygienic environments, robotics and automated technology have a transforming effect in lowering manual labour. Robots are utilized automatically for media preparation, reagent addition, and sample collecting in upstream operations. They handle chores like column packing, filtration setup, and sample transport in downstream processing. In biomanufacturing cleanrooms, robotic arms and automated guided vehicles (AGVs) are increasingly employed to move items, therefore avoiding human-generated contamination. Maintaining regular processes and thorough digital logs helps these systems also improve compliance with Good Manufacturing Practices (GMP). One prominent use is in fill-finish processes, in which robotic devices guarantee exact filling of syringes or vials and apply seals without human touch, therefore reducing contamination hazards and guaranteeing dose accuracy.

Table 2. Key automation technologies in biomanufacturing

Technology	Functionality	Applications in Biomanufacturing
SCADA	Real-time process monitoring and centralized control	Monitoring bioreactors and utilities
DCS	Distributed real-time control of unit operations	Integrated control in continuous production
Robotics	Automated handling of materials and aseptic operations	Fill-finish, media preparation
PAT	In-line and real-time quality attribute monitoring	Real-time release testing (RTRT)
AI/ML	Predictive analytics, anomaly detection	Yield prediction, process optimization

This table shows Key technologies in Automation in Bio-manufacturing, (Lang, Meyer, & Smith, 2020).

Benefits and Impact on Manufacturing

Integration of automation technology in biomanufacturing offers many advantages that together improve the regulatory compliance, scalability, and production process resilience.

Here are some impactful benefits -

Improved Process Consistency and Quality

By standardizing running processes and lowering manual interventions, automation lowers human error. Tight control of process variables made possible by real-time data collecting and feedback control guarantees homogeneous batch product quality. In biomanufacturing, where small variations in pH, temperature, or oxygen levels can greatly impact production and product properties, this is particularly critical.

Enhanced Scalability and Throughput

From pilot to commercial size, automation lets processes be smoothly scaled. DCS and SCADA are modular and flexible control systems that help to incorporate additional unit functions without completely revamping the infrastructure. Faster development cycles and lower time-to--market are achieved in part via high-throughput screening, robotic medium preparation, and automated inoculation systems.

Reduced Operational Costs

Although the initial outlay in automation technology can be significant, over time lower labour expenses, less material waste, and lower utility usage will pay off. By means of real-time monitoring, automation also promotes predictive maintenance, therefore preventing unplanned downtime and expensive repairs.

Regulatory Compliance and Data Integrity

Automation systems help one comply with rules established by organizations as the FDA and EMA. Essential for regulatory filings and inspections, data is complete, consistent, and correct thanks in part to features such electronic batch records, audit trails, and alert management. Often including 21 CFR Part 11 compliance elements, SCADA and DCS systems fit GMP environments.

Support for Continuous Manufacturing and PAT

Real-time analysis and control in Process Analytical Technology (PAT) systems mostly depends on automation. Advanced analytics combined with sensors helps to continuously monitor important quality attributes (CQAs), hence supporting flexible process control techniques. This provides the basis for ongoing manufacturing, which provides more solid supply chains, faster reaction to demand changes, and improved resource economy.

ADVANCED CONTROL SYSTEMS IN BIOMANUFACTURING

Advanced control systems that improve precision, consistency, and efficiency have fundamentally changed biomanufacturing. Real-time monitoring and management of important processes made possible by these technologies guarantees product quality and regulatory compliance by themselves. Key advanced control systems-process analytical technology (PAT), model predictive control (MPC), artificial intelligence and machine learning (AI/ML), and their interaction with digital manufacturing systems-are discussed in this chapter.

Process Analytical Technology (PAT)

By means of timely measurements of important quality and performance traits of raw and in-process materials, Process Analytical Technology (PAT) is a tool for designing, assessing, and managing manufacturing. It complements the Quality by Design (QbD) paradigm pushed by regulatory bodies such as the FDA and helps to enable real-time quality assurance. PAT instruments comprise spectroscopic techniques (e.g., NIR, Raman, UV-Vis), chemometric models, multivariate data analysis (MVDA), and real-time sensors. These instruments let biomanufacturers real-time monitor important quality characteristics (CQAs) and essential process parameters (CPRs). In upstream bioprocesses, for example, PAT lets real-time monitor variables including pH, dissolved oxygen, glucose levels, and biomass concentration. By means of PAT, batch variability is lowered, process understanding is enhanced, and dependency on end-product testing is minimized. Integration of PAT into bioprocesses allows producers to take a proactive approach to process control, therefore guaranteeing constant quality and regulatory compliance, (FDA, 2004; Rathore & Jesubalan, 2022).

Model Predictive Control (MPC)

An advanced process control method called model predictive control (MPC) optimizes control operations by using dynamic models to forecast future process behaviour. In biomanufacturing, MPC provides a strong method for controlling intricate, multivariable processes under time limits and limitations, (FDA, 2006). MPC's capacity to employ real-time data and predictive models to ascertain ideal control inputs while considering operational restrictions and process disruptions defines its main strength. In bioprocesses as fermentation, where several interacting factors affect output and product quality, (Ghasemi & Behzadnia, 2018), MPC is very useful. In biomanufacturing, MPC calls for the construction of precise process models based on either hybrid techniques, empirical data, or first-principles. These models enable the controller to foresee process results and modify inputs, hence preserving stability and performance even with variation. Moreover, compatible with PAT tools, MPC allows dynamic control depending on real-time measurements. For example, MPC can help to maximize glucose feeding in a fed-batch culture so preserving goal growth rates and product titers.

Artificial Intelligence and Machine Learning Applications

By allowing data-driven decisions and process optimization, artificial intelligence (AI) and machine learning (ML) are revolutionizing biomanufacturing. These systems build prediction models and sophisticated control techniques using vast amounts of historical and real-time data, (EMA, 2020). Support vector machines (SVM), random forests, neural networks, and deep learning models are applied in bioprocessing for problems including:

- Forecasting bioreactor performance and product production.
- spotting anomalies and process deviations.
- improving medium composition and process parameters.
- increasing equipment predictive maintenance

By analysing data from several sources—PAT tools, sensors, previous batch records—AI/ML systems can find trends and correlations do not clear from conventional analysis. These realizations support speedier troubleshooting and proactive control plans, (Yin et al., 2021). Furthermore, under investigation are adaptive control techniques and reinforcement learning to create self-learning bioprocess systems able to independently modify operations to satisfy performance criteria and quality requirements. Integration of AI/ML requires proper data infrastructure, including data lakes, cloud computing, and secure data pipelines to ensure availability, integrity, and privacy of manufacturing data.

Integration with Digital Manufacturing

Digital manufacturing is the application of digital technologies to produce a virtual manufacturing model. Digital manufacturing offers a foundation for real-time monitoring, modelling, and bioprocessing optimization when coupled with sophisticated control systems, (Levine et al., 2019).

Technologies central to digital manufacturing include:

- Digital twins
- Industrial Internet of Things (IIoT)
- Cloud computing and big data analytics
- Manufacturing Execution Systems (MES)
- Enterprise Resource Planning (ERP)

A digital twin is a virtual replica of a real-time, operational condition, performance-oriented physical bioprocess reflecting its state. Coupling digital twins with PAT and MPC enables predictive analytics, proactive maintenance, and ongoing development, (Lang, Meyer, & Smith, 2020).

While cloud platforms support scalable data storage and advanced analytics, IIoT lets equipment, sensors, and control systems communicate seamlessly. Systems for MES and ERP offer integration across compliance, supply chains, manufacturing, and quality.

Combining artificial intelligence/machine learning, PAT, and MPC with digital manufacturing produces an intelligent, flexible, resilient whole biomanufacturing ecosystem. This confluence helps the biopharmaceutical sector's Industry 4.0 goal come to pass.

CASE STUDIES AND INDUSTRIAL APPLICATIONS

Real-world case studies enable one to more value the effective application of modern control systems in biomanufacturing. Companies in the pharmaceutical and biotechnology industries have used technologies such Process Analytical Technology (PAT), Model Predictive Control (MPC), Artificial Intelligence (AI), and Machine Learning (ML) to increase production, compliance, and product quality. Emphasizing Amgen, Genentech, and other trailblazing companies that have successfully implemented these technologies into their manufacturing processes, this chapter provides a comprehensive and broad analysis of various important industrial applications.

Amgen: Next-Generation Biomanufacturing

Amgen's Next-Generation Biomanufacturing (NGB) facility in Singapore is one amazing illustration of how clever control systems may change biomanufacturing techniques. Opening in 2014, this structure highlights adaptability, digital innovation, and embrace of cutting-edge technologies, (Hosinski, 2022).

Key Innovations and Technologies:

- Modular and Single-Use Systems: Using modular, flexible cleanroom pods and single-use bioreactor technology, Amgen's plant Eliminating the need for complex cleaning validation processes lets these technologies turn around manufacturing batches quickly.
- Model Predictive Control (MPC): In bioprocessing, MPC guarantees best nutritional availability in fed-batch systems. It projects system behaviours using mathematical models, therefore enhancing the control of significant process parameters (CPPs).
- Real-Time PAT Integration: Combining Raman spectroscopy and Near-Infrared (NIR) gives spectroscopic-based PAT equipment real-time detection of metabolites, viable cell density, and significant medium components.
- Data Analytics, AI, and Machine Learning: Advanced data analytics provide predictive maintenance, process anomaly detection, and real-time modifications to enhance output of production, (Bakeev, 2010).

Operational Advantages:

- Efficiency Gains: Comparatively to conventional production, the facility reduced its footprint by 75% and its running expenses by roughly 50%.
- Sustainability Improvements: Smart facility design and single-use solutions' adoption help to save water and energy consumption.
- Regulatory Alignment: The data-driven control system and real-time monitoring help to enable improved FDA and EMA regulatory framework compliance.

Genentech: Real-Time Monitoring with PAT

Now a member of Roche Group, Genentech has long been known for innovatively using PAT in mass biopharmaceutical production. Genentech changed the way bioprocesses were managed and optimised by including sophisticated monitoring technology, (Qin & Badgwell, 2003).

PAT Strategies Implemented:

- Raman Spectroscopy and NIR: - Designed for ongoing, non-invasive bioreactors' essential analyte measurements-glucose, lactate, ammonia, and viable cell density.
- Multivariate Data Analysis (MVDA): Using past data, MVDA models are constructed to forecast and regulate product quality parameters including glycosylation patterns, charge variations, and aggregation, (Camacho & Bordons, 2007).
- Automated Feedback Control Systems: MVDA models are built from prior data to forecast and control product quality factors including glycosylation patterns, charge changes, and aggregation, (Camacho & Bordons, 2007).
- Enhanced Product Consistency: Higher batch-to- batch consistency-which is vital for therapeutic proteins-was obtained by Genentech by constant monitoring CPPs and CQAs.
- Decreased Batch Failures: Early process deviation identification helped to lower the batch failure rate and related economic loss rate.
- Faster Process Development: Faster creation of strong processes during scale-up made possible by PAT technologies greatly reduces time to market for novel treatments.
- Real-World Applications: Genentech used Raman-based PAT to automatically adjust feed methods in commercial mAb manufacturing, therefore enhancing cell viability and final titer by up to 20%.

Other Notable Examples

Advanced control systems have also been effectively included into operations of several other biopharmaceutical enterprises.

Pfizer

Digitalisation in Manufacturing of COVID-19 Vaccine Accelerated production of the BNT162b2 COVID-19 vaccination by Pfizer presents a historic case of digital manufacturing excellence:

Digital Twin Technologies

Using digital twin models, Pfizer simulated manufacturing techniques, therefore optimising production parameters without interfering with current operations.

- AI and Predictive Analytics: Advanced algorithms controlled worldwide supply chains, inventory, and expected supply concerns.
- IoT and PAT: I Real-time tracking of temperature, pressure, and product quality throughout manufacturing and cold chain logistics made possible by integration of IoT sensors.

Impact

With these projects, Pfizer was able to reach an unheard-of scale-up and generate billions of doses in eighteen months, (Camacho & Bordons, 2007; Ghosh et al., 2020).

Biogen

MPC in Monoclonal Antibody Manufacturing Biogen has been a leader in adopting MPC and PAT to streamline mAb production:

- Real-Time Adaptive Control: Oxygen uptake rate (OUR) and biomass concentration were used to adjust feed rates dynamically, maintaining optimal growth conditions.
- Yield Improvement: Implementation of MPC improved final product yield by approximately 15% compared to traditional control methods.
- Process Robustness: Reduced intra-batch and inter-batch variability during scale-up, (Lee et al., 2015).
- Merck & Co.: MES and PAT Integration for Digital Manufacturing Merck's "Digitally Enabled Manufacturing" initiative epitomizes the fusion of Manufacturing Execution Systems (MES), Enterprise Resource Planning (ERP), and PAT:
- Real-Time Process Monitoring: MES platforms provided operators with real-time dashboards showing process health indicators sourced from PAT systems.
- Closed-Loop Manufacturing: Automated closed-loop controls adjusted critical process parameters in real-time based on PAT data streams.
- Compliance and Traceability: Integrated systems ensured data integrity, enhanced traceability, and compliance with regulatory demands such as FDA's 21 CFR Part 11, (Levine et al., 2019; Srai et al., 2020).
- GSK: Use of AI in Vaccine Production GlaxoSmithKline (GSK) has successfully employed AI and ML algorithms to enhance vaccine manufacturing:
- Predictive Quality Assurance: AI models predict potential deviations in production well before they occur, enabling proactive interventions.
- Automation of Process Development: Machine learning tools automatically screen cell lines and optimize growth media, significantly reducing the time needed for process development, (Tao et al., 2019).
- Sanofi: Continuous Bioprocessing and PAT Sanofi's Framingham facility represents a leading example of continuous bioprocessing supported by PAT:
- Continuous Perfusion Systems: Continuous monitoring of CPPs allowed automatic adjustment of perfusion rates.
- Real-Time Release Testing (RTRT): Integrated PAT systems enabled real-time product release decisions, cutting down traditional QC testing timelines, (Amgen, 2021).

CHALLENGES AND LIMITATIONS

Although the use of sophisticated control systems in biomanufacturing offers many advantages in compliance, uniformity, and efficiency, businesses still have to negotiate certain difficulties. One can classify these difficulties mostly into technological constraints and expenses, personnel and skill needs, and data management and cybersecurity hazards. Every one of these domains reflects important factors influencing the scalability, dependability, and regulatory fit of these advanced systems.

Technological Barriers and Costs

One of the biggest problems with modern control systems is that they are very complicated and cost a lot of money. These systems often need complicated hardware, the ability to work with multiple software platforms, and a lot of testing, which raises both operational (OPEX) and capital (CAPEX) costs. To use PAT, MPC, AI, or ML, you need to spend a lot of money up front on spectroscopic sensors, data processing units, and automation infrastructure. Also, the cost goes up because of the software development needed for real-time monitoring and predictive control. Small and medium-sized businesses (SMEs) might not be able to afford these costs, which makes it harder for them to get access, (Walsh, 2018).

System integration problems: Advanced control systems need to work together smoothly across platforms like Enterprise Resource Planning (ERP), Distributed Control Systems (DCS), and Manufacturing Execution Systems (MES). It is hard and takes a lot of resources to make things work together, especially with old infrastructure, (FDA, 2004). Another problem is scalability, especially when moving from pilot to full-scale production. Some methods work well in the lab, but when they are used on a large scale, they often have problems like sensors not being accurate, feedback taking too long, and data lagging, (Kewaunee International Group, 2023).

Regulatory frameworks like FDA's 21 CFR Part 11 or EMA's Annex 11 also require strict validation and qualification before new technologies can be used. Good Automated Manufacturing Practice (GAMP) says that each system must follow certain rules, which means longer timelines and more paperwork.

Workforce and Skill Requirements

Adopting these technologies is greatly hampered by the dearth of qualified experts with multidisciplinary knowledge spanning biotechnology, control engineering, computer science, and data analytics, (Pfizer, 2021). Conventional pharmaceutical education courses mostly stress chemistry and biology, paying no attention to control theory, automation, or software integration. Consequently, the present workforce lacks the necessary skills to implement and maintain modern control systems, (Biogen, 2020). Effective application calls for those who grasp both the operational logic of control systems and the biological features of the process. Developing and testing a Raman-based PAT model, for instance, calls for process engineering, spectroscopy, and chemometrics, (Merck & Co., 2019). Companies must heavily commit in ongoing education and training initiatives to equip employees with fresh skills. Though they demand long-term commitment, initiatives such industry-academia partnership, certifications from companies like ISPE, and digital simulation platforms assist close the skills gap. Many companies, particularly those with established processes, may have cultural opposition to implementing automated and artificial intelligence-driven systems. Clear explanation of the advantages and progressive adoption plans including operators in the transformation process will help one overcome this.

Data Management and Cybersecurity

As biomanufacturing moves to data-rich environments, the volume, variety, and speed of process data make it harder to manage data, keep it safe, and follow the rules. Advanced control systems make large databases that include sensor readings at high frequencies, control loop data, and metadata from software platforms, (Acharya, 2025). To handle such large amounts of data, you need storage solutions that are strong, scalable, redundant, and always available.

Integrity of Data and Traceability

Pharmaceutical manufacturing needs data that is correct, can be traced, and can be audited. Audit trails, secure access controls, and system validation are all ways to make sure that data is correct. If you don't do this right, you could face legal penalties, recalls, or not following the rules, (GSK, 2021).

Combining IoT, cloud computing, and networked control systems makes cybersecurity much worse. This includes stealing intellectual property, ransomware, and getting into systems without permission. The U.S. Department of Health and Human Services (HHS) (Sanofi, 2020) says that cyber threats have been on the rise in the pharmaceutical industry for the past ten years. Regulators now want businesses to include specific cybersecurity plans in their Quality Management Systems (QMS). FDA guidelines on cybersecurity in the making of medical devices are also having a big impact on what drug companies expect.

Mitigation Strategies

Firewall implementation, MFA multi-factor authentication, and encryption methods application. Security Information and Event Management (SIEM) systems enable real-time system log and network activity monitoring.

Regular audits, penetration testing, staff cybersecurity training.

Another difficulty is the absence of standardising in data formats among many equipment and programs. This compromises interoperability and results in data analysis and decision-making inefficiencies. Open data standards like OPC-UA (Rathore, 2009) (Open Platform Communications-Unified Architecture) can assist solve these issues but demand industry-wide cooperation.

FUTURE TRENDS AND OPPORTUNITIES

As biomanufacturing develops, the incorporation of innovative technologies is determining its course forward. Transformational change is being facilitated by new paradigms including Smart Biomanufacturing under the Industry 4.0 umbrella, the use of Digital Twins, and regulatory advancements promoting automation. These potential developments are discussed in this chapter together with the chances they bring for the biomanufacturing industry.

Smart Biomanufacturing and Industry 4.0

Smart biomanufacturing is the application of advanced sensors, data analytics, cyber-physical systems, and autonomous control systems to real-time optimisation and automation of bioprocesses. Industry 4.0 ideas, which stress connection, data-driven decision-making, and system-wide integration (GAMP 5, 2022) greatly impact it.

Key Technologies

The Internet of Things (IoT) is based on collecting data in real time from connected sensors and devices. Big data analytics is the process of looking at large datasets in a systematic way to find useful information, (Davis, 2023). AI and machine learning (ML) make it possible to do things like predictive maintenance, finding problems, and adaptive control. Cloud computing lets you store, process, and work together on data from afar. 3D printing and additive manufacturing have the potential to make personalized medicine and custom bioreactor parts.

Effect on Biomanufacturing

Smart biomanufacturing can greatly improve process control, lower production variability, and raise the quality of the products. For example, Pfizer has used AI to test smart bioprocessing systems that can change the conditions of fermentation on the fly, increasing output by up to 15%, (Narayanan et al., 2021).

Collaboration between ecosystems is important for smart biomanufacturing in the future. More and more, biomanufacturers work with universities and tech companies to come up with new ideas together. The U.S. Department of Defense supports programs like BioFabUSA that speed up smart manufacturing by sharing knowledge and funding pilot projects, (ISPE, 2020).

For smart systems to work well, there need to be global standards for sharing data and making systems work together. Using protocols like OPC UA (Open Platform Communications Unified Architecture) makes it easier for equipment and software to work together all over the world.

Smart biomanufacturing has a lot of potential, but it also has some problems that make it hard to adopt. These include getting the right regulatory approvals, making sure that data can be shared between systems, and protecting against cyberattacks.

Digital Twins and Predictive Modelling

Digital twins are virtual copies of a physical bioprocess or manufacturing system updated in real-time depending on sensor data. It lets companies replicate, forecast, and maximise processes without interfering with real-world output, (FDA, 2018; OPC Foundation, 2021).

Parts of Digital Twins

Data Acquisition Layer: gathers sensor real-time data.

Layer of modelling combines data-driven and physics-based models, (FDA, 2018).

Analytics Layer: Via simulations and optimisations offers practical insights.

Figure 2. Schematic showing a digital twin model in biomanufacturing. It integrates real-time data input, predictive modelling, and feedback control loops to optimize fermentation and purification processes

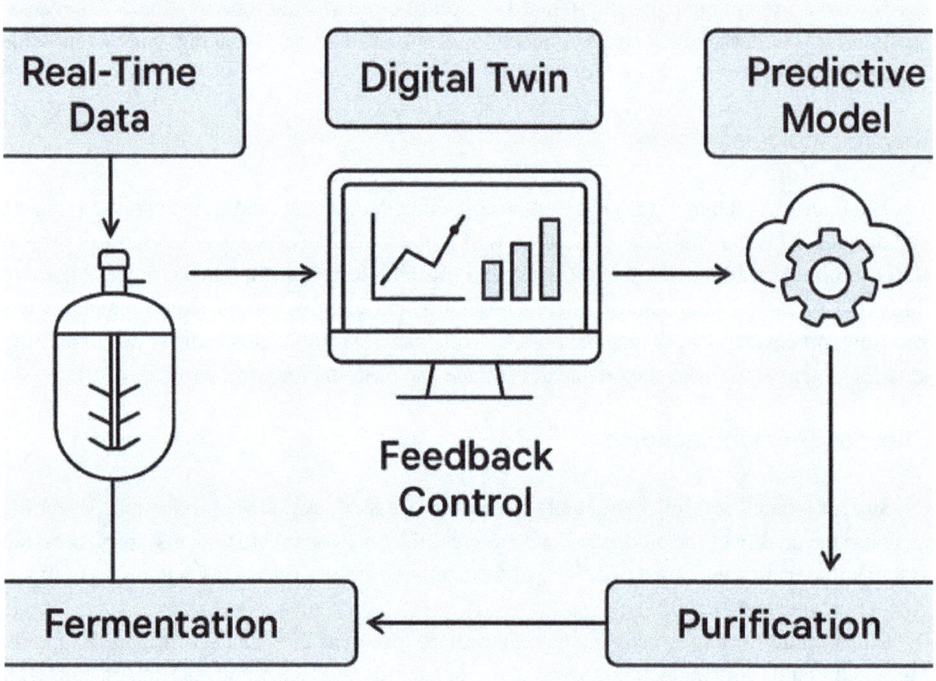

(Tao et al., 2018)

Applications in Biomanufacturing

Predictive models help to find ideal running conditions for processes. Digital twins help to forecast equipment breakdown before they happen, hence lowering downtime, (OPC Foundation, 2021).

Operators can be taught on virtual systems prior to working on live systems. Design of Experiments (DoE): Virtual experimentation employing Digital Twins lowers the requirement for physical experimentation, therefore saving time and money and strengthening data robustness, (Ramaswamy et al., 2020).

Digital twins track system behaviour over time and enable traceability of deviations, maintenance requirements, and performance trends thereby supporting lifecycle management. This long-term awareness enables more intelligent choices about capacity increases and improvements.

Case Studies

Digital twins for vaccine manufacture allow GSK to replicate scale-up from lab to production level, hence drastically lowering tech transfer delays.

Biogen uses predictive algorithms to maximise monoclonal antibody generation, therefore lowering costs and improving quality of output.

Creating correct Digital Twins calls both dependability from many sources and great topic knowledge. Furthermore, computational resource needs can be really high.

Regulatory Innovations Supporting Automation

Regulatory authorities are progressively in favour of the move towards data-driven, automated manufacturing. Globally, ideas like Quality by Design (QbD), continuous manufacturing, and real-time release testing (RTRT) are underlined, (Lee et al., 2018; HHS, 2022).

Key Regulatory Initiatives

Emerging Technology Program (ETP) of FDA helps companies implementing new technology, (HHS, 2022).

The EMA Guideline on PAT promotes integration of analytical technology for improved process understanding and control.

The ICH Q13 Guideline offers a structure for ongoing pharmaceutical manufacture, (Lee, Bagheri, & Kao, 2015). Advantages of Regulatory Innovation.

Enhanced Approvals

Faster decisions and approvals can result from real-time data. Automation and advanced analytics help to lower human error, hence supporting data integrity standards.

Constant quality is guaranteed by means of feedback loops and ongoing monitoring, (BioFab-USA, 2021). Globally harmonisation of automated process standards is being given top priority as regulatory bodies such the FDA, EMA, and PMDA (Japan) co-operate more and more. This helps businesses to simplify filings to several markets.

Regulatory Sandboxes and Try Beds

Agencies are increasingly looking at the use of regulatory "sandboxes"-safe settings where businesses may try new technologies under guided control, therefore enabling innovation without the immediate risk of non-compliance. These sandboxes let authorities better grasp novel tools before official approval routes are set by means of real-time feedback, (Pfizer, 2021).

Regulatory Compliance Challenges

Companies must negotiate rigorous validation, plenty of documentation, and changing expectations even while regulatory authorities are increasingly receptive to creativity. Particularly regarding validation of AI models, authorities demand openness and explainability, therefore posing a yet unresolved issue. Prospects for Cooperation: Initiatives like the National Institute for Innovation in Manufacturing Biopharmaceuticals (NIIMBL) and public-private partnerships (e.g., BioPharma Operations Group) offer venues for businesses to cooperatively collaborate on regulatory scientific issues, (BioFabUSA, 2021).

SUSTAINABILITY AND GREEN BIOMANUFACTURING

Biomanufacturing, which uses live cells or enzymes to make biologics and other products, has changed the pharmaceutical and biotechnology industries. But its effect on the environment, especially when it comes to waste, resource use, and energy use, is becoming more and more of a worry. As more and more people around the world become aware of climate change, environmental damage, and the depletion of non-renewable resources, the industry is under more and more pressure to adopt sustainable practices that protect the environment while ensuring long-term viability.

In biomanufacturing, sustainability means being socially, financially, and environmentally responsible throughout the entire production process, from getting raw materials to shipping and throwing away products. Green biomanufacturing focuses on using resources wisely, cutting down on emissions, using renewable inputs, and following the principles of a circular economy. These are in line with the United Nations' Sustainable Development Goals (SDGs), especially SDG 12 (Responsible Consumption and Production) and SDG 13 (Climate Action), (FDA, 2004).

Companies now know that being environmentally friendly is not only the right thing to do, but it is also good for business. It can help save money, lower risks, come up with new ideas, and improve the reputation of your brand. This chapter talks about important sustainability issues in biomanufacturing, such as ways to lower the carbon footprint, use less energy, and recycle waste.

Reducing Carbon Footprint in Bioprocessing

Carbon Footprint in Biomanufacturing

Introduction Biomanufacturing's carbon footprint consists in greenhouse gas (GHG) emissions from energy consumption, raw material use, transportation, and waste disposal all through the product lifetime. Although biotechnology is sometimes considered as a greener substitute for petrochemical-based manufacturing, the energy-intensive character of bioreactors, fermentation techniques, and downstream purifying operations can cause major carbon emissions. Emissions Sources of Carbon In bioprocessing, key sources of emissions include:

- Energy use for temperature regulation, aeration, and agitation.
- In sterilization-in-place (SIP) and cleaning-in-place (CIP) systems, steam and cold-water usage.
- Using solvents and feedstocks derived from fossils in cell culture medium and purification
- Cold chain logistical biopharmaceutical transportation emissions.

According to a Biogen analysis, almost 80% of operational carbon emissions in monoclonal antibody manufacture came from facility energy use, (Pfizer, 2021). Approaches for Minimising

Carbon Footprint Process Optimisation Main levers to lower resource use and waste are raising yields and lowering batch failures. By removing the resource loss and downtime related with batch manufacturing, adoption of continuous bioprocessing can improve efficiency. Renewable Energy Use To run their biomanufacturing plants, many top pharmaceutical companies are moving to solar, wind, and biomass-based energy sources. Amgen's Singapore facility, for example, depends less on the grid since solar energy powers it in part. Carbon Accounting and Lifecycle Analysis (LCA), LCA tools find hotspots in the carbon lifetime of a product. SimaPro and GaBi let firms model cradle-to-grave carbon footprints and apply focused reductions. Digitalisation and artificial intelligence Digital twins and predictive analytics assist to maximise energy consumption and lower waste. Real-time data from SCADA systems, for instance, can point up HVAC or CIP cycle inefficiencies.

Energy-Efficient Technologies in Biomanufacturing

Biomanufacturing uses a lot of energy for things like HVAC systems, sterilization methods, and bioreactor operation. Companies are using energy-efficient technologies to lower their costs and the damage they do to the environment. HVAC systems can use up to 65% of all the energy used, especially in cleanrooms. Variable Air Volume (VAV), demand-controlled ventilation, and Energy Recovery Ventilation (ERV) are examples of advanced control strategies that keep airflow and temperature at their best while still following the rules. Integration with Building Management Systems (BMS) makes control and efficiency even better.

Cleaning and sterilizing in a way that saves energy: Traditional SIP and CIP processes use a lot of resources. New technologies like microwave-assisted sterilization and ozonated water for CIP cut down on the need for heat and chemicals. Cleaning products that use enzymes and work at room temperature also use less hot water and energy.

New bioreactors use less energy to mix things and have better insulation. Single-use bioreactors (SUBs) don't need to be steam sterilized and are easier to clean, which saves 20–30% energy. Model Predictive Control (MPC) lets you optimize aeration and agitation in real time.

Heat Recovery and Integration

Using thermal loops, steam recovery, and heat exchangers to capture heat from exhaust or fermentation lowers overall energy use. Biogen and Roche have saved 10–15% each year by using waste heat recovery in their European facilities.

Waste Management and Circular Economy Approaches

Biomanufacturing waste covers biomass, used media, single-use system plastics, solvents, and packaging materials. Environmentally damaging and expensive are conventional disposal techniques include incineration or landfill. Ideas of the circular economy seek to minimise, recycle, and reuse resources all through the product life.

Waste Types Used in Biomanufacturing

- Biological waste: contaminated cultures, cell trash, biomass.

- Chemical waste: cleaners, buffers, and solvents.
- Plastic trash includes single-use bioreactor bags, filters, and tubing.

Cardboard, foam, and dry ice are examples of waste from packaging and shipping that harms the environment.

Biomass Value-Adding

Microbial or cell culture biomass that has already been used and is often thrown away can be anaerobically digested to make useful things like animal feed, biofertilizers, or biogas. This lowers the cost of disposal and helps keep energy in a circle.

Recycling and Using Single-Use Systems Again:

Single-use technologies use less water and energy, but they also make a lot of plastic waste. Companies now work together with recyclers to Collect and recycle plastic film and tubing using machines Use pyrolysis and other thermochemical methods to turn plastic trash into energy. In some countries, Millipore Sigma has started a recycling program that makes a closed-loop supply chain for its single-use systems. Using green solvents (like ethanol and supercritical CO_2) and setting up distillation units makes solvent-heavy downstream processes more environmentally friendly. Novo Nordisk was able to recover 80% of the solvent used in making insulin by using multi-stage distillation and adsorption. Planning for Circularity: Including end-of-life factors in the design of equipment and facilities helps with recycling and reuse. You can use modular equipment for different things, and packaging that can be recycled or broken down into natural materials cuts down on trash in landfills. ISO 14001-certified Environmental Management Systems (EMS) encourage ongoing progress in reducing waste and designing things that last, (OPC Foundation, 2021; Ramaswamy et al., 2020; Lee et al., 2018; HHS, 2022; Lee, Bagheri, & Kao, 2015; BioFabUSA, 2021).

CONCLUSION

Summary of Key Points

The Technological Change in Biomanufacturing Automated systems and advanced controls are changing the way things are made in biotechnology and pharmaceuticals. The shift is from manual, batch-based processes to integrated, intelligent, and continuous operations. This is because people want things to be more efficient, of higher quality, able to grow, follow rules, and be good for the environment.

The Biomanufacturing Landscape and Its Problems

The industry is growing because of more health needs and biologics like monoclonal antibodies, gene therapies, and vaccines. But traditional biomanufacturing has high costs, batch variability, long lead times, and a need for skilled workers. Regulatory requirements for quality and consistency make real-time monitoring and strong process control even more important, (GSK, 2022).

What Automation Does Automation helps make sure that things are done the same way every time, reduces mistakes, and helps with following the rules. Key technologies are: • SCADA, which lets you control everything from one place and keep track of data.

- DCS lets you control operations from different places but still keep them all in sync.
- Robotics makes it easier to handle materials, package them, and process them in a sterile way, (FDA, 2017).

When used together, these technologies make biomanufacturing environments safer and more efficient. Advanced Control and Optimization in Real Time Today's systems use:

- PAT lets you check the quality of something while it's being made with sensors and chemometric models.
- MPC controls more than one variable at a time to keep things from going wrong.
- AI/ML finds patterns in data to improve things, find problems, and plan maintenance ahead of time.

These make it possible to control things in real time and adaptively, which means less testing of the final product.

Adoption by the Industry

Amgen and Genentech's case studies show how these drugs can help people in the real world. Amgen's next-generation biomanufacturing (NGB) uses modular, continuous platforms to speed up product release and cut down on energy and water use, (Tao et al., 2018). Genentech uses real-time PAT to make things more consistent and cut down on mistakes, showing that automation is a useful and effective answer.

Things to Think About When it Comes to Regulations

Automation helps meet the standards set by the FDA, EMA, and ICH. It makes it easier to find things and validate them. The FDA's "Pharmaceutical Quality for the 21st Century" program encourages innovation by supporting PAT and QbD, (Fuller et al., 2020). Digital tools make sure that records are safe and ready for an audit under 21 CFR Part 11.

Problems and Limitations

Smart biomanufacturing has a lot of potential, but it also has a lot of problems to deal with, such as: • High costs of implementation • Outdated legacy systems • Lack of skills in automation and data science • Cybersecurity threats

To deal with these, you need to make smart investments, build up your IT infrastructure, and train your workers.

The Road Ahead in Automated Biomanufacturing

Biomanufacturing is clearly moving toward models that are smarter, more flexible, and more sustainable. New technologies, global health priorities, flexible regulations, and the merging of biotechnology with information and material sciences are all pushing this change.

Industry 4.0 and Smart Biomanufacturing Smart biomanufacturing combines traditional manufacturing with new technologies from Industry 4.0, such as IoT, cyber-physical systems, and cloud computing. This combination makes it possible: Analytics in real time Control that predicts Sharing data across the whole business without any problems Making decisions automatically, (ICH Q13 Expert Working Group, 2021). Sensors check things like pH, oxygen, and metabolites at different points in the production process. AI uses this information to change the agitation or nutrient feeds on its own, which means less work for people. This digital change makes resource orchestration smarter and makes systems that optimize themselves. Digital twins and virtual modelling

Digital twins are virtual models of real-world processes that use design-of-experiment (DoE) inputs and past data to predict what will happen. With the help of machine learning, they support: Optimization in silico Less need for repeated physical tests, (EMA, 2019). Companies like Siemens and Dassault Systems are making digital twin applications for biopharma better by connecting real-time sensor data to process models that change over time. Edge and Cloud Computing Edge computing works with cloud systems by letting you do real-time analytics right at the site. Devices on bioreactors or skids process data on site and only send important information to the cloud. This hybrid model makes things more resilient and uses less bandwidth, (NIIMBL, 2022). Using AI and Machine Learning for Quality Control Advanced machine learning keeps learning from process data, finding problems that traditional methods miss and suggesting new ways to control them. Computer vision improves quality checks on labels, aseptic fills, and closures. This lowers the risk of contamination and makes sure that everything is up to code. Changes to the rules Automation helps meet regulatory goals. Innovators can get involved early through the FDA's Emerging Technology Program (ETP), (Anastasopoulou et al., 2020). In Europe and Asia, regulatory sandboxes let people safely test new digital technologies. ICH Q13 encourages continuous manufacturing and helps make sure that regulations are the same around the world. Biomanufacturing that is good for the environment Automation makes things more sustainable by giving you real-time control, which cuts down on waste and makes the best use of resources. Tools that help keep track of energy, water, and emissions support environmentally friendly production and circular economy practices. Training and the Future Workforce Bioengineers of the future need to know how to use GxP systems, data tools, and program equipment. It is very important to get training in biology, engineering, and data science all at once. To build this skilled workforce, academia, industry, and government need to work together.

REFERENCES

. **Acharya, A. (2025, March 12).** *Closing the skills gap with industry-academia partnerships.* Millennium Post.

Amgen. (2021). *Amgen's Next-Generation Biomanufacturing.* https://www.amgen.com/stories/2021/06/next-generation-biomanufacturing

Anastasopoulou, A.. (2020). Environmental impact assessment of monoclonal antibody manufacturing using Life Cycle Assessment. *Biotechnology Progress, 36*(2), e2924.

Bakeev, K. A. (Ed.). (2010). *Process Analytical Technology: Spectroscopic Tools and Implementation Strategies for the Chemical and Pharmaceutical Industries.* Wiley.

BioFabUSA. (2021). *Enabling Next-Generation Biomanufacturing. Advanced Regenerative Manufacturing Institute.* ARMI.

Biogen. (2020). *Innovation in Biomanufacturing.* https://www.biogen.com/en_us/responsibility/manufacturing.html

Camacho, E. F., & Bordons, C. (2007). *Model Predictive Control.* Springer.

. **Davis, L. (2023, November 22).** *Revolutionizing data insights: The impact of IoT in big data analytics.* MetaPress.

EMA. (2019). Guideline on the Use of Process Analytical Technology (PAT) in the Manufacture of Medicinal Products.

EMA. (2020). Guideline on process validation for the manufacture of biotechnology-derived active substances and data to be provided in the regulatory submission.

EMA. (2020). Guideline on process validation for the manufacture of biotechnology-derived active substances and data to be provided in the regulatory submission.

European Commission. (2015). EudraLex - Volume 4 - Good Manufacturing Practice (GMP) guidelines. https://ec.europa.eu/health/documents/eudralex_en

European Commission. (2015). EudraLex - Volume 4 - Good Manufacturing Practice (GMP) guidelines. https://ec.europa.eu/health/documents/eudralex_en

. FDA. (2004). *Guidance for Industry: PAT — A Framework for Innovative Pharmaceutical Development, Manufacturing, and Quality Assurance.*

FDA. (2006). Guidance for Industry: Q8(R2) Pharmaceutical Development. U.S. Food and Drug Administration. https://www.fda.gov

FDA. (2017). *Advancement of Emerging Technology Applications for Pharmaceutical Innovation and Modernization.* U.S. Food and Drug Administration.

FDA. (2018). *Cybersecurity for Networked Medical Devices Containing Off-the-Shelf (OTS) Software.* U.S. Food and Drug Administration.

. OPC Foundation. (2021). OPC Unified Architecture Specification.

Fuller, A., Fan, Z., Day, C., & Barlow, C. (2020). Digital twin: Enabling technologies, challenges and open research. *IEEE Access : Practical Innovations, Open Solutions*, *8*, 108952–108971.

. GAMP 5. (2022). A Risk-Based Approach to Compliant GxP Computerized Systems. ISPE.

Ghasemi, R., & Behzadnia, N. (2018). Real-time monitoring and control strategies in biopharmaceutical manufacturing. *Journal of Industrial Microbiology & Biotechnology*, *45*(7), 593–606.

Ghasemi, R., & Behzadnia, N. (2018). Real-time monitoring and control strategies in biopharmaceutical manufacturing. *Journal of Industrial Microbiology & Biotechnology*, *45*(7), 593–606.

Ghosh, R.. (2020). Artificial intelligence and machine learning in biomanufacturing: A review. *Biotechnology Journal*, *15*(9), 1900566.

Ghosh, R.. (2020). Artificial intelligence and machine learning inbiomanufacturing: A review. *Biotechnology Journal*, *15*(9), 1900566.

Gronemeyer, P., Ditz, R., & Strube, J. (2014). Trends in Upstream and Downstream Process Development for Antibody Manufacturing. *Bioengineering (Basel, Switzerland)*, *1*(4), 188–212. PMID: 28955024

GSK. (2021). *Artificial Intelligence and Machine Learning in Biomanufacturing*. Retrieved from https://www.gsk.com/en-gb/media/press-releases/gsk-uses-ai-in-manufacturing

GSK. (2022). *Digital Transformation in Vaccine Manufacturing*. GSK Innovation Reports.

HHS. (2022). *Healthcare Cybersecurity and Risk Mitigation Guide*. Department of Health and Human Services.

Hosinski, G. **(2022).** *IoT at Amgen – Evaluating and piloting Industry 4.0 technology in biomanufacturing* (Master's thesis, Massachusetts Institute of Technology).

. ICH Q13 Expert Working Group. (2021). Continuous Manufacturing of Drug Substances and Drug Products.

ISPE. (2020). *Pharmaceutical Workforce of the Future: Education and Training for Advanced Manufacturing*. International Society for Pharmaceutical Engineering.

. Kewaunee International Group. (2023, November 29). Scaling up from pilot plants to large-scale production.

Kroll, P.. (2017). Model Predictive Control of Bioprocesses: A Review. *Journal of Process Control*, *56*, 1–14.

Lang, D. A., Meyer, T., & Smith, C. D. (2020). Robotics in Biopharmaceutical Fill-Finish Operations: Benefits and Considerations. *Pharmaceutical Engineering*, *40*(3), 58–65.

Lang, D. A., Meyer, T., & Smith, C. D. (2020). Robotics in Biopharmaceutical Fill-Finish Operations: Benefits and Considerations. *Pharmaceutical Engineering*, *40*(3), 58–65.

Langer, E. S. (2015). Biopharmaceutical Manufacturing Trends. *BioProcess International, 13*(4), 24–30.

Lee, J.. (2018). Industrial big data analytics and cyber-physical systems for future manufacturing systems. *Annual Reviews in Control, 45*, 1–10.

Lee, J., Bagheri, B., & Kao, H. A. (2015). A cyber-physical systems architecture for Industry 4.0-based manufacturing systems. *Manufacturing Letters, 3*, 18–23.

Lee, J., Lapira, E., Bagheri, B., & Kao, H. A. (2020). *Industrial AI: Applications with Sustainable Performance*. Springer.

Lee, S. L.. (2015). Modernizing pharmaceutical manufacturing: From batch to continuous production. *Journal of Pharmaceutical Innovation, 10*(3), 191–199.

Levine, H. L.. (2019). Continuous Biomanufacturing: Modern Approaches and Technologies. *BioProcess International, 17*(4), 42–49.

Merck & Co. (2019). *Digital Transformation in Manufacturing*. Retrieved from https://www.merck.com/news/digital-manufacturing-initiatives

Narayanan, H.. (2021). Industry 4.0 in pharmaceutical manufacturing: A systematic review. *Journal of Industrial Information Integration, 24*, 100224.

. NIIMBL. (2022). Accelerating Innovation in Biopharmaceutical Manufacturing.

Pfizer. (2021). *Pfizer's Manufacturing Response to COVID-19*. https://www.pfizer.com/news/hot-topics/manufacturing-response-covid-19

. Pfizer. (2021). Smart Manufacturing Initiatives at Pfizer. Pfizer Reports.

Qin, S. J., & Badgwell, T. A. (2003). A survey of industrial model predictive control technology. *Control Engineering Practice, 11*(7), 733–764.

Qin, S. J., & Badgwell, T. A. (2003). A survey of industrial model predictive control technology. *Control Engineering Practice, 11*(7), 733–764.

. Ramaswamy, R. et al. (2020). Big data analytics in pharmaceutical manufacturing. Pharmaceutical Engineering, 40(3).

Rathore, A. S. (2009). Roadmap for implementation of quality by design (QbD) for biotechnology products. *Trends in Biotechnology, 27*(9), 546–553. PMID: 19647883

Rathore, A. S., & Jesubalan, N. G. (2022). Perspectives on Process Analytical Technology. *Biopharm International, 35*(5), 31–35.

Rathore, A. S., & Saxena, N. (2023). Digitalization: The Route to Biopharma 4.0. *Biopharm International, 36*(11), 25–29.

Rathore, A. S., & Winkle, H. (2009). Quality by Design for Biopharmaceuticals. *Nature Biotechnology, 27*(1), 26–34. PMID: 19131992

Sanofi. (2020). *Digital Factory of the Future*. Retrieved from https://www.sanofi.com/en/our-stories/our-people/our-digital-factory-of-the-future

Shukla, A. A., & Thömmes, J. (2010). Recent advances in large-scale production of monoclonal antibodies and related proteins. *Trends in Biotechnology, 28*(5), 253–261. PMID: 20304511

Srai, J. S.. (2020). Digitalisation in pharmaceutical manufacturing: State-of-the-art review and future perspectives. *Computers in Industry, 117*, 103213.

Tao, F.. (2019). Digital twin in industry: State-of-the-art. *IEEE Transactions on Industrial Informatics, 15*(4), 2405–2415.

Tao, F., Qi, Q., Liu, A., & Kusiak, A. (2018). Data-driven smart manufacturing. *Journal of Manufacturing Systems, 48*, 157–169.

Walsh, G. (2018). *Biopharmaceuticals: Biochemistry and Biotechnology* (3rd ed.). Wiley-Blackwell.

Walsh, G. (2018). Biopharmaceutical benchmarks 2018. *Nature Biotechnology, 36*(12), 1136–1145. PMID: 30520869

Yin, J., Li, G., Liu, Y., & Wang, J. (2021). Application of SCADA Systems in Biopharmaceutical Manufacturing. *Journal of Biotechnology Advances, 39*(5), 210–225. DOI: 10.1016/j.biotechadv.2021.107581

Chapter 7
Bioprocess Optimization Strategies:
Enhancing Efficiency and Yield in Bio-Manufacturing

Deepak Kumar Jha
https://orcid.org/0000-0002-1979-7940
Karnataka College of Pharmacy, India

S. Archana
https://orcid.org/0009-0000-0814-3282
Ahmedabad University, India

Zohreh Elyasi
https://orcid.org/0009-0004-9537-1935
University of Eastern Piedmont, Novara, Italy

ABSTRACT

With the increasing global demand for biopharmaceuticals and industrial biologics, optimizing biomanufacturing processes become imperative. The optimization of bioprocesses aims to maximize the efficiency and yield in biomanufacturing while maintaining cost-effectiveness. This chapter discusses the key strategies employed for bioprocess optimization and scale-up for the efficient production of biological products. It also discusses the importance of bioreactor configuration refinements, dynamic media optimization, process parameter refinement and real-time monitoring via advanced PAT. The integration of AI and ML in predictive modelling, efficiency enhancement and minimizing operational risks are also presented. Furthermore, the transition from batch to continuous manufacturing and the implementation of QbD as key drivers of efficiency and consistency are emphasized. Optimizing downstream processing are equally crucial to enable higher product recovery. Finally, addressing key bottlenecks such as scale-up and regulatory constraints are also reviewed.

DOI: 10.4018/979-8-3373-2873-7.ch007

INTRODUCTION

Bioprocess technology, also known as fermentation technology, is loosely defined as any process that utilizes living source such as bacteria, yeast, fungi or mammalian cells for the production of high value biopharmaceuticals including vaccines, monoclonal antibodies and/or antibiotics and other industrial products such as biofuels, enzymes and specialty chemicals. With the increasing demand for these products, it is imperative to optimize the bioprocess system for ensuring high product yield and quality, while reducing production costs and environment impact. Bioprocess optimization involves refinement at various stages of the biomanufacturing process.

The optimization often begins with fine tuning the composition of the growth media conditions followed by optimizing the critical process parameters (CPPs) such as dissolved oxygen and pH to achieve optimum growth and productivity. A combination of classical, statistical and mathematical approaches and high throughput screening are often employed to identify the optimum medium components that supports the cell growth or productivity. With the advent of advanced sensor technologies, often integrated with machine learning algorithms, allow for real time monitoring and adjustments of CPPs efficiently, thereby maximizing product yield and quality (Galbraith et al., 2018, Mandenius & Brundin, 2008).

Improvement in the strains used in the biomanufacturing is a core aspect to enhance productivity, stability and specificity of a typical bioprocess system. This can be achieved through classical mutagenesis, recombination, protoplast fusion and genetic recombination technology. Integrating the omics technologies: genomics, transcriptomics, proteomics and metabolomics can make the bioprocess optimization more explicit by providing insights into the phenotypic trait of the strain used in the bio production, understand the changes in the cell metabolism to achieve the best state of biomass growth as well as identify the bottlenecks associated with the metabolic pathways, thereby guiding optimization processes efficiently (Parekh et al., 2000, Lee et al., 2005).

Scaling up bioprocesses from lab bench to the market is one of the major challenges that has to be tamed. Bioreactors represent the heart of any bioprocess technology. They are specialized vessels designed to support the growth of cells/microorganisms under optimum conditions to enable the large-scale production of the desired products with high efficiency and reproducibility. Physical factors such as bioreactor type and configuration can influence mixing efficiency, mass transfer, oxygen transfer rates, agitation speed, shear stress and heat dissipation. Selecting the desired operating conditions such as optimum temperature, pH, feed supply and other chemicals such as pH buffering agents and antifoam agents, all can impact the bioreactor process efficiency which in turn can impact biomass growth, yield and quality. Therefore, translating the optimized conditions developed in a laboratory scale to an industrial scale is very crucial. Developing innovative bioreactor configurations and implementing the application of 'Design of Experiments (DoE), a mathematical model for designing the experiment and identifying the optimal process parameters' and 'Process Analytical Technology (PAT), a tool encompassing various analytical instruments and sensors (both in-line and on-line) allowing for continuous process monitoring and control of CPPs' can help achieve an efficient production processes (Reisman, 1993).

Optimization strategies for the downstream processing is equally important as that of upstream activities. Downstream processes focus on the recovery, concentration, purification and formulation of the desired product. Techniques like filtration, centrifugation, precipitation, adsorption and various chromatographic technologies can be optimized for the purpose of improving product yield and quality while maintaining reduced production costs. Evolutionary algorithms and mathematical process modelling are powerful tools for optimizing various steps of downstream processing and to gain a deeper understanding of the overall system and also identify areas for improving the yield and quality of the product at a faster rate. Additionally, various computational tools help in simulating complex biochemical and metabolic pathways, thus aiding in manipulation of these pathways so as to maximize the product yield and quality (Baumann & Hubbuch, 2017, Rathore et al., 2021).

Biological variability such as microorganism specific differences and environmental factors, can directly impact the reproducibility of a bioprocess system, especially for high volume production applications. This drives the need for the transition from batch to continuous bioprocess system, producing higher productivity and quality with minimum variability (Rathore et al., 2015).

Addressing the environmental impact of bioprocessing early in the developmental stages is crucial for achieving a more sustainable manufacturing. Therefore, optimizing resources, energy use and waste reduction are significant factors for achieving a sustainable bioprocess system. Sustainable/Green biotechnology integrates green technologies and practises to produce environmental friendly products while meeting the quality of the product, minimizing the environmental impact and production costs. Strategies such as utilizing renewable sources (for example, agricultural residues), energy-efficient sources (for example, solar, wind or biomass), single-use technologies and waste valorisation can be implemented to produce eco-friendly products and improving the overall process efficiency (Tang et al., 2020).

Adhering to the regulatory frameworks in the bioprocessing industry is important to ensure the production of safe and effective products. Several national and international regulatory agencies, oversee every stage of bioprocessing i.e., research development to manufacturing, environmental release and post-market surveillance. These agencies will ensure that the biologics meet the regulatory standards before its reach to the public (Narhi & Nordstrom, 2005).

The objectives of this chapter will cover the fundamentals of the bioprocess technology, various strategies for optimizing the bioprocess in order to achieve maximum productivity and yield and finally cover the regulatory bodies involved in the production of safe and effective biologics.

FUNDAMENTALS OF A BIOPROCESS SYSTEM

A typical bioprocess system is divided into 3 major categories (**Moser, 1988**):

(a) Upstream processing (preparation phase)
(b) Bioreaction (production phase) and
(c) Downstream processing (purification phase) (**Figure 1**).

Upstream processing involves nutrient media preparation, preculture preparation for inoculation in large bioreactors and bioreactor preparation including equipment, feed lines and sensor sterilization, medium addition, connection of the bioreactor to the control units and defining the process parameter set points in the software.

Bioreaction / fermentation is the process where the source (mammalian cells/microorganisms) produces the desired product. This can be done through 4 major types of operation modes classified based on the type of product being produced: batch, fed-batch, continuous and perfusion culture. During the cultivation period, the process parameters (agitation, pH, temperature and dissolved oxygen) are controlled at set points. In addition, sampling and culture feeding are done based on the requirement of the specific bioprocess system. At the end of the bioreaction, the culture is harvested at the end of the growth phase or when it enters the stationary phase, as the desired product concentration would be the maximum in this phase.

Downstream processing (DSP) focuses on: (a) product recovery from cell, broth (or both), (b) product concentration and purification, (c) packaging of the purified product and (d) quality control of the purified product. In addition, proper disposal and treatment of the waste streams is an integral part of DSP thus ensuring proper resource recycling and reducing environmental impact effectively.

Figure 1. Fundamental stages of bioprocess technology: The three fundamental steps of bioprocess technology include upstream (preparative phase), bioreaction (production phase) and downstream (purification phase) respectively

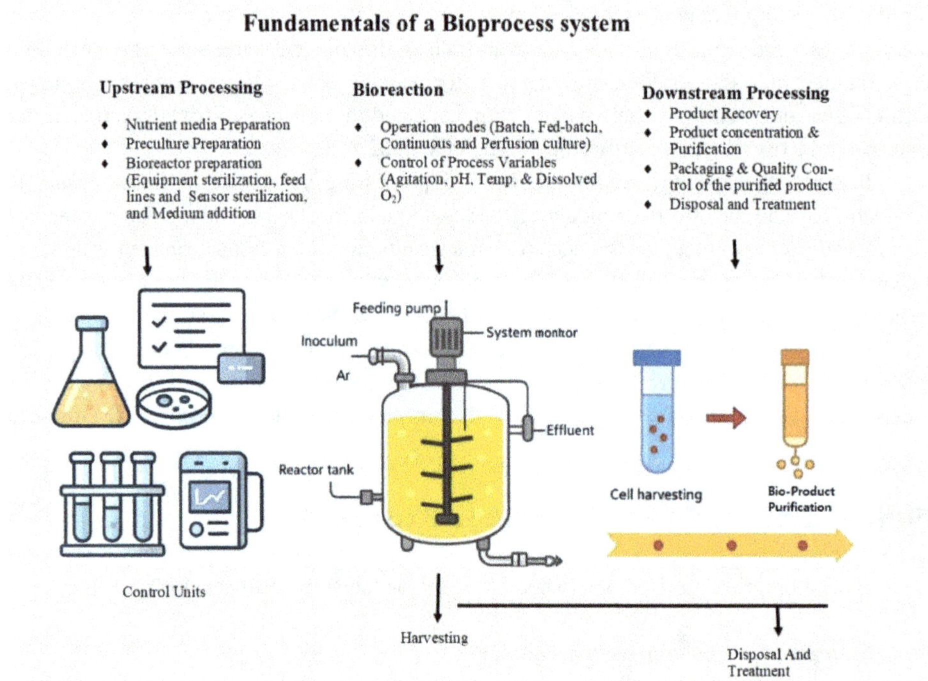

STRATEGIES FOR ENHANCING BIOPROCESS YIELD

To enhance bioprocess yield and productivity, various optimization strategies must be implemented across all the 3 stages of bioprocessing: upstream processing, fermentation/ bioreaction and downstream processing.

Strategies for Optimizing Upstream Bioprocessing

Media development, strain improvement, bioreactor or design optimization and process control strategies form the basis of upstream bioprocessing. Upstream bioprocessing needs to be improved because it directly impacts growth, productivity, quality and production costs. Additionally, a well optimized upstream bioprocess can improve downstream efficiency, yield and quality of the target product effectively.

Medium Optimization

Medium optimization is a process which involves refining the composition and concentration of the growth medium in order to enhance the biomass growth with the best physiological state for higher productivity. Classical and statistical / mathematical are two distinct approaches that can be utilized to improve the efficiency of the production medium.

Classical. Classical method is further divided into open and close-ended system. In an open-ended system, any number and type of components (carbon/nitrogen source, minerals and growth factor to name a few) and conditions can be tested for improving the efficiency of the growth medium, whereas a close-ended system involves systematic variation of predefined set of components (two or more levels) and conditions in a controlled manner, allowing for assessment of interactions between the factors that will eventually result in identifying the optimal medium composition. The former system is more advantageous because it allows for a more comprehensive exploration of different variables and conditions simultaneously, thereby identifying the effective media formulation. Additionally, this system does not make any assumptions as to which variables are best suited for the bioreaction process. Although the latter system is simpler, it does not consider other variables/ parameters that could be beneficial in the production medium. Therefore, for optimizing the production medium, it would be an ideal strategy to start with an open-ended approach which identifies promising parameters and then moving to the close-ended system to optimize those promising parameters for achieving an optimal production medium (Singh et al., 2017).

Open-ended approaches include (Galbraith et al., 2018, Singh et al., 2017, Radzun et al., 2024):

(a) Borrowing
(b) Component Replacement
(c) Supplementation

Borrowing is a simple and easy method where medium components and process conditions to grow the experimental cells / microorganisms are acquired from the existing literature. Although this method shortens the development time required for media optimization, it would be challenging to select the most appropriate ones for the bioprocess from many options available in knowledge database.

Component replacement is an iterative process where only a specific type of component in the fermentation media (for example: different sources of carbon, nitrogen or other essential minerals) are compared and studied for their effect on cell growth and productivity. However, this method does not provide an insight into the component interactions.

Supplementation experiments involve testing different potential supplements of carbon or nitrogen sources on cell growth and metabolite production. Because it is again an iterative process, it is extremely time consuming in order to achieve a more refined media.

Close-ended approaches include:

(a) Biological mimicry, and
(b) One-factor-at-a-time (OFAT)

Biological mimicry: In this approach, the biomass growth would reach its maximum if mass balance strategy is followed i.e., the media is formulated based on the elemental composition (micro and macro elements) of the cells/microorganisms that would produce the highest yield. The major disadvantage associated with this method is that it is very challenging and complex to analyse each elemental composition. Additionally, they are expensive, time-consuming and does not provide any information on component interactions (Singh et al., 2017).

One-factor-at-a-time (OFAT) approach has been the most popular experimental strategy for optimizing the medium components. OFAT experiments involve varying one independent variable while holding all other parameters constant at a certain level across trials. This approach allows to observe the direct effect of that individual variable on the cell growth and productivity. Although this method is easy, simple and straightforward, it is extremely time consuming and is limited by optimizing only a small number of variables because for more variables, a relatively large number of experimental runs are required which often becomes expensive. Additionally, this method does not determine component interactions. Multiple OFAT is a more structured process than the traditional OFAT in that it involves sequential optimization of multiple independent factors that will allow for a more efficient bioprocess in terms of quality and yield (Jana et al., 2019, Gupta & Edula., 2021).

Case Study

Objective: To improve the yield of recombinant human insulin variant production in *Escherichia coli* using the OFAT approach (**Jing et al., 2018**).

Methodology: Various carbon sources (glycerol/glucose/sucrose) and nitrogen sources (yeast extract/tryptone) were tested individually and studied its effect on the cell density and expression of the recombinant protein using optical density (OD600) and protein assays (SDS-PAGE).

Results: (1) The ratio of 3% yeast extract to 1% tryptone resulted in the maximum cell density. (2) The addition of glycerol in the medium led to an increase in the OD600 from 5.0 to 7.0 compared to glucose and sucrose. This was also reflected in terms of the expression levels of the recombinant protein.

From the above approaches it can be concluded that classical method of medium optimization though simple and straightforward, it suffers from several limitations such as time-consuming, expensive, iterative experimentation with less accuracy, resource intensive, overlook interactions among the components in the medium and not easily scalable when many variables require optimization to develop an efficient bioprocess system.

Statistical/Mathematical

Modern statistical/mathematical techniques can overcome the limitations of the classical method of medium optimization by allowing the researchers to design the experiments, optimize variables simultaneously, evaluate the component interactions and predict their response value effectively. The utilization of these techniques can improve process efficiency and the overall economics in the bioprocess. Some of the major statistical/mathematical tools for optimizing the medium components include:

(a) Factorial design
(b) Plackett and Burman's design
(c) Taguchi design
(d) Central composite design (CCD),
(e) Artificial neural network (ANN)

Factorial Design: This method helps in understanding the responses of multiple variables that are changed simultaneously at two levels (e.g., low, high) effectively. A mathematical equation (polynomial equation) is then employed from the experimental results to understand the response value as a function of the level of the factors tested. There are two major types of factorial design: (a) Full factorial design, and (b) Partial/ Fractional factorial design (Hunt et al., 2014, Kalil et al., 2000, Hamid et al., 2018).

In a full factorial design, every possible combinations of the levels of each factor are tested in an experiment, whereas in a partial/fractional factorial design, only a representative subset of a full factorial design is tested in an experiment. The latter is chosen when the experimental runs required for a large number of variables (considering each combination of factor levels) are impracticable (Hunt et al., 2014, Kalil et al., 2000, Hamid et al., 2018).

The advantage of factorial designs is that they provide a comprehensive information on the interactions among factors that produces the most desirable outcome (Hunt et al., 2014, Kalil et al., 2000, Hamid et al., 2018).

Plackett-Burman Design (PBD): PBD (a two-level (either low or high) fractional factorial design) is utilized when the researchers want to screen out the most significant physicochemical factors that influence the biomass growth and yield. This method is suitable when more than 5 independent variables are involved i.e., it enables to screen 'n' variables using 'n+1' experiments, where 'n' indicates the number of variables to be tested and 'n+1' must be the multiple of 4. Therefore, the number of variables that can be included in this design can be 7, 11, 15 etc. The only concern associated with this method is that they do not clearly distinguish the interaction effects among factors, as it only detects the main effects (Wasko et al., 2010, Ghaderi et al., 2018).

Case Study

Objective: To improve the production of full-length recombinant tocilizumab (TCZ) in *Pichia pastoris* (Das et al., 2025).

Methodology: (a) Various carbon and nitrogen sources (mannitol, glycine, histidine, K2SO4, KH2PO4, CaSO4.2H2O, sorbitol and ammonium sulphate) were tested for their ability to enhance the production of full length TCZ using a 2-level PBD. (b) The screened medium components were further optimized for their optimum concentrations using box-behnken design and ANN.

Results: (1) Mannitol and glycine were suitable for the enhanced production of full length TCZ from *P.pastoris.* ANN model compared to box-behnken design improved the prediction and showed a remarkable increase in the full length TCZ from the screened medium components (0.35mg/L and 0.42g/L in shake-flask culture and 0.44mg/L and 0.45g/L in batch culture respectively).

Taguchi Design: This method overcomes the problems associated with PBD in that this design employs an orthogonal array system to determine how multiple factors at different levels affect the yield and quality in a small number of experiments rather than testing all possibilities which would be time consuming like factorial design (Das et al., 2014, Chenthamarakshan et al., 2017, Darvishi & Abolhasan Moghaddami, 2019).

It is a three-phase approach encompassing:

(a) System strategy: Helps in defining the objective

(b) Parameter design: Designing factors that influence the outcome and helps in specifying the experimental levels of those factors. Additionally, in this step, an appropriate predefined orthogonal array is selected based on the number of factors and their levels.

For example, the table below represents an orthogonal array with 3 parameters and 2 levels (**Table 1**).

Table 1. L4 orthogonal array

Trial No	Factor A	Factor B	Factor C
1	L	L	L
2	L	H	H
3	H	L	H
4	H	H	L

'L' indicates low-level of the selected factor and 'H' indicates high level of the selected factor. The above table is called L4 orthogonal array i.e., L4 indicates 4 trials. Similarly, there are other predefined orthogonal arrays that covers upto 50 variables. This design provides the paramount effects of different factors on the response value.

(c) Tolerance design: It aims to create a design that are less sensitive to uncontrollable factors (noise factor) (for e.g., environmental conditions and changes in the material properties with time and use to name a few) and eventually maximizing the signal.

Although this method is fully developed with the advantage of reduced experimental runs, cost and resources, it has the limitation in that it does not indicate what factor has the highest effect on the outcome.

Central Composite Design (CCD): It is a 2 factor five level experimental design that estimates the main effects and interaction between the factors (variables). Additionally, this design also helps in studying the response value at levels beyond the usual (i.e., low/high), thus making this model suitable to understand both linear and quadratic effects of factors, leading to the formulation of a more optimal media. This type of design is used for the production of the complex and chemically defined media. The figure below represents a classic CCD for 2 factors at 5 levels (Figure 2) (Ibrahim et al., 2005, Wasli et al., 2009).

Figure 2. A classic CCD for 2 factors at 5 levels: The level of the factors is represented by: -α (Lowest), -1 (Low), 0 (Middle point), +1 (High), +α (Highest). The four corner points of the design space indicates main effects and interactions. The four-star points beyond the design space indicates the response value at the extreme levels of the factors (possibility of quadratic effects) and the centre point indicates the non-linear response

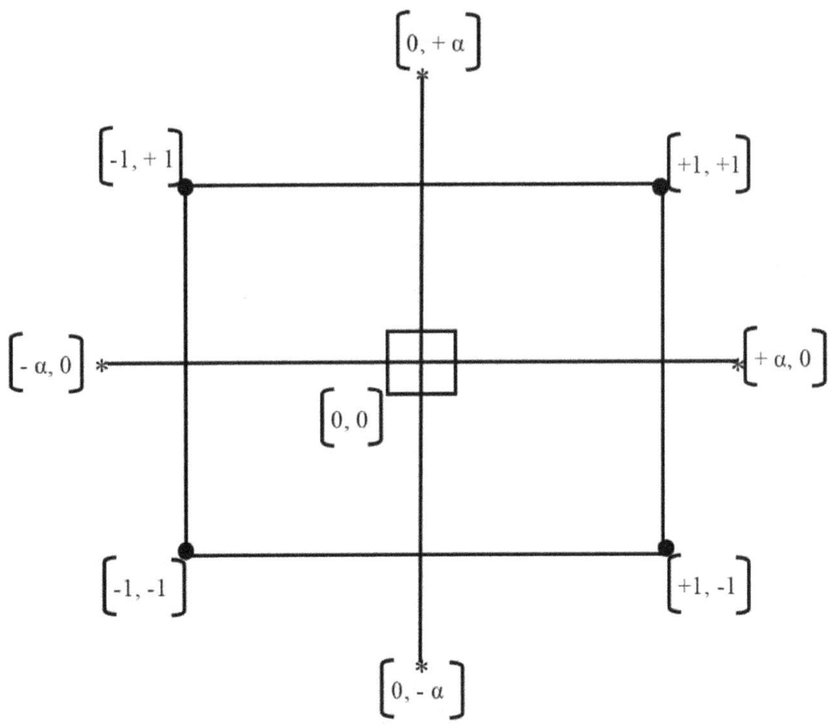

Artificial Neural Network (ANN): It is a mathematical/computational model that helps find the optimum media composition from the best combination of a given set of data inputs to achieve a desirable outcome (**Sewsynker-Sukai et al., 2017**).

Bioreactor Design and Process Control Strategies

Efficient bioreactor operation is the key to achieve improved product yield and quality. A spectrum of strategies should be implemented determined by benefit to cost ratio to improve the overall process performance and ensuring reliability of outcomes (**Figure 3**).

Figure 3. Bioreactor design and process control strategies. The figure represents various strategies to improve the bioprocess efficiency in terms (a) selecting an appropriate bioreactor type based on the application, (b) fine-tuning the operational parameters and (c) implementing real-time process monitoring and control

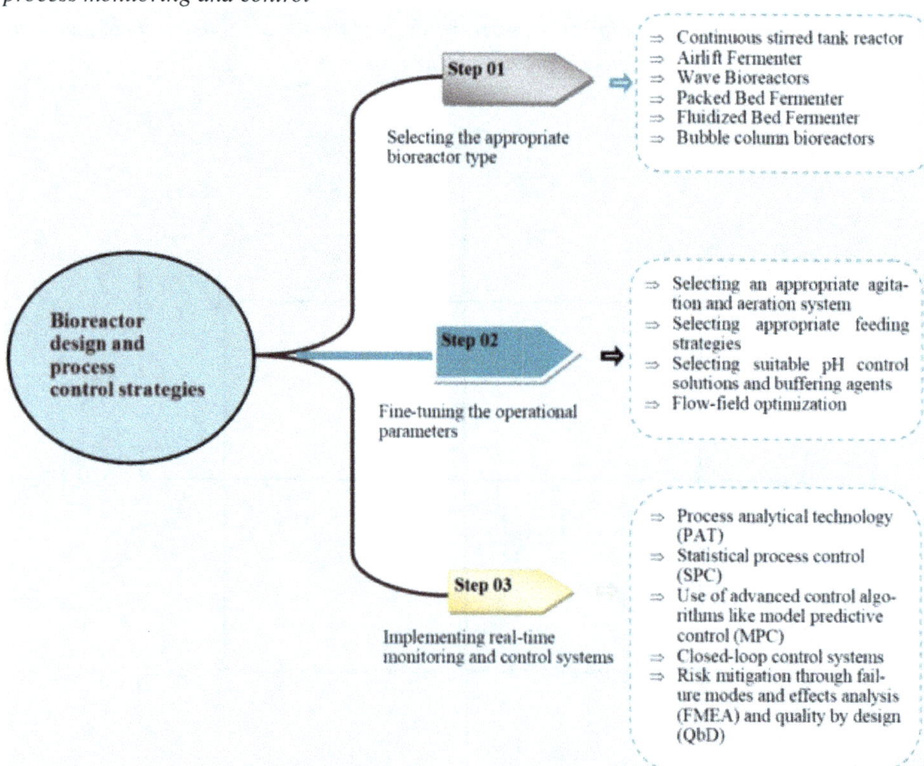

Selecting an Appropriate Bioreactor Type

Selection of the right bioreactor type, size and mode of running is crucial because these factors affect the yield and quality of the desired product immensely. The table below provides characteristics features of different bioreactor types that has been exploited and developed for different applications (**Table 2**). Each bioreactor type varies in design and performance attributes, offering distinct advantages and limitations. The choice of the bioreactor largely depends on the operational characteristics and target product specifications in terms of yield and quality. Therefore, comparing the bioreactor types are often impractical as their effectiveness is determined by the end-product requirements.

Table 2 describes the characteristic features of the different types of the bioreactors suitable for the application along with its associated advantages and disadvantages that can impact the quality and yield of the product.

Table 2. Different bioreactor types and its characteristic features

Type of Bioreactor	Characteristic Features	Advantages	Disadvantages	Applications
Continuous stirred tank reactor (CSTR) (**Sinner et al., 2020, Malcata, 1989**)	• Steady state operating conditions. • Continuous operation • Feed assumes uniform composition throughout the reactor. • Output stream composition identical to the composition of the material inside the reactor. • Ideal for liquid phase reaction.	• Easy to control temperature. • Easy to operate. • Low labour expenses. • Less expensive and easier to construct. • CSTR behaviour well understood. • Possibility for cascade operation.	• Low overall throughput per unit volume (due to short residence time of the reactants inside the reactor). • Single units are not suitable for slow reactions.	• Food and beverage industry. • Chemical and pharmaceutical industry for the production of polymers and plastics and active pharmaceutical ingredient. • Bioremediation and Waste water treatment. • Biofuel production. • Cosmetic Industry.
Airlift fermenter (Tower Reactor) (**Moresi, 1981, Chen, 1990**)	• A two-zone system (riser and down comer tube). • Pneumatically agitated device i.e., the gas – liquid mixture in the riser tube creates a density difference between the two tubes that drives the circulation of the liquid and thereby improves the oxygen transfer inside the fermenter. (Gas-liquid mass transfer and mixing) • Suitable for shear- sensitive cultures.	•High-yield coupled with low energy requirement due to absence of mechanical agitation. • Simple structure and low installation cost. • Easier to scale-up due to simple design. • Easy to sterilize the fermenter. • Uniform mixing and oxygenation.	• Possibility of formation of dead zones. • Support costs (For e.g., gas compression costs). •Difficulty in flow rate control.	• Food and beverage industry. • Production of biotechnological and pharmaceutical products. • Waste water treatment. • Bio-fuel production.
Wave bioreactor (**Dutta et al., 2024, Yuk et al., 2011**)	• Wave induced motion (Rocking motion of the culture at a specified angle and frequency). • Generation of the waves by rocking promotes efficient mixing and greater volumetric oxygen transfer. • Employs single use plastic bag for cultivation. • Suitable for shear- sensitive cultures.	• Wave bioreactors are typically single use reactors, eliminating the need of washing and sterilization after each use. • Simple, safe and flexible production. • Suitable for culturing various cell types (mammalian cells, plant cells and insect cells).	• Smaller scale operations due to the size limit of the cell bags. • Requires trained personnel to optimize the rocking angle, speed and gas flow for different applications.	• Production of biopharmaceuticals i.e., monoclonal antibodies and vaccine production. • Bio-fuel and nutraceutical development.
Packed bed fermenter (**Bakkivaraj et al., 2016, Polakovic et al., 1993**)	• Consists of a packing bed material containing catalyst/ immobilized enzymes or microbes or other adsorbents to improve the contact between 2 phases. • Chemical reaction happens on the surface of the material or within the matrix as the reactant (gas/liquid) flows through the bed to generate the product. • Follow a continuous mode of operation but these reactors can also operate in a batch and fed batch mode.	• Low construction and operating costs. • High conversion rate. • No back mixing of the substrate stream. • Ability to work in high temperatures and pressure.	• Potential for pressure drop. • Considerations to be taken for the residence time of the substrate in the bed. • Low heat transfer coefficient • Blockage of the reactor due to excessive cell growth, density and nutrients.	• Chemical industry. • Wastewater treatment. • Environmental engineering.

continued on following page

Table 2. Continued

Type of Bioreactor	Characteristic Features	Advantages	Disadvantages	Applications
Fluidized Bed Fermenter (**Andrews & Przezdziecki, 1986, Kang et al., 2024**)	• A type of catalytic reactor where solid catalysts are fluidized during the reaction unlike packed bed reactor. • High gas flow or fluid velocity allows for efficient contact between reactants and catalysts resulting in an enhanced mass transfer rate. • Operates in continuous mode.	•Improved temperature control and heat transfer rates unlike packed bed reactor • High mass transfer rates. • Easy control of pH. • Good mixing is achieved. • Easy to scale up.	• Potential for back mixing. • Difficult to predict fluidization patterns. • Loss of particles during the process can be expected which results in sudden changes in the flow rate. •High operational costs • Possibility for erosion and wear of the reactor components.	• Biomass conversion and biofuel production. • Chemical and petroleum Industry.
Bubble Column Bioreactor (**Gonzalez-Gloria et al., 2022, Abufalgha et al., 2020**)	• Employs gas bubbles to achieve mixing and aeration within the fermenter. • High interfacial surface area to volume ratio allow for an efficient gas-liquid and gas–(liquid-solid) catalyst interaction efficiently.	• Excellent heat and mass transfer rates. • Simple to construct. • Easy to maintain and operate. •Low power consumptions.	• Significant back mixing. • Potential for pressure drop. • Challenging to optimize the ideal gas hold up volume based on the system in study. • Coalescence of the gas substrates.	• Chemical, petrochemical, biochemical Industry

Fine Tuning the Operational Parameters

Fine tuning the process conditions in the bioprocess industry is critical to ensure maximum yield and quality of the desired product and also ensuring batch consistency and efficiency of the product produced. Fine tuning the CPPs such as pH, temperature, dissolved oxygen, nutrient concentrations, by-product levels and agitation systems can result in an increased productivity, reproducibility and efficiency of the bioprocess system.

Selecting an Appropriate Aeration-Agitation System

Choosing a good aeration and agitation system is important as it directly impacts the oxygen and nutrient availability throughout the culture which in turn reflects in the overall process efficiency.

The two major structural components of the aeration and agitation system includes:

(a) The agitator
(b) The aeration system

The Agitator

Depending on the type of bioprocess, culture properties and reactor type, size and geometry, appropriate agitators and their agitation speed are selected. In a typical bioreactor system, agitation can be achieved by mechanical stirring, liquid recirculation (pumping or through external loops), gas injection or biogas recirculation (pneumatic mixing in the case of anaerobic digestion) (**Alves & Vasconcelos, 1996**). Agitation in fermentation processes improves:

(a) Oxygen transfer rate
(b) Heat and mass transfer
(c) Uniform mixing and nutrient distribution
(d) Preventing cell clumping and sedimentation
(e) Accelerating reaction rates and improving product yield.

To optimize the agitator system, several key factors must be carefully considered (based on the content processed) in order to achieve improved product yield and quality (**Esmeralda-Guzman et al., 2024**). These include:

(a) Agitator type (impeller type: axial-flow impellers (for low viscous liquids), radial-flow impellers (for gas dispersion and solid suspension) and hydrofoil impellers (for shear sensitive application systems)
(b) Optimizing the motor and speed (based on the viscosity of the liquid)
(c) Tank height and diameter (influence the impeller diameter and the need for multi-level impellers)

The Aeration System

Aeration refers to the process of supplying oxygen into a submerged culture for its metabolic requirements (Jenkins, 2013). Diffused aeration is the most common type of aeration in bioreactors and sparges are specific device used to facilitate aeration.

Majorly, fine-bubble diffusers and coarse-bubble diffusers are employed within a bioreactor to introduce oxygen into the liquid medium where they convert the gaseous form of oxygen into fine bubbles within the liquid medium. The choice between both the systems is based on the requirements of the bioreaction process. For example, in activated sludge aeration tanks, chemical industries or any other industrial processes, fine-bubble diffuser system are adopted as they maximize the oxygen transfer by generating smaller bubbles that provides an efficient gas-liquid contact. Coarse-bubble diffusers on the other hand, produce a larger diameter bubbles that are effective in displacing, churning and mixing the liquid effectively as seen most commonly in sludge storage tanks. Surface aeration are also used in a bioreactor but less frequently and they work by creating turbulence on the liquid surface majorly by employing rotating blades, rotors or brushes. This turbulence facilitates aeration during the process. This kind of aeration system was employed majorly in the wastewater treatment effectively (Roman & Muresan, 2015, Desai & Zimmerman, 2023).

Depending on the oxygen requirements of the specific bioprocess, mixing needs and energy efficiency considerations and removal of unwanted gases (especially carbon dioxide) during the process, the aeration and agitation systems are chosen.

Selecting an Appropriate Feeding Strategy

Selecting an appropriate bioprocess operation mode namely: batch, fed-batch and continuous cultures, is key in bioprocess development because optimizing the nutrient supply can directly affect the cell density and viability and as a result the product titre and quality respectively. Based on the application, either of the three operation modes can be selected.

In a batch fermentation, the nutrients are administered at the start of the bioprocess, with no further additions during the entire process. This bioprocess lasts until the feed is consumed by the culture. Because this fermentation occurs under closed system, there is minimal control over the growth conditions and therefore might result in the potential variations in the product quality across batches. Additionally, the turnover rate (product yield) will also be less due to limited nutrient availability and other control conditions inside the bioreactor. This type of operation mode is well suited for the production of secondary metabolites such as antibiotics because production often happens at the stationary phase of the microbial growth. Also, the short culture period in batch fermentation minimizes the risk of contamination or genetic mutation, thereby making this system suitable to produce the products where these factors become critical in terms of product consistency and quality. This strategy has also been used commonly for strain characterization and optimization of the nutrient medium. Despite the ease to manage and low maintainence costs, they have lower productivity levels due to frequent cleaning and sterilizing the reactor (Constantinides et al, 1970, Gopalakrishnan et al., 2024).

Unlike batch fermentation where nutrient supply is a limiting factor, a fed-batch process overcomes this limiting factor by the systematic addition of nutrients during cultivation. It is carried out in a partly open system and has more control over the microbial/cell growth and the desired product. The major advantage of this type of fermentation over batch fermentation is that it prevents the accumulation of inhibitory agents/toxic by-products by feeding with less substrate at the start of the cultivation, followed by its addition in small doses during the entire process. This will eventually improve the cell growth during the entire bioprocess. Therefore, this type of fermentation is suitable for the production of recombinant proteins from mammalian cell systems where higher biomass yield is required. Additionally, this type of system is preferred for the production of baker's yeast over batch fermentation due to substrate inhibition and ethanol production of the latter system. Moreover, the substrates can be switched at different stages during the process, enabling switch on/off the specific genes, thereby controlling the product formation effectively (Chang et al., 1998, Ko & Wang, 2006). Some disadvantages that has to be considered while choosing this feeding strategy are:

(1) Pose risk of contamination and mutation (due to semi-closed system)
(2) Because harvesting the biomass/product is carried out only at the end of the process, removal of the by-products from the reactor is not possible.
(3) The setup and control methods of this type of fermentation are complex and time consuming.

In a continuous culture, fresh culture medium (nutrients) are added to the bioreactor when the system reaches steady-state conditions and at the same time equal volume of the culture broth (containing cells, products and by-products) are removed from the reactor. In other words, the nutrients consumed by the culture and toxic by-products produced by the culture are replaced and removed at a constant rate. As the name suggests, it is carried in an open system and therefore there is an increased risk of contamination and mutation (Nieto-Taype et al., 2020).

Selecting an Appropriate pH Control Solutions and Buffering Agents

In bioprocess industry, maintaining narrow pH range is very important to ensure optimal cell growth and product quality. There is always a change in the pH in bioreactor due to the following (Simutis & Lubbert, 2015):

(a) Exponential growth phase of the culture generates large amounts of carbon dioxide and lactate as a metabolic waste product which can make the culture acidic, and
(b) Temperature can influence ionization of water and buffer components that can eventually result in significant pH shift in the system.

In order to achieve an effective pH control system, it requires the use of:

(a) Accurate pH sensors
(b) pH control strategies, and
(c) Bioprocess control software.

pH Sensors

There are three types of pH sensors that can be employed in the bioreactor. These include:

(a) Electrochemical pH sensors
(b) Optical pH sensors, and
(c) Digital pH sensors.

Electrochemical pH Sensors. These are glass membrane pH sensors that measures the hydrogen ion concentration in the media by detecting the potential difference generated across the two electrodes (potentiometric) or by detecting the current generated when a potential is applied across a 3-electrode system (voltametric) which then corresponds to changes in pH. These glass pH sensors can be applied in various bioreactor conditions as it can measure a wide pH range, but if not carefully managed, it can lose its accuracy over time. Hence frequent calibration is a requirement if these sensors are utilized in the industry (Backer et al., 2011).

Optical pH Sensors. These sensors are mainly optimized for culture media and physiological solutions. It consists of a fluorescent dye which emits light at a specific wavelength upon excitation from a blue light. The changes in the hydrogen ion concentration result in the wavelength shift, which is then measured using a detector (Ulber et al., 2003). The benefits of optical pH sensors include:

(a) Inexpensive and disposable, ideal for single use applications.
(b) No shelf-life restrictions.
(c) No calibrations required prior to use.

Optical pH sensors are also associated with certain disadvantages which include:

(a) Can measure a relatively limited pH range (4.5-8)
(b) Highly sensitive to organic solvents as they can damage the fluorescent dye.

Digital pH Sensors. They are more advanced and reliable pH sensors which work by converting the analogue signal into a digital signal in the sensor itself (contains an electronic chip in the sensor head) (Rathore et al., 2022).

pH Control Strategies

In mammalian cell cultures, carbon dioxide is considered as an acid component, therefore bicarbonate buffer/HEPES buffer is added as a base to maintain the pH. Bicarbonate buffer is preferred over HEPES as the former is the most physiological one. Sometimes a two-sided pH control system is used in mammalian cell cultures where the sodium bicarbonate addition is coupled with carbon dioxide sparging. That is, the dissolved carbon dioxide lowers the pH by becoming carbonic acid and concentrated bicarbonate solution is mixed with the medium to increase the pH (Zhang, 2010).

In microbial cultures, a wide variety of basic solutions (sodium hydroxide, potassium hydroxide and ammonium hydroxide) and acidic solutions (phosphoric acid or sulphuric acid) can be used to increase or decrease the pH as these cultures are typically harder than mammalian cell cultures. Although HCl is an acid, it is not preferred to be used in the industry as it can damage the stainless-steel components in the bioreactor. Selection of an appropriate pH control solution should be based on the chemical resistance of the pump tubing (Osman et al., 2016).

Bioprocess Control Software

Two major software's that are commonly used in the industry include SCADA and PID respectively.

SCADA (Supervisory Control and Data Acquisition) is a software that allows for process monitoring, control and automation respectively (Kakes, 2008).

PID (Proportional-Integral-Derivative) controller reads inputs from sensors, calculates the difference between the measured value and the set point and adjusts the process control variables accordingly (**Roeva & Slavov, 2012**).

Flow Field Optimization

Flow field optimization in bioprocess industry refers to the control of the fluid flow paths within the bioreactor with the goal to improve nutrient distribution and hence the mass transfer. This in turn affects the overall process efficiency of the system.

Computational Fluid Dynamics (CFD) is a widely used tool in bioprocess industry to predict the fluid flow and assess the mixing efficiency and also helps identify dead zones and shear spots that could impact the process efficiency in terms of yield and product consistency.

DoE is also a powerful methodology that uses various mathematical models to optimize the flow field parameters such as channel geometry and flow rates and predict their response before any physical experiments (Kumar et al., 2014).

Implementing Real Time Monitoring and Control Systems

Implementing real time monitoring and control technologies in bioprocessing is integral as it can enhance the process efficiency, improve product yield and quality and ensure reproducibility of the process. Some of the systems employed in the industry are described below:

(a) Process Analytical Technology: It is a system that covers a range of tools to design, analyse and control the CPPs and critical quality attributes (CQAs) effectively. Additionally, PAT also aims to reduce process costs, process cycle time and facilitate regulatory acceptance.
(b) Statistical Process Control (SPC): It uses statistical techniques to monitor and control the process method. It also plays a pivotal role in detecting common cause variation (stemming within the process) and special cause variation (stemming from external sources and indicating that the process is out of statistical control) effectively (Dassau et al., 2006).
(c) Model Predictive Control (MPC): It is a multiple-input-multiple-output (MIMO) control algorithm that provides a future trajectory of the batch based on multiple measured process variables. That is, the model aims to minimize the error between the future trajectory and desired trajectory. Additionally, this algorithm can handle complex interactions and adjust the process variables smoothly (Eslami & Jungbauer, 2024).
(d) Closed look control systems: Closed loop control refers to the system that automatically corrects the process variables by measuring the actual value and the desired set value (e.g., PID controller) (Monteiro et al., 2023).
(e) Risk mitigation through 'Failure Modes and Effects Analysis (FMEA)' and 'QbD': FMEA in one hand is a preventive tool that has been increasingly used in the pharmaceutical industry to help identify potential failure modes, effects and causes of failures. Additionally, it points out the risk priority levels based on 'S': Severity (consequence of the failure), 'O': Occurrence (probability of failure) and 'D': Detection (probability of detecting the failure). On the other hand, QbD prevents the failure by designing the process development from the beginning (Mollah, 2005).

Strain Improvement Strategies

It refers to the process that focuses on modifying the strain in order to enhance the traits of the strain so as to improve the yield, productivity, stability and efficiency of the bioprocess. Some of the examples of the outcomes of strain improvement include:

(a) Enhanced enzyme production such as fructosyltransferase (Food industry)
(b) Improved utilization of low-cost substrates thereby making bioprocess system more economical.
(c) Production of biofuels from renewable resources (Green Technology)
(d) Production of novel products.

Strain improvement can be achieved through 4 major techniques (Han & Parekh, 2005, Parekh et al., 2000):

(a) Mutagenesis

(b) Genetic Recombination
(c) Recombinant DNA Technology, and
(d) Metabolic engineering

Mutagenesis

This method involves inducing mutations either through physical (X-rays/γ-rays/UV rays) or chemical (mutagens such as bromouracil/chlorouracil/nitrous acid/hydroxylamine) methods to create unique strains with desired biotechnological characteristics.

Genetic Recombination

It is the process of combining genetic information from 2 genotypes potentially resulting in unique strains with superior characteristics compare d to the original strains. This can be achieved by 3 major techniques:

(a) Protoplast fusion: Fusion of 2 closely related protoplasts.
(b) Transformation: Direct uptake of the exogenous DNA by the recipient cell/protoplasts.
(c) Conjugation: Unidirectional transfer of the genetic material from one strain to another through cell-to-cell contact.

Recombinant DNA Technology

This technique involves targeted modifications of the genome such as gene amplification, deletion, genome editing using CRISPR/Cas9 and introduction of new genes into the host organism via cloning in order to create strains that can produce products of commercial value. For example, insulin and interferon production in bacterial species via cloning.

CRISPR/Cas9 Technology in Strain Improvement

This technology has emerged as a revolutionary method for editing the genome with high precision, speed and flexibility. This method creates site-specific double strand breaks in the genome, which are then followed by host mediated repair mechanisms and thus enabling gene knockouts, insertions or replacements.

Through this process, the technology can aim at:

(a) Eliminating undesired metabolic pathways/ by-product formation.
(b) Improve substrate utilization
(c) Over-expression of the key synthetic genes
(d) Enhance stress resistance, and
(e) Introducing new biosynthetic pathways to boost the production of target molecule.

Additionally, this technology is more accurate, has minimal off-target effects and allows for multiplex gene-editing efficiently. This kind of technology has been successfully applied to improve strains of *E. coli, S. cerevisiae* and *C.glutamicum* used in biopharmaceutical manufacturing.

Metabolic Engineering

This technique also involves recombinant DNA technology which aims in manipulating the metabolic pathways of the host organism in order to produce an enhanced amount of the desired protein. Metabolic flux analysis (MFA) is an important analytical tool which determines the intracellular fluxes of metabolites thereby providing insights into the pathway bottlenecks and areas of optimization.

Case Studies

1. Objective: To enhance the production of erythromycin through the strain improvement technique (Devi et al., 2013).

Methodology: *Saccharopolyspora erythraea* exposed to random UV mutagenesis.

Result: Mutant strain showed a 40% increase in erythromycin in the production medium compared to the wild type strain.

2. Objective: To enhance the production of cephalomycin C (Chen et al., 1988).

Methodology: Cloning of a gene cluster (29.3kb) from *Streptomyces cattleya* into a heterologous host *Streptomyces lividans*.

Result: The amplification of the entire pathway in the heterologous host resulted in 2.3-fold increase in the production of Cephalomycin C.

Strategies for Optimizing Downstream Processing

Downstream processing involves a series of unit operations after upstream processes that aims to isolate, concentrate, purify and formulate the product efficiently. Optimizing the downstream processing is critical as it can directly impact the yield, product quality, total production costs and market competitiveness (**Figure 4**).

There are 4 major vital steps in downstream processing (Baumann & Hubbuch, 2017). This includes:

(1) Removal of insoluble (Solid-liquid separation)
(2) Product isolation and enrichment
(3) Product refinement/purification
(4) Final product processing (Finishing and formulation)

If the product is intracellular, then an additional step of cell disruption is required.

Figure 4. Overview of the downstream processing steps. This diagram represents an overview of the DSP steps that requires optimization for a better yield and quality of the desired bioproduct: This includes (a) removing the insolubles, (b) isolating the desired bioproduct, (c) purifying the isolated bioproduct and (d) formulating the bioproduct

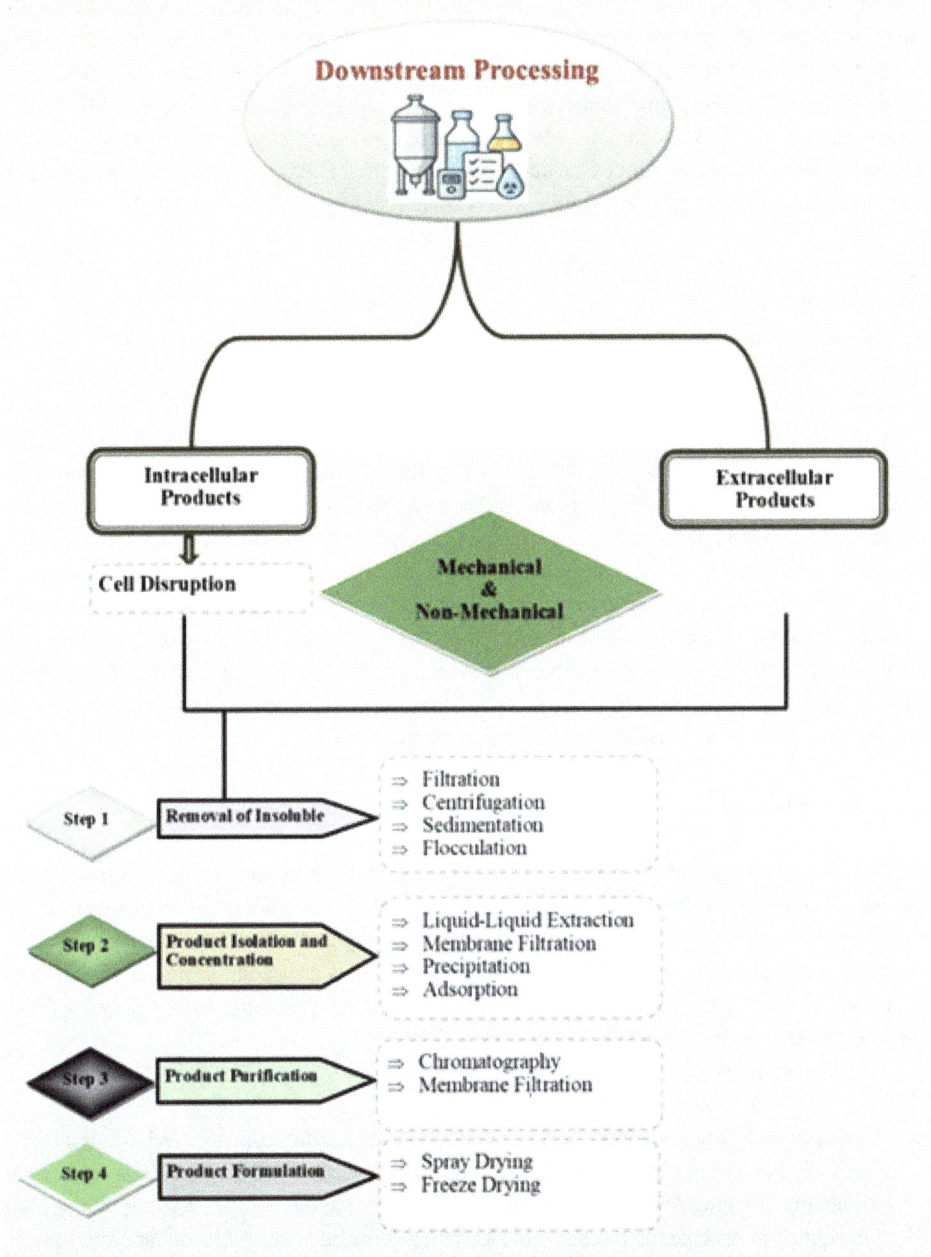

Removal of Insoluble

The type of insoluble that are common in bioprocess industry include: cells (if the product is extracellular), cell debris (if the product is intracellular) and particulate matter (suspended solids/ undissolved salts). To remove the insoluble, techniques like filtration, centrifugation, sedimentation and flocculation can be employed. The type of these techniques must be selected carefully based on the product sensitivity and scale of operation so as to improve the product yield, quality, production costs and also meet the regulatory compliance set by the bodies like FDA, EMA etc.

Filtration. It is the primary clarification step that is employed to separate debris from a liquid or gas phase. It is a technique where a particle containing medium when passed through a porous matrix/material separates particulate matter from the fermentation broth based on size. The commonly used 3 types of filtration at this stage includes:

(a) Depth filtration
(b) Microfiltration, and
(c) Acoustic field flow separation.

Depth Filtration

The filters of this type of filtration process are usually composed of cellulose fibres combined with inorganic filter aids such as activated carbon, perlite or diatomaceous earth and a resin binder that enhances the wet strength of the filter. Additionally, there are also charged depth filters where they contain charged polymers or ion-exchange particles within the filters. They serve two main functions: (a) exclusion of large particles trapped within the membrane, (b) particle adsorption due to amine chemistry and (c) removal of residual DNA, viruses and endotoxins (if positively charged depth filters are employed during the process). Optimizing the media selection (i.e., employing two different depth filter media), the flow rate (due to the possibility for clogging and pressure drop) and design of depth filter (incorporating charged polymers) can improve the impurity clearance efficiently (Nejatishahidein & Zydney, 2021).

Microfiltration

It is another most commonly used technique to remove the particulate matter from the liquid medium. It has a large pore size (0.1-5µm) that enables to operate under relatively low pressures which in turn enhances the membrane life, reduces fouling and provides an additional benefit of minimal energy and cost requirements. These membranes are generally made of polymeric membranes such as polysulfone (PSU), polyethersulfone (PES), polyamide (PA), polyvinylidene fluoride (PVDF) and cellulose acetate to name a few.

There are two types of membrane filtration:

(a) Static filtration: In static filtration (also known as dead end filtration), the feed flow is directed vertically into the membrane causing the particles to accumulate on the filter's surface and eventually clogging the membrane quickly. To overcome this issue, a booster pump might be required to provide the force so as to keep the flow rate intact or the membranes must be cleaned or replaced at fixed intervals for optimal performance. Another way to overcome the limitation of this filtration system is to switch to cross flow filtration system (Raghunath et al., 2012).

(b) Cross flow filtration: In cross flow filtration, the feed flow is directed across the membrane which reduces the chance of clogging and helps the system maintain constant flow rate over a longer period of time (Raghunath et al., 2012).

In applications where the feed contains more particulate matter, depth filtration is preferred over microfiltration as the former is capable of removing large impurities effectively while the latter will have clogging issues quickly. Optimizing the material for the filters, choosing the right configuration of the filter (hollow-fibre, flat sheet etc.), flow rate, minimizing the fouling of the membrane and real time monitoring will ensure product purity and yield effectively.

Acoustic Field Flow Separation

It is an emerging technique which leverages the ultrasound waves to move a target cell/particle from one feed stream into a new feed stream for the separation of next particle population (Kausley et al., 2022).

Centrifugation. It is one of the major techniques adopted in bioprocessing that uses centrifugal force to separate the particle debris from liquid phase based on density and size. Each centrifuge type has its own specific operational characteristics such as rotation speed (indicative of separation efficiency), capacity and shear force, that must be carefully considered based on the nature of the product (i.e., cell type, size and sensitivity) in order to improve the product quality and yield.

In recent years, there has been an increasing demand for continuous flow industrial centrifuges wherein there will be continuous feeding of the fermentation broth and collection of the clarified liquid with removal of insoluble performed intermittently.

Most commonly used centrifuges in the industrial applications include:

(a) Disc stack centrifuge
(b) Tubular bowl centrifuge
(c) Scroll bowl (decanter) centrifuge, and
(d) Multi chamber centrifuge

Disc Stack Centrifuge. It is the most widely used centrifuge to separate biomass from liquid. It has also been successfully utilized in liquid-liquid separation by using high centrifugal forces (6000-12000G). It can be operated under batch, semi-continuous and continuous modes. This centrifuge is characterized by closed spaced conical discs within the centrifuge bowl. When the suspended cultures arrive through the intake port, and when subjected to high centrifugal force, the suspended solids (denser particles) move from the bowl base towards the rotating bowl wall whereas the clarified liquid (or less dense particles) are displaced in the centre. The particulates can be removed continuously or intermittently based on the volume of the solids accumulated. Although it provides a good separation efficiency, it is not ideal for shear sensitive products. Additionally, the energy demand to operate this centrifuge is very high which adds to the total production costs (Esmaeilnejad-Ahranjani & Hajimoradi, 2022).

Tubular Bowl Centrifuge. It is a simple centrifuge that is also used to separate solid-liquid and liquid-liquid-solid effectively. It is less scalable and is applicable for processing smaller volumes. This is a type of centrifuge that can achieve a fine separation due to high centrifugal forces (15000G). Apart from clarifying the culture medium, it is also suitable for extracting and concentrating the product. It contains a single rotating bowl that has a single inlet feed and a two outlet streams. Once the liquid mixture experiences the centrifugal force, the very fine particles sediment near the inner walls of the bowl and the two liquid phases (light and heavy fraction) are removed simultaneously from the two streams. The solid particles that were retained in the bowl can be removed manually once the machine is stopped for cleaning. This type of centrifuge would be ideal for applications like: (a) separating 2 immiscible liquids and (b) purification of vaccines and food products such as oils/fruit juices etc (Esmaeilnejad-Ahranjani & Hajimoradi, 2022).

Multi-Chamber Centrifuge. It is an advanced version of a tubular bowl centrifuge that consists of a series of tubular bowls arranged coaxially with increasing diameter to achieve an enhanced separation efficiency. Each chamber in this centrifuge experiences a variation in the centrifugal force with the highest force in the periphery chambers and the lowest in the small diameter chambers. When the feed is fed into the small diameter chamber (central spindle), they progress through to the outer chambers in a zig-zag fashion and get separated based on the density. That is, the heavier particles get deposited in the smallest diameter bowl and the smallest particles settle down in the periphery chambers due to a higher centrifugal force experienced by them. The major advantage of this type of centrifuge is that, it has a greater solids capacity with no loss of efficiency as the chamber fills with solid particles. These types of systems are found commonly in the food industry to clarify fruit juices, beer etc (Udayan et al., 2022).

Scroll (Decanter) Centrifuge. Scroll centrifuge, also known as rotating bowl centrifuge, works on the principle of sedimentation to separate solid material from liquid. It is commonly used in the wastewater treatment of biosolids but they are also suitable for a wide range of applications in pharmaceuticals, food and beverage industry, chemical industry and biofuel production. The primary principle is similar to that of a static container/sedimentation tanks which exploits the differences in the specific gravities of the particulate matter and fluid in order to facilitate their separation. These older technologies take a considerable amount of time for the gravitational separation to occur (based on 1X G-force) whereas this newer technology enhances the sedimentation rate by spinning the bowl at high speed rotation (3000 times than that of normal gravitational acceleration). Under the influence of high centrifugal acceleration, the larger and denser solids settle in the bowl's inner wall, whereas the liquid moves towards the centre and gets discharged at the opposite end of the centrifuge via the centrate outlet. This type of centrifuge is a choice of selection which contains a higher content of biomass. The advantage of this type of centrifuge is that it is easy to maintain and eliminates the need for any replacement parts such as filter cloths. Additionally, the operation can also be automated thereby reducing labour requirements and enhancing productivity effectively (Udayan et al., 2022).

Flocculation. It is the process where fine/suspended particles clump together to form large aggregates that can be easily separated from the liquid medium. The particles can be brought together either by neutralizing the surface charges or by bridging the surface ions between the particles and making the average particle size bigger that eventually comes out of the liquid in the form of flocs or flakes. Additionally, two other modes of flocculation: patching (neutralization of localized surface charge) and sweeping (mechanical entrapment of fine/dispersed particles) are also employed.

It is achieved by the addition of various types of flocculants (chemical/biological/physical/physicochemical/auto flocculation). The greatest advantage of flocculation is that it is a low cost, employ nontoxic inexpensive flocculants, low energy consumption, easy operation and highly efficient technique (effective at even low doses). Additionally, these flocculants remain attached to the particulate matter they generate and therefore there are no additional steps required to remove them. Flocculation finds its use mainly to remove cells from the broth and also to remove the cell debris. Flocculation is generally preferred to be used prior to filtration because of the ability of the flocculants to coagulate the finer particles effectively and yields a more porous filter cake which can be easily removed from the membrane (Gervais & Wang, 2025, Yasarla & Ramarao, 2012).

Product Isolation and Concentration

Once the particulate matter/ suspended particles/ colloidal particles are removed, the following step is aimed to isolate the desired product from the remaining solution or from the cells (if the product is intracellular). This often involves techniques such as liquid-liquid extraction, membrane filtration, precipitation and adsorption. The choice of isolation method will greatly impact on the recovery, purity and product stability. Additionally, it will also influence the scalability, process time and cost of the overall downstream processing.

If the desired product is located within the cell such as vitamins/ enzymes, such molecules have to be released from the cells (with maximum recovery and in active form) for further processing. Cell disruption methods can be categorized into non-mechanical (physical, chemical and enzymatic) and mechanical methods respectively. The table below describes various non-mechanical and mechanical methods of cell disruption with their associated advantages and disadvantages that will eventually help in selecting the choice of method for breakage of the cells with the goal to recover maximum product in active form (Table 3) (Kakko et al., 2016, Gomes et al., 2020).

Based on the nature of the product to be isolated from the cells, a variety of strategies both mechanical and non-mechanical are presented, along with their associated advantages and disadvantages that will help in choosing the appropriate method of cell disruption.

Table 3. Various types of cell disruption methods

A. Mechanical methods of cell disruption			
Techniques	**Description**	**Advantages**	**Disadvantages**
• Bead Mill	• Use of grinding beads (glass/ceramic) to crack open the cells.	• Adapted for small- and large-scale production. • Ability to achieve uniform particle sizes. • Effective for viscous samples. • Can operate in continuous or batch mode. • Works well with complex tissues	• Choice of bead size and weight, concentration of the beads and agitation speed should be decided based on the cell type. • High power consumption • Generates heat that could damage intracellular proteins. • Potential risk for contamination
• Ultrasonication	• Uses high frequency sound waves to generate tiny bubbles (cavitation) which collapse to produce local shockwave that disrupt the cells in suspension.	• Ideal for any cell type. • High lysing efficiency.	• High cost. • Not scalable. • Very loud process. • Generate heat, requires cooling system.
• Liquid Homogenization	• Cells are lysed by forcing the cell suspension through a small orifice.	• Uniform particle size reduction. • Ensures stability and reproducibility.	• Not scalable. • Use of Dounce homogenizer may vary in reproducibility.

continued on following page

Table 3. Continued

A. Mechanical methods of cell disruption			
Techniques	**Description**	**Advantages**	**Disadvantages**
• French press / High pressure homogenization	• Cell suspension is forced through a narrow gap under very high pressure (1500 bar) and cells break open upon discharge when the pressure drops to atmospheric.	• Most widely used methods for cell disruption.	• Small scale method but can be scalable. • Factors like heat generation, operating pressure and number of passes affect the protein release.
B. Non- Mechanical Methods of Cell Disruption			
Physical methods			
• Thermolysis (Microwave treatment)	• Breakage of the cells when they are subjected to short high temperature shocks.	• Easy to operate. • Suitable for large scale production.	• Suitable for only heat stable intracellular proteins/products.
• Decompression	• Involves subjecting the cell suspension to a pressurized supercritical gas for a specified time (depending on the cell type). During the incubation time, the gas enters the cell and upon release, the cell expands rapidly and results in cell rupture.	• Gentle on cells. • Easy removal of large debris and facilitating the extraction of the desired product easily.	• Suitable only for small scale laboratories.
• Osmotic shock	• This method initially involves suspending the cells in high/low salt concentrations and then subjecting them to opposite conditions immediately resulting in osmotic pressure and cell lysis.	• Easy to perform.	• Low efficiency. • Enzymatic pre-treatment would be a requirement for efficient disruption. • Dependency on high amounts of salts and water. • May add on to the DSP costs due to product dilution during the process.
Chemical and enzymatic methods			
• Detergents	• Widely used cell lysis method which works by disrupting protein-lipid interactions effectively. • Can be anionic (SDS), non-ionic (Triton X-100) and cationic (CTAB)	• Effective for laboratory experiments (for example: extraction of DNA, RNA or proteins from cells).	• Potential for denaturation of many proteins in lysis process. • Hinder subsequent purification steps.
• Solvents	• Solvents like alcohols, DMSO and toluene can extract lipid components from cell wall/membrane and thereby releasing the intracellular components.	• Rapid and simple method. • Easy recovery of the target molecules.	• Possibility of some other proteins to get denatured. • Caution must be exercised for their potential ignitability nature.
• Enzymes	• Enzymes work by selective interaction with the component of the cell wall/ membrane, modify the cell boundary and allow the intracellular compounds to seep out. • Lysozyme (for bacteria), zymolase (for yeast and fungi), cellulases, chitinases, glucanases and xylanases are the most commonly used for cell disruption.	• Gentle method of cell disruption.	• Limited only to small scale industries due to high cost of the enzyme. • May complicate further DSP steps.

Liquid-Liquid Extraction. Liquid-liquid extraction (LLE), also known as solvent extraction/ partitioning, is a process where the solutes in the mixture of a liquid solution separate based on the difference in their solubility when they come in contact with another phase. It is mainly used to extract antibiotics or enzymes from the fermentation broths. The two liquid phases will be generally immiscible or partially miscible (one phase is aqueous while the other will be an organic phase). The efficiency of extraction is based on the partition coefficient/distribution coefficient (p). It is a measure of how a compound in a mixture distributes itself in the two immiscible phases (Mazzola et al., 2008).

Partition coefficient is defined as the ratio of the solute between the organic phase and the aqueous phase at equilibrium.

(p) = Concentration of the solute in organic phase/concentration of the solute in aqueous phase.

The choice of the solvent should be such that it has a higher 'p' i.e., the desired solute should be in the organic phase and a low 'p' for the impurities.

The extraction of the compound can be based on (Muller et al., 2000):

(a) Physical property of the solute
(b) Dissociation property of the solute, and
(c) Reactive property of the solute, i.e., the extraction of the desired compound can be done by allowing it to react to a carrier molecule and then extracted into the organic solvent.

Other factors which will affect the extraction efficiency include (Muller et al., 2000):

(a) pH and ionic strength of the solution
(b) Temperature
(c) Contact time between the two phases.

The advantages of LLE include (Muller et al., 2000):

(a) Highly efficient
(b) Versatile, applicable for azeotropic mixtures and also heat sensitive compounds.
(c) Can be operated in continuous mode
(d) Low cost and energy requirements, and
(e) Easily scalable.

It also has multiple disadvantages such as (Muller et al., 2000):

(a) Solvent recovery after product extraction may add on to the cost in further DSP steps.
(b) Possibility for degradation of heat sensitive compounds during the solvent recovery process.
(c) Might not be efficient to extract highly polar compounds.
(d) The amount of solvent used can interfere with the chromatographic analysis.
(e) Time-consuming
(f) Potential loss of sample due to its adsorption onto glassware, and
(g) The solvents if not recovered or recycled after the process, might pose serious environmental concerns.

Membrane Filtration. As previously mentioned, membrane filtration uses a semi-permeable membrane of specific pore size to selectively retain the molecules larger than the pore size, while allowing the smaller molecules to pass through the pores. This system can serve 3 major functions:

(a) Separation of the biomolecules from complex mixtures

(b) Concentrating the product
(c) Purifying the product.

The two major types of pressure-driven membrane filtration processes include:

(a) Ultrafiltration, and
(b) Reverse osmosis.

Ultrafiltration (UF). This type of membrane filtration effectively fractionates molecules ranging from 1000-50000 Da. It requires a pressure of 1-7 bar or a centrifugal force of 2000G. They are commonly used in the research and industry to concentrate protein solutions or extracellular vesicles and also to isolate low/high molecular weight compounds from different solvents used. Although the process is simple, scalable and not time consuming, few considerations to be considered include (Jonsson & Tragardh, 1990, Cheang & Zydney, 2004):

(a) UF might not be highly effective if different substance with similar properties are to be separated.
(b) Product yield will be much superior if centrifuge-driven UF is used instead of pressure-driven UF
(c) Chances of membrane fouling quickly (if dead-end filtration is chosen)
(d) Cannot separate monovalent/divalent ions from the product effectively, therefore require additional filtration step to purify the product.

Reverse Osmosis (RO). Unlike UF, RO process is able to filter out the tiniest contaminants. This treatment system uses extremely small pores (pore size ranging from 0.0001 to 0.001 microns) to eliminate dissolved ions (monovalent/multivalent) and various other small molecules and particles including salts, minerals, viruses, bacteria, organic compounds and endotoxins. It is primarily used in water purification for various applications like pharmaceutical industry for drug manufacturing and preparing injectable drugs, in the food and beverage sector such as fruit and vegetable juices concentration, milk and whey concentration and wine dealcoholisation (Kilduff et al., 2004).

RO is a very efficient process as it can fractionate, concentrate and also purify the product effectively in a single unit operation. Additionally, this system will have minimal impact on the quality of the product as there is no heat, pH or chemical changes involved during the process. Furthermore, it is an energy efficient process with respect to it concentrating the product as there is no phase change requirement unlike evaporative concentration which requires thermal energy (heat) for the water removal. When using RO systems, the energy cost is variable and it depends on the size and usage of the system, ionic content of the fluid sample and volume of the fluid sample respectively. There are few factors that has to be considered when selecting RO systems (**Tomczak & Gryta, 2022**). These include:

(a) Scaling of the membrane
(b) Membrane fouling
(c) Chemical nature of the membrane, as it affects the permeation of the constituents from the fluid mixture through the porous membranes.

Precipitation. It is a well-established and widely used method for large scale recovery of the proteins from complex mixtures. It is also used in the industry for the isolation of antibiotics and citric acid from fermentation broths, and in addition it may also be used to remove unwanted contaminants such as nucleic acids, pigments etc. from complex mixtures. With respect to protein applications, proteins can be recovered and precipitated based on their properties such as ionic strength, pH, dielectric constant, size, temperature and hydrophobicity of the protein. The precipitation techniques aimed to recover the proteins are such that they do not lose their biological function. Some of the major precipitation methods employed in the industry for the recovery of the proteins are described in the below table (Table 4) (Pennell, 1960, Zala et al., 2012).

Table 4. Various precipitation methods: This table indicates the various types of precipitation methods employed in the industry to isolate the proteins along with the key considerations for each technique

Precipitation technique	Principle	Technique considerations
Salting out	• Reducing the solubility of the protein in the solution of high ionic strength i.e., at high concentration of the salts, hydration barriers of the protein molecules are disrupted because these salts compete with target molecule for the water molecules and thus resulting in the exposure of hydrophobic patches of the protein surface, thus tending to aggregate and precipitate.	• Heat of solution should be minimal. • Desalting required for further purification of the protein.
Isoelectric precipitation	• Reducing the solubility of the protein by adjusting the pH to their isoelectric point where they have zero charge.	• No desalting required • Extraction pH and time should be optimized carefully for maximal recovery of the protein. • Filtration/centrifugation might be a requirement if the extracted protein contains seed material.
Organic solvents	• Solvents such as ethanol, acetone and 2-propanol reduce the dielectric constant of the medium and thereby enhancing the attractive forces between the proteins that results in their precipitation. • Additionally, the organic solvents reduce the hydration levels that can also result in their aggregation due to the exposure of the interactive sites	• Required the operation to be performed at lower temperatures to avoid denaturation problems. • Because the addition of the organic solvents results in temperature rise due to 'heat of mixing', efficient cooling systems are required. • Flammability of the organic solvents to be considered when using it in large scale industries.
Precipitation with non-ionic polymers (Polyethylene glycol)	• Works similar to that of organic solvents i.e., PEG reduces the availability of water molecules for protein solvation and thus precipitates protein.	• PEG does not denature the proteins instead the proteins become stabilized upon interaction with PEG. • Need an additional step to remove the PEG from the precipitate such as UF/adsorption.
Precipitation with ionic polymers (polyacrylic acid and polyethyleneimine)	• Ionic polymers complex with charged protein molecules, result in their charge neutralization and precipitation.	
Affinity precipitation	• Employs the use of ligands (attached to an insoluble matrix/solid) that selectively and reversibly binds the target molecules and precipitates it from the solution. • Commonly used ligands include: lectins, antibodies and p-amino benzamidine	• Can generate high purity homogenous protein product with yield greater than 90%. • Ligands can be easily separated from the precipitate and can be recycled for further use. • High cost is a key consideration when employing it in large scale operations.

Some of the limitations associated with precipitation methods include:

(a) Possibility of co-precipitation of impurities along with the target proteins.
(b) Certain precipitation methods are difficult to scale-up.
(c) Possibility of irreversible denaturation (due to harsh precipitation conditions) and,
(d) May complicate further downstream processing steps if the precipitants (solvents/salts) are a part of the target protein.

Adsorption. Adsorption is the process that relies on the adhesion of the target molecules to the solid material (adsorbent) embedded in the column while allowing the other components in the mixture to pass through. It is again mainly employed in protein applications. The major properties of the protein that can be used for adsorption include:

(a) Electrostatic interaction
(b) Hydrophobicity of the protein
(c) Surface energy, and
(d) Intermolecular forces.

Activated charcoal was the most commonly used adsorbent in earlier days but now fibrous adsorbents such as cellulose based fibres, wool based fibres and synthetic polymeric fibres are gaining much attention in biomanufacturing due to cost effectiveness, wide range of available options of surface chemistries (functional groups, surface charge, hydrophilicity or hydrophobicity) and physical and chemical robustness of the adsorbent (Schneider et al., 2022).

Some of the limitations associated with adsorption technique include:

(a) Adsorbents may bind to both the desired product and impurities of similar nature, thereby reducing the purification efficiency.
(b) May lead to difficulty in desorption of the target product from the adsorbents, thereby affecting the product quality, and
(c) May face scale-up challenges due to the difficulty in maintaining uniform distribution and binding capacity of the adsorbent throughout the process.

Purification of the Product

The biological products (proteins, enzymes etc.) isolated in the previous stage can very well be purified by a versatile separation and purification technique known as chromatography. The type of chromatography to be employed for the purification is dependent on the nature of the product and the impurities present. Additionally, considerations such as processing of larger volumes of the isolated product, reducing process steps and cost, and ability to improve the purification yield have to be considered when selecting a specific chromatographic technique for the purification process.

Chromatography in general, exploits the ability of the analytes in the mobile phase to separate based on their affinities towards the stationary phase. The below table will highlight the various types of chromatographic methods that are employed frequently in the industry for product purification (Table 5) (Freitag, 2013, Rathore et al., 2018).

Table 5. Various chromatographic techniques: This table depicts a variety of chromatography types that can be chosen to isolate and purify the desired bioproduct based on the nature of the bioproduct

Chromatographic technique	Key feature	Application
Ion exchange chromatography	Separation of the molecules based on charge	Proteins, nucleic acids, enzymes and vaccines.
Size exclusion chromatography	Separation of the molecules based on the size and shape	Particularly useful to remove salts and low molecular weight compounds.
Affinity chromatography	Separation of the molecule based on the interaction of the molecule and the ligand	mAb, fusion proteins
Hydrophobic interaction chromatography	Separation of the molecules with subtle hydrophobic variations.	Proteins, mAb
Multimodal chromatography	Separation of the molecules from complex mixtures based on multiple interaction modes	Proteins and metabolites.
High performance liquid chromatography	High resolution technique to separate molecules based on either polarity/charge.	Peptides and small molecules
Simulated moving bed chromatography	Continuous separation of the molecules from the complex mixtures.	Large volume separation of pharmaceuticals.

Apart from chromatography, membrane-based filtration (UF and RO) are also commonly employed to purify the product. It is seen utilized majorly in biopharmaceutical manufacturing for the removal of viruses from biologics.

Formulation of the Product

Crystallization and drying are the most common approaches in formulating many products (Ishwarya et al., 2015, Abdul-Fattah & Truong, 2010, Hekmat, 2015).

Crystallization: It is the most common method employed in the pharmaceutical industry (>90%) to synthesize active pharmaceutical ingredients (APIs). Crystallization process is achieved by 4 major steps:

(a) Preparation of the supersaturated solution
(b) Inducing nucleation by solvent evaporation or cooling
(c) Growth of the crystals, and
(d) Harvesting and drying of the crystals.

Crystallization Challenges: Although it is the predominant type used in the industry, it has several challenges which includes:

(a) Attaining a uniform particle size distribution i.e., wide particle size distribution and shape can affect the filtration and drying process immensely.
(b) The final crystal size obtained directly impact the quality of the final product with smaller particles having enhanced solubility and dissociation characteristics.

Factors to be considered to achieve a good crystallization include:

(a) Solvent selection, and
(b) Controlling nucleation and crystal growth by selecting the optimum temperature.

Drying: It is a process which basically involves the removal of moisture from the product by the process of heat transfer to the product. Because most of the products are heat sensitive, drying process must be performed carefully. The drying process is achieved by either of the two methods: (a) Spray drying and (b) Freeze drying.

Spray Drying: It is a choice of method for drying a large volume of liquid. In this process, the solution to be dried are atomized and directed over a hot gas stream (150-250^{0}C) for the water to evaporate while leaving behind the solid particles. This is a preferred method for enzymes, antibiotics and food products because of the rapid drying while maintaining the temperature of the particles low.

Freeze Drying: This is the gentle method of drying as it does not cause loss of biological activity and is used for many pharmaceutical products such as vaccines, enzymes etc. It works based on the principle of sublimation of the frozen product directly into vapour, bypassing the liquid phase. Although it is a time-consuming process and requires specialized equipment and expertise, it is still employed in the industry due to its ability to produce a more stable product.

Challenges in DSP

The major challenges that needs to be optimized and co-ordinated include:

(a) Processing of complex mixtures
(b) Maintaining the stability of the product throughout the process
(c) Cost involved in DSP
(d) Reducing the environmental impact throughout the process, and
(e) Adhering to the regulatory standards.

SCALE UP AND INDUSTRIAL APPLICATIONS

Challenges in Scaling Up Bioprocess

One of the major concerns and a challenge in the bioprocess industry is to scale up the laboratory bioprocesses to industry. Some of the major challenges that has to be tamed for efficient scale up include (Figure 5) (Marques et al., 2010, Du et al., 2022):

(a) Biological variability: Shear stress, altered pH, nutrient over gradients, O2 gradients.
(b) Problems of mass and heat transfer: Uniform mixing, effective heat dissipation that will ultimately have an impact on cell growth and product formulation.
(c) Constraints in reactor design: Balancing of equipment mixing, aeration as well as scale-specific physical parameters.
(d) Reproducibility of process: It is hard to preserve product quality, yield and consistency of a process across scales.

(e) Regulatory and Validations: Adherence to GMP and regulatory requirements is increased at industrial scale.
(f) Cost and Resource Intensiveness: Scale-up is a high-capital require high-quality labour, and sourcing adequate raw materials.
(g) Complexity of Instrumentation and Automation: Increased bioreactors, sophisticated sensors, control systems to control and maintain desirable conditions.

Strategies for Seamless Transition From Batch-To-Continuous Biomanufacturing

Some of the major strategies that can be applied for the transition from batch-to-continuous biomanufacturing include (Figure 5) (Challener, 2023, Zydney, 2016, Xu & Zydney, 2023):

(a) Process Intensification:
- In high cell density cultures and perfusion to make sure that they maximize their products at low volumes.
- One-use technology to be more flexible and reduce contamination consequences.

(b) Monitoring and Control:
- PAT tool and Raman spectroscopy offer current analytics that can be monitored in place of critical process parameters.
- Automation of continuous processes is made to stabilise through feedback control loops.

(c) Scalable and Modular Reactor Design:
- Multiple tasks can be pruned in parallel by simply transitioning scales using modular systems.
- Microbial or mammalian cell systems and plug-and-play bioreactors might be adapted to each other.

(d) Intrinsic Upstream and Downstream Processes:
- The two upstream (fermentation/bioreactor) and downstream (purification) processes are interconnected to enable continuous flow.
- Technologies like simulated moving bed chromatography and tangential flow filtration (TFF) can be used.

(e) Modelling Tools and Digital Twin:
- Use of computational models and digital twins to show scale-up behaviour and optimize parameters the parameters before the physical realisation. Integration does not only make processes more efficient, but it saves an enormous amount of time that could have been dedicated to development and optimisation. Consequently, researchers are able to quickly accommodate alternative requirements in biopharmaceutical manufacturing and finally resulting into more responsive and flexible production solutions.

(f) Lifecycle and regulatory harmonisation approaches:
- The Quality by Design (QbD) approaches guarantee the development of products where quality is prioritized at initial stages, leading to easier approvals by the regulators and uniformity in terms of products dealing with their entire life cycle. When these principles are embedded, the manufacturers will enjoy a stronger ver-

sion of compliance and at the same time promote innovation in the processes they undertake.

Figure 5. Challenges and strategies for efficient scale up in the bioprocess industry

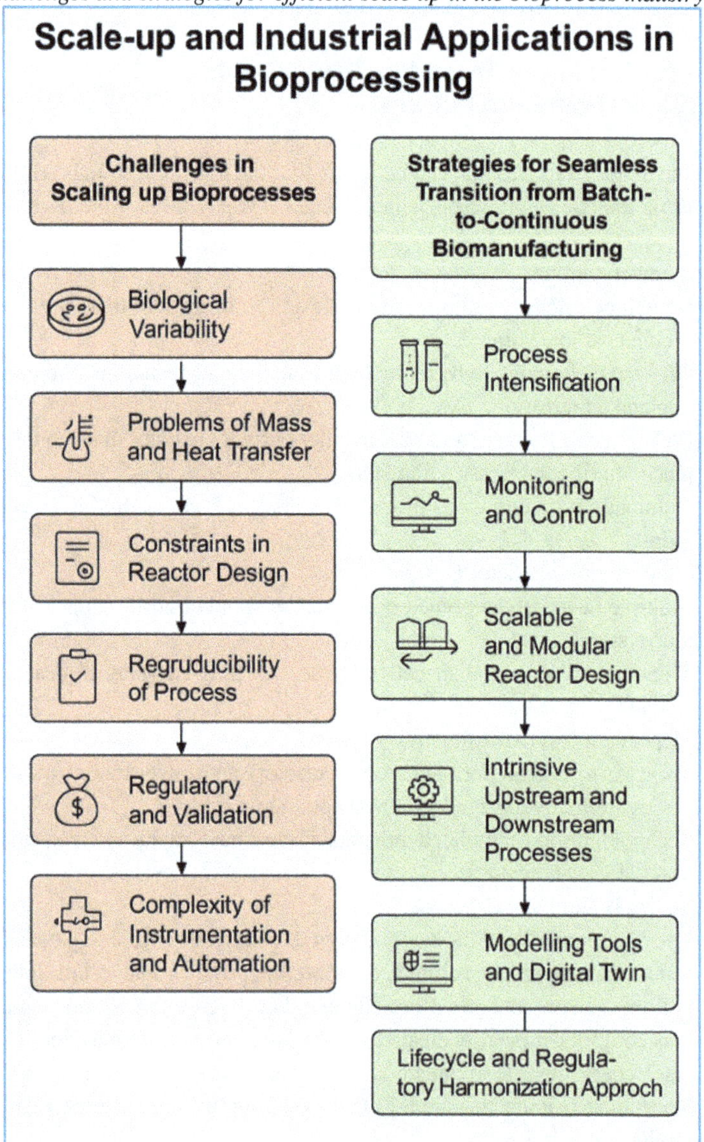

REGULATORY CONSIDERATIONS AND COMPLIANCE IN THE BIOPROCESS OPTIMIZATION

The biopharmaceutical sector is experiencing an upward trend of migrating to continuous biomanufacturing and digital innovation, with advanced technologies and strengthened regulatory guidance. Continuous biomanufacturing presents unique challenges in validation, real-time monitoring, and product consistency, prompting regulators worldwide to reassess existing guidelines. The Regulatory agencies like; FDA have long been proponents of continuous processing of small and large molecule drugs. The action of legislation like the Prescription Drug User Fee Act (PDUFA VII) promoted in 2022 and the Food and Drug Omnibus Reform Act (FDORA) as part of Consolidated Appropriations Act 2023 and the 2022 Executive Order on the National Biotechnology and Biomanufacturing Initiative issued by President Biden all served to facilitate in the creation and use of advanced manufacturing methods. In 2023, a major regulatory milestone was the publication of the ICH Q13 (Continuous Manufacturing of Drug Substances and Drug Products) guideline on continuous manufacturing that offers principles of the development of drug products and drug substances along with commercial manufacturing. An example of an acceptable guideline in FDA and EMA, it may be considered as a major stride towards harmonization of regulations internationally since it allows the manufacturers a chance to define specific methods of implementation (Table 6) (Fisher et al., 2023, Dahlgren & Hausner, 2023).

Table 6. Global regulatory bodies and their role in the bioprocess industry

Regulatory Body	Region	Focus Area	Key Guidance
FDA	USA	Drug Manufacturing	cGMP, QbD, PAT
EMA	Europe	Biologics and Biosimilars	EU-GMP Annexes
ICH	Global	Quality by Design	ICH Q8, Q9, Q10
WHO	Global	Global GMP Harmonization	WHO GMP Guidelines
CDSCO	India	Schedule M Compliance	GMP under Drugs Act

Moreover, the ICH Q9 (R1) guideline of January 2025 focuses on quality risk management, particularly in relation to supply chains and equipment, supporting effective manufacturing systems and the introduction of continuous processes even more. Industry processes like BioPhorum have been instrumental in assisting with regulatory and technical issues, through providing road-maps, risk assessment template, and practical advice in the area of continuous downstream processing of therapeutic proteins. Though initially the rate of continuous bioprocessing was slow to take off, now even the industry is catching the motion. According to surveys conducted by BioPlan Associates and by EMD Millipore, a significant number of biomanufacturers (up to 70 percent) are considering or are in fact planning to use continuous chromatography and perfusion technologies in the next two years, joined by intensified fed-batch process goals, cell line and media optimization and enhanced buffer management. Such tendencies signify the intensification of the process commitment over the board (Pathodiya, 2025, Silva et al., 2023).

The central Drugs standard control organization (CDSCO) and the World Health Organization (WHO) are important in providing standards and control of bioprocessing to maintain safety, quality, and effectiveness of biological products. WHO is an international regulating body in that it promotes internationally harmonised Good Manufacturing Practice (GMP) guidelines which are specifically prepared with regard to the pharmaceutical and biological products. It happens also to operate a Prequalification Program to evaluate and clear biopharmaceuticals including vaccines and biosimilars to be used in public health programs and specifically in low- and middle-income countries. WHO assists with capacity building through regulatory technical training, guidance papers and international harmonization through its Technical Report Series (TRS). Conversely, CDSCO is the national regulatory body in India that issues approval, monitors and controls the quality of drugs and biologicals. It promotes Good Manufacturing Practices under the Schedule M under the Drugs and Cosmetics Act and manages clinical trials, licensing of imports and post marketing surveillance of bioproducts. CDSCO also undertakes inspection of facilities and it has collaborated with WHO and ICH to bring the regulatory environment of India in line with international best practices especially in the area of vaccines and advanced biologics (**Figure 6**). In India, CDSCO is gradually incorporating GMP standards and encouraging innovation via schemes like the New Drugs and Clinical Trials Rules (2019). On the need for adaptive regulatory models that support real-time release testing (RTRT), Process Analytical Technology (PAT), and digital twins. This harmonization is crucial to streamline to reduce the development timelines and access the high-quality products.

Figure 6. Roles of WHO and CDSCO

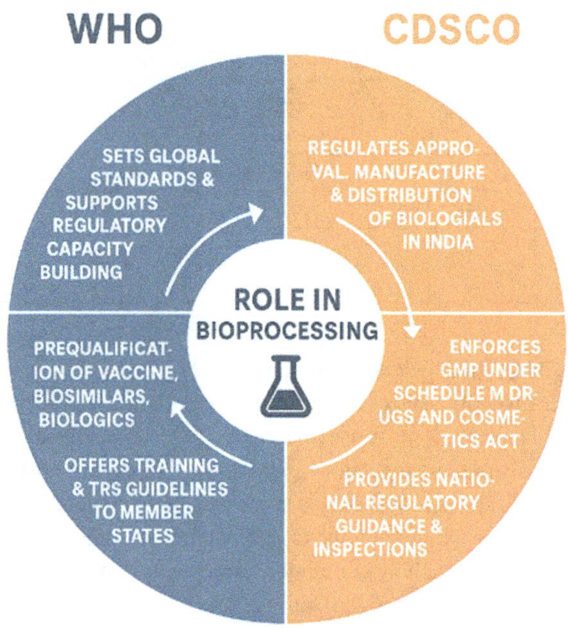

There are approximately 80 companies currently engaged in the development and supply of equipment towards continuous biomanufacturing. Large and mid-sized biotech and pharmaceutical companies have been the most adopting, with a low adoption by biosimilar manufacturer. Both new facilities and new products can have continuous processes applied to novel products and second-generation formulations at both facilities. The combination of both single-use and stainless-steel systems are commonly found in commercial operations, but those commercial-size processes are usually found on the clinical scale side of the spectrum with disposable technologies.

Market predictions indicate that the worldwide continuous bioprocessing market is increasing in compound annual growth rate between 6.4-22 percent. Further development of process analytical technologies (PAT), data management, and merger of up/downstream unit operation are likely to lead to an even faster pace of adoption. Consecutively, continuous biomanufacturing has become a major prospect of modern pharmaceutical production that brings improved efficiency, flexibility, and quality of the products.

FUTURE TRENDS AND INNOVATIONS IN BIOPROCESSING OPTIMIZATION

The development of bioprocessing technology new bio-products are being produced with more complex structure and functions requiring new production platforms.

Role of Digital Biomanufacturing in Bioprocessing

Digital biomanufacturing incorporates data science, automation, artificial intelligence (AI), and cyber-physical systems both to improve dynamic control and flexibility of bioprocesses and to increase the efficiency of the biomanufacturing system as a whole. It converts traditional manufacturing into an intelligent, predictable and adaptive system (Figure 7) (Estevez & Navarro, 2017).

Figure 7. Functions of digital biomanufacturing

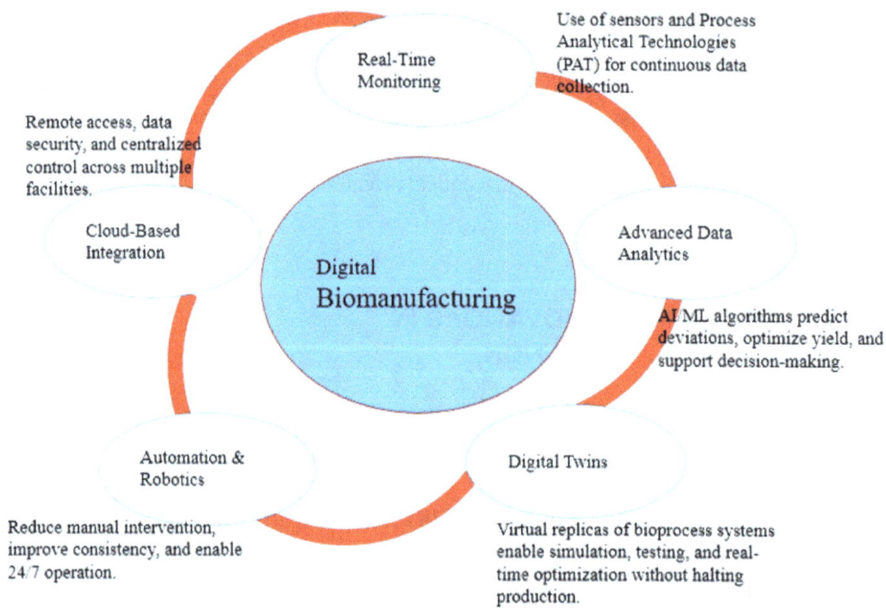

Role of Artificial Intelligence in Bioprocess

Artificial Intelligence (AI) is rapidly becoming a revolutionary solution to bioprocess optimization, especially with the role it can play in predictive analytics. Allowing the AI systems to combine machine learning (ML) algorithms and large amounts of data on bioprocess status (e.g., sensor outputs, process parameters, and omics samples), it will be possible to detect unseen trends and predict deviations and recommend beforehand action plans to control processes. These predictive models are used to improve real-time decision-making and increase the robustness of the processes as well as reduce the number of batch failures because anomalies would be detected early. As an example, multivariate training could provide predictions on cell growth, product yield, or even metabolic shift with high accuracy with AI to adjust dynamic processes appropriately. Moreover, the combination of AI and 'digital twins, virtual representations of the bioprocess environment collector, allows continuous simulation, optimization, and test scenarios without affecting production. With regulatory organizations increasingly recognizing the potential of both AI in Process Analytical Technology (PAT) and Real-Time Release Testing (RTRT) systems, it is becoming increasingly likely to play a core role in the future of an intelligent biomanufacturing environment. With the development of this bioprocessing technology we are also seeing rising presence of next-generation bio-products, which are increasingly more complex, targeted, and potentially therapeutic. The innovations require the creation of new and flexible production platforms to fit the needs of the contemporary healthcare and the biotechnology industries.

Role of Gene Editing Technologies in Bioprocessing

A potentially even more revolutionary field is that of synthetic biology and genome editing, in which genetically engineered mammalian and microbial cell lines (which frequently make use of products like CRISPR/Cas9, ZFNs, TALENs) are created to synthesize bespoke therapeutic proteins, enzymes, and cell-based medicines.

Benefits

- Faster development with high yield
- Ability to degrade or remove immunogenic products or proteins
- Enhance the development of Gene therapies, cellular therapies and Biosimilars.
- Ability to enhance Quality control and regulatory compliance by precise genetic control.

Role of Cell-Free biomanufacturing in Bioprocessing

Cell-free biomanufacturing is another innovation, using living cells rather than the enzymes or cell lysates. The advantage of this strategy is the possibility of acceleration of the development cycle, the reduction of biosafety risks, and better control over the quality of products; it is a perfect choice when it comes to diagnostic reagents, vaccines, and on-demand therapeutics. The introduction of modular and single-use bioreactors has contributed to a great extent towards enhancing flexibility of manufacturing. Such systems minimize the chances of cross-contamination, reduce costs of cleaning and validation, and are especially appropriate in multi-producing plants and low production capacities. Continuous manufacturing is also becoming more and more used, with traditional batch moving aside in favor of its continuous equivalents, thereby leading to greater efficiency in the process. Such systems allow building of a stable-state production with improved consistency, increased throughput, and decreased time-to-market, which are essential features of biologics scale-up and supply to the global market. Lastly, the bioproducts landscape is also broadening as next-generation biologics (bispecific antibodies, gene therapies, mRNA vaccines, and microbiome-based therapeutics) are becoming common. These products have sophisticated mechanisms of action, targeted delivery, and potential resolution to quote intractable diseases, which means that there is a necessity of having robust, flexible, and creative bioprocessing technologies (Rogers & Jensen, 2019, Su et al., 2019).

CONCLUSION

In summary, this chapter has systematically presented the overview of the bioprocess system, followed by outlining various in-depth optimization strategies across both upstream and downstream processes. It further discussed the challenges for scale up and reviewed various strategies to address them. Lastly, it emphasized the role of regulatory agencies in assuring the product quality and safety prior to the environmental release.

REFERENCES

Abdul-Fattah, A. M., & Truong, V. L. (2010). Drying process methods for biopharmaceutical products: an overview. *Formulation and process development strategies for manufacturing biopharmaceuticals*, 705-738.

Abufalgha, A. A., Clarke, K. G., & Pott, R. W. (2020). Characterisation of bubble diameter and gas hold-up in simulated hydrocarbon-based bioprocesses in a bubble column reactor. *Biochemical Engineering Journal*, *158*, 107577.

Alves, S. S., & Vasconcelos, J. M. T. (1996). Optimisation of agitation and aeration in fermenters. *Bioprocess Engineering*, *14*(3), 119–123.

Andrews, G. F., & Przezdziecki, J. (1986). Design of fluidized-bed fermentors. *Biotechnology and Bioengineering*, *28*(6), 802–810. PMID: 18555396

Bäcker, M., Delle, L., Poghossian, A., Biselli, M., Zang, W., Wagner, P., & Schöning, M. J. (2011). Electrochemical sensor array for bioprocess monitoring. *Electrochimica Acta*, *56*(26), 9673–9678.

Baumann, P., & Hubbuch, J. (2017). Downstream process development strategies for effective bioprocesses: Trends, progress, and combinatorial approaches. *Engineering in Life Sciences*, *17*(11), 1142–1158. PMID: 32624742

Challener, C. A. (2023). *The future is continuous: Accelerating the shift in biomanufacturing*. Pharma's Almanac.

Chang, C. C., Ryu, D. D. Y., Park, C. S., Kim, J. Y., & Ogrydziak, D. M. (1998). Recombinant bioprocess optimization for heterologous protein production using two-stage, cyclic fed-batch culture. *Applied Microbiology and Biotechnology*, *49*(5), 531–537. PMID: 9650251

Cheang, B., & Zydney, A. L. (2004). A two-stage ultrafiltration process for fractionation of whey protein isolate. *Journal of Membrane Science*, *231*(1-2), 159–167.

Chen, C. W., Lin, H. F., Kuo, C. L., Tsai, H. L., & Tsai, J. F. Y. (1988). Cloning and expression of a DNA sequence conferring cephamycin C production. *Bio/technology*, *6*(10), 1222–1224.

Chen, N. Y. (1990). The design of airlift fermenters for use in biotechnology. *Biotechnology & Genetic Engineering Reviews*, *8*(1), 379–396.

Chenthamarakshan, A., Parambayil, N., Miziriya, N., Soumya, P. S., Lakshmi, M. K., Ramgopal, A., & Nambisan, P. (2017). Optimization of laccase production from Marasmiellus palmivorus LA1 by Taguchi method of design of experiments. *BMC Biotechnology*, *17*(1), 12. PMID: 28193272

Constantinides, A., Spencer, J. L., & Gaden, E. L.Jr. (1970). Optimization of batch fermentation processes. I. Development of mathematical models for batch penicillin fermentations. *Biotechnology and Bioengineering*, *12*(5), 803–830. PMID: 5489784

Dahlgren, G., & Hausner, D. B. (2023). *ICH Q13 and what is next for continuous manufacturing*. Pharmaceutical Engineering.

Darvishi, F., & Abolhasan Moghaddami, N. (2019). Optimization of an industrial medium from molasses for bioethanol production using the Taguchi statistical experimental-design method. *Fermentation (Basel, Switzerland)*, *5*(1), 14.

Das, P. K., Sahoo, A., & Veeranki, V. D. (2025). Modeling and Optimization of Recombinant Tocilizumab Production From Pichia pastoris Using Response Surface Methodology and Artificial Neural Network. *Biotechnology and Bioengineering*. PMID: 40371610

Das, S. P., Das, D., & Goyal, A. (2014). Statistical optimization of fermentation process parameters by Taguchi orthogonal array design for improved bioethanol production. *Journal of Fuels*, *2014*(1), 419674.

Dassau, E., Zadok, I., & Lewin, D. R. (2006). Combining six-sigma with integrated design and control for yield enhancement in bioprocessing. *Industrial & Engineering Chemistry Research*, *45*(25), 8299–8309.

Desai, P. D., & Zimmerman, W. B. (2023). Microbubble Intensification of Bioprocessing: The role of direct microorganism and bubble interactions. *Johnson Matthey Technology Review*, *67*(4), 371–401.

() Devi, C. S., Saini, A., Rastogi, S., Naine, S. J., & Mohanasrinivasan, V. (2013). Strain improvement and optimization studies for enhanced production of erythromycin in bagasse based medium using Saccharopolyspora erythraea MTCC 1103. *3 Biotech, 5*(1), 23.

Du, C., Zhang, Y., Gao, X., Liu, Q., & Wang, X. (2022). Model-based optimization in large-scale fermentation: Recent advances and future prospects. *Bioengineering (Basel, Switzerland)*, *9*(9), 473. PMID: 36135019

Dutta, D., Kumar, P., Singh, A., & Khade, S. (2024). Bioprocess strategies for enhanced performance in single-use bioreactors for biomolecule synthesis: A biokinetic approach. *Food Bioengineering*, *3*(3), 337–351.

Eslami, T., & Jungbauer, A. (2024). Control strategy for biopharmaceutical production by model predictive control. *Biotechnology Progress*, *40*(2), 3426. PMID: 38199980

Esmaeilnejad-Ahranjani, P., & Hajimoradi, M. (2022). Optimization of industrial-scale centrifugal separation of biological products: Comparing the performance of tubular and disc stack centrifuges. *Biochemical Engineering Journal*, *178*, 108281.

() Esmeralda-Guzmán, M., Juan, J. B. F., Aguilar, C. N., Juan, A. A. V., & Sepúlveda, L. (2024). Parameters that influence the fermentation submerged process: bioprocess development in biotechnology. *Bioresources and Bioprocess in Biotechnology for a Sustainable Future*, 179-200.

Estevez, A. T., & Navarro, D. (2017). Biomanufacturing the future: Biodigital architecture & genetics. *Procedia Manufacturing*, *12*, 7–16.

() Fisher, A. C., O'Connor, T., Welch, J., & Lee, S. (2023). Removing regulatory hurdles for continuous pharmaceutical manufacturing. *Pharmaceutical Engineering, 43*(14).

Freitag, R. (2013). Chromatographic techniques in the downstream processing of proteins in biotechnology. In *Animal Cell Biotechnology* (pp. 419–458). Methods and Protocols.

Galbraith, S. C., Bhatia, H., Liu, H., & Yoon, S. (2018). Media formulation optimization: Current and future opportunities. *Current Opinion in Chemical Engineering, 22*, 42–47.

Gervais, J., & Wang, C. (2025). Flocculation and Filtration. *BioProcess International, 23*, 3.

Ghaderi, H., Arasteh, J., & Hesampour, A. (2018). Using response surface methodology in combination with Plackett–Burman design for optimization of culture media and extracellular expression of Trichoderma reesei synthetic endoglucanase II in Escherichia coli. *Molecular Biology Reports, 45*(5), 1197–1208. PMID: 30032381

Gomes, T. A., Zanette, C. M., & Spier, M. R. (2020). An overview of cell disruption methods for intracellular biomolecules recovery. *Preparative Biochemistry & Biotechnology, 50*(7), 635–654. PMID: 32074000

González-Gloria, K. D., Rodríguez-Jasso, R. M., Saxena, R., Sindhu, R., Ali, S. S., Singhania, R. R., & Ruiz, H. A. (2022). Bubble column bioreactor design and evaluation for bioethanol production using simultaneous saccharification and fermentation strategy from hydrothermally pretreated lignocellulosic biomass. *Biochemical Engineering Journal, 187*, 108645.

() Gopalakrishnan, A. V., Suresh, H., Mariappan, G., Kanagaraja, A., & Raman, P. (2024). Industrial Microbial Bioprocess Development: A Comprehensive Overview. *Industrial Microbiology and Biotechnology: A New Horizon of the Microbial World*, 89-154.

() Gupta, P. K., & Edula, J. R. (2021). Strategies for Enhancing Product Yield: Design of Experiments. *Fermentation: Processes, Benefits and Risks*, 15.

Hamid, K. A., Elsayed, E. A., El Enshasy, H. A., Esawy, M., & Malek, R. A. (2018). Bioprocess optimization for levan production by Bacillus subtilis B58. *Journal of Scientific and Industrial Research, 77*, 386–393.

() Han, L., & Parekh, S. R. (2005). Development of improved strains and optimization of fermentation processes. *Microbial processes and products*, 1-23.

Hekmat, D. (2015). Large-scale crystallization of proteins for purification and formulation. *Bioprocess and Biosystems Engineering, 38*(7), 1209–1231. PMID: 25700885

Hunt, M. M., Meng, G., Rancourt, D. E., Gates, I. D., & Kallos, M. S. (2014). Factorial experimental design for the culture of human embryonic stem cells as aggregates in stirred suspension bioreactors reveals the potential for interaction effects between bioprocess parameters. *Tissue Engineering. Part C, Methods, 20*(1), 76–89. PMID: 23668683

Ibrahim, H. M., Yusoff, W. M. W., Hamid, A. A., Illias, R. M., Hassan, O., & Omar, O. (2005). Optimization of medium for the production of β-cyclodextrin glucanotransferase using Central Composite Design (CCD). *Process Biochemistry, 40*(2), 753–758.

Ishwarya, S. P., Anandharamakrishnan, C., & Stapley, A. G. (2015). Spray-freeze-drying: A novel process for the drying of foods and bioproducts. *Trends in Food Science & Technology, 41*(2), 161–181.

Jana, S. C., Madhusree, C., & Utpal, R. (2019). Optimization of media and culture conditions for improved production of bacteriocin by using conventional one-factor-at-a-time (OFAT) method. *EC Microbiology, 15*, 251–258.

Jenkins, T. E. (2013). *Aeration control system design: a practical guide to energy and process optimization.* John Wiley & Sons.

Jing, J., Chen, Y., Sheng, L., & Wu, M. (2018). Optimized production of insulin variant, a recombinant platelet aggregation inhibitor, by high cell-density fermentation of recombinant Escherichia coli. *Protein Expression and Purification, 152*, 7–12. PMID: 30033357

Jönsson, A. S., & Trägårdh, G. (1990). Ultrafiltration applications. *Desalination, 77*, 135–179.

() Kakes, E. (2008). SCADA Systems for Bioreactors. *Practical Fermentation Technology*, 289-322.

Kakko, N., Ivanona, N., & Rantasalo, A. (2016). Cell disruption methods. *CHEM-E3140. Bioprocess Technology, II*, 11–13.

Kalil, S. J., Maugeri, F., & Rodrigues, M. I. (2000). Response surface analysis and simulation as a tool for bioprocess design and optimization. *Process Biochemistry, 35*(6), 539–550.

Kang, H. J., Yu, H. H., Cho, C. W., Rhee, Y. K., Kim, T. W., & Chin, Y. W. (2024). Optimization of medium composition and fluidized bed drying conditions for efficient production of dry yeast. *Microorganisms, 13*(1), 22. PMID: 39858790

() Kausley, S. B., Dastane, G. G., Patil, R. A., Jadhav, A. J., Desai, K. S., & Pandit, A. B. (2022). Applications of ultrasound in separation processes. *Sustainable separation engineering: materials, techniques and process development*, 155-197.

Kilduff, J. E., Mattaraj, S., Wigton, A., Kitis, M., & Karanfil, T. (2004). Effects of reverse osmosis isolation on reactivity of naturally occurring dissolved organic matter in physicochemical processes. *Water Research, 38*(4), 1026–1036. PMID: 14769423

Ko, C. L., & Wang, F. S. (2006). Run-to-run fed-batch optimization for protein production using recombinant Escherichia coli. *Biochemical Engineering Journal, 30*(3), 279–285.

Kumar, V., Bhalla, A., & Rathore, A. S. (2014). Design of experiments applications in bioprocessing: Concepts and approach. *Biotechnology Progress, 30*(1), 86–99. PMID: 24123959

Lee, S. Y., Lee, D. Y., & Kim, T. Y. (2005). Systems biotechnology for strain improvement. *Trends in Biotechnology, 23*(7), 349–358. PMID: 15923052

Malcata, F. X. (1989). CSTR's in Biochemical Reactions: An Optimization Problem. *Chemical Engineering Education, 23*(2), 112–128.

Mandenius, C. F., & Brundin, A. (2008). Bioprocess optimization using design-of-experiments methodology. *Biotechnology Progress, 24*(6), 1191–1203. PMID: 19194932

Marques, M. P. C., Fernandes, P., & Cabral, J. M. S. (2010). Bioreactor design for microbial and cell cultures: A review on the major scale-up issues. *Journal of Chemical Technology and Biotechnology*, *85*(10), 1184–1194.

Mazzola, P. G., Lopes, A. M., Hasmann, F. A., Jozala, A. F., Penna, T. C., Magalhaes, P. O., & Pessoa, A.Jr. (2008). Liquid–liquid extraction of biomolecules: an overview and update of the main techniques. *Journal of Chemical Technology & Biotechnology: International Research in Process. Environmental & Clean Technology*, *83*(2), 143–157.

Mollah, A. H. (2005). Application of failure mode and effect analysis (FMEA) for process risk assessment. *BioProcess International*, *5*, 12–20.

Monteiro, M., Fadda, S., & Kontoravdi, C. (2023). Towards advanced bioprocess optimization: A multiscale modelling approach. *Computational and Structural Biotechnology Journal*, *21*, 3639–3655. PMID: 37520284

Moresi, M. (1981). Optimal design of airlift fermenters. *Biotechnology and Bioengineering*, *23*(11), 2537–2560.

Moser, A. (1988). The principles of bioprocess technology. In *Bioprocess Technology* (pp. 13–65). Kinetics and Reactors.

Müller, E., Berger, R., Blass, E., Sluyts, D., & Pfennig, A. (2000). *Liquid–liquid extraction.* Ullmann's Encyclopedia of Industrial Chemistry.

Närhi, M., & Nordström, K. (2005). Manufacturing, regulatory and commercial challenges of biopharmaceuticals production: A Finnish perspective. *European Journal of Pharmaceutics and Biopharmaceutics*, *59*(3), 397–405. PMID: 15760720

Nejatishahidein, N., & Zydney, A. L. (2021). Depth filtration in bioprocessing—New opportunities for an old technology. *Current Opinion in Chemical Engineering*, *34*, 100746.

Nieto-Taype, M. A., Garcia-Ortega, X., Albiol, J., Montesinos-Seguí, J. L., & Valero, F. (2020). Continuous cultivation as a tool toward the rational bioprocess development with Pichia Pastoris cell factory. *Frontiers in Bioengineering and Biotechnology*, *8*, 632. PMID: 32671036

Osman, Y., Elrazak, A. A., & Khater, W. (2016). Bioprocess optimization of microbial biopolymer production. *Journal of Biobased Materials and Bioenergy*, *10*(2), 119–128.

Parekh, S., Vinci, V. A., & Strobel, R. J. (2000). Improvement of microbial strains and fermentation processes. *Applied Microbiology and Biotechnology*, *54*(3), 287–301. PMID: 11030563

Parekh, S., Vinci, V. A., & Strobel, R. J. (2000). Improvement of microbial strains and fermentation processes. *Applied Microbiology and Biotechnology*, *54*(3), 287–301. PMID: 11030563

Pathodiya, M. (2025). Quality Risk Management: Degree of formality, Formal and Informal QRM. *Journal of Drug Delivery and Therapeutics*, *15*(2).

PENNELL. R. B. (1960). Fractionation and isolation of purified components by precipitation methods. In *The plasma proteins*, 9-50.

Polakovič, M., Báleš, V., Dluhý, M., & Štefuca, V. (1993). Optimization of a packed bed bioreactor with immobilized cells using experimental design. *Bioprocess Engineering*, *9*(5), 225–230.

Radzun, K. A., Agha, H. M., Abdullah, N. F. F., Ahmad, M. I., Ivanovski, I., Mohammed, A. A., & Alkamil, A. A. (2024). Media optimization techniques for microalgae through technological advancements: A mini review. *AUIQ Complementary Biological System*, *1*(1), 7.

Raghunath, B., Bin, W. A. N. G., Pattnaik, P. R. I. Y. A. B. R. A. T. A., & Janssens, J. E. R. O. E. N. (2012). Best practices for optimization and scale-up of microfiltration TFF processes. *Bioprocess. J*, *11*(1), 30–40.

Rathore, A. S., Agarwal, H., Sharma, A. K., Pathak, M., & Muthukumar, S. J. P. B. (2015). Continuous processing for production of biopharmaceuticals. *Preparative Biochemistry & Biotechnology*, *45*(8), 836–849. PMID: 25674930

Rathore, A. S., Kumar, D., & Kateja, N. (2018). Recent developments in chromatographic purification of biopharmaceuticals. *Biotechnology Letters*, *40*(6), 895–905. PMID: 29700726

Rathore, A. S., Mishra, S., Nikita, S., & Priyanka, P. (2021). Bioprocess control: Current progress and future perspectives. *Life (Chicago, Ill.)*, *11*(6), 557. PMID: 34199245

Rathore, A. S., Nikita, S., & Jesubalan, N. G. (2022). Digitization in bioprocessing: The role of soft sensors in monitoring and control of downstream processing for production of biotherapeutic products. *Biosensors & Bioelectronics: X*, *12*, 100263.

Reisman, H. B. (1993). Problems in scale-up of biotechnology production processes. *Critical Reviews in Biotechnology*, *13*(3), 195–253. PMID: 8221898

Roeva, O., & Slavov, T. (2012). PID controller tuning based on metaheuristic algorithms for bioprocess control. *Biotechnology, Biotechnological Equipment*, *26*(5), 3267–3277.

Rogers, L., & Jensen, K. F. (2019). Continuous manufacturing–the Green Chemistry promise? *Green Chemistry*, *21*(13), 3481–3498.

Roman, M. D., & Muresan, M. V. (2015). Process optimization of aeration in the biological treatment using fine bubble diffusers. In *Proc., 6th Int. Conf. on Modern Power System.* Cluj-napoca, Romania: EBSCO Information Services.

Schneider, A., Herlevi, L. M., Guo, Y., & Fernandez Lahore, H. M. (2022). Perspectives on adsorption technology as an effective strategy for continuous downstream bioprocessing. *Journal of Chemical Technology and Biotechnology*, *97*(9), 2305–2316.

Sewsynker-Sukai, Y., Faloye, F., & Kana, E. B. G. (2017). Artificial neural networks: An efficient tool for modelling and optimization of biofuel production (a mini review). *Biotechnology, Biotechnological Equipment*, *31*(2), 221–235.

() Silva, R. C., Almeida, R., Ferreira, P., Menezes, J. C., & Martinho, Â. (2023). Agile, data-driven life cycle management for continuous manufacturing. *Pharmaceutical Engineering*, 24.

Simutis, R., & Lübbert, A. (2015). Bioreactor control improves bioprocess performance. *Biotechnology Journal*, *10*(8), 1115–1130. PMID: 26228573

Singh, V., Haque, S., Niwas, R., Srivastava, A., Pasupuleti, M., & Tripathi, C. (2017). Strategies for fermentation medium optimization: An in-depth review. *Frontiers in Microbiology*, *7*, 2087. PMID: 28111566

Sinner, P., Herwig, C., & Kager, J. (2020). Time scale analysis and optimization of a continuous microbial bioprocess. *Computer-Aided Chemical Engineering*, *48*, 1603–1608.

Su, Q., Ganesh, S., Moreno, M., Bommireddy, Y., Gonzalez, M., Reklaitis, G. V., & Nagy, Z. K. (2019). A perspective on Quality-by-Control (QbC) in pharmaceutical continuous manufacturing. *Computers & Chemical Engineering*, *125*, 216–231. PMID: 36845965

Tang, D. Y. Y., Yew, G. Y., Koyande, A. K., Chew, K. W., Vo, D. V. N., & Show, P. L. (2020). Green technology for the industrial production of biofuels and bioproducts from microalgae: A review. *Environmental Chemistry Letters*, *18*(6), 1967–1985.

Tomczak, W., & Gryta, M. (2022). The application of cellulose acetate membranes for separation of fermentation broths by the reverse osmosis: A feasibility study. *International Journal of Molecular Sciences*, *23*(19), 11738. PMID: 36233037

Udayan, A., Sirohi, R., Sreekumar, N., Sang, B. I., & Sim, S. J. (2022). Mass cultivation and harvesting of microalgal biomass: Current trends and future perspectives. *Bioresource Technology*, *344*, 126406. PMID: 34826565

Ulber, R., Frerichs, J. G., & Beutel, S. (2003). Optical sensor systems for bioprocess monitoring. *Analytical and Bioanalytical Chemistry*, *376*(3), 342–348. PMID: 12728296

Waśko, A., Kordowska-Wiater, M., Podleśny, M., Polak-Berecka, M., Targoński, Z., & Kubik-Komar, A. (2010). The Plackett-Burman design in optimization of media components for biomass production of Lactobacillus rhamnosus OXY. *Acta Biologica Hungarica*, *61*(3), 344–355. PMID: 20724280

Wasli, A. S., Salleh, M. M., Abd-Aziz, S., Hassan, O., & Mahadi, N. M. (2009). Medium optimization for chitinase production from Trichoderma virens using central composite design. *Biotechnology and Bioprocess Engineering; BBE*, *14*(6), 781–787.

Xu, S., & Zydney, A. L. (2023). Strategies for integration of perfusion-based upstream with continuous downstream purification. *Frontiers in Bioengineering and Biotechnology*, *11*, 1211410.

Yasarla, L. R., & Ramarao, B. V. (2012). Dynamics of flocculation of lignocellulosic hydrolyzates by polymers. *Industrial & Engineering Chemistry Research*, *51*(19), 6847–6861.

Yuk, I. H., Baskar, D., Duffy, P. H., Hsiung, J., Leung, S., & Lin, A. A. (2011). Overcoming challenges in WAVE bioreactors without feedback controls for pH and dissolved oxygen. *Biotechnology Progress*, *27*(5), 1397–1406. PMID: 21987370

Zala, S. P., Patel, K. P., Patel, K. S., Parmar, J. P., Sen, D. J., Parmar, J. P., & Scopus, C. (2012). Laboratory techniques of purification and isolation. *Int. J. Drug Dev. Res*, *4*(2), 41–55.

Zhang, J. (2010). Mammalian cell culture for biopharmaceutical production. *Manual of industrial microbiology and biotechnology*, 157-178.

Zydney, A. L. (2016). Continuous downstream processing for high value biologics: A review. *Biotechnology and Bioengineering*, *113*(3), 465–475. PMID: 26153056

KEY TERMS AND DEFINITIONS

Medium Optimization: It is defined as a process which involves refining the composition and concentration of the growth medium in order to enhance the biomass growth with the best physiological state for higher productivity.

Artificial Neural Network (ANN): It is defined as a mathematical/computational model that helps find the optimum media composition from the best combination of a given set of data inputs to achieve a desirable outcome.

Aeration: It is defined as the process of supplying oxygen into a submerged culture for its metabolic requirements.

Flow Field Optimization: It is defined as the process of controlling the fluid flow paths within the bioreactor with the goal to improve nutrient distribution and hence the mass transfer.

Process Analytical Technology (PAT): It is defined as a system that covers a range of tools to design, analyse and control the critical process parameters and critical quality attributes (CQAs) effectively.

Genetic Recombination: It is defined as the process of combining genetic information from 2 genotypes.

Flocculation: It is defined as the process of clumping suspended particles together to form large aggregates in the liquid medium.

Partition Coefficient: Partition coefficient is defined as the ratio of the solute between the organic phase and the aqueous phase at equilibrium.

Chapter 8
Biotechnology in the Food and Beverage Industry:
Fermentation and Beyond – Innovations, Applications, and Future Prospects

Muhammad Anas
https://orcid.org/0000-0001-5127-8043
Selçuk University, Turkey

Sameel Hassan
University of Tuscia, Italy

Aliza Falak
Independent Researcher, Pakistan

Erdogan E. Hakki
Selcuk University, Turkey

Javed Iqbal
https://orcid.org/0000-0002-9032-2622
Bacha Khan University, Pakistan

ABSTRACT

Biotechnology in the food and beverage industry has revolutionized production by enhancing nutritional value, sustainability, and waste valorization. Plant-based beverages, agro-industrial by-products, and food waste are utilized in microbial fermentation, enzyme technologies, and genetic engineering to produce high-value products such as bioactive compounds, organic acids, bioplastics, and nutraceuticals. Microbial enzymes improve texture, taste, shelf life, and economic efficiency in food processing. Enzyme functionality is further enhanced through immobilization and protein engineering. However, biotechnology faces challenges in safety, regulation, ethics, and consumer acceptance. Regulatory systems, like GRAS norms in the U.S. and EU pre-market

DOI: 10.4018/979-8-3373-2873-7.ch008

assessments, vary globally. Ethical concerns include environmental risks, socio-economic factors, and cultural sensitivities. Transparency, labeling, and risk management are crucial in building trust and balancing innovation with responsibility.

INTRODUCTION

The involvement of biotechnology in the food and beverage industry is considered to be a revolutionary period which has brought modernization in food production, processing and innovation (Mirsalami & Mirsalami, 2025). With twofold pressure of surging population in the world, accelerating climate change, environmental destruction and shifting consumption habits, the versatile and resilient set of strategies and approaches offered by biotechnology will offer a myriad of solutions to these multi-dimensional problems. It enhances the quality of food, increases safety, strengthens the nutrition value, the reduction of waste, generates sustainable solutions to traditional processes through the deployment of living organisms, enzymes and cellular systems. Biotechnology has been revolutionizing how food is produced and consumed in a microbial fermentation and gene editing enzyme engineering and synthetic bio-technology (Bibra et al., 2021).

The historical predecessor of biotechnological food manipulations dates back to the ancient period of time when humans employed the method of fermentation to obtain such products as bread, cheese, wine, and yogurt- products produced through the use of the natural capabilities of bacteria. These methods of production in history were errors trial and were embedded in the art and craft activity (Warda et al., 2025). Nevertheless, together with the emergence of molecular biology, genetic engineering, and omics technologies, they have shifted the definition of the mentioned methodologies towards the high-precision, efficient, and scale-up ability into industrial scale. Recent advances in food biotechnology have enabled one to produce the designed microbial strains, optimize the metabolic pathway to attain the desired production of particular compound, and develop the controlled fermentation conditions that may prove useful in the achievement of predictable products. Because of this, heterogeneity of raw materials and other conventional ways of production have therefore been significantly opposed (Ajayeoba & Ijabadeniyi, 2025).

Another major offering of the biotechnology is development of functional foods and nutraceuticals- the products which incorporate the health-promoting additives (probiotics, bioactive peptides, antioxidants, and vitamins) (Singh & Negi, 2025). These compounds are produced by engineered microbial strains in the downstream fermentation processes, thus providing consumers with foods that do not only satisfy physiological needs but also play immunological protecting, maintenance of gut integrity, and management of chronic diseases. Running synchronously to all of this was a progress in enzyme technology, which in food processing, provides highly specific, efficient, and environmentally friendly alternatives to chemical treatments (Ngongolo & Mmbando, 2024).

There is also a revolution in the food industry in terms of sustainability with the help of biotechnology. Historically, microbial bioconversion creates value by converting agro-industrial by-products and waste streams that were previously considered as environmental liabilities into valuable products (organic acids, bioplastics, single-cell proteins, and bioethanol) (Mohamed et al., 2021). Such valorizing corresponds to the model of the circular economy, diminishes the production of green house-gasses and popularizes zero-waste processing paradigms. At the same time, precision fermentation and synthetic biology are enabling the production of animal-free proteins, fats and dairy alternatives, reducing land, water and animal product reliance and supplying more scalable and climate adaptable production pipelines (Tarafdar et al., 2022).

Regulation and security are essential elements of a biotechnology innovation. International standards, strict approved quality-control measures, and disciplined risk-assessment mechanisms ensure safety and ethical manufacture of foods produced through biotechnology (Okpala & Korzeniowska, 2023). In addition to that, public opinion, openness, and fashionable labels support the maintenance of consumer confidence, specifically in the areas of genetically modified organisms (GMOs) or synthetic-biology applications (Ajayeoba & Ijabadeniyi, 2025; Shetty & Sarkar, 2020).

The chapter is intended to give an in-depth but concentrated discussion of biotechnology in the food and beverage sector and its relationship with ancient fermentation and the current technological advances that improve the quality of products, sustainability as well as their marketing value. It describes the principles and advantages of the classical fermentation, clarifies the use and progress of enzyme technologies and investigates the evolution of probiotics and functional foods. It also covers the issue of sustainability and valorization of waste showing the biotechnological pathways of turning by-products into renewable energy, bioactives, and biodegradable wrappings as part of the circular economy models. New technologies like precision fermentation, synthetic biology, and microbial engineering are described and the challenges around them with regards to technical, economic, regulatory, and ethical concerns involved in the industry are explained. The emerging trends and future considerations conclude the chapter and arm the readers with the scientific perception and practice-related context to know and interact with the present and future biotechnological methods of food production.

CLASSICAL FERMENTATION IN THE FOOD INDUSTRY

Fermentation is one of the earliest biotechnological processes used by man that dates back to over 10,000 years as studied archaeologically. It was initially created to preserve food before refrigeration became an option, but quickly found additional use in providing different flavor profiles, textures, and overall healthier profiles to foodstuffs (Mujahid et al., 2024). classical fermentation takes advantage of the endogenous metabolic coupling of carbohydrates and other natural substrates with microorganisms such as bacteria, yeasts and molds to produce simpler products like alcohols, organic acids, carbon dioxide and other gases. These microbial transformations are the basis of many well-known foods and beverages that are consumed throughout the globe such as bread, cheese and yogurt, wine, beer, kimchi, sauerkraut, miso, tempeh and vinegar among others (Praveen & Brogi, 2025).

In classical fermentation central microorganisms tend to be strain-specific and environment-specific. The fermentation of dairy products, vegetables, and meat is impossible without lactic acid bacteria (LAB), which, in particular, are species belonging to Lactobacillus, Leuconostoc, and Streptococcus. Their main role is the breakdown of sugars to lactic acid, which at the same time reduces pH causing inhibition of pathogenic microorganisms and providing the typical acidic taste of fermented goods (Vinderola et al., 2019). A yeast species known as Saccharomyces cerevisiae has been central to alcoholic fermentation, converting glucose to ethanol and carbon dioxide which has centrally played a role in the baking industry and brewery industry. The soy-based and mold-fermentation products owe their ability to hydrolyze a complex substance, e.g.

proteins and polysaccharides to filamentous fungi, e.g. *Aspergillus oryzae*, *Rhizopus oligosporus* and *Penicillium camemberti* (Zhang et al., 2025).

The main benefit of classical fermentation is that it enriches foods by the bioactive compounds: B vitamins, essential amino acids, short-chain fatty acids (SCFAs), and antimicrobial peptides (Lim & Abd Rahim, 2025). At the same time, it reduces the antinutrients like phytic acid, tannins and trypsin inhibitors and increases the bioavailability of minerals and protein digestibility aut rusten of special interest to populations subsisting on plant-based foods. Moreover, the flavor, aroma, mouthfeel, which is produced by microbial metabolism, is the point of consumer preferences and cultural food identity (Hidalgo-Fuentes et al., 2024).

Despite its pioneering origins, classical fermentation is historically limited on its ability to be consistent, scaleable and safe. Conventional processes normally use spontaneous fermentation using native micro soil that can cause batch to batch inconsistencies in the product quality. Microbial succession and metabolite production have also been shown to be heavily dependent on such environmental factors as temperature, humidity, and composition of the raw materials (Zhu et al., 2022). Such variability increases the potential of spoilage organisms or pathogens contamination. Furthermore, regular fermentation does not possess the real-time control of the process and it is still heavy on craft knowledge whose cultural foundation is complex, but not easy to standardize in the industry (Niyigaba et al., 2025).

In order to overcome these drawback classical fermentation has increasingly incorporated the scientific technology such as pure starter cultures, strain selection, and precise formulated media. The standardization of inocula allows consistent fermentation kinetics, predictable flavor accretion and an increase in food safety (Vinicius De Melo Pereira et al., 2020). Starter cultures are chosen based on functionality, e.g. high acidification rate, antimicrobial production, textural enhancement, as well as their overall stability towards different processing conditions. The mutualistic association between *Lactobacillus delbrueckii* subsp. *bulgaricus* and *Streptococcus thermophilus* is used as a model in the production of yogurt given that it is consistent and compatible (Vinicius De Melo Pereira et al., 2020).

Molecular techniques have advanced our understanding of the classical fermentation further in the past several decades. Mapping of the microbial communities, metabolic pathways and volatile compound production in fermented foods have been done by the use of techniques like 16S rRNA sequencing, metagenomics, metabolomics. Such data enable logical advancements in starter culture design and control of fermentation (Singh & Kumar, 2025). While classical fermentation remains a cornerstone of the food industry, modern biotechnology particularly enzyme technologies has expanded the possibilities for improving efficiency, sustainability, and product diversity

Enzyme Technologies in Food and Beverage Biotechnology

Enzymes are biological catalysts with two major types (primarily proteins) that activate or speed up another biochemical reaction without being permanently changed in the process. They are valuable tools in the food and beverage industry due to their outstanding substrate specificity and their capability (under mild conditions of temperature and pH) to deliver yields without producing significant amounts of unwanted side-products, characteristics that render them far superior to traditional chemical catalysts (Chandrasekaran et al., 2015). Not only do these properties help maintain sensory properties of foods (e.g. flavor, aroma and texture), they also help improve efficiency of the process, save energy and water and generate clean-label foods. Enzyme applications are broad in the level of processing and the type of products. In brewing, amylases break down starch in the brew to more accessible sugars that can be fermented thus leading to greater efficiency in brewing, hence making sure that the alcoholic content is constant (Gomaa, 2018). Dairy processing uses lactase to hydrolyse lactose to glucose and galactose to manufacture lactose-free milk and to value-add to whey into fermentation raw materials used in other value-added products (i.e. rennet (containing chymosin) used in cheese-making to coagulate milk). In bread, amylases enhance dough manipulation and loaf volume and inhibit loaf staling and proteases alter gluten to increase bread extensibility/softness (Acharya et al., 2023). Juice and wine industry Enzyme In the juice and wine industry, pectin degrading enzymes called pectinases are used to hydrolyze pectin in cell walls in order to enhance juice production and clarity and the ability to filter the juice. The use of proteases to tenderize meat through the use of papain and bromelain with the aim of improving their texture and consumer acceptability has been used (Yang et al., 2021).

Improvement of the stability, reusability and catalytic activity of enzymes in industrial conditions has been among the recent achievements of the enzyme technology. Techniques of immobilization which attached enzymes to solid supports, entrapped them in gels or cross-linked them into aggregates allow the repeated use of enzymes, continuous processing and a higher heat, pH and inhibitor tolerance. The capability of enzyme cocktails, or mixtures of complementary enzymes, means that several components can be broken down in the complex food matrices simultaneously in a more efficient process (Noori et al., 2019). The recombinant DNA technology has made it possible to produce enzymes in large quantities at a low cost and on a genetically engineered microbial host which includes Bacillus, Aspergillus and Kluyveromyces among others ensuring high yields and good quality. Techniques of protein engineering such as directed evolution and rational design are used to change the amino acid sequences to improve thermal stability, change pH optima, increase substrate specificity and resistance against processing inhibitors (Kumar et al., 2025).

In the future, the changing trends are giving enzymes a new path in the food and beverage industry. Computational enzyme design employing the principles of artificial intelligence reduces the cost and time of enzyme development by facilitating modelling of the needed structural modifications to achieve a better functioning enzyme (Singh et al., 2021). Similarly, genome editing through CRISPR/Cas9 is underway to generate species-specific mutants via microbial strains optimized morphology, and metabolic flux aimed at a vastly enhanced yield of enzymes, limited by-products with a specific activity profile. Collectively, such innovations mean that enzyme technology has become an important way to be at the forefront of becoming not only a sustainable food production practice but also an efficient way of doing so by connecting traditional understanding and practices in processing with the most advanced biotechnology to satisfy changing consumer demands and challenges in the industry (Basaran, 2024).

MODERN BIOTECHNOLOGICAL TOOLS IN FERMENTATION

The catch-all practice of contemporary biotechnology has changed the nature of fermentation, the systems that sustained human societies through millennia. Use of genetic engineering, synthetic biology, optimization of metabolic pathways, and sophisticated analytical tools now support fermentation processes that are increasingly precise, predictable, and readily scaled: once the domain of artisanal and semi-controlled processes, they are becoming increasingly precise, predictable and highly scalable (Botta et al., 2024). These advances do not only increase efficiency and the quality of products, but also enlarge the range of operations producing new bioactive substances synthesis, new flavor profile design, and the creation of customized metabolites. Therefore, fermentation is no more an exclusively preservative strategy or flavor addition, it has become a bio-manufacturing technology (Shokoohi & Attar, 2024).

Genetic engineering is one of such powerful tools. The recombinant DNA technologies allow the controlled alteration of microbial genomes, such that the organisms can produce large quantities of specific enzymes or inhibit unwanted metabolic activities or survive extreme industrial environments; high concentration of ethanol, osmotic pressure and acidic pH (Khan et al., 2016). In fermentation of alcohol industrially, the Saccharomyces cerevisiae strains have been modified to increase the ethanol production and minimize the by-products like glycerol and acetic acid. Other concomitant activities have adjusted Lactobacillus plantarum in vegetable fermentation to increase folate content to overcome micronutrient deficiency among people in need (Dhiman et al., 2025).

Genome editing with the CRISPR genome editing tool CRISPR/Cas9 has also accelerated strain improvement, providing specific, speedy, and multiplexed gene modification with relatively low off-target outcomes. Food fermentation Enzymes With CRISPR, yeast and bacteria strains are developed to produce more desirable aroma compounds, break down antinutritional compounds, or secrete more nitrogen in vitamin and amino acids (Dhiman et al., 2025). Further, CRISPR interference(CRISPRi) allows an engineer to silence individual genes without permanent changes in the genome, which can be particularly useful in a regulatory context, where genetically modified organisms (GMOs) face popular or legal opposition in many jurisdictions (Hassane et al., 2025).

Metabolic engineering, more than single-gene edits, optimizes complete biosynthetic pathways and networks. Rewiring of the metabolism has allowed researchers to capture the precursors and channel them towards intended end-product production with reduced intermediates and unwanted side-products (Bommer et al., 2020). The latter includes metabolic tuning (in the directed-evolution of lactic acid fermentation to produce both greater product yield and higher optical purity by reducing ethanol and carbon dioxide formation), and pathway engineering (of Acetobacter species to increase acetic acid production, and minimize premature oxidation that would intrude on flavor) (Hoff et al., 2021).

Synthetic biology builds on this fermentation capability to engineer and construct new gene circuit and regulatory modules to program cellular behavior. Examples of appliances are the development of microbial communities of which each with distinctive functionality- one strain breaks down complex carbohydrates, another breaks down the sugars generated and produces the target metabolic products (Satari et al., 2023). The affected communities, often engineered, are often more complex and more effective than monocultures, and can resemble more closely traditional fermentation successions, but be more predictable and controllable. Synthetic biology can also be used to express pathways that are not native to common cell factories e.g. Escherichia coli or Bacillus subtilis to produce natural flavoring agents e.g. vanillin, nootkatone, pharmacological compounds e.g. GABA, and rare bioactives that are hard to extract in the original sources e.g. plants or animals (Nikoloudaki et al., 2024).

Modern fermentation research cannot ignore omics-based profiling, that is, genomics, transcriptomics, proteomics, and metabolomics. These systems allow systems-level characterization of gene expression, protein synthesis and metabolic output, allowing investigators to optimize environmental conditions, substrate composition and co-culture combinations in order to achieve better results. As an example, metabolomic cheese ripening studies have clarified the metabolic processes of amino acid degradation which produce certain flavors; this has informed supplement culture choice (Wen et al., 2024).

Strain improvement is further boosted by high throughput screening and adaptive laboratory evolution (ALE). In the case of ALE, by exerting selective pressure on microbial cultures over a series of generations, some naturally evolved features are obtained like tolerance to stresses or improved substrate utilization (Hirasawa & Maeda, 2022). After target phenotypes being desirable are obtained, the mutations that cause them can be sequenced and applied to other strains through genome editing methods. This strategy has been used to prepare hyper-tolerant starter cultures which can be used in high temperature or low pH fermentation thus increasing the possibilities of developing non-conventional conditions or extreme situations (Mariyes et al., 2024).

Fermentation has also been enhanced by bio process modelling and real-time observation. Simulation of metabolic flux and optimization of reactor conditions to increase productivity can be performed by using computational tools. pH, temperature, oxygen levels and nutrient levels are all monitored through automatic systems connected to sensors and feedback systems to ensure product standardization, reduced occurrences of failed batches and ease of regulatory compliance- especially in food grade applications (Gargalo et al., 2020).

Modern fermentation is used in the functional foods sphere to produce powerful food active compounds in optimized form such as antioxidants, probiotics, vitamins and phytochemicals. Example of which being engineered *Lactococcus lactis* which can manufacture therapeutic proteins as well as antimicrobial peptides directly in the gastrointestinal tract (Plavec & Berlec, 2019). Similar developments concern natural sweeteners (e.g. tagatose produced by fermentation), flavor enhancing compounds (e.g. kokumi peptides), and mood-stimulating substances (e.g. tryptophan metabolites), which are all developed through tailor-made fermentation processes (Sun et al., 2022).

Figure 1. Summary of advanced biotechnological tools and their specific applications in enhancing fermentation processes for improved productivity, precision, and scalability

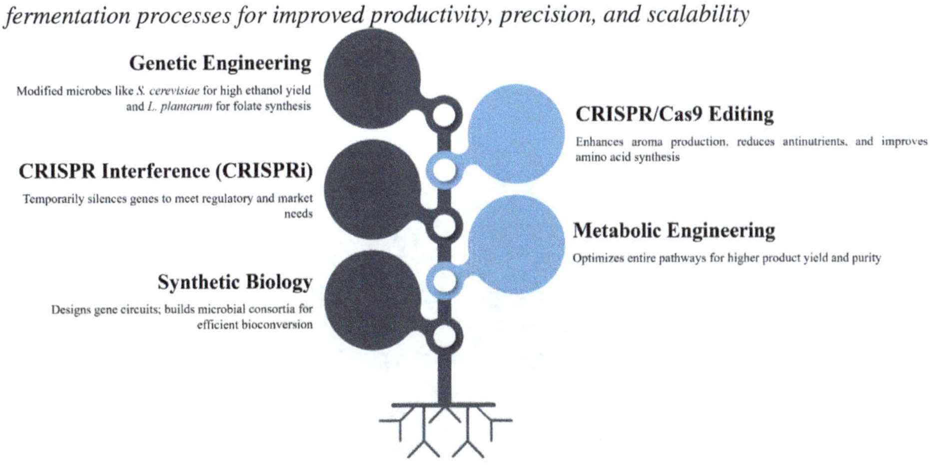

FUNCTIONAL FOODS AND PROBIOTICS

During the recent years, demand of functional foods has also increased significantly all across the world due to the increased attention of consumers to their health, immune support as well as disease prevention. In this context, the functional food movement has revolved around probiotics and prebiotics. The stability, selective delivery, and careful design of such elements are engineering aspects and biotechnology has played a central role in these areas making functional food innovation another most important subset of food biotechnology of today (Donato et al., 2023).

Probiotics and Their Health Implications

Probiotics are live microorganisms that can have quantifiable health benefits to their human host when said microorganisms are consumed in reasonable amounts. Examples of representative genera are *Lactobacillus, Bifidobacterium,* and *Saccharomyces (*Voidarou et al., 2020*).* These communities of microbes inhabit the gastrointestinal tract, regulate the microbiota present in the host and enhance mucosal immunity. Probiotic consumption has shown numerous empirical relations with a reduced prevalence of irritable bowel syndrome (IBS), lactose intolerance, inflammatory bowel diseases (IBD), allergies, and respectively, enhanced mental health conditions through the use of a gut-brain axis (Pejcz, 2024).

Modern biotechnological innovations have narrowed down the methods of screening and the selection of strains, the main priorities of which are increased survivability, high adhesion properties, and higher resistance to bile salts. Genomic sequencing, comparative genomics, allows the discovery of probiotic candidates that could have favorable gene repertoires of stress tolerance and those that have clinically relevant functional gene clusters. Furthermore, metabolic engineering offers a chance of increasing outputs of useful metabolites, a short-chain fatty acids (SCFAs), bacteriocins, and neurotransmitters, like GABA and serotonin (Terpou et al., 2019).

Figure 2. Overview of key biotechnological innovations supporting probiotic development and functional food formulation to improve gut health, immunity, and therapeutic outcomes

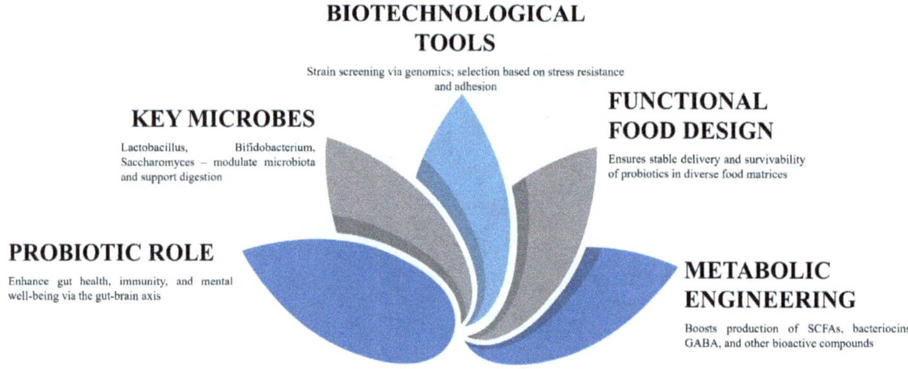

Prebiotics, Synbiotics, and Postbiotics

Prebiotics are characterized as non-digestible food constituents (e.g. inulin, fructooligosaccharide) to have a selective stimulatory impact to dedicated helpful gut microorganisms. Modern biotechnology allows intentional synthesis of new prebiotics through the bio synthesis of plant polysaccharides, algal extracts or agro-industrial by-products, thus matching the molecular structure to the enzyme profile of probioticity bacteria of interest and, therefore, establishing synergistic associations (Nascimento & Barros, 2025). The current research agenda has shed light on the role of synbiotics i.e., a combination of probiotics and prebiotics that have been designed to improve therapeutic efficacy. In vitro models and computational methods help to develop such systems rationally; e.g. the combination of Bifidobacterium breve with suitable xylo oligosaccharides can be formally proven to afford greater colonization and immune modulation in the gastro intestinal apparatus (Beltrán-Velasco & Clemente-Suárez, 2025).

Postbiotics is an emerging area of research, consisting of the vast bioactive compounds formed during microbial metabolism that still hold therapeutic activity even when the microbial cells lose that viability. They are products of the metabolome that can be extracted, purified, and integrated into the food system by metabolomic experiments and optimized fermentation approaches (short-chain fatty acids, extracellular polysaccharides (e.g., boviccarbonate), vitamins (e.g., B12, K2), and antimicrobial peptides) (Prajapati et al., 2023).

Encapsulation and Delivery Technologies

The characteristics of probiotics, especially their survival during processing and storage, and their survival in the gastrointestinal tract, are an enduring problem. Therefore, superior microencapsulation methods have been devised to keep microorganisms safe against environmental forces; such methods are spray-drying, freeze-drying, and coacervation, among others (Meena et al., 2023). Modern biotechnology has facilitated the production of new encapsulation systems, e.g. alginate-chitosan combinations, protein-polysaccharide mixtures, and phosphate-sensitive intelligent hydrogels. Microencapsulating does not only increase the shelf life of probiotics but also promotes specific actions throughout the intestine (Ramos et al., 2018). Some of the preparations use engineered bacterial spores (e.g., *Bacillus coagulans*) or carrier that are lipid-based to deliver viable cells to the gastrointestinal tract. These technologies have an added advantage in the fields of beverage systems and dairy substitutes, where pH, oxygen and temperature changes can wipe out probiotic survivability (Yoha et al., 2022).

Functional Fermented Foods

The development of biotechnological innovation has spawned new categories of useful fermented foods, plant-based yogurts, probiotics-enriched juices, fermented cereals, and new strains of kombucha-like probiotics whose microbial cocktail has undergone bio engineering. As an example, lactobacillus plantarum strains have been designed to produce soymilk fermentation thus enriches the product with vitamin B complex, hydrolyzed peptides and isoflavone aglycones possessing antioxidant potential. The kefir grains have also been inoculated with special culture to yield lactose-free, immune-enhancing drinks (Dhiman et al., 2025).

Those are the fermented functional foods that also support micronutrient fortification. Bioengineering Specific strains of the Lactobacillus genus have been developed to produce unusually high quantities of folate, riboflavin, or iron-binding compounds during fermentation. These kinds of engineered tissue are particularly important in developing countries where the shortage of such micronutrients persists. The biotechnological methods are, thus, a sustainable and socially acceptable mode through which the situation of hidden hunger can be resolved (Dhiman et al., 2025).

Clinical Evidence and Regulatory Landscape

The clinical effectiveness of functional foods is progressively supported as empirical evidence by randomised controlled trials (RCTs) and by meta-analyses. Aspirin and Lactobacillus rhamnosus GG have been shown to reduce the rate of antibiotic-related diarrhoea and Bifidobacterium infantis 35624 to benefit patients with inflammatory bowel disease (IBD) and irritable bowel syndrome (IBS). However, the regulatory circles vary significantly between jurisdiction. In the European Union (EU) health claims cannot be given to probiotics without prior approval by the EFSA, and are treated as a dietary supplement by the Food and Drug Administration (FDA) in the United States (Mukherjee et al., 2022). As a result biotechnology companies are compelled to spend on intensive scientific validation, safety testing and extensive strain characterization in an attempt to meet these conflicting requirements. Sequencing and protein expression (genomic/proteomic) techniques are also being used to confirm lack of antibiotic resistance gene, virulence factors and toxins in industrial probiotic strains (Abdul Manan, 2025).

Table 1. Usage of Biotechnological tools by category and usage

S. No.	Category	Application/Detail	Biotechnological Tool/Strategy	Reference
1	Probiotics	Gut microbiota modulation	Probiotic strain engineering	(Jiang et al., 2025)
2	Probiotics	Anti-inflammatory effects in IBD	Genetically enhanced *L. plantarum*	(Wu et al., 2022)
3	Probiotics	GABA production for neurological benefits	Metabolic engineering	(Luo et al., 2021)
4	Probiotics	Lactose intolerance alleviation	Use of *Lactobacillus acidophilus*	(Masoumi et al., 2021)
5	Probiotics	Cholesterol reduction	*Lactobacillus reuteri* with BSH activity	(Puttarat et al., 2021)
6	Probiotics	Immune modulation	*Bifidobacterium breve*	(Choi et al., 2022)
7	Prebiotics	Gut-selective carbohydrate utilization	Enzymatic modification of oligosaccharides	(Stern & Brenner, 2018)
8	Prebiotics	Enhancement of *Bifidobacteria* growth	Fructooligosaccharide (FOS) production	(Mao et al., 2018)
9	Synbiotics	Improved colonization in GI tract	Rational strain-substrate pairing	(Parhi et al., 2022)
10	Postbiotics	Bioactive peptide production	Controlled fermentation	(Singh, 2025)
11	Encapsulation	Protecting probiotics from gastric acid	Alginate-chitosan microcapsules	(Călinoiu et al., 2019)

continued on following page

Table 1. Continued

S. No.	Category	Application/Detail	Biotechnological Tool/Strategy	Reference
12	Encapsulation	Targeted intestinal release	pH-sensitive hydrogels	(Suhail et al., 2022)
13	Functional Foods	Probiotic dairy alternatives	Fermentation of plant milks	(Shori & Al Zahrani, 2021)
14	Functional Foods	Enhanced folate production	Engineered *L. lactis*	(Lu et al., 2019)
15	Functional Foods	Bioactive isoflavones in soy beverages	Fermentation using *L. plantarum*	(Skrzypczak et al., 2024)
16	Clinical Outcomes	IBS symptom relief	*Bifidobacterium infantis* 35624	(Sabaté & Iglicki, 2022)
17	Clinical Outcomes	Diarrhea reduction post-antibiotics	*L. rhamnosus* GG	(Daisley & Allen-Vercoe, 2024)
18	Regulatory	EU probiotic claim restrictions	EFSA health claim guidelines	(Garg et al., 2024)
19	Regulatory	U.S. supplement classification	GRAS status and labeling requirements	(Frestedt, 2018)
20	Genetic Screening	Selection of robust strains	Genomic and proteomic profiling	(Soonsanga et al., 2025)
21	Delivery Systems	Spores for improved shelf life	Use of *Bacillus coagulans*	(Poshadri et al., 2022)
22	Metabolite Enhancement	SCFA production	Pathway engineering	(Wang et al., 2019)
23	Consumer Products	Kombucha with enriched antioxidants	Fermentation with engineered yeast-bacteria consortia	(Ferremi Leali et al., 2022)
24	Consumer Products	Fortified fruit juices	Probiotic addition and bioactive metabolite enhancement	(Naseem et al., 2023)
25	Industrial Process	Consistency in fermentation outcomes	Biosensor and pH monitoring	(Goldrick et al., 2019)
26	Personalized Nutrition	Tailored probiotic recommendations	Microbiome sequencing	(Bianchetti et al., 2023)
27	Stabilization	Freeze-drying of probiotics	Cryoprotectants optimization	(Romyasamit et al., 2022)
28	Sustainable Biotech	Use of agro-industrial residues for prebiotics	Bioconversion via enzyme hydrolysis	(Ravindran et al., 2018)
29	Quality Control	Removal of antibiotic resistance genes	Genetic screening tools	(Feldgarden et al., 2019)
30	Future Trends	Designer synbiotics for disease-targeted therapy	Systems biology and AI modeling	(Kang et al., 2020)

BIOPROCESS OPTIMIZATION AND SCALE-UP IN FOOD FERMENTATION

In the food and beverage industry, application of the technology to fermentation in an industrial environment requires not only the organization, but also optimization of the bioprocess and its subsequent upscale (Formenti et al., 2014). The conventional operations were commonly identified by manual methods of technique and open operations process; whereas biotechnology today is enabling high-regulated procedures and predictable production by structural design of engineered bioprocesses. The main goals of this undertaking are maximization of product yield, minimization of the cost of production, maintenance of product consistency and long-scale viability as well as functionality of the microbes in the course.

Bioreactor Design and Fermentation Systems

The bioreactor principle represents the center of industrial fermentation as a designed containment system that is utilized to support microbial or enzyme transformations with specific physicochemical environments. In food biotechnology application, these reactors should ensure sterility, effective gas exchange, homogeneous mixing as well as effective delivery of nutrients. Therefore, the type of operation (batch, fed-batch or continuous) is chosen depending on the need of the product (Mitra & Murthy, 2022).

Batch fermentation has continued to be the most usual in manufacturing dairy products and alcohol beverages: a defined amount of substrate is inoculated and left to ferment without any additional input. Simple and cost-effective, it is, however, restrictive to large scale production (Al-Maqtari et al., 2019). Fed-batch removes this by providing substrate sequentially, which provides more biomass build-up and longer production periods, which is beneficial in production of probiotics and enzymes. In fermentations used to make vinegar and kombucha (continuous fermentation), new substrate is added continually and product drawn off, maintaining a constant production rate, which requires vigorous monitoring to avoid contamination (Mahmoodi & Nassireslami, 2022).

The configuration of bioreactor is also varied. STRs are very common in the fermentation of beverages, although airlift fermenters, PBRs and MBRs have each proven useful in some microbial systems and product classes. The example is PBRs, which are appropriate to immobilized probiotics and beverage fermentation is dominated by STRs (HD & Vijayan P. U, 2025).

Other important parameters in fermentation control are parameters that need to be optimized in order to get maximum microbial activity and yield of product. Modern biotechnology enables real time pH, temperature, dissolved oxygen (DO), agitation, foam formation among others to be monitored and automated (Palladino et al., 2024). The typical feature of modern fermentation plants are data streams gathered with biosensors, programmable logic controllers (PLCs) and supervisory control and data acquisition (SCADA) systems to facilitate fully automated control, quick response times to faults and ensure uniform product quality, which is essential to food grade systems (Chai et al., 2022).

Downstream Processing and Product Recovery

On completion of the fermentation, down stream processing is the next step in which the desired product is extracted and the product is purified. Processing layout depends on what is targeted: probiotics cells, enzymes, organic acids or functional metabolites. With probiotics the task usually follows the route of centrifugation, filtering, and then spray drying, before encapsulation. On the contrary, beverages and metabolites require processes like clarification, pasteurization, solvent extraction, chromatography and freeze drying (Agarwal et al., 2020).

- The stand-out problem in this phase is how to preserve the biological activity of the functional parts during recovery and storage afterwards. The maintenance of activity of enzymes, or probiotic viability, e.g. requires careful control of dry conditions, water content, and follow-on packaging.

- The development of bio-technology has made a variety of contributions to this phase including:
- Energy-friendly purification Membrane separation (ultrafiltration, nanofiltration);
- Freeze dried probiotic cryoprotectant formulation; and
- Preservatives made of bio substances to increase shelf life after recovery.

Cost Optimization and Yield Enhancement

Cost to yield ratio is a key aspect to the economic viability in industrial fermentation. Recent biotechnological development has made four main strategies possible that together strengthen the process economics, enhance sustainability and reduce impact on the environment: (Lokko et al., 2018) (1) Strain improvement by mutagenesis or genetic engineering to raise product titers; (2) Medium optimization using low-cost feedstock, e.g. molasses or whey or agricultural waste; (3) Modelling metabolism to cut out by- product formation and concentrate carbon flux towards the target chemical; (4) In situ product recovery (ISPR) processes, which filter inhibitory compounds out of the fermentation, thereby raising Taken together, the measures will enhance the profitability of the processes and allow reducing the environmental impact of fermentation-based industries (Ajayeoba & Ijabadeniyi, 2025; Macwan et al., 2025).

Case Studies and Industrial Applications

- **Yogurt and fermented milk:** With the dairy industrial fermentation, implicit in the production of yogurt and the fermentation of other fermented milk products is the existence of temperature-pH control during fed-batch fermentation to achieve both the formation of lactic acid and the required textural behavior (Chen & Hang, 2019).
- **Kombucha production:** The integrated platform of process optimization is given by using the continuous fermentation systems which utilize symbiotic cultures of bacteria and yeast (SCOBY) and the real-time measurements of pH value and sugar concentrations (Yee et al., 2025).
- **Ethanol production:** Fermentation is done on a large scale using genetically-improved strains of Saccharomyces cerevisiae strains and raised ethanol tolerance (da Silva Fernandes et al., 2022).
- **Probiotic powders:** Cultured microorganisms are then further fermented in a high-density medium then removed after centrifugation and over freeze-drying process done under cryoprotectant (Cui et al., 2022).

Table 2. Biotechnological tools by application and category

S. No.	Category	Application/Detail	Biotechnological Tool/Strategy	Reference
1	Bioreactor Type	Batch fermentation in yogurt and kimchi production	Fixed volume substrate inoculation	(Yee et al., 2025)
2	Bioreactor Type	Fed-batch system for high biomass in probiotics	Incremental nutrient feeding	(Malvido et al., 2019)
3	Bioreactor Type	Continuous kombucha fermentation	Simultaneous feed and removal	(Błaszak et al., 2024)
4	Bioreactor Design	Stirred tank reactor (STR) for dairy fermentation	Uniform mixing and oxygenation	(Kaur & Sharma, 2021)
5	Bioreactor Design	Airlift fermenter for low shear environments	Gas lift-driven circulation	(Johnson et al., 2018)
6	Bioreactor Design	Packed-bed reactors for immobilized probiotics	Cell entrapment system	(Patarroyo et al., 2020)
7	Process Control	pH optimization for lactic acid bacteria	Real-time pH monitoring	(Muncan et al., 2020)
8	Process Control	Temperature control in yeast fermentation	Automated bioreactor temperature regulation	(Chai et al., 2022)
9	Process Control	Oxygen control in aerobic fermentations	DO sensors with oxygen sparging	(Phillips, 2020)
10	Process Control	Foam control during microbial fermentation	Antifoaming agents and sensors	(Agarwal et al., 2022)
11	Process Control	Agitation rate optimization	Agitator design and impeller selection	(Benz, 2022)
12	Fermentation Monitoring	SCADA for real-time process monitoring	Supervisory control and data acquisition	(Lisci, 2023)
13	Fermentation Monitoring	Biosensor-based sugar monitoring	Glucose/lactose biosensors	(Rout & Chakraborty, 2020)
14	Downstream Processing	Centrifugation of probiotic biomass	Solid-liquid separation	(Agrawal, 2024)
15	Downstream Processing	Spray drying for commercial probiotic powder	Rapid dehydration with encapsulants	(Wang & Zhong, 2024)
16	Downstream Processing	Freeze drying of enzymes and probiotics	Cryoprotectant addition	(Krunic & Osmokrovic, 2025)
17	Product Stabilization	Moisture control in storage of dried probiotics	Vacuum packaging	(Jannah et al., 2022)
18	Product Stabilization	Shelf-life extension using bio-preservatives	Nisin and other bacteriocins	(Katakhade et al., 2023)
19	Cost Optimization	Use of molasses and whey as substrates	Substrate substitution	(Kumar et al., 2018)
20	Cost Optimization	Bioconversion of agro-waste	Enzymatic hydrolysis and microbial digestion	(Ravindran et al., 2018)
21	Strain Improvement	Mutant selection for high-yield *Lactobacillus*	UV mutagenesis	(Jeyachandran et al., 2024)
22	Strain Improvement	Genetic engineering of yeasts for ethanol tolerance	Recombinant DNA technology	(Adebami et al., 2022)
23	Metabolic Engineering	Redirection of carbon flux to reduce by-products	Knockout of side-product genes	(Nguyen, 2018)
24	ISPR	Removal of ethanol during fermentation	In situ extraction system	(Santos et al., 2021)

continued on following page

Table 2. Continued

S. No.	Category	Application/Detail	Biotechnological Tool/Strategy	Reference
25	Industrial Case Study	High-density fermentation for probiotic powders	Optimized fed-batch with microaeration	(Martin & Chan, 2024)
26	Industrial Case Study	Kombucha process intensification	Use of starter culture and pH control	(Fabricio et al., 2023)
27	Industrial Case Study	Ethanol from corn using engineered *S. cerevisiae*	CRISPR/Cas9-modified yeast	(de Mélo et al., 2023)
28	Sustainability	Fermentation using food industry by-products	Circular bioprocessing	(Minervini et al., 2022)
29	Energy Efficiency	Ultrafiltration in metabolite recovery	Low-energy downstream purification	(Janković et al., 2024)
30	Future Trends	AI for process optimization in fermentation	Machine learning for parameter prediction	(Z. Wang et al., 2025)

BIOTECHNOLOGY IN THE BEVERAGE INDUSTRY

Contemporary biotechnology has triggered a significant change in the beverage industry. According to recent technological development in the area of optimizing the fermentation process, developing flavor, and engineering product functionality, the classical categories like beer, wine, and cider have been metamorphosed, and, at the same time, enabled the emergence of non-alcoholic functional beverages that satisfy the health-conscious needs of consumers (Giri et al., 2023). The classical systems of fermentation may also be improved using biotechnological methods, which increase the yield, quality, consistency and nutritional profile. This consumer preference is reflected in the appearance of the wide range of non-alcoholic beverages, one of which is kombucha, probiotic juices, and various fermented goods (Malakar et al., 2020).

Production of alcoholic beverages, especially in the brewing and wine industries, is still under the impact of genetically optimized strains of *Saccharomyces cerevisiae* and *Oenococcus oeni*. These strains provide an increased resistance to stress, higher alcohol productivity and enhanced flavor compound complex. Metabolic engineering allows control of fermentation by-products, such as acetaldehyde and hydrogen sulfide, but also allows excess production of esters and higher alcohols which are also important flavor and aroma compounds (Hirst & Richter, 2016). As an example, using CRISPR/cas9-based editing, yeast strains have been designed to express higher concentrations of isoamyl acetate, a compound which confers a fruity flavor to beer and sake. Similar progress in transcriptomics and proteomics has revealed how yeast gene expression relates to fermentation performance under different stress conditions, to make bespoke strains to suit the characteristics of specific beverages and local taste preferences (Adebami et al., 2022).

Biotechnological innovations have also enhanced the process of wine fermentation. In addition to increasing ethanol fermentation, concepts have shifted towards tempering malolactic fermentation and microbial succession as a way of alleviating spoilage and streamlining sensory characteristics. Using non-*Saccharomyces* yeasts such as *Torulaspora delbrueckii* and *Lachancea thermotolerans*, most often as mixed or sequential cultures, has increasingly become a distinctive practice as well (He et al., 2024). The yeasts increase both complexity and acidity, but not drastically to alcohol content, where there are worries with climatic changes pushing the sugar content of grapes. The use of biotechnological approaches has also been used in resolving and preventing Brettanomyces-related spoilage through fast PCR-based detection and specific antimicrobial peptides (Cosme et al., 2024).

Fermentation of fruits, cereals as well as various plant materials has played an important role in the world of non-alcoholic beverages and has contributed to the production of bioactive compounds to support health with organic acids, polyphenols, vitamins, and short-chain fatty acids. A more specific case is that of kombucha production which entails a complicated symbiotic culture of bacteria and yeast (SCOBY) which can be profiled and optimized towards higher productivity of glucuronic acid, and more consistent flavor profiles (Ray et al., 2024). The incorporation of Lactobacterium and Bifidobacterium in fruit and vegetable juices has made it possible to introduce the probiotic juices to be consumed by lactose intolerant consumers and those who are interested in taking alternative food products that are free of dairy products. Biotechnology can be used to select an acidic and oxygen-rich matrix-only strains with abnormally high viability, or encapsulation or mechanical stress-resistance engineering can be used to stabilize against leakage during gastrointestinal processing and storage (Gonçalves et al., 2025).

Other fermentation that has also undergone fermentation optimization are plant-based drinks like oat milk, soy milk, almond milk among others. Transformation of anti-nutritional factors by biotechnological tools (e.g., phytate, oligosaccharides) and increase of protein assimilation and micronutrient bioavailability has been achieved. Engineered lactic acid bacteria fermentation can help to increase the level of folate and riboflavin, as well as of produce antioxidant or even antihypertensive peptides. Synthetic biology even in some cases inserts biosynthetic path into microbes that process the extracts of the plants, leading to the production of new beverages based on health enhancement as such without relying on the traditional extraction of the plants (Dhiman et al., 2025).

Biotechnology also promotes sustainability of beverage manufacture by valorization of agro-industrial by-products. Microbial fermentation can be used to convert fruit pomace, spent grains, and peels into functional beverages/ ingredient products thus minimizing waste and promoting circular economy models. The strategy would be particularly relevant in juice and wine industries, where large volumes of organic wastes are normally being disposed off. The translation of high value products quickly and cheaply has been enabled through the engineering of microbes which are able to degrade complex polysaccharides and could generate bioactive metabolites, out of pre-underappreciated resources (Barcelos et al., 2020).

Quality assurance and safety services are established with molecular diagnostic tests, high throughput screening and fermentation monitoring systems. Biosensors, which have the capacity to detect contaminants, spoilage organism or off flavor substances in real time, have improved operation accuracy and responsiveness. Tracy Mechanisms such as microbial fingerprinting and genomic barcoding based traceability also assist in authenticity, verification as well as brand protection, in premium wine and craft beverage industries (Niyigaba et al., 2025).

ENZYME TECHNOLOGY IN FOOD AND BEVERAGE PROCESSING

In the modern food and beverage biotechnology, enzyme technology has a leading role as it facilitates the accomplishment of a certain, efficient, and environmentally friendly transformation of the food components. During the last few decades, microbial enzymes produced using standard fermentation methods have increasingly replaced their animal and plant-derived equivalents, mainly due to microbial systems having a much better scalability range, a lower price of production, and due to a widened functionality range (Dhiman et al., 2025). Thus the enzymes have become important tools to enhance texture, flavor, shelf stability, digestibility, and nutritional cost of a diversified food and beverage products. Advances in biotechnology are not only helpful to discover new enzymes, but also to systematically improve them, either by genetic and protein engineering, enzyme immobilization, or by optimizing fermentation procedures (Singh & Kumar, 2019).

Role and Types of Microbial Enzymes in Food Processing

In the food industry, enzymes are used as biocatalysts, or accelerating the biochemical conversions, but are not part of the product. Microbial enzymes rule by their diversity and salient adaptive qualities. The various types of enzymes used in pretty much any food system such as amylases, proteases, lipases, cellulases, pectinases, lactases, and glucose oxidases have very particular consequences on starch molecules, protein molecules, or even the lipid or dietary-fiber molecules (Bilal & Iqbal, 2020).

In the food processing industry, amylases are essential, especially in baking and brewing, because of their catalytic ability to hydrolyse starch into simple sugars. Amylases in baking enhance crust color and crust improvement, and by altering starch architecture retarding staling (Fallahi et al., 2018). During brewing cereal starches are hydrolyzed to fermentable sugars by amylases, and this affects alcohol yield and flavor. Proteins that breakdown proteins to peptides and amino acids are essential in meat tenderization, production of cheese and enhancement of flavour in fermented products. Microbial rennets, especially Mucor miehei protease, are now being heavily used to replace traditional calf rennet in most applications by vegetarians in cheese-making (Philipps-Wiemann, 2018).

Genetic Engineering of Enzyme-Producing Microorganisms

Conventional production of enzymes depended on wild-type microbial cells; the essence of gene engineering has allowed production of enzymes with improved characteristics through overproduction in engineered microbial cells. It is possible to insert genes that code high-activity enzymes in fast-growing cells like Escherichia coli, Bacillus subtilis or Aspergillus niger. Such hosts can be modified such that enzyme expression, secretion and stability is enhanced. Transcriptional efficiency can also be improved by adding certain promoters and signal peptides that improve export of enzyme into the media, to facilitate downstream purification (Deckers et al., 2020).

One practice that has been frequently used is called site-directed mutagenesis, where single amino acids in a given protein structure are affected to enhance thermostability, pH tolerance or specificity towards a certain substrate. To take another instance, in the case of baking where high temperature activity is needed, engineered xylanases that are more thermophilic are available. Directed evolution (also called directed mutation), which simulates natural selection in the laboratory, is another method, in which libraries of enzyme variants are created and desirable traits are chosen. These modes do not only increase the utility of known enzymes, but also result in the discovery of completely different functions (Watanabe et al., 2021).

Immobilized Enzyme Systems

The enzyme immobilization refers to the process of immobilizing the enzymes onto solid phases relatively without loss of the enzyme catalytic activity. This strategy leads to the reuse of enzymes and an increase in the process stability. Application Immobilized enzyme systems are coming in use more frequently in continuous processes in food applications such as juice clarification, high-fructose corn syrup production and lactose hydrolysis of milk. Methods used to immobilize go as entrapment of the enzymes in alginate beads, covalent attachment to grafted silica or resins, and adsorption of the enzymes to porous carriers, (Taheri-Kafrani et al., 2021).

Immobilized enzymes have the following major advantages, namely: increased stability to denaturation, long working life, and better ease of product recovery. An example is where immobilized glucose isomerase is a vital part of carbohydrate conversion of glucose to fructose in the industrial production of sweeteners; use of continuous column reactor provides economies of scale production. Similarly, the lactase immobilized system has also been developed to continue production of lactose-free milk during inline treatment of milk resulting in minimal loss of enzyme (Taheri-Kafrani et al., 2021).

Applications in Specific Food and Beverage Products

Enzyme preparation is the mandatory element in the baking industry, which is aimed at reinforcing the strength of the dough, shortening the mixing time, increasing the level of crumb softness and extending shelf-life. To be more particular, a combination of amylases, xylanases, lipases, and oxidoreductases have synergistic effects to improve the quality of bread, most often included in formulations. Also, we can add proteases in a bid to reduce gluten strength in cookies and crackers (Sheikholeslami et al., 2021).

Proteinases and glucanases are used in the brewing industry to initiate the hydrolisis of cell wall polyssacharides and proteins with the aim of simplifying the filtration progress and ensuring the haze resistance. Adjuncts like rice or corn require external amylases to make conversion of starch at low levels especially in low-malt formulation. On the same note, enzyme cocktails in the manufacture of beer without alcoholic content are used to make changes in fermentation pathways but importantly maintain the mouthfeel of the beverage (Fallahi et al., 2018).

Sustainability and Waste Valorization

Large quantities of by-products of the food and beverage industry include whey products arising through milk processing, spent grain during brewing, peels of fruit and vegetables during manufacture of fresh juices, and nutritive wastewater. Unless controlled, these streams have led to environmental pollution by posing high biochemical oxygen demand and emission of greenhouse gases. The requirements of the targeted solutions of bio-technology to utilize such residues to value-added products is consistent with the sustainability and circular economy concepts (Das et al., 2022). Through fermentation the wastes which are rich in carbohydrates are changed into bioethanol or biogas rich in methane acting as renewable on site power and eliminating the usage of fossil fuels. Bioactive ingredients, including polyphenols in grape pomace, carotenoids in carrot or tomato peels, and dietary fiber in fruit pulps, have been recovered using enzymatic and microbial extraction methods as a functional food ingredient, natural food colorant and nutraceuticals blend product (Panahi et al., 2022). Whey and starch-rich residues can be converted into lactic acid, a source product of PLA bioplastics, that can also be used to provide a compostable, alternative to petroleum based packaging materials. Compared to standard treatment routes, enzyme-based treatment uses less energy consumptions and it does not use harmful chemicals which makes it environmentally friendly both in terms of managing waste and generation of the value added products (Bhat, 2021).

Intended use of waste valorization can be illustrated with actual examples of valorization: breweries produce high protein animal feed out of spent grain; citrus peels are fermented to cultivate probiotic ferments and dairy processing plants can be used to produce lactose-free syrups or fermentation media into high value microbial products (Silva et al., 2025). Most of the time, these plans are deeply embedded in the circular economy paradigm where once product is finished being used in one process; it can be used in another process- e.g. installing anaerobic digesters to feed energy back to the processing facilities (Hussain et al., 2020).

The advent of enzymatic biorefineries explains how enzyme technology can go beyond incremental product improvement and become fully integrated into the circular economies, transforming a wide variety of waste streams into nutraceuticals, bioethanol and functional ingredients (Shankar et al., 2024).

Challenges and Regulatory Aspects

Even though enzymes give major benefits to food processing, the application of the enzymes is strictly regulated as it should ensure safety of consumers and guarantee transparency of information. The regulatory bodies, The EFSA and FDA require the enzyme preparations to be free of contaminants, allergens and toxic metabolites. Moreover, genetically modified microorganisms (GMMs) may be used in most jurisdictions, although this has to be disclosed openly and the product of the enzyme (which, in most cases, will be an enzyme product) must contain no living GMMs or DNA (Trump et al., 2023).

Another obstacle is the perception of the people. Though the enzyme-treated products are mostly acceptable there is a tendency to panic which may be developed when genetic engineering is involved. Manufacturers thus emphasize on the natural sources as well as particularity of enzymes and invest in awareness of consumers regarding the safety and advantages of the enzymes (Ojeih et al., 2024).

BIOTECHNOLOGY FOR WASTE VALORIZATION AND BY-PRODUCT UTILIZATION

The increased demand of green food production has drawn the interest into disposal reduction and the greatest possible value of food industry by-products. Bioeconomy can be created through the use of efficient and sustainable approaches provided by Biotechnology to convert food and beverage processing foodwaste into high-value products, generating the circular bioeconomy. The concept is also called waste valorization, and in addition to mitigating environmental load, it makes the economy resilient by increasing the product streams and lessening dependence on raw materials (Sharma et al., 2021).

The food and beverage sector produces massive amounts of waste materials- fruit pulp, vegetable scraps, brewers grain, whey, molasses and crustacean shells being a few of them. These by-products have always been considered low-value or disposable materials but currently have been highlighted as having great amounts of carbohydrates, proteins, lipids, and bioactives. Biotechnological innovations change these residues to functional food components, enzyme, organic acid, biofuel, bioplastics, and nutraceuticals (Pinela et al., 2024).

One of the most known is the bio-conversion of peel of fruits and vegetables who are rich in polyphenols, dietary fiber and essential oils. Cellulases and pectinases (listed by name under Enzymes that hydrolyze cell walls) depolymerize cell wall material, producing soluble sugar and bioactive which may be fermented by lactic acid bacteria or yeasts to produce organic acids, flavor posits, or potentially ethanol (Al-Maqtari et al., 2019). Microbial fermentation has implemented Apple pomace, oblong skin and grape skin to create probiotic drinks, antioxidant extracts, and enhancers of flavor. Examples of such as engineered Lactobacillus plantarum strains have been characterized by high efficiency to convert waste rich in pectin to lactic acid and simultaneously enrich the medium with health promoting compounds (Toy et al., 2022).

Another primary target of valorization is whey that is a by-product of cheese production. Whey contains a lot of lactose and proteins which can be fermented to yield bioethanol, single-coll proteins or probiotic cultures. Whey is transformed to value added products using recombinant microbes that can metabolize lactose. As well, whey proteins are hydrolyzed by microbial protease to produce peptides used in formulating functional foods with antioxidant, antihypertensive or Antimicrobial activity (Singh & Negi, 2025).

The main byset of brewing and distilling is spent grain which contains high fiber, protein and remaining starch. Its breakdown using enzyme and microbial processes can be done through biotechnology and results into fermentable sugars that are used as ethanol or organic acid or enzyme production. Some fungal species like aspergillus niger and rhizopus oryzae have been employed in conversion of spent grain to citric acid or lipases and some filamentous fungi have also helped in producing animal feed supplement during solid-state fermentation (Puligundla & Mok, 2021).

Juice and wine industries always dispose of grapes pomace and fruit press cakes although they are rich in phenolic compounds and fermentable sugars. These by-products are fermented in specialized microbial consortia to create acetic acid, gluconic or flavored vinegar. Moreover, tannin-containing residues could be enzymatically or microbially treated to obtain hydrolysates that could be used as food additives (natural food preservatives and nutraceuticals) (Abreu et al., 2024). One possible area of potential innovation is in utilizing as feedstock chitin-containing shellfish waste products like shrimp and crab shells, currently land-filled or burned. Chitin can be transformed into chitosan biological polymer through microbial fermentation or enzymatic hydrolysis, and has been used in food packaging, water purification and drug release, and is biodegraded. This is facilitated further by chitinases and de-acetylases which are enzymes present in genetically modified strains, enhancing both efficiency and specificity of this process (Shetranjiwalla & Ononiwu, 2025).

Used cooking oils and fats are also valorized in a biotechnological manner, being converted by lipase producing microbes to biodiesel or specialty fatty acids. Such processes do not only produce alternative fuels, but also minimize pollution, associated with disposal. In order to beat the challenges of high fat content conversion, it has been engineered that enzymes like lipases or esterases would be very active in non-polar conditions so that high conversion could be achieved even with high fat waste streams (Bezbradica et al., 2017). The lignocellulosic residues of Agro-industries such as sugarcane bagasse, rice husk, and corn stover are being processed more and more using the consolidated bioprocessing (CBP) in which the cellulolytic microbes can break up and ferment these without delay. This method which is in its research and pilot scale use promises to create bioethanol, biopolymers and organic acids via recalcitrant biomass (Blasi et al., 2023).

Microbial engineering is the field that is at the core of strain design to valorize wastes. It is possible to design microbes to convert complex waste substrates to well defined and targeted end-products using metabolic pathway optimization, synthetic operons, and gene cluster integration. An example is the *Corynebacterium glutamicum* which has been genetically modified to use glycerol in biodiesel wastes and to manufacture glutamic acid and bioplastics. A lipid-accumulating yeast, *Yarrowia lipolytica*, is used to convert cooking oil waste to microbial lipids to be converted into biodiesel or Omega-3 fatty acids (Aggarwal et al., 2024).

SAFETY, REGULATORY, AND ETHICAL CONSIDERATIONS IN FOOD BIOTECHNOLOGY

With biotechnology so deeply penetrating the food and beverage industry, issues pertaining to safety, regulatory rules and ethical considerations have come into the fore. Even though there are many benefits related to the application of biotechnology, not only in the production of products that become higher in terms of quality and nutriment level but also in relation to their sustainability (Wu et al., 2014), and minimization of wastes, measures of applying biotechnology should be subject to strict standards to ensure that it does not compromise the safety of the consumers, healthy populations alike, and to avoid abuse (Singh). Here we are going to discuss the safety measures, the regulatory policies and the ethical controversies of applying biotechnology in the food sector.

Safety Assessment of Biotechnological Products

The microorganisms used, the process of production and the end product are well scrutinized in assessing the safety of the food product derived by means of biotechnology. The regulators insist on using Generally Recognized as Safe (GRAS) microorganisms such as lactic acid bacteria, yeasts, and even some fungi, whose safety of use has a history older than production of food. Extra testing is placed when genetically modified microorganisms (GMMs) are applied to ensure that there are no negative genes, allergens, toxins, and antibiotic-resistance markers within the final product (Voeikova et al., 2020).

The genetic strategies are used to determine the stability and identity of the microbial strains: molecular characterization (whole-genome sequencing, PCR, and proteomics). Simultaneously, toxicological experiments determine mutagenicity, immunogenicity, and the by-products of the metabolism. In the case of enzymes manufacture, it is vital to eliminate all traces of DNA, living GMMs, and fermentation by-products, particularly, when the enzyme shall be used in infant foods or in medical nutrition (Bari & Zaman, 2021).

International Regulatory Frameworks

The different regulatory regimes governing the different regions of the world have continued to govern the biotechnological products in the different regions and at most instances these regulatory regimes are based on difference in perception of the citizens, the legal systems, and risk tolerance. In the United States, food ingredients and additives, as well as enzymes and probiotics are regulated by Food and Drug Administration (FDA) as food ingredients with the GRAS system (Stazi & Jovine, 2022). The Environmental Protection Agency (EPA) and the U.S. department of agriculture (USDA) can come into play especially where the genetic alteration of organisms are used in agricultural production. Within the European Union the regulation is even tighter and centralized with the authority of the European Food Safety Authority (EFSA). Any enzyme, microbial culture, food additive produced through the biotech process should have their pre-market approval. Regulation (EC) No 1829/2003 places regulations on GMOs and GMMs and has labeling requirements in case they find presence above 0.9% in the final product. EU policy is subject to precautionary principle and so any uncertainty or absence of scientific opinion is likely to mean limiting permission (Eckerstorfer et al., 2019).

Labeling and Consumer Transparency

One of the most controversial areas of modern food governance is formed by biotechnological processing of foods. On one hand, pro-side of the question argues that these products are equally safe as the conventional ones and, as such, do not require mandatory labeling, and, on the other hand, consumer organisations demand transparency and the possibility of informed choice. The compulsory labeling of genetically modified (GM) ingredients exists in the EU and many countries of Asia, regardless of there being no live modified organisms present in the final product (Evans, 2019). In comparison, the 2022 National Bioengineered Food Disclosure Standard in the United States allows disclosure by a digital link, such as a QR code, open to criticism owing to accessibility restrictions. The probiotics and other functional foods are also considered under labeling regulation where its claimed properties are supposed to be developed with hard scientific data. The use of health-related claims like, e.g., a product is capable of enhancing digestion, or strengthens the immune system, is limited and, most likely, enables the submission of randomized clinical trials and a whole dossier before being granted. Different labeling of variables within and across nations creates more confusion and possibly undermine consumer confidence (Goodman, 2019).

Ethical Considerations in Food Biotechnology

Some of the questions about ethics in food biotechnology are the acceptable genetic modification, socio-economic effects on farmers and consumers among others. Consumer freedom is one of the major concerns overtly the right of a consumer not to take biotechnologically engineered foodstuffs in situations whereby there is vagueness or no labeling whatsoever. This autonomy is of paramount importance and transparency and traceability are the key ethical principles that are to be maintained to support such autonomy (Singh, 2025).

Naturalness of food is also a question. The usage of synthetic biology and fake genetic structures is perceived as an attempt to violate the conventional food identities although the use of enzymes and microbes in the fermentation process is old. There might be also the effect of cultural and religious beliefs on the acceptability of the population. As another example, some religiously inspired dietary requirements (e.g. halal, kosher) might not sanction the use of enzymes made using forbidden genetic resources and cells (Siegrist & Hartmann, 2020).

In a wider perspective, equity and access might be of concern because of the utilization of biotechnology. High-tech biotechnological devices are largely in the hands of multinational companies, which are accused of the monopolization of the situation, the loss of independence of farmers, and high prices of inputs. Survival of small-scale food producers depends on their resources, and subsequently adoption of biotech-based innovations may further widen the inequality associated with the global food system (Torrorey-Sawe, 2025).

Issue also exists concerning whether the use of GMMs in food and environmental systems are supposed to be ethical or not. Despite the stringent containment measures, there is fear that modified strains may accidentally escape into the natural environment and there is possibility of horizontal gene transfer as well as long term ecological effects. Although risk assessment determines that GMMs utilized in food are safe, it is necessary to continue this process based on the ethical principle of precaution to be exercised (Deckers et al., 2020).

Public Perception and Communication

The factors that create the acceptances of food biotechnologies among the people are related to the complex interaction of scientific literacy, the cultural context, media reporting as well as trust in the regulatory bodies. The information that is not true as well as the fear-based stories can crush awareness, even regarding scientifically proven products. An example is that genetically modified yeasts strains used in wine fermentation or, recombinant enzymes in cheese production might be banned, even though there has been decades of safe use (Overton & Yang, 2023).

Science communication plays an important role in enabling the solution to the gap between innovation and consumer acceptance. Informed choice can be encouraged through educational programs, easy-to-read disclosures, wide availability of safety information, as well as stakeholders involvement. There should be cooperation among scientists, industry players and regulatory bodies to de-mystify biotechnology and deal with such issues before they arise (Broad, 2023).

FUTURE TRENDS AND INNOVATIONS IN FOOD AND BEVERAGE BIOTECHNOLOGY

Biotechnology will presumably remain at the limelight of all things in the food beverage sector as the food security/world ambivalence, degrading environment, population growth and global warming increasingly force their way to the fore (Panda & Shetty, 2018). The field (as evidenced by the current trends) is getting narrower, sustainable, and personal as new tools such as omics techniques, synthetic biology, artificial intelligence and biomanufacturing come into use that plays a significant role. Collectively, they will transform the agricultural, processing and consumption model and are bringing about the era of precision fermenting, designer microbes and intelligent food systems (Sahu & Panda, 2018).

Precision Fermentation and Synthetic Biology

One massive leap in the field of biotechnology is precision fermentation, which allows microorganisms to be programmed directly to make proteins, vitamins, enzymes, and flavor molecules with extreme accuracy. Rather than using the full length of a naturally occurring microbial pathway one utilizes the method of precision fermentation which uses the science of synthetic biology to introduce, regulate, or shut down individual and specific genes of a host organism (Mirsalami & Mirsalami, 2025).The strategies enable production of molecules that are either hard to find in nature or those that consume large-scale agricultural inputs.

The use of casein and whey proteins (microbial in their origins) is now used to formulate animal free dairy foods; heme, a flavoring agent, is grown through modified bacteria, and vitamin B12 is manufactured in genetically altered bacteria. *Pichia pastoris*, *Yarrowia lipolytica* and *Bacillus subtilis* have become choice hosts of cost effective production of the biomolecules in industrial and academic research laboratories worldwide (Jayakrishnan et al., 2024). Equally, synthetic biology has led to creation of new, designed, or even artificial biosynthetic pathways and the creation of an entirely synthetic cell factory that can be used to manufacture foodstuffs, food colorants and health beneficial metabolic products.

The current research is also devoted to the modular mixes of engineered microorganisms that aim to mimic the complexity of natural fermentation systems, simultaneously granting more instruments of control and operational efficiency (Nguyen et al., 2018).The idea behind this modular approach is to allow the carrying out of fermentations by using more than a single strain thereby allowing them to co-ferment and give desirable flavors, nutritional improvements or process stabilization at the same time.

AI and Data-Driven Optimization

The next revolution of artificial intelligence (AI), machine learning (ML) and big data analytics is redefining the bioprocess optimization, strain selection, and predictive modelling paradigms in the food biotechnology sector. One of the ways in which those methods help is the possibility to access trends in large datasets through genomics, proteomics, metabolomics and process-analytical methods, to identify key bottlenecks and find correlations that would otherwise have gone undetected (Umoga et al., 2024).

During fermentation, the AI based algorithms can be used as a microbial growth models, to predict the nutrient requirements, to optimize yields and to hasten the production by shortening the time. In product development, ML is used to make new products by predicting the effects of molecular structure on textural, sensory and stabilizer properties (Selvarajan, 2021). Moreover, AI-based technologies allow simulating preferences of consumers and regional flavor varieties, thus they make the production consistent with these market peculiarities.

The use of digital twins (digital replicas of bioreactors and other fermenting systems) is augmented with AI, and thus, enables real-time monitoring, specific correcting measures and predictive maintenance (Udugama et al., 2021). The smart control systems improve the consistency of the processes, minimize the resource consumption, and cut the use of energy and emissions into the environment, so that they lead to more sustainable production models.

Cell-Free Systems and Biomanufacturing

Traditionally, the traditional fermentation depended on the metabolic activities inherent in the live organisms to produce certain metabolites. The gaining of cell-free biosynthesis is a paradigmatic development, where native enzymes or metabolic pathways are removed out of their parental cells and then utilized in carefully specified extracellular microenvironments (Vilkhovoy et al., 2020). The resulting scale and company change allows it to remove the strains of bacterial growth, expand on the flexibility of the experiments, shorten contamination hazard, and the acceleration of reaction kinetics.

Research in modern times concerns the use of cell-free platform in speeding up the production of flavor compounds, rare sugars, food pigments, and nutraceuticals. As an example, the fruit peels or crop wastes that are by-products of the agricultural industry can be turned into high value additions by the enzymatic cocktails that result out of the metabolic engineering of microbial strains without involving the large-scale fermentation technologies (Rollin et al., 2013). At the same time, modular biomanufacturing architectures where the nature of the bioreactors is miniaturized and continuous-flow are arising and are being adapted to deployment beyond centralized biomanufacturing plants (Dudley et al., 2015). Such portable facilities (and they can be in restaurants, local farms, and community facilities) will enable just-in-time manufacture of fermented foods, enzymes, or probiotics. De-centralized production powers up local food systems, achieves a reduction in transport emissions and equips producers with a greater level of quality and freshness control.

Personalized Nutrition and Microbiome Engineering

Personalized nutrition has become a no longer farfetched idea in the science of microbiome, basing on empirical data. By interrogating the particular structure of microbiota within the gut and genetic potential as well as the nutritional requirements of an individual in a systematic manner, the current nutritional approaches can be adjusted to optimize the health-related functionalities. The essence of this breakthrough is biotechnology, which will allow the personal compilation of individual probiotics, prebiotics, and postbiotics to alleviate a deficit of microbiome diversity (Bashiardes et al., 2018). In some situations, living probiotics in form of biosynthetic strains, which produce therapeutic factors, including anti-inflammatory peptides, antioxidants, or short-chain fatty acids, provide a direct way of modifying the intestine. At the same time, the artificial-intelligence platforms are being used to develop individual synbiotic blends that focus on the person specific gut profile and consequently suggest specific pre-biotic / strain combinations that may result in maximum efficacy (Asar et al., 2025).

In the future, it would be expected that the synergistic implementation of wearable functioning smart garments and in-home laboratory diagnostic technologies in combination with digital-nutrition systems would lead to real-time adjustment of diets by recalibrating meals depending on health signs, stress levels, and changes in microbiome functions (Wang et al., 2025). The overlapping of biotechnology and digital health is an indication of a transition of universal dietary standards to bio-personalized nutrition.

Sustainable Packaging and Edible Coatings

On the side of green packaging of foodstuffs, there is also the technological advance in that regard, with the invention of biodegradable, edible and active packaging material. Plastic containers, wrappings and films are also likely to switch to polymers obtained by microbial fermentation such as polyhydroxyalkanoates (PHAs), polylatic acid (PLA) and bacterial cellulose as renewable alternatives to petroleum-based plastics. Meanwhile they are also in the progress of edible coating which has been enriched with antimicrobial peptides, probiotics, or antioxidants in order to introduce perishable products to dual purposes; serving them with shelf life extension as well as with functional benefits (Bremenkamp & Sousa Gallagher, 2025). These coatings can either be used directly on fruits, vegetables, meat or dairy products and therefore avoid spoilage and also the build up of waste materials in wrapping of these food products.

Further, there is evolution of studies that interface biosensor incorporated smart-packaging system. These developments make use of biotechnological components like pH sensitive markers, enzyme driven color change, DNA barcode to offer real time information of quality of the product (i,e how fresh it is, whether contaminated or whether genuine) (Zhou et al., 2025). The biosensors integrated enhance food supply safety and reflect the increasing demand of the consumers in the sense of transparency, as well as traceability.

Food Security, Climate Resilience, and Global Impact

Biotechnology is now being accepted as one of the major plans to curb food insecurity and adapt to climatic changes. The discipline offers scalable, climate-smart options that might revolutionize the global food system, especially the engineering of microorganisms that make crops drought and salt tolerant as crop inoculants, and further development of sources of protein generated using fermentation that require insignificant agricultural land and water (Toromade et al., 2024). Single-cell proteins (also known as microbial proteins) are normally grown on alcohols, like methane, carbon dioxide and agricultural waste products as their carbon source; they show potential as animal feeds, meat alternatives and in the second order, to provide a higher nutritional and lower energetic footprint than conventional production of livestock (García Martínez et al., 2022). Similar attempts to use fermentation to create alternatives to fats, dairy, and egg products are gaining ground, especially in areas where traditional food production is logistically difficult due to climate change, separating food production and food-growing land and increasing resilience to weather disturbances and facilitating food predictability, including equitable access to healthy food.

Challenges, Regulatory Framework, and Consumer Acceptance

Large investments, special hardware and optimization are needed to scale processes up from the laboratory to industry to protect the product quality and safety and flavors and aroma. Another issue is the strain stability because engineered or genetically modified microorganisms might lose their performance on prolonged usage in industry. Besides, the mistrust of the consumers particularly in regard to the genetically modified organisms (GMOs) and new ingredients is another obstacle even where safety is well established (Dederer, 2016; Naveen & Sontakke, 2024).

There is regional variation of the regulation requirements. The European Union has the novel foods regulation in force which requires prior authorization before marketing food and afterwards intensive examination of their safety and labeling of GMOs with a threshold of more than 0.9 percent. In the United States, bioengineered foods have labeling requirements that are stipulated in the National Bioengineered Food Disclosure Standard (NBFDS) and safety evaluation which is done using the Generally Recognized as Safe (GRAS) system under the Food and Drug Administration (FDA) (Howell, 2023). The Codex Alimentarius internationally gives guidelines, which have harmonizing shape on national policies. The negotiations through these frameworks are a necessary part of the business but may be resource-consuming especially to the producers who operate in more than one market (Fink, 2023). Ethical factors also inform on the acceptance such as open labeling and fair intellectual property on the microbial strains as well as consumer data under the personalized nutrition systems. New products such as animal-free dairy proteins have brought to the fore the discussion of terminology used in labels and consumer understanding.

To enhance acceptance, the following needs to be done; active communication, education and openness. Through good communication of science, stressing on sustainability and nutritional advantage, and making sure that this supply chain is traceable, any industry player can create confidence among consumers to promote the overall use of food biotechnology.

CONCLUSION

Biotechnology has become a key force of innovation in the food and beverage industry, not only fuelling significant innovations along the entire value chain such as the transformation of raw materials, product development, preservation, and sustainability. Enzymatic engineering, genetic modification, data-driven fermentation optimization and forms of microbial systems enable biotechnology to not only supplement functional, nutritional and sensory properties of foods but also reshapes the food production landscape under the rising population and environmental limits.

A review of traditional fermented processes which has formed the backbone of food preservation and a part of food cultures since ancient times was introduced in the discussion. The practices have been made sophisticated, well controlled and scaling by the reality of biotechnology but the practices have also become a refinement of simple practices. The more recent advancements with CRISPR, omics approaches and synthetic biology in turn have transformed conventional microbial species into high performance cell factories specifically engineered to produce desired bioactives, enzymes and flavor compounds with improved precision. As an important acceleration of this process, precision fermentation allows producing animal-free proteins, functional lipids, and other rare micronutrients fully in vivo that previously could be derived solely via agriculturally demanding pathways.

The next topic of focus was the emergence of functional foods and probiotic, which serve as evidence on how the designed microbial strains and encapsulation techniques enable the provision of health-giving foodstuffs that meet the specific physiological needs of the individual. Digital platforms and artificial intelligence are attaining uniform quality, efficiency of operation and cost control of the industrial fermentation ventures, as bioprocess engineering and scale-up techniques are being enabled. These types of combinations in the beverage industry have resulted in the emergence of new consumer types of drinks and alcohol-free beverages that have high health properties, customized taste, and longer shelf life.

More focus was put on enzyme technology which simplifies food processing through lesser chemical input and also enhances more variety of the product. At the same time, biotechnological waste valorization approaches provide economically and environmentally circular-sustainable approaches, manufacturing value-added products (organic acids, flavor, biopolymers, and functional ingredients) out of agro-industrial by-products.

Notably, application of biotechnology in the sector is limited by rigid safety and regulatory environments set to protect the health of the consumers. Such ethical aspects as a label transparency, equal access and environment should be considered as ethical aspects of the biotechnological innovation and not taken out of the process of such innovation development resulting in irresponsible development that would erode the public acceptance and social traditions.

The final appraisal sketched the tendencies emerging, namely precision fermentation, cell-free systems, AI-enhanced bioprocess optimization, intelligent packaging as well as microbiome-informed personalized nutrition, and suggested that the next decade will be marked by a re-conceptualization of food systems and food delivery. As biotechnology evolves, it is expected that it will not only supplement what is already there in the food systems, but it will write new paradigms which are sustainable, inclusive and would be resistant to shocks of the future.

REFERENCES

Abdul Manan, M. (2025). Progress in Probiotic Science: Prospects of Functional Probiotic-Based Foods and Beverages. *International Journal of Food Sciences*, *2025*(1), 5567567.

Abreu, T., Sousa, P., Gonçalves, J., Hontman, N., Teixeira, J., Câmara, J. S., & Perestrelo, R. (2024). Grape pomace as a renewable natural biosource of value-added compounds with potential food industrial applications. *Beverages*, *10*(2), 45.

Acharya, P., Fasim, A., More, V. S., Shivaram, A. K., & More, S. S. (2023). Enzyme technology in value addition of dairy and milk production. In *Value-addition in beverages through enzyme technology* (pp. 77–96). Elsevier.

Adebami, G. E., Kuila, A., Ajunwa, O. M., Fasiku, S. A., & Asemoloye, M. D. (2022). Genetics and metabolic engineering of yeast strains for efficient ethanol production. *Journal of Food Process Engineering*, *45*(7), e13798.

Agarwal, A., Jaiswal, N., Tripathi, A. D., & Paul, V. (2020). Downstream processing; applications and recent updates. In *Bioprocessing for Biofuel Production: Strategies to Improve Process Parameters* (pp. 29-55). Springer.

Agarwal, A., Liu, Y., Dooley, L., McDowell, C., & Thaysen, M. (2022). Large-scale industrial fermenter foaming control: Automated machine learning for antifoam prediction and defoaming process implementation. *Industrial & Engineering Chemistry Research*, *61*(15), 5227–5238.

Aggarwal, N., Pham, H. L., Ranjan, B., Saini, M., Liang, Y., Hossain, G. S., Ling, H., Foo, J. L., & Chang, M. W. (2024). Microbial engineering strategies to utilize waste feedstock for sustainable bioproduction. *Nature Reviews Bioengineering*, *2*(2), 155–174.

Agrawal, R. (2024). Downstream Processing. In *Textbook of Industrial Microbiology* (pp. 279–295). Springer.

Ajayeoba, T. A., & Ijabadeniyi, O. A. (2025). Transforming Food for the Future: Precision Fermentation as a Key to Sustainability, Nutrition, and Health. *Nutrition and Health (Berkhamsted, Hertfordshire)*.

Al-Maqtari, Q. A., Waleed, A., & Mahdi, A. A. (2019). Microbial enzymes produced by fermentation and their applications in the food industry-A review. *International Journal of Agriculture Innovation and Research*, *8*(1), 2319–1473.

Asar, R., Erenler, S., Devecioglu, D., Ispirli, H., Karbancioglu-Guler, F., Ozturk, H. I., & Dertli, E. (2025). Understanding the Functionality of Probiotics on the Edge of Artificial Intelligence (AI) Era. *Fermentation (Basel, Switzerland)*, *11*(5), 259.

Barcelos, M. C., Ramos, C. L., Kuddus, M., Rodriguez-Couto, S., Srivastava, N., Ramteke, P. W., Mishra, P. K., & Molina, G. (2020). Enzymatic potential for the valorization of agro-industrial by-products. *Biotechnology Letters*, *42*(10), 1799–1827.

Bari, M. L., & Zaman, S. (2021). Microbial biotechnology in food and health: present and future food safety regulation. In *Microbial Biotechnology in Food and Health* (pp. 1–20). Elsevier.

Basaran, P. (2024). Plant Molecular Farming for the Bulk Production of Industrial Enzymes. In *Applications of Plant Molecular Farming* (pp. 69–110). Springer.

Bashiardes, S., Godneva, A., Elinav, E., & Segal, E. (2018). Towards utilization of the human genome and microbiome for personalized nutrition. *Current Opinion in Biotechnology, 51*, 57–63.

Beltrán-Velasco, A. I., & Clemente-Suárez, V. J. (2025). Harnessing gut microbiota for biomimetic innovations in health and biotechnology. *Biomimetics, 10*(2), 73.

Benz, G. T. (2022). *Agitator Design Technology for Biofuels and Renewable Chemicals*. John Wiley & Sons.

Bezbradica, D., Crovic, M. J., Tanaskovic, S., Lukovic, N., Carevic, M., Milivojevic, A., & Knezevic-Jugovic, Z. (2017). Enzymatic syntheses of esters-Green chemistry for valuable food, fuel and fine chemicals. *Current Organic Chemistry, 21*(2), 104–138.

Bhat, R. (2021). Valorization of agri-food wastes and by-products: recent trends, innovations and sustainability challenges.

Bianchetti, G., De Maio, F., Abeltino, A., Serantoni, C., Riente, A., Santarelli, G., Sanguinetti, M., Delogu, G., Martinoli, R., & Barbaresi, S. (2023). Unraveling the gut microbiome–diet connection: Exploring the impact of digital precision and personalized nutrition on microbiota composition and host physiology. *Nutrients, 15*(18), 3931.

Bibra, M., Krishnaraj, R. N., & Sani, R. K. (2021). Fermentation strategies in the food and beverage industry. *Biomolecular Engineering Solutions for Renewable Specialty Chemicals: Microorganisms, Products, and Processes*, 141-164.

Bilal, M., & Iqbal, H. M. (2020). State-of-the-art strategies and applied perspectives of enzyme biocatalysis in food sector—Current status and future trends. *Critical Reviews in Food Science and Nutrition, 60*(12), 2052–2066.

Blasi, A., Verardi, A., Lopresto, C. G., Siciliano, S., & Sangiorgio, P. (2023). Lignocellulosic agricultural waste valorization to obtain valuable products: An overview. *Recycling, 8*(4), 61.

Błaszak, B., Dorawa, P., Sudoł, P., Fabiszak, K., Świadek, M., Witucka, K., Zimnicka, J., Brudnicki, M., Maciejewski, B., & Bovkun, D. (2024). Kombucha fermentation in coffee: Application of constant air flow reactor. *Processes (Basel, Switzerland), 12*(10), 2159.

Bommer, G. T., Van Schaftingen, E., & Veiga-da-Cunha, M. (2020). Metabolite repair enzymes control metabolic damage in glycolysis. *Trends in Biochemical Sciences, 45*(3), 228–243.

Botta, C., Tsoureki, D., Gautam, A., Patz, S., Pissaridi, K., Ferrocino, I., Franciosa, I., Cocolin, L., Huson, D. H., & Rantsiou, K. (2024). The pros and cons of tracking the microbial contamination in infant food processing chain through amplicon sequencing and metagenomics. In *Food System Microbiomes* (pp. 1–161). Abstracts Book.

Bremenkamp, I., & Sousa Gallagher, M. J. (2025). Edible coatings for ready-to-eat products: Critical review of recent studies, sustainable packaging perspectives, challenges and emerging trends. *Polymers, 17*(3), 376.

Broad, G. M. (2023). Improving the agri-food biotechnology conversation: Bridging science communication with science and technology studies. *Agriculture and Human Values*, *40*(3), 929–938.

Călinoiu, L.-F., Ştefănescu, B. E., Pop, I. D., Muntean, L., & Vodnar, D. C. (2019). Chitosan coating applications in probiotic microencapsulation. *Coatings*, *9*(3), 194.

Chai, W. Y., Teo, K. T. K., Tan, M. K., & Tham, H. J. (2022). Fermentation process control and optimization. *Chemical Engineering & Technology*, *45*(10), 1731–1747.

Chandrasekaran, M., Basheer, S. M., Chellappan, S., Krishna, J. G., & Beena, P. (2015). Enzymes in food and beverage production: An overview. *Enzym Food Beverage Process CRC Press*, *25*, 133–154.

Chen, W., & Hang, F. (2019). Lactic acid bacteria starter. In *Lactic Acid Bacteria: Bioengineering and Industrial Applications* (pp. 93-143). Springer.

Choi, Y. J., Shin, S.-H., & Shin, H. S. (2022). Immunomodulatory Effects of Bifidobacterium spp. and Use of Bifidobacterium breve and Bifidobacterium longum on Acute Diarrhea in Children. *Journal of Microbiology and Biotechnology*, *32*(9), 1186.

Cosme, F., Nunes, F. M., & Filipe-Ribeiro, L. (2024). *Winemaking: Advanced Technology and Flavor Research* (Vol. 13). MDPI.

Cui, S., Hu, M., Sun, Y., Mao, B., Zhang, Q., Zhao, J., Tang, X., & Zhang, H. (2022). Effect of trehalose and lactose treatments on the freeze-drying resistance of lactic acid bacteria in high-density culture. *Microorganisms*, *11*(1), 48.

da Silva Fernandes, F., de Souza, É. S., Carneiro, L. M., Alves Silva, J. P., de Souza, J. V. B., & da Silva Batista, J. (2022). Current ethanol production requirements for the yeast Saccharomyces cerevisiae. *International Journal of Microbiology*, *2022*(1), 7878830.

Daisley, B. A., & Allen-Vercoe, E. (2024). Microbes as medicine. *Annals of the New York Academy of Sciences*, *1541*(1), 63–82.

Das, D., Panesar, P. S., Panesar, G., & Timilsena, Y. (2022). Sources, composition, and characterization of agro-industrial byproducts. In *Valorization of Agro-Industrial Byproducts* (pp. 11–30). CRC Press.

de Mélo, A. H., Nunes, A. L., Carvalho, P. H., da Silva, M. F., Teixeira, G. S., & Goldbeck, R. (2023). Evaluation of Saccharomyces cerevisiae modified via CRISPR/Cas9 as a cellulosic platform microorganism in simultaneously saccharification and fermentation processes. *Bioprocess and Biosystems Engineering*, *46*(8), 1111–1119.

Deckers, M., Deforce, D., Fraiture, M.-A., & Roosens, N. H. (2020). Genetically modified microorganisms for industrial food enzyme production: An overview. *Foods*, *9*(3), 326.

Dederer, H.-G. (2016). The challenge of regulating genetically modified organisms in the European Union: trends and issues. In *Contemporary Issues in Environmental Law: The EU and Japan* (pp. 139-168). Springer.

Dhiman, S., Kaur, S., Thakur, B., Singh, P., & Tripathi, M. (2025). Nutritional Enhancement of Plant-Based Fermented Foods: Microbial Innovations for a Sustainable Future. *Fermentation (Basel, Switzerland)*, *11*(6), 346.

Donato, K., Medori, M., Stuppia, L., Beccari, T., Dundar, M., Marks, R., Michelini, S., Borghetti, E., Zuccato, C., & Seppilli, L. (2023). Unleashing the potential of biotechnology for sustainable development. *European Review for Medical and Pharmacological Sciences*, *27*(6, Suppl), 100–113.

Dudley, Q. M., Karim, A. S., & Jewett, M. C. (2015). Cell-free metabolic engineering: Biomanufacturing beyond the cell. *Biotechnology Journal*, *10*(1), 69–82.

Eckerstorfer, M. F., Engelhard, M., Heissenberger, A., Simon, S., & Teichmann, H. (2019). Plants developed by new genetic modification techniques—Comparison of existing regulatory frameworks in the EU and non-EU countries. *Frontiers in Bioengineering and Biotechnology*, *7*, 26.

Evans, H. M. (2019). A New Age of Evolution: Protecting the Consumer's Moral and Legal Right to Know through the Clear and Transparent Labeling of All Genetically Modified Foods. *Journal of Law and Health*, *33*, vi.

Fabricio, M. F., Vargas, B. K., Tischer, B., Wagner, R., Ribeiro, S. R., Cordeiro, N., Flôres, S. H., & Ayub, M. A. Z. (2023). Revamping kombucha production: Achieving consistency and probiotic potential through a tailor-made microbial consortium. *International Journal of Gastronomy and Food Science*, *34*, 100844.

Fallahi, P., Habte-Tsion, H.-M., & Rossi, W. (2018). Depolymerizating enzymes in human food: bakery, dairy products, and drinks. In *Enzymes in human and animal nutrition* (pp. 211–237). Elsevier.

Feldgarden, M., Brover, V., Haft, D. H., Prasad, A. B., Slotta, D. J., Tolstoy, I., Tyson, G. H., Zhao, S., Hsu, C.-H., & McDermott, P. F. (2019). Validating the AMRFinder tool and resistance gene database by using antimicrobial resistance genotype-phenotype correlations in a collection of isolates. *Antimicrobial Agents and Chemotherapy*, *63*(11), 00483–00419. DOI: 10.1128/aac

Ferremi Leali, N., Binati, R. L., Martelli, F., Gatto, V., Luzzini, G., Salini, A., Slaghenaufi, D., Fusco, S., Ugliano, M., & Torriani, S. (2022). Reconstruction of simplified microbial consortia to modulate sensory quality of kombucha tea. *Foods*, *11*(19), 3045.

Fink, B. A. (2023). Codex Alimentarius at home and abroad: the regulatory costs of developing and implementing international and national food-safety standards. In *Research Handbook on International Food Law* (pp. 347–367). Edward Elgar Publishing.

Formenti, L. R., Nørregaard, A., Bolic, A., Hernandez, D. Q., Hagemann, T., Heins, A. L., Larsson, H., Mears, L., Mauricio-Iglesias, M., & Krühne, U. (2014). Challenges in industrial fermentation technology research. *Biotechnology Journal*, *9*(6), 727–738.

Frestedt, J. L. (2018). Foods, food additives, and generally regarded as safe (GRAS) food assessments. *Food control and biosecurity*, 543-565.

García Martínez, J. B., Pearce, J. M., Throup, J., Cates, J., Lackner, M., & Denkenberger, D. C. (2022). Methane single cell protein: Potential to secure a global protein supply against catastrophic food shocks. *Frontiers in Bioengineering and Biotechnology, 10*, 906704.

Garg, V., Velumani, D., Lin, Y.-C., & Haye, A. (2024). A comprehensive review of probiotic claim regulations: Updates from the Asia-Pacific regions, the United States, and Europe. *PharmaNutrition*, •••, 100423.

Gargalo, C. L., Udugama, I., Pontius, K., Lopez, P. C., Nielsen, R. F., Hasanzadeh, A., Mansouri, S. S., Bayer, C., Junicke, H., & Gernaey, K. V. (2020). Towards smart biomanufacturing: A perspective on recent developments in industrial measurement and monitoring technologies for bio-based production processes. *Journal of Industrial Microbiology & Biotechnology: Official Journal of the Society for Industrial Microbiology and Biotechnology, 47*(11), 947–964.

Giri, N. A., Sakhale, B. K., & Nirmal, N. P. (2023). Functional beverages: an emerging trend in beverage world. *Recent Frontiers of Phytochemicals*, 123-142.

Goldrick, S., Duran-Villalobos, C. A., Jankauskas, K., Lovett, D., Farid, S. S., & Lennox, B. (2019). Modern day monitoring and control challenges outlined on an industrial-scale benchmark fermentation process. *Computers & Chemical Engineering, 130*, 106471.

Gomaa, A. (2018). Application of enzymes in brewing. *J. Nutr. Food Sci. Forecast, 1*(5).

Gonçalves, G. C. V., Weis, C. M. S. C., Wolff, É. R., Alves, V., Sanches, F. L., Tormen, L., Treichel, H., & Bertan, L. C. (2025). Vegan fermented drinks as an alternative to milk: Trend or challenge? *Food Science and Engineering*, 1-26.

Goodman, A.-L. (2019). A Natural Stand Off between the Food and Drug Administration and the Courts: The Rise in Food-Labeling Litigation & the Need for Regulatory Reform. *BCL Rev., 60*, 271.

Hassane, A. M., Obiedallah, M., Karimi, J., Khattab, S. M., Hussein, H. R., Abo-Dahab, Y., Eltoukhy, A., Abo-Dahab, N. F., & Abouelela, M. E. (2025). Unravelling fungal genome editing revolution: Pathological and biotechnological application aspects. *Archives of Microbiology, 207*(7), 150.

HD, A., & Vijayan P. U, H. (2025). Bio-green Evolution: The Journey of Microalgae Products from Lab to Market—An Overview of Microalgae-Based Processes and Products—Part I. *Microalgae Horizons: Fundamentals, Innovations, and Industrial Applications*, 185-275.

He, Y., Degraeve, P., & Oulahal, N. (2024). Bioprotective yeasts: Potential to limit postharvest spoilage and to extend shelf life or improve microbial safety of processed foods. *Heliyon, 10*(3).

Hidalgo-Fuentes, B., de Jesús-José, E., Cabrera-Hidalgo, A. J., Sandoval-Castilla, O., Espinosa-Solares, T., González-Reza, R. M., Zambrano-Zaragoza, M. L., Liceaga, A. M., & Aguilar-Toalá, J. E. (2024). Plant-based fermented beverages: Nutritional composition, sensory properties, and health benefits. *Foods, 13*(6), 844.

Hirasawa, T., & Maeda, T. (2022). Adaptive laboratory evolution of microorganisms: Methodology and application for bioproduction. *Microorganisms, 11*(1), 92.

Hirst, M. B., & Richter, C. L. (2016). Review of aroma formation through metabolic pathways of Saccharomyces cerevisiae in beverage fermentations. *American Journal of Enology and Viticulture*, *67*(4), 361–370.

Hoff, B., Plassmeier, J., Blankschien, M., Letzel, A. C., Kourtz, L., Schröder, H., Koch, W., & Zelder, O. (2021). Unlocking nature's biosynthetic power—Metabolic engineering for the fermentative production of chemicals. *Angewandte Chemie International Edition*, *60*(5), 2258–2278.

Howell, J. (2023). Regulatory considerations of encapsulation used in the food industry. In *Microencapsulation in the Food Industry* (pp. 419–425). Elsevier.

Hussain, Z., Mishra, J., & Vanacore, E. (2020). Waste to energy and circular economy: The case of anaerobic digestion. *Journal of Enterprise Information Management*, *33*(4), 817–838.

Janković, T., Straathof, A. J., & Kiss, A. A. (2024). Eco-efficient downstream processing of 1, 3-propanediol applicable to various fermentation processes. *Process Biochemistry*, *143*, 210–224.

Jannah, S. R., Rahayu, E. S., Yanti, R., Suroto, D. A., & Wikandari, R. (2022). Study of Viability, Storage Stability, and Shelf Life of Probiotic Instant Coffee Lactiplantibacillus plantarum Subsp. plantarum Dad-13 in Vacuum and Nonvacuum Packaging at Different Storage Temperatures. *International Journal of Food Sciences*, *2022*(1), 1663772.

Jayakrishnan, A., Wan Rosli, W. R., Tahir, A. R. M., Razak, F. S. A., Kee, P. E., Ng, H. S., Chew, Y.-L., Lee, S.-K., Ramasamy, M., & Tan, C. S. (2024). Evolving paradigms of recombinant protein production in pharmaceutical industry: A rigorous review. *Sci*, *6*(1), 9.

Jeyachandran, S., Vibhute, P., Kumar, D., & Ragavendran, C. (2024). Random mutagenesis as a tool for industrial strain improvement for enhanced production of antibiotics: A review. *Molecular Biology Reports*, *51*(1), 19.

Jiang, J., Ma, Y., Zhou, L., Han, W., Liang, Y., Dong, J., Ding, Y., Li, W., Lei, Q., & Li, J. (2025). Synergistic Genetic and Chemical Engineering of Probiotics for Enhanced Intestinal Microbiota Regulation and Ulcerative Colitis Treatment. *Advanced Materials*, •••, 2417050.

Johnson, T. J., Katuwal, S., Anderson, G. A., Gu, L., Zhou, R., & Gibbons, W. R. (2018). Photobioreactor cultivation strategies for microalgae and cyanobacteria. *Biotechnology Progress*, *34*(4), 811–827.

Kang, M., Choe, D., Kim, K., Cho, B.-K., & Cho, S. (2020). Synthetic biology approaches in the development of engineered therapeutic microbes. *International Journal of Molecular Sciences*, *21*(22), 8744.

Katakhade, R., Sahoo, S., Anerao, K., & Poshadri, A. (2023). Bacteriocin as a bio-preservative and its applications in food products. *Pharma Innov. J*, *12*, 2226–2231.

Kaur, I., & Sharma, A. D. (2021). Bioreactor: Design, functions and fermentation innovations. *Res. Rev. Biotechnol. Biosci*, *8*, 34–43.

Khan, S., Ullah, M. W., Siddique, R., Nabi, G., Manan, S., Yousaf, M., & Hou, H. (2016). Role of recombinant DNA technology to improve life. *International Journal of Genomics*, *2016*(1), 2405954.

Krunic, T., & Osmokrovic, A. (2025). Effect of pretreatment, lyophilization parameters and different cryoprotectants on the efficiency of probiotic freeze-drying immobilization. *Hemijska Industrija*.

Kumar, M. U., Jeyasundar, P. G. S. A., Das, M. A., Azeem, M., Mani, V. M., & Ayswaria, R. (2025). *Recombinant DNA Technology in the Improvement of Microbial Enzyme Production*. Microbial Enzymes.

Kumar, V., Kothari, R., Pathak, V. V., & Tyagi, S. (2018). Optimization of substrate concentration for sustainable biohydrogen production and kinetics from sugarcane molasses: Experimental and economical assessment. *Waste and Biomass Valorization*, *9*(2), 273–281.

Lim, E. J., & Abd Rahim, M. H. (2025). Fermentation for Enhanced Biosynthesis and Bioavailability of Micronutrients, Prebiotics, Bioactive Peptides and Functional Fatty Acids in Food Products. *International Journal of Advanced Research in Food Science and Agriculture Technology*, *4*(1), 9–27.

Lisci, S. (2023). Development of monitoring and control systems for biotechnological processes.

Lokko, Y., Heijde, M., Schebesta, K., Scholtès, P., Van Montagu, M., & Giacca, M. (2018). Biotechnology and the bioeconomy—Towards inclusive and sustainable industrial development. *New Biotechnology*, *40*, 5–10.

Lu, C., Liu, Y., Li, J., Liu, L., & Du, G. (2019). Engineering of biosynthesis pathway and NADPH supply for improved L-5-methyltetrahydrofolate production by Lactococcus lactis. *Journal of Microbiology and Biotechnology*, *31*(1), 154.

Luo, H., Liu, Z., Xie, F., Bilal, M., Liu, L., Yang, R., & Wang, Z. (2021). Microbial production of gamma-aminobutyric acid: Applications, state-of-the-art achievements, and future perspectives. *Critical Reviews in Biotechnology*, *41*(4), 491–512.

Macwan, A., Desai, D., Vandra, N., Mishra, K. K., & Jha, Y. (2025). Biotechnology for Global Sustainability: Innovations, Applications, and Challenges. *Int. Res. J. Adv. Eng. Manag*, 59-65.

Mahmoodi, M., & Nassireslami, E. (2022). Control algorithms and strategies of feeding for fed-batch fermentation of Escherichia coli: A review of 40 years of experience. *Preparative Biochemistry & Biotechnology*, *52*(7), 823–834.

Malakar, S., Paul, S. K., & Pou, K. J. (2020). Biotechnological interventions in beverage production. In *Biotechnological progress and beverage consumption* (pp. 1–37). Elsevier.

Malvido, M. C., González, E. A., Bazán Tantaleán, D. L., Bendaña Jácome, R. J., & Guerra, N. P. (2019). Batch and fed-batch production of probiotic biomass and nisin in nutrient-supplemented whey media. *Brazilian Journal of Microbiology : Publication of the Brazilian Society for Microbiology*, *50*(4), 915–925.

Mao, B., Gu, J., Li, D., Cui, S., Zhao, J., Zhang, H., & Chen, W. (2018). Effects of different doses of fructooligosaccharides (FOS) on the composition of mice fecal microbiota, especially the Bifidobacterium composition. *Nutrients*, *10*(8), 1105.

Mariyes, T. C., Ju, E.-J., & Lee, J.-H. (2024). Enhancing microbial resilience: The role of adaptive laboratory evolution in industrial biotechnology. *Journal of Life Science*, *34*(10), 730–743.

Martin, G. J., & Chan, S. (2024). Future production of yeast biomass for sustainable proteins: A critical review. *Sustainable Food Technology*.

Masoumi, S. J., Mehrabani, D., Saberifiroozi, M., Fattahi, M. R., Moradi, F., & Najafi, M. (2021). The effect of yogurt fortified with Lactobacillus acidophilus and Bifidobacterium sp. probiotic in patients with lactose intolerance. *Food Science & Nutrition*, *9*(3), 1704–1711.

Meena, K. K., Taneja, N. K., Ojha, A., & Meena, S. (2023). Application of spray-drying and freeze-drying for microencapsulation of lactic acid bacteria: A review. *Annals of Phytomedicine*, *12*(1), 706–716.

Minervini, F., Comitini, F., De Boni, A., Fiorino, G. M., Rodrigues, F., Tlais, A. Z. A., Carafa, I., & De Angelis, M. (2022). Sustainable and Health-Protecting Food Ingredients from Bioprocessed Food by-Products and Wastes. *Sustainability*, *14*(22), 15283.

Mirsalami, S. M., & Mirsalami, M. (2025). Advances in genetically engineered microorganisms: Transforming food production through precision fermentation and synthetic biology. *Future Foods : a Dedicated Journal for Sustainability in Food Science*, *11*, 100601.

Mitra, S., & Murthy, G. S. (2022). Bioreactor control systems in the biopharmaceutical industry: A critical perspective. *Systems Microbiology and Biomanufacturing*, *2*(1), 91–112.

Mohamed, H., Shah, A. M., & Song, Y. (2021). Conversion of agro-industrial wastes into value-added products. In *Conversion of renewable biomass into bioproducts* (pp. 197–217). ACS Publications.

Mujahid, M., Wakeel, M., Ali, A. M., Saeed, S., Nawaz, A. S., & Hafeez, K. (2024). Food fermentation: Traditional practices and modern applications in food industry. *International Journal of Food and Fermentation Technology*, *14*(1), 239–273.

Mukherjee, A., Gómez-Sala, B., O'Connor, E. M., Kenny, J. G., & Cotter, P. D. (2022). Global regulatory frameworks for fermented foods: A review. *Frontiers in Nutrition*, *9*, 902642.

Muncan, J., Tei, K., & Tsenkova, R. (2020). Real-time monitoring of yogurt fermentation process by aquaphotomics near-infrared spectroscopy. *Sensors (Basel)*, *21*(1), 177.

Nascimento, A. P. S., & Barros, A. N. (2025). Sustainable Innovations in Food Microbiology: Fermentation, Biocontrol, and Functional Foods. *Foods*, *14*(13), 2320.

Naseem, Z., Mir, S. A., Wani, S. M., Rouf, M. A., Bashir, I., & Zehra, A. (2023). Probiotic-fortified fruit juices: Health benefits, challenges, and future perspective. *Nutrition (Burbank, Los Angeles County, Calif.)*, *115*, 112154.

Naveen, A. K., & Sontakke, M. (2024). A review on regulatory aspects, challenges and public perception in acceptance of genetically modified foods. *Food Science and Biotechnology*, *33*(4), 791–804.

Ngongolo, K., & Mmbando, G. S. (2024). Harnessing biotechnology and breeding strategies for climate-resilient agriculture: Pathways to sustainable global food security. *Discover Sustainability*, *5*(1), 431.

Nguyen, D. M. N. (2018). Understanding the redox metabolism of pyrococcus furiosus for efficient metabolic engineering.

Nguyen, P. Q., Courchesne, N. M. D., Duraj-Thatte, A., Praveschotinunt, P., & Joshi, N. S. (2018). Engineered living materials: Prospects and challenges for using biological systems to direct the assembly of smart materials. *Advanced Materials*, *30*(19), 1704847.

Nikoloudaki, O., Aheto, F., Di Cagno, R., & Gobbetti, M. (2024). Synthetic microbial communities: A gateway to understanding resistance, resilience, and functionality in spontaneously fermented food microbiomes. *Food Research International*, *192*, 114780.

Niyigaba, T., Küçükgöz, K., Kołożyn-Krajewska, D., Krolikowski, T., & Trząskowska, M. (2025). Advances in fermentation technology: A focus on health and safety. *Applied Sciences (Basel, Switzerland)*, *15*(6), 3001.

Noori, R., Perwez, M., & Sardar, M. (2019). Cross-linked enzyme aggregates: current developments and applications. *Biocatalysis: Enzymatic basics and applications*, 83-112.

Ojeih, C. A., Ogidan, O., Oluwajobi, Y. F., & Adebayo, B. O. (2024). Biotechnology Regulatory Conundrum: Balancing Innovation and Oversight. *Journal of Sustainable Development Law and Policy (The)*, *15*(3), 120–144.

Okpala, C. O. R., & Korzeniowska, M. (2023). Understanding the relevance of quality management in agro-food product industry: From ethical considerations to assuring food hygiene quality safety standards and its associated processes. *Food Reviews International*, *39*(4), 1879–1952.

Overton, H. K., & Yang, F. (2023). Do information disputes work: The effect of perceived risk, news disputes and credibility on consumer attitudes and trust toward biotechnology companies. *Journal of Communication Management (London)*.

Palladino, F., Marcelino, P. R. F., Schlogl, A. E., José, Á. H. M., Rodrigues, R. C. L. B., Fabrino, D. L., Santos, I. J. B., & Rosa, C. A. (2024). Bioreactors: Applications and innovations for a sustainable and healthy future—a critical review. *Applied Sciences (Basel, Switzerland)*, *14*(20), 9346.

Panahi, H. K. S., Dehhaghi, M., Guillemin, G. J., Gupta, V. K., Lam, S. S., Aghbashlo, M., & Tabatabaei, M. (2022). Bioethanol production from food wastes rich in carbohydrates. *Current Opinion in Food Science*, *43*, 71–81.

Panda, S. K., & Shetty, P. H. (2018). *Innovations in technologies for fermented food and beverage industries*. Springer.

Parhi, P., Song, K. P., & Choo, W. S. (2022). Growth and survival of Bifidobacterium breve and Bifidobacterium longum in various sugar systems with fructooligosaccharide supplementation. *Journal of Food Science and Technology*, *59*(10), 3775–3786.

Patarroyo, J. L., Florez-Rojas, J. S., Pradilla, D., Valderrama-Rincón, J. D., Cruz, J. C., & Reyes, L. H. (2020). Formulation and characterization of gelatin-based hydrogels for the encapsulation of Kluyveromyces lactis—Applications in packed-bed reactors and probiotics delivery in humans. *Polymers*, *12*(6), 1287.

Pejcz, E. (2024). Biotechnological approach of technological advancements for sustainable probiotic bread production. *Sustainability*, *16*(8), 3275.

Philipps-Wiemann, P. (2018). Proteases—human food. In *Enzymes in human and animal nutrition* (pp. 267–277). Elsevier.

Phillips, J. A. (2020). "Novel" sensors for the monitoring of fermentation processes. In *Computer control of fermentation processes* (pp. 15-72). CRC Press.

Pinela, J., Añibarro-Ortega, M., & Barros, L. (2024). Food waste biotransformation into food ingredients: A brief overview of challenges and opportunities. *Foods*, *13*(21), 3389.

Plavec, T. V., & Berlec, A. (2019). Engineering of lactic acid bacteria for delivery of therapeutic proteins and peptides. *Applied Microbiology and Biotechnology*, *103*(5), 2053–2066.

Poshadri, A., HW, D., UM, K., & SD, K. (2022). Bacillus coagulans and its spore as potential probiotics in the production of novel shelf-stable foods. *Current Research in Nutrition and Food Science*, *10*(3).

Prajapati, N., Patel, J., Singh, S., Yadav, V. K., Joshi, C., Patani, A., Prajapati, D., Sahoo, D. K., & Patel, A. (2023). Postbiotic production: Harnessing the power of microbial metabolites for health applications. *Frontiers in Microbiology*, *14*, 1306192.

Praveen, M., & Brogi, S. (2025). Microbial fermentation in food and beverage industries: Innovations, challenges, and opportunities. *Foods*, *14*(1), 114.

Puligundla, P., & Mok, C. (2021). Recent advances in biotechnological valorization of brewers' spent grain. *Food Science and Biotechnology*, *30*(3), 341–353.

Puttarat, N., Ladda, B., Kasorn, A., Tanasupawat, S., & Taweechotipatr, M. (2021). Cholesterol-lowering activity and functional characterization of lactic acid bacteria isolated from traditional Thai foods for their potential used as probiotics. *Songklanakarin Journal of Science and Technology*, *43*(5).

Ramos, P. E., Cerqueira, M. A., Teixeira, J. A., & Vicente, A. A. (2018). Physiological protection of probiotic microcapsules by coatings. *Critical Reviews in Food Science and Nutrition*, *58*(11), 1864–1877.

Ravindran, R., Hassan, S. S., Williams, G. A., & Jaiswal, A. K. (2018). A review on bioconversion of agro-industrial wastes to industrially important enzymes. *Bioengineering (Basel, Switzerland)*, *5*(4), 93.

Ray, R. C., Paramithiotis, S., Thekkangil, A., Nethravathy, V., Rai, A. K., & Martin, J. G. P. (2024). Food fermentation and its relevance in the human history. In *Trending topics on fermented foods* (pp. 1–57). Springer.

Rollin, J. A., Tam, T. K., & Zhang, Y.-H. P. (2013). New biotechnology paradigm: Cell-free biosystems for biomanufacturing. *Green Chemistry*, *15*(7), 1708–1719.

Romyasamit, C., Saengsuwan, P., Boonserm, P., Thamjarongwong, B., & Singkhamanan, K. (2022). Optimization of cryoprotectants for freeze-dried potential probiotic Enterococcus faecalis and evaluation of its storage stability. *Drying Technology*, *40*(11), 2283–2292.

Rout, P., & Chakraborty, C. (2020). The commercial application of biosensors as an analytical device. *International Journal of Current Microbiology and Applied Sciences*, *9*(5), 864–880.

Sabaté, J.-M., & Iglicki, F. (2022). Effect of Bifidobacterium longum 35624 on disease severity and quality of life in patients with irritable bowel syndrome. *World Journal of Gastroenterology*, *28*(7), 732.

Sahu, L., & Panda, S. K. (2018). Innovative technologies and implications in fermented food and beverage industries: an overview. *Innovations in technologies for fermented food and beverage industries*, 1-23.

Santos, A. G., de Albuquerque, T. L., Ribeiro, B. D., & Coelho, M. A. Z. (2021). In situ product recovery techniques aiming to obtain biotechnological products: A glance to current knowledge. *Biotechnology and Applied Biochemistry*, *68*(5), 1044–1057.

Satari, L., Iglesias, A., & Porcar, M. (2023). The microbiome of things: Appliances, machines, and devices hosting artificial niche-adapted microbial communities. *Microorganisms*, *11*(6), 1507.

Selvarajan, G. (2021). Leveraging AI-enhanced analytics for industry-specific optimization: A strategic approach to transforming data-driven decision-making. *International Journal of Enhanced Research in Science Technology and Engineering*, *10*, 78–84.

Shankar, A., Saini, S., & Sharma, K. K. (2024). Fungal-integrated second-generation lignocellulosic biorefinery: Utilization of agricultural biomass for co-production of lignocellulolytic enzymes, mushroom, fungal polysaccharides, and bioethanol. *Biomass Conversion and Biorefinery*, *14*(1), 1117–1131.

Sharma, P., Gaur, V. K., Sirohi, R., Varjani, S., Kim, S. H., & Wong, J. W. (2021). Sustainable processing of food waste for production of bio-based products for circular bioeconomy. *Bioresource Technology*, *325*, 124684.

Sheikholeslami, Z., Mahfouzi, M., Karimi, M., & Ghiafehdavoodi, M. (2021). Modification of dough characteristics and baking quality based on whole wheat flour by enzymes and emulsifiers supplementation. *Lebensmittel-Wissenschaft + Technologie*, *139*, 110794.

Shetranjiwalla, S., & Ononiwu, A. (2025). Identifying barriers to scaled-up production and commercialization of chitin and chitosan using green technologies: A review and quantitative green chemistry assessment. *International Journal of Biological Macromolecules*, •••, 305.

Shetty, K., & Sarkar, D. (2020). *Functional Foods and Biotechnology: Biotransformation and analysis of functional foods and ingredients*. CRC Press.

Shokoohi, M., & Attar, T. (2024). Biomanufacturing for a sustainable future: Unleashing the potential of biotechnology in pharmaceutical raw material production. [IJHES]. *International Journal of New Findings in Health and Educational Sciences*, *2*(2), 142–153.

Shori, A. B., & Al Zahrani, A. J. (2021). Non-dairy plant-based milk products as alternatives to conventional dairy products for delivering probiotics. *Food Science and Technology (Campinas)*, *42*, e101321.

Siegrist, M., & Hartmann, C. (2020). Perceived naturalness, disgust, trust and food neophobia as predictors of cultured meat acceptance in ten countries. *Appetite*, *155*, 104814.

Silva, S. O., Mafra, A. K. C., Pelissari, F. M., Rodrigues de Lemos, L., & Molina, G. (2025). Biotechnology in Agro-Industry: Valorization of Agricultural Wastes, By-Products and Sustainable Practices. *Microorganisms*, *13*(8), 1789.

Singh, A., & Kumar, S. (2025). Exploring the Functionality of Microbes in Fermented Foods: Technological Advancements and Future Directions. *Fermentation (Basel, Switzerland)*, *11*(6), 300.

Singh, A., & Negi, P. S. (2025). Biotechnological application of health-promising bioactive compounds. In *Biotechnological Intervention in Production of Bioactive Compounds: Biosynthesis, Characterization and Applications* (pp. 73-94). Springer.

Singh, B. P. (2025). Harnessing probiotic fermentation for the generation of food-derived bioactive peptides: Current status and prospects. *European Food Research and Technology*, •••, 1–16.

Singh, N., Malik, S., Gupta, A., & Srivastava, K. R. (2021). Revolutionizing enzyme engineering through artificial intelligence and machine learning. *Emerging Topics in Life Sciences*, *5*(1), 113–125.

Singh, P., & Kumar, S. (2019). Microbial enzyme in food biotechnology. In *Enzymes in food biotechnology* (pp. 19–28). Elsevier.

Skrzypczak, K., Teterycz, D., Gustaw, W., Domagała, D., Mielczarek, P., & Kasprzyk-Pochopień, J. (2024). The possibility of using Lactobacillus plantarum 299v to reinforce the bioactive properties of legume-derived beverages. *Applied Sciences (Basel, Switzerland)*, *14*(12), 5187.

Soonsanga, S., Rungrod, A., Utamatho, M., Trakulnaleamsai, C., Paenpong, P., Pootakham, W., Phaonakrop, N., Roytrakul, S., & Promdonkoy, B. (2025). Integrated genomic and proteomic analysis of local Bacillus thuringiensis isolates for targeted insect pest control and functional insight. *Archives of Microbiology*, *207*(9), 1–12.

Stazi, A., & Jovine, R. (2022). Food traceability in Europe, the US and China: comparative law and regulatory technology. *BioLaw Journal*(2).

Stern, E. K., & Brenner, D. M. (2018). Gut microbiota-based therapies for irritable bowel syndrome. *Clinical and Translational Gastroenterology*, *9*(2), e134.

Suhail, M., Shao, Y.-F., Vu, Q. L., & Wu, P.-C. (2022). Designing of pH-sensitive hydrogels for colon targeted drug delivery; characterization and in vitro evaluation. *Gels (Basel, Switzerland)*, *8*(3), 155.

Sun, W., Shahrajabian, M. H., & Lin, M. (2022). Research progress of fermented functional foods and protein factory-microbial fermentation technology. *Fermentation (Basel, Switzerland)*, *8*(12), 688.

Taheri-Kafrani, A., Kharazmi, S., Nasrollahzadeh, M., Soozanipour, A., Ejeian, F., Etedali, P., Mansouri-Tehrani, H.-A., Razmjou, A., Yek, S. M.-G., & Varma, R. S. (2021). Recent developments in enzyme immobilization technology for high-throughput processing in food industries. *Critical Reviews in Food Science and Nutrition*, *61*(19), 3160–3196.

Tarafdar, A., Pandey, A., Sirohi, R., Soccol, C. R., & Dussap, C.-G. (2022). *Current Developments in Biotechnology and Bioengineering: Advances in Food Engineering*. Elsevier.

Terpou, A., Papadaki, A., Lappa, I. K., Kachrimanidou, V., Bosnea, L. A., & Kopsahelis, N. (2019). Probiotics in food systems: Significance and emerging strategies towards improved viability and delivery of enhanced beneficial value. *Nutrients*, *11*(7), 1591.

Toromade, A. S., Soyombo, D. A., Kupa, E., & Ijomah, T. I. (2024). Reviewing the impact of climate change on global food security: Challenges and solutions. *International journal of applied research in social sciences, 6*(7), 1403-1416.

Torrorey-Sawe, R. (2025). *Global Bioethics: Addressing Current Challenges*. Innovations, and the Needs of Underserved Populations.

Toy, J. Y. H., Lu, Y., Huang, D., Matsumura, K., & Liu, S.-Q. (2022). Enzymatic treatment, unfermented and fermented fruit-based products: Current state of knowledge. *Critical Reviews in Food Science and Nutrition*, *62*(7), 1890–1911.

Trump, B., Cummings, C., Klasa, K., Galaitsi, S., & Linkov, I. (2023). Governing biotechnology to provide safety and security and address ethical, legal, and social implications. *Frontiers in Genetics*, *13*, 1052371.

Udugama, I. A., Lopez, P. C., Gargalo, C. L., Li, X., Bayer, C., & Gernaey, K. V. (2021). Digital Twin in biomanufacturing: Challenges and opportunities towards its implementation. *Systems Microbiology and Biomanufacturing*, *1*(3), 257–274.

Umoga, U. J., Sodiya, E. O., Ugwuanyi, E. D., Jacks, B. S., Lottu, O. A., Daraojimba, O. D., & Obaigbena, A. (2024). Exploring the potential of AI-driven optimization in enhancing network performance and efficiency. *Magna Scientia Advanced Research and Reviews*, *10*(1), 368–378.

Vilkhovoy, M., Adhikari, A., Vadhin, S., & Varner, J. D. (2020). The evolution of cell free biomanufacturing. *Processes (Basel, Switzerland)*, *8*(6), 675.

Vinderola, G., Ouwehand, A., Salminen, S., & von Wright, A. (2019). *Lactic acid bacteria: microbiological and functional aspects*. Crc Press.

Vinicius De Melo Pereira, G., De Carvalho Neto, D. P., Junqueira, A. C. D. O., Karp, S. G., Letti, L. A., Magalhães Júnior, A. I., & Soccol, C. R. (2020). A review of selection criteria for starter culture development in the food fermentation industry. *Food Reviews International, 36*(2), 135–167.

Voeikova, T., Zhuravliova, O., & Debabov, V. (2020). Comparative analysis of legal regulation of industrial use of genetic-engineering-modified microorganisms in the united states, European Union, and Russian Federation. *Molecular Genetics, Microbiology and Virology, 35*(2), 69–77.

Voidarou, C., Antoniadou, M., Rozos, G., Tzora, A., Skoufos, I., Varzakas, T., Lagiou, A., & Bezirtzoglou, E. (2020). Fermentative foods: Microbiology, biochemistry, potential human health benefits and public health issues. *Foods, 10*(1), 69.

Wang, A., & Zhong, Q. (2024). Drying of probiotics to enhance the viability during preparation, storage, food application, and digestion: A review. *Comprehensive Reviews in Food Science and Food Safety, 23*(1), e13287.

Wang, C., Fu, L., Ametefe, D. S., Wang, S., & John, D. (2025). E-textiles in healthcare: A systematic literature review of wearable technologies for monitoring and enhancing human health. *Neural Computing & Applications, 37*(4), 2089–2111.

Wang, F., Bi, Y., Diao, J., Lv, M., Cui, J., Chen, L., & Zhang, W. (2019). Metabolic engineering to enhance biosynthesis of both docosahexaenoic acid and odd-chain fatty acids in Schizochytrium sp. S31. *Biotechnology for Biofuels, 12*(1), 141.

Wang, Z., Zeng, D., Zhu, Y., Zhou, M., Kondo, A., Hasunuma, T., & Zhao, X. (2025). Fermentation design and process optimization strategy based on machine learning ML-BASED FERMENTATION DESIGN AND OPTIMIZATION. *Biodesign Research*, •••, 100002.

Warda, M., Tekin, S., Khafaga, N., Sengul, E., Çelebi, F., & Laçin, B. B. (2025). *Comprehensive Insights Into Genetically Modified Foods: Technological Advances, Nutritional Benefits, Therapeutic Applications, and Health Implications*. Food Safety and Health.

Watanabe, S., Ito, M., & Kigawa, T. (2021). DiRect: Site-directed mutagenesis method for protein engineering by rational design. *Biochemical and Biophysical Research Communications, 551*, 107–113.

Wen, L., Yang, L., Chen, C., Li, J., Fu, J., Liu, G., Kan, Q., Ho, C.-T., Huang, Q., & Lan, Y. (2024). Applications of multi-omics techniques to unravel the fermentation process and the flavor formation mechanism in fermented foods. *Critical Reviews in Food Science and Nutrition, 64*(23), 8367–8383.

Wu, G., Fanzo, J., Miller, D. D., Pingali, P., Post, M., Steiner, J. L., & Thalacker-Mercer, A. E. (2014). Production and supply of high-quality food protein for human consumption: Sustainability, challenges, and innovations. *Annals of the New York Academy of Sciences, 1321*(1), 1–19.

Wu, Y., Jha, R., Li, A., Liu, H., Zhang, Z., Zhang, C., Zhai, Q., & Zhang, J. (2022). Probiotics (Lactobacillus plantarum HNU082) supplementation relieves ulcerative colitis by affecting intestinal barrier functions, immunity-related gene expression, gut microbiota, and metabolic pathways in mice. *Microbiology Spectrum, 10*(6), e01651–e01622.

Yang, H., Cai, G., Lu, J., & Gómez Plaza, E. (2021). The production and application of enzymes related to the quality of fruit wine. *Critical Reviews in Food Science and Nutrition, 61*(10), 1605–1615.

Yee, C. S., Zahia-Azizan, N. A., Abd Rahim, M. H., Mohd Zaini, N. A., Raja-Razali, R. B., Ushidee-Radzi, M. A., Ilham, Z., & Wan-Mohtar, W. A. A. Q. I. (2025). Smart Fermentation Technologies: Microbial Process Control in Traditional Fermented Foods. *Fermentation (Basel, Switzerland), 11*(6), 323.

Yoha, K., Nida, S., Dutta, S., Moses, J., & Anandharamakrishnan, C. (2022). Targeted delivery of probiotics: Perspectives on research and commercialization. *Probiotics and Antimicrobial Proteins, 14*(1), 15–48.

Zhang, Y., Zhu, X., Wang, N., Liu, X., Wang, L., & Ning, K. (2025). Synergy of traditional practices and modern technology: Advancing the understanding and applications of microbial resources and processes in fermented foods. *Trends in Food Science & Technology*, •••, 104891.

Zhou, X., Tang, J., Jacobs, T. L., & Saguy, I. S. (2025). Transforming Food Supply Chains Through Digital Tracking and Monitoring Technologies. *Trends in Food Science & Technology*, •••, 105142.

Zhu, M., Zheng, J., Xie, J., Zhao, D., Qiao, Z.-W., Huang, D., & Luo, H.-B. (2022). Effects of environmental factors on the microbial community changes during medium-high temperature Daqu manufacturing. *Food Research International, 153*, 110955.

Chapter 9
Biomanufacturing of Biofuels and Bioplastic: Innovations for a Sustainable Future

M. Divya
Sacred Heart College, Tirupattur, India

P. Prakathi
Sacred Heart College, Tirupattur, India

L. Yuvalakshmi
Sacred Heart College, Tirupattur, India

B. Lokeshwari
https://orcid.org/0009-0005-6612-5134
Sacred Heart College, Tirupattur, India

P. Saranraj
https://orcid.org/0000-0002-5052-6532
Sacred Heart College, Tirupattur, India

ABSTRACT

Bioplastics are derived from renewable resources, such as microorganisms, biowaste, or plants, rather than non-renewable resources like fossil fuels or petroleum. Algal bioplastics provide a renewable alternative to Petroleum-based polymers. Various microalgae strains grown in different environments can produce a wide range of biopolymers, including proteins, cellulose-based polymer compounds, starch-based polymers, polyhydroxybutyrate, polyurethane, and polylactic acid. Bioplastics are one of the most innovative environmentally sustainable materials developed today. Using bioplastics will put the country on the path of development and sustainability and will help to reduce waste biomass and solid waste greenhouse gases from the environment. Bioplastics are an important alternative because they are sustainable, environmentally sustainable, and highly adaptable. Biomass, or biofuels, will be used to refer to products that result as intended from biomass or the by-products (vegetable oil, synthetic biofuels, biogas, biodiesel, bioethanol, and biohydrogen).

DOI: 10.4018/979-8-3373-2873-7.ch009

INTRODUCTION

Plastics can be made from natural gas, coal, petrochemicals, or oil. Carbon-based polymers have transformed plastics for the population growth and technological advances that have resulted in enormous applications in plastic production over recent years (Peng *et al.,* 2021). They possess numerous superior-quality properties like strength, stability, clarity, lightness, flexibility, durability, affordability, and corrosion resistance. Due to biodegradation and hydrophobicity, fossil fuel-based polymers hurt the environment, leading to pollution, global warming, and a decrease in the availability of fossil fuels (Sudhakar *et al.,* 2024). Synthetic plastics emit toxic compounds into the atmosphere, contaminating ecosystems and water sources (Bhatia *et al.,* 2019). To address these issues, plastics are made from natural, renewable biomass sources. Bioplastics are polymers that are produced from naturally occurring polymers derived from microbes, plants, or animals. Microorganisms are a great source for the manufacturing of bioplastics because of their cultivation, high output, quick growth rate, ease of gene manipulation, etc. (Rahman & Bhoi, 2021).

Bioplastics provide a green alternative to traditional plastic derived from petroleum-based plastic since they are biodegradable and can be composted. Biobased and biodegradable categories are used to categorize bio-plastics. Proteins, starch, cellulose, and other renewable biomass resources are used to make bioplastics. Microbial polyesters examples include PLA, or Polylactic acid, and Poly Hydroxy Alkenoates (PHA) (Fig1). Under specific circumstances, microbes can break down polymers that degrade into organic molecules like carbon dioxide, water, and biomass. Natural source-based polymers and both polymers made from petroleum have the potential to biodegrade (Di Bartolo *et al.,* 2021). The decrease in petroleum consumption, renewable resources, and combating the increasing environmental issues related to conventional plastics are the reasons for bioplastics. Lower greenhouse gas emissions, biodegradation, reduced demand for fossil fuels, and waste reusability are some of the benefits of bioplastics. That plant-based bioplastics possess good mechanical and chemical properties; they are harmful to the future as they compete with human food. The alternative source of renewable plastic polymer is the major source of bioplastics (Rosenboom *et al.,* 2022).

Figure 1. Taxonomy of common bioplastics

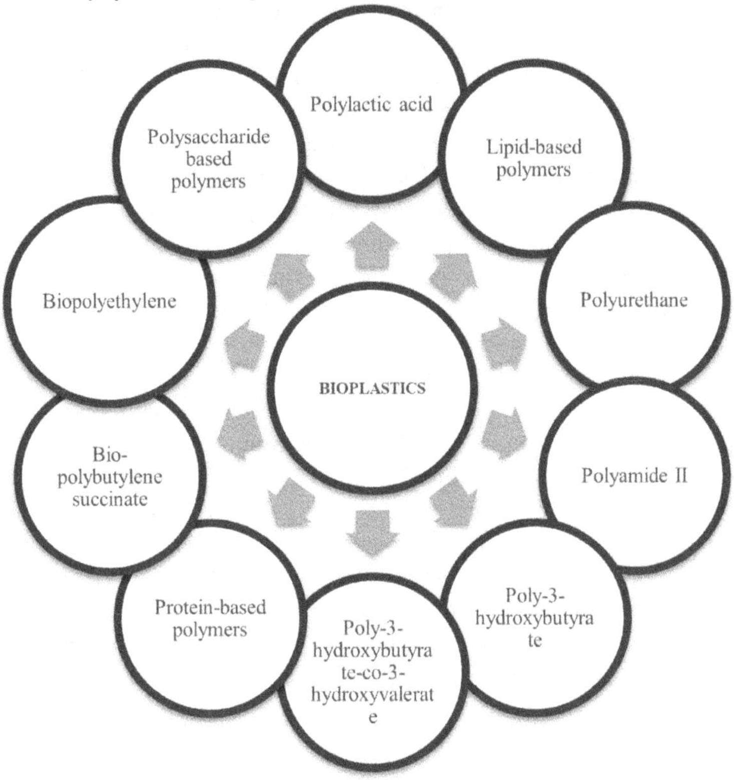

Biofuels, which are renewable energy sources derived from biological carbon fixation, are an essential part of new energy sources. Therefore, a great deal of technological research and development is needed to produce biofuel. However, because the biomasses used to produce biofuels absorb CO2 during their growth, the carbon released during combustion is a part of a closed carbon cycle, which can help reduce these emissions. Biofuels, which are derived from renewable biomass sources, are a good alternative to finite fossil fuels because they emit carbon dioxide that is either recycled by new plants during their photosynthesis process or is much lower than that which harms the environment. Conversely, biofuels are made from inexpensive and plentiful bioresources, including woody biomass, energy crops, agricultural residues, and organic fractions of municipal solid waste that are rich in carbon that can be replenished and renewed. Thermochemical conversion uses high temperatures, pressures, and catalysts to transform biomass into specific solid, liquid, and gaseous biofuels through processes like pyrolysis, liquefaction, and gasification. Pyrolysis is the process of heating biomass without oxygen to create biochar and bio-oil, which can then be converted into fuels for vehicles. These biomasses need to be properly converted into halophilic lipid-based biofuels, algae, Fischer-Tropsch (FT) fuel, biobutanol, bioethanol, bio methanol, bio-dimethyl ether, biomethane, and biohydrogen. Biodegradable polymer production capacity is monitored annually using device dynamics modelling and conventional procedures. The word "Biofuel" signifies a range of products produced out of biomasses or their residuals, including vegetable oils, synthetic biofuels, biogas, biodiesel, biofuel, bio-methanol, bio-ethers, and biohydrogen (Ghobashy *et al.,* 2021). The potential for green materials to be utilized in industries such as packaging, biomaterials, and construction is required to speed up their adoption and development. The transition to a circular economy by the environmental impact of plastic waste and greenhouse gas emissions, emphasizing recycling and reuse as key strategies to minimize waste and non-renewable resources (Adeniyi *et al.,* 2018).

Biofuels, particularly liquid biofuels, offer numerous significant benefits as renewable energy sources. They provide a readily storable, portable energy source that may be used whenever needed. In contrast to fossil fuels, they can significantly reduce carbon dioxide, micropollutant, and particulate emissions. They may support countries in balancing energy markets, improving energy security, and distinguishing their energy supply. The cycle of renewable energy sources like photovoltaic and wind-based folic systems could be utilized to create a new circular economy, involving manufacturing, waste biomass recovery, and energy crop cultivation, despite the challenges of the large amounts of electricity without powerlines or inefficient batteries (Dalton *et al.,* 2022). Liquid biofuels, due to their lightweight nature and energy density, are used to serve as a bridge fuel while switching from burning fossil fuels to alternative energy sources or evolve as an energy source. It is referred to as a "Food versus fuel" conflict when first-generation biofuel platforms use food commodities such as feedstock, corn, cane, starch, or vegetable oil because there is a significant pressure on food prices and availability. Although lignocellulosic-based biofuel, also referred to as second-generation biofuels, has a low amount of fermentable sugar and is expensive to pretreat for biomass, it may be a viable substitute (Dang *et al.,* 2022). Third-generation liquid biofuels are made from microalgae biomass, which can be refined using conventional techniques to create a range of renewable, green fuels, such as diesel, gasoline, and jet fuel. All of the biofuel and chemical production processes (second and third generations especially) have yet to be commercialized because most of their sales prices and relative lack of ultimately being profitable with petroproducts. Bioenergy is a sustainable and low-carbon energy source that can be easily integrated into current transportation and fuel storage systems. Biofuels currently account for 2% of all transportation fuels, and as science and technology advance, it is anticipated that this percentage will rise quickly.

TYPES AND PROPERTIES OF BIOPLASTICS

Microbes or plants are the sources of bioplastics. When bio-based plastics are released into the environment, they can decompose and break down organically over time. The first synthetic bioplastic manufactured from cellulose was parkesine, which was created in 1862. The damage to the environment caused by plastic waste, including greenhouse gas emissions, ecosystem damage, and marine contamination. This conundrum is increasing the need for novel, eco-friendly alternatives to conventional plastics. Because of their possible biodegradability and innocuousness, biodegradable polymers have emerged as a novel means of avoiding the harm brought on by the growing usage of plastics. But further research or commercialization is required, as biodegradable plastics now only account for a small percentage of the worldwide plastics industry. Bioplastics are used in similar applications because they are of good quality and are similar to ordinary plastics because of stability, strength, resilience to wear and tear, and light weight. It is advantageous to increase the use of bioplastics since it will reduce environmental issues and human dependency on fossil fuels (Chong et al., 2022). Bioplastics also have additional benefits, such as being clearer and more transparent, biodegradable, low emissions of greenhouse gases, energy efficient, byproduct reclamation, decreased carbon footprint, reduced litter, greater surface quality, greater vapor permeability, clarity or transparency, and decreased likelihood to change the product's flavor as it is being stored.

A wide range of materials, each with unique features and compositions, are included in the topic of bioplastics. A biobased polymer is called a bioplastic (derived from microorganism or renewable raw materials), biodegradable (decomposes spontaneously in the right environmental circumstances), or both. As a result, bioplastics fall into one of three groups. Plastics made of biodegradable polymers from fossil fuels decompose naturally in the environment. This group includes polyesters like polycaprolactone, polybutylene succinate, polybutylene adipate-co-terephthalate, and polyglycolic acid. These plastics are unstable and biodegradable due to their ester linkage. Polyvinyl chloride and polyethene are examples of bio-based and non-biodegradable polymers that fall under this category. Chemically, these plastics are comparable to those in category 1. Nonetheless, they have a smaller carbon footprint because they don't emit more carbon dioxide when they are burned. This group includes bio-derived plastics like polyethylene (PE) or polyethylene terephthalate (PET), as well as polymers like polyamides (PA) and polymers (PUR). Bio-based and biodegradable plastics are made from natural polymers such as proteins, polysaccharides, lipids from plants, or animal sources (Razzak *et al.,* 2017). Microorganisms, including polyhydroxybutyrate, are used to make plastics. This category includes compostable plastics like polylactic acid (PLA), polyhydroxyalkanoates (PHA), polypropylene succinate (PBS), and starch blends.

The mechanical characteristics of bioplastics include tensile strength, flexibility, and impact resistance. The polymer mix, manufacturing procedures, and additives are some of the factors influencing these characteristics. Among the most important elements of the de Customizing the properties of bioplastics to satisfy the requirements of certain applications is one of most important parts of their development. The kind of polymer and the intended application have an impact on boiling point of bio plastics and the glass temperature of transition. The development of bioplastics involves modifying their properties to satisfy the requirements of particular uses. The kind of polymer and the intended application have an impact on the melting point of bioplastics and the glass transition temperature. It is necessary to comprehend these features in order to design processing and applications. Some bioplastics might not withstand heat as well as traditional plastics. One of the main advantages of bioplastics is their biodegradability. Under the correct circumstances, they can decompose into innocuous molecules, lessening their influence on the environment. However, different bioplastic forms may have different rates and rates of biodegradability, necessitating particular disposal settings (Ramos *et al.,* 2019).

Simple monomers are produced when polymers with a high molecular weight depolymerize as a result of bacteria adhering to polymer surfaces and then secreting extracellular enzymes for hydrolysis attack. This process is referred to as bioproduction and biological degradation of bioplastics. Although anaerobic as well as aerobic environments are typically used for microbial biodegradation, the aerobic procedure is more effective with respect to of energy gain. Microbes employ oxygen during aerobic digestion to create water and carbon dioxide as byproducts. In anaerobic digestion, which occurs without oxygen (anaerobic and methanogenic microorganisms), polymers biodegrade to produce methane, carbon dioxide, water, and other metabolites.

SOURCES OF BIOPLASTICS

Bioplastics are environmentally friendly substitutes for conventional plastics because they can be produced from diverse renewable materials fossil-based and non-biodegradable, biodegradable as well as biobased, with non-biodegradable and biobased are the primary categories of bioplastics (Dang et al., 2022) (Figure 2). Bioplastics (such as PHAs) are produced and stored by a range of microbes, including bacteria, fungus, yeasts as well as microalgae, as an origin of energy and carbon. The amount of polymer produced depends on the type of microbe and substrate, the organisms' physiology, and the availability of appropriate physicochemical and nutritional conditions. *Citrobacter, Pseudomonas, Enterobacter, Klebsiella, Rhizobium, Azotobacter,* and *Alcaligenes* are among the bacteria that have been found to be viable for the production of bioplastics. These bacteria's ability to survive may be hampered by both the availability of nutrients and their inability to produce enough PHA. For instance, *Halomonas alkaliantarctica* generated the most PHA (0.42 g/L) when carbon was derived from dairy waste. Additionally, it was shown that *Bacillus megaterium* released 0.98 g PHA/carbon when cocoa fruit residue was present. Low-molecular-weight PHB is also produced by several bacteria and yeasts that use polyphosphate complex in their membrane transport, including *Ralstonia eutropha, Candida krusei, Rhodotorula glutinis, Kluyveromyces africans,* and *Saccharomyces cerevisiae.* Microalgae is a viable, reasonably priced, and environmentally friendly bio-factory to produce bioplastics. This can be accomplished by using algae biomass alone or in combination with other materials. *Ulva armoricana*, *Laminaria japonica*, *Chlorella* sp., *Spirulina* sp., and *Enteromorpha crinite* are among the microalgae that are reportedly suitable for the production of bioplastics. It has been demonstrated that 30–80% of PHB is produced by cyanobacteria such as *Muscorum* sp., *Synechococcus* sp., and *Synechocystis* sp. *Calothrix scytonemicola* also synthesizes PHA. Other well-known microalgae that produce bioplastics include *Phaeodactylum tricornutum*, *Scenedesmus almeriensis*, *Neochloris oleoabundans*, *Nannocloropsis gaditana*, and *Chlorogloea fritschii.* Nonetheless, among the most recognized and effective microalgae for the synthesis of biobased bioplastics are *Chlorella* sp.

Figure 2. Classification and characteristics of bioplastics

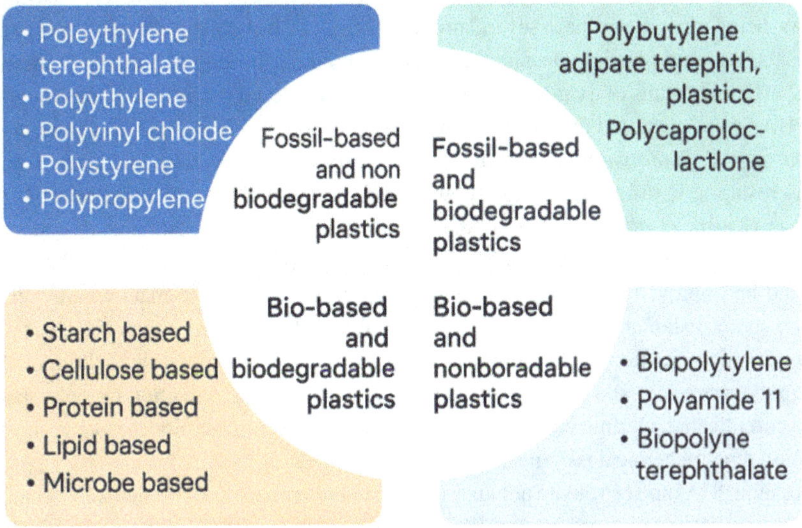

Polyhydroxyalkanoates (PHAs)

A heterogeneous population of PHA-producing microbes is a family of carbon-based biodegradable polyesters in conditions of nutrient scarcity (Pandey *et al.,* 2022). They have been internationally known as eco-friendly substitute for petroleum-based non-biodegradable polymers owing to their total biodegradability and comparable mechanical and thermal properties. PHAs with short chain lengths are often used in throwaway food packaging and goods due to their isolated carbon-based chains (Chong et al., 2022). Productivity potential of PHAs from Microalgae and Cyanobacteria. PHAs are widely applied across the majority of industries. They are viable for a variety of uses as they have physical characteristics with petrochemical polymers and are biodegradable. Their modifiable biodegradability and biocompatibility enabled them to control the medicinal applications of systems for medication delivery and tissue engineering. They are used in agriculture to fabricate biodegradable films, which cut plastic wastage and labor expenses. PHAs contribute a lot towards the advancement of sustainable agriculture (Razzak *et al.,* 2017).

PHAs are used in container manufacturing, disposable tableware, and packaging material. They have even been used to make biodegradable fishing nets to eliminate one of the major causes of plastic marine pollution. Production of PHA is still more costly compared to polypropylene, mainly because of the substrate cost. Microalgae that can synthesize and accumulate PHA is an affordable and environmentally friendly way of producing bioplastics in carbon- and energy-storing polyesters (Ramos *et al.,* 2019). Microalgae absorb CO2 from the environment when they grow to reduce the effects of global warming by producing bioplastics and carbon sequestration. These may be stored and banked by microalgal species such as *Synechococcus, Arthrospira platensis,*

Scenedesmus sp., *Dunaliella tertiolecta*, and *Chlorella vulgaris* cell interiors during times of low nitrogen and phosphorus availability.

PHAs, being monomeric, have several properties that allow them to be applied as elastomers, adhesives, and thermoplastics. Despite the great potential of oil-derived plastics as alternatives to PHAs, efficient means of extraction and reducing production costs have remained out of their reach. PHAs were extracted and purified from *Synechococcus elongatus, Oscillatoria salina, Chlorella* sp and *Leptolyngbya valerian.* Cell-disruptive biological, chemical, and physical processes resulting in instability, recovery, and purification must be used to recover PHAs from microalgae (Kartik *et al.,* 2021). Microalgal PHAs are recovered, destabilized, and purified using physical, chemical, and even biological processes (Hoang *et al.,* 2022). The yield of PHA could be improved by optimizing culture conditions and genetic manipulation so that it becomes a more sustainable source in comparison to petroleum-based polymers. Their process can make the identification of the optimal methods for the highest possible yield in extraction from biopolymers easier and the process between alternatives for extracting biopolymers from cells less complicated. Optimized PHA production or their potential as biodegradable substitutes for traditional petrochemical polymers (Vasile *et al.,* 2019).

Microalgal PHAs and petroleum polymer-derived polymers have both strengths and weaknesses in biodegradable alternative production. PHAs are used on disposable items and food packaging, and economic feasibility can be improved and a circular economy fostered using cost-effective and renewable feedstocks like microalgae. Microalgae also provide a green way of manufacturing bioplastics in that they are able to develop under different conditions and conventional cultivation for freshwater or cultivable land (Ali *et al.,* 2023). Genetic modification and better techniques like the hybrid integer non-linear model can increase PHA production, minimizing plastic waste and reliance on non-renewable resources with greater sustainability.

Polylactic Acid (PLA)

PLA is a polyester thermoplastic that is unsaturated that comes from renewable resources and is therapeutic and biodegradable (Chong *et al.,* 2022). PLA is an alternative to conventional plastics since it is biodegradable. They are produced using renewable resources like sugarcane, tapioca roots, chips, cornstarch, and algae, PLA requires two to three times more feedstock than other biopolymers. It can be generated using equipment initially used for petroleum-based plastics, lowering production costs. PLA is soluble in under three years and is commonly used in 3D printing and thermoforming in thin film form, making it an environmentally friendly material (Colwill *et al.,* 2012).

PLA is a permeable bioplastic, that degrades rapidly when exposed to UV light. To improve its mechanical properties and degradability, PLA is blended with hydrophilic and hydrophobic polymers. This strategy is sensitive and enhances its biodegradability. Microalgae are seen as an environmentally sustainable and safe source of lactic acid and PLA synthesis for the potential of these two bioplastic species (Wichard *et al.,* 2015). PLA becomes increasingly biodegradable when blended with microalgae biomass and the PLA-green algal mixture degrades completely through aerobic degradation in five to six weeks.

PLA and green algae blends lose tensile strength as algae concentration increases, affecting biodegradability. PLA is blended with biomass microalgae to improve biodegradability, making it weaker to environmental microbes (Yap *et al.,* 2023). Microalgae biomass in PLA synthesis reduces tensile strength and microplastic contamination risk. PLA degrades easily into harmless byproducts, reducing microplastics. Produced from crops like maize or sugarcane, microalgae can be cultivated in diverse sites, biodiversity and releasing resources for food production (Lakshmi *et al.,* 2020). Microalgae can be used as a renewable PLA feedstock, reducing agricultural and environmental pressures. Polymer mixes are required to address major problems like penetrating and UV deterioration, and efforts are underway to enhance PLA's properties.

Ulvan

Ulva species are a form of green microalgae with special qualities and the potential to be a source of bio plastics. They are frequently found in salty and marine habitats. Because Ulvan makes up 45% of their cell walls, these algae produce more polysaccharides than land crops. Ulvan is a polyanionic sulfate polysaccharide with hydrophobic or hydrophilic functional groups that can provide thermos-reversible coatings. It can be isolated from Ulva species through various synthetic processes, such as solvent casting, carboxymethylation, cross-linking, Soxhlet extraction, acid, enzymatic extraction, water extraction, and precipitation (Kanagesan *et al.,* 2022). Chitosan, poly vinyl chloride (PVC), polyvinyl alcohol (PVA), polyethylene (3,4-ethylenedioxythiophene) (PEDOT), and polyethylene oxide (PEO) are among the polymers that Ulvan can be used with. Ulva species also contain starch that can be employed as feedstock for *Lactobacillus plantarum* fermentation and PLA films. Ulvan has major properties that allow for its use in many applications, including bioplastics, cosmetics, and medicinal purposes. The extraction of Ulvan is dependent upon pH solubility and potential interactions between molecules.

Alginate

Alginate, a highly valuable bioresource due to its biocompatibility, non-toxicity, and biodegradable nature, is found in the cell walls of brown seaweed. In recent years, many bioplastics based on brown seaweed, including alginates, have been studied and suggested as alternatives for conventional plastics because of the potential benefits for our environment. Alginate bioplastics containing varying amounts of Inverted Sugars (IS) have demonstrated flexibility and complete breakdown within four days in soil disposing tests (Mohammed *et al.,* 2023). The extraction and pH of productions have a considerable effect on alginate properties that are versatile in drug delivery and tissue engineering applications. *Sargassum natans* is an invasive brown seaweed in the Caribbean that could make renewable alginate-composite bioplastics to replace plastic packaging. These alginate composite bioplastics possess high tensile modulus, strong water vapor barrier, and extremely high oxygen barrier properties for both oxygen-degradable perishables and low-humidity food packaging. The viability of alginates from different brown seaweed species to be utilized in making biodegradable sheets for packaging. The formulation contained sago starch and alginate. The most effective solution for the water barrier properties but had more mechanical characteristics of regular plastic bag attributes (Jayakody *et al.,* 2022), alginate composite bioplastics, more specifically from macroalgae, provides the alternative to plastic packaging.

Carrageenan

Red seaweed polysaccharides such as agar and carrageenan have developed into powerful and useful materials for biomedical, food, and cosmetics applications. There are three forms of carrageenan with different concentrations of sulfate ester groups. The development of bioplastics from cellulose and carrageenan as the major materials have allowable certification for food packaging possibilities, due to their strength, thermal stability, and breakdown (Wang *et al.,* 2022). Carrageenan is also hydrophobic and could be considered for use in resistant packaging. Carrageenan's yield can vary depending upon the seaweed, extraction methods, and amount of sulfate groups. Carrageenan coatings can inhibit ripening and firmness increasing the shelf life of fruit and those same coatings can preserve fish fillets as well and have preserved for up to 30 days once in storage. The solubility of carrageenan can differ based on the quantity and location of sulfate groups in ester and then 3,6-anhydrogalactose.

Carrageenan has potential as a material for producing bioplastic. This can be attributed to its mechanical strength, thermal conductivity, and biodegradability (Kakadellis & Harris, 2020). Research is being done on carrageenan as a sustainable substitute for traditional polymers in food product coating. Biopolymers also enhance the viability of carrageenan influencing bioplastic manufacturing and effective sustainable packaging. Additional factors of carrageenan and extraction technique can also affect the properties and functionalities of carrageenan-based bioplastics (Kim *et al.,* 2020).

LIFE CYCLE OF BIOPLASTICS

By evaluating the full life cycle, Life cycle assessment offers a comprehensive, quantitative, and qualitative understanding of bioplastics effects on the environment using metrics such as acidification potential, eutrophication, ecotoxicity, human toxicity, and global warming potential, among others. It is employed to evaluate a process or product's sustainability. Many analytical methods are used, such as gate-to-grave (use and end-of-life stage), cradle-to-gate (acquisition of resources and manufacturing processes), and cradle-to-grave (acquisition, manufacturing steps, usage, and end-of-life). Bioplastics reduce greenhouse gas emissions and do away with hazardous production techniques. It has been demonstrated that the production of bio-PE results in greenhouse gas emissions of roughly 0.75 kgCO2eq/kg PE meaning they are 140% lower than the emissions from PE made from fossil fuels. The amount of non-renewable energy used is reduced by almost 65% as a result. After evaluating the life cycle of a number of bioplastics according to the risks they pose to the environment and human health. These risks included feedstock genetic modification, energy and water efficiency, exposure to hazardous chemicals and solvents during manufacturing, and the emission of hazardous byproducts. In comparison to petrochemical polymers, the authors documented sustainable improvements for PLA and PHA biobased polymers. Harding et al., (2017) described a workable cradle-to-gate method for PHB biosynthesis. In comparison to the production of polypropylene, this method was found to be environmentally friendly and sustainable because it significantly reduced levels of toxicity, acidification, ozone layer depletion, and abiotic depletion.

Rueda et al. (2023) performed a life cycle assessment for PHB formation by *Synechocystis* species R2020 in order to assess the sustainability of the bioplastic synthesis. The detrimental environmental consequences of the production process were significantly decreased (67–75%) by raising the PHB concentrations in the microalgal biomass. The ecology was negatively impacted by the usage of chemicals and building materials (like using chloroform to purify PHB). Bioplastics end-of-life is regarded as a crucial component of life cycle assessment. It comprises using a variety of techniques to manage and get rid of bioplastics effectively. These consist of anaerobic digestion, composting, incineration, recycling, and landfilling. Mechanical recycling is thought to be the best option for managing bioplastics due to its low cost, low carbon footprint, and inability to emit harmful gases. Rosenboom et al. (2022) for example, found that the mechanical reuse of PLA produced less CO2 (0.62 kg) than landfilling, anaerobic digestion, composting, and incineration. The gathering of raw materials, biomass processing, fermentation, distribution, use, end-of-life adoption, bio-refining, material extraction, injection or blow molding and transportation are all included in the life cycle.

Figure 3. Bioplastics categories

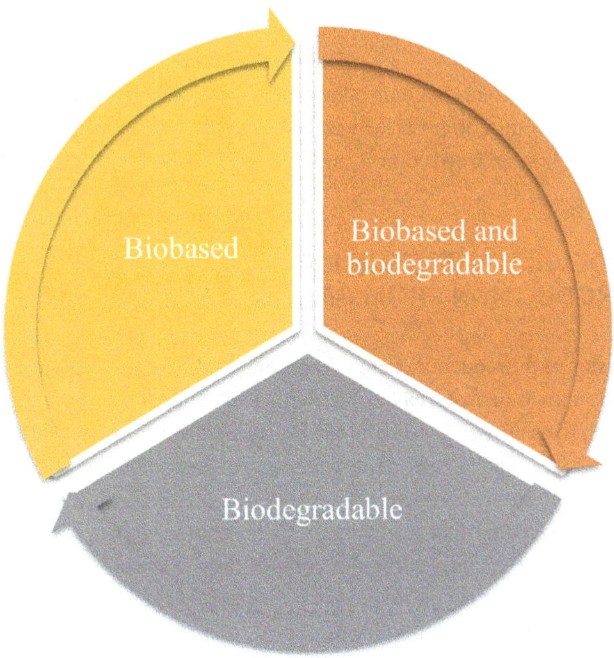

Sustainability

Sustainable growth and environmental concerns are increasingly recognized by multilateral organizations and governments. Economic growth often determines the ecological infrastructure, and environmental degradation can hinder economic growth. Sustainable development is defined as development and output can be influenced by environmental degradation and natural resource depletion (Hopewell *et al.,* 2009). The fastest-growing market category for bio-oriented commodities worldwide is bioplastics. A sustainable company generated through bio-plastic use and communicates with suppliers and customers.

Recycling

Plastics can be recycled through two methods: substituting the end product after processing, washing, and redistributing, and replenishing and re-melting thermoplastics (Hong *et al.,* 2021). Recycling is crucial for addressing environmental issues, but it requires more sorting than metals, glass, and separation based on type. Different plastics may appear like water and oil when coated and set in distinct phases. Due to material structure weakness, these combinations can only be used in limited recycling schemes. Recycling includes the accumulation of colorants and pollutants, and biodegradable polymers have superior properties and melting points compared to petroleum plastics, making recovered material non-recyclable (Papong *et al.,* 2014). Despite its simplicity, recycling plastics is challenging due to its complexity and potential environmental issues.

Compostable

Biodegradable solid products degrade completely to biomass and particulate within a predetermined time frame, forming compost (Jariyasakoolroj *et al.,* 2020). This natural fertilizer aids in miniaturization, recuperation, weed control, and soil erosion, promoting a healthier environment.

INNOVATIVE DEVELOPMENTS IN BIOPLASTIC AND BIOFUELS PRODUCTION FROM ORGANIC WASTE

These days, using and producing energy from renewable sources is crucial. Among the options, biofuels have shown themselves to be a viable substitute for fossil fuels. A tested method for gathering and storing biomass waste is necessary before a full-scale biofuel plant can be established to process organic waste. Strong legislative measures for enhancing the garbage collection and storage system should be implemented in order to overcome this obstacle. Furthermore, for waste-derived biofuels to maintain their position in the energy market over time, government subsidies and incentives for the construction of biofuel plants based on organic waste must be beneficial. Furthermore, industry-driven initiatives are essential for advancing the development of organic waste-based biofuels processes. For instance, a number of strategic alliances between major biofuel producers and aircraft manufacturers were established in the aviation industry to expedite commercial deployment. These programs primarily help achieve regulatory goals like lowering emissions, enhancing fuel security, and—above all—keeping the country from suffering from changes in the price of oil. Additionally, enhanced technologies lead to greater value addition in terms of process optimization and cost control. Biofuels can be produced from organic waste in three different ways: (i) thermochemical, (ii) physiochemical, and (iii) biochemical techniques (Figure 4). These technologies include (i) the hydrolysis and fermentation of agricultural residues to produce ethanol, (ii) the anaerobic fermentation process to produce biogas, and (iii) the transesterification process to produce biodiesel.

Figure 4. Biofuel conversion pathways from organic waste

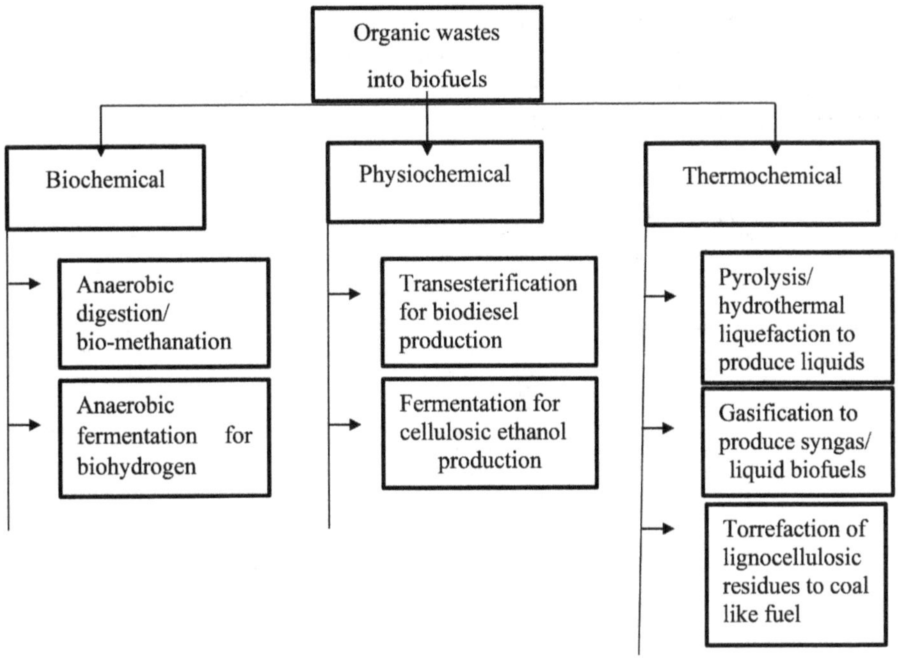

Technological advancements are essential for the effective production of biofuels in order to reduce the use of fossil fuels in global production and infrastructure applications and guarantee future energy security. Therefore, rapid advancements in sustainable biofuel production are essential to meeting the world's future energy needs. the persistent issues with waste management, such as the increased use of land and water for trash processing and handling. The appealing option of converting waste into energy is a viable solution to this problem. However, these technologies need to be continuously improved, and policies need to support their market adoption, in order to guarantee the viability of turning organic waste into biofuels. Examining technological advancements for turning organic waste into usable biofuels is the aim of this paper. Furthermore, it is evident that biodiesel is an excellent biofuel with a lot of potential for use in the transportation sector as a stand-alone fuel. The process intensification processes used to produce biodiesel from organic matter in order to achieve environmentally friendly and profitable development are covered in greater detail in this paper (Agarwal *et al.,* 2017).

Particular kinds of polymeric materials derived from bioresources are known as bioplastics, and they are thought to be competitively priced and environmentally friendly substitutes for traditional petrochemical plastics. One important development that can help expand the bioeconomy and reduce reliance on fossil fuels is the use of bio-based polymers. Commercial or industrial goods (apart from food or feed) that contain biological substances in one or more significant quantities are referred to as bio-based products. The activity of living things is the main source of renewable materials used to create bio-based bioplastics. As mentioned earlier, polyhydroxyalkanoate, or polylactic acid, poly-3-hydroxybutyrate, polyamide 11, polyhydroxyurethanes, cellulose-based, starch-based, protein-based, and lipid-based bio polymers are some of the promising biopolymers used in the bioplastic industries. Because of their biocompatibility and biodegradability, bioplastics are regarded as superior polymers to synthetic ones. As a result, they are ideal for high-value industrial applications such as packaging and biomedicine. Bioplastics usually take three to six months to completely biodegrade, whereas plastics based on petrochemicals take centuries (Azad *et al.,* 2015) (Table 1).

Table 1. Distinction between conventional plastics and bioplastics

Attribute	Conventional Polymers (Petro plastics)	Biopolymers (Bioplastics)
Feedstock & Origin	Predominantly derived from fossil fuel reserves and petrochemical feedstocks.	Sourced from renewable biological materials, such as plant biomass, algae, or microorganisms.
Environmental Impact	Persistent environmental pollutants; contribute significantly to ecosystem degradation and microplastic accumulation.	Designed to be environmentally benign, often featuring biodegradability or compost ability under specific conditions.
Primary Applications	Ubiquitous in packaging, consumer goods (e.g., bottles, grocery bags, footwear), construction, textiles, electronics insulation, and automotive components.	Employed in specialized applications including biodegradable food packaging, compostable service ware, biomedical devices (e.g., sutures, implants), bio-composites for automotive interiors, and edible films.
Carbon Footprint	Production and incineration generate substantial greenhouse gas emissions, directly contributing to atmospheric carbon dioxide levels.	Emissions are significantly lower; often considered carbon-neutral as the plants used for production sequester atmospheric CO_2 during growth.
Exemplary Materials	High-density polyethylene (HDPE), Low-density polyethylene (LDPE), Polyethylene terephthalate (PET), Polyvinyl chloride (PVC), Polystyrene (PS), Polypropylene (PP).	Polyhydroxyalkanoates (PHA), Polylactic acid (PLA), Polyhydroxybutyrate (PHB), Polyamide 11 (PA11), advanced polyhydroxy urethanes, and biopolymers derived from cellulose, starch, proteins, and lipids.

CLASSIFICATION OF BIOFUELS

Based on where their raw materials come from, biofuels are divided into four categories: First generation (1G), Second generation (2G), Third generation (3G), and Fourth generation (4G) are the three generations (Table 3). Fatty Acid Methyl Esters (FAME) in sugar are the source of (n = 1–4) bio-alcohol, starch, vegetable oils, lipids, and first-generation biofuel. The total amount of carbon dioxide in our atmosphere, which is necessary for the production of biofuel of the second generation, is mostly determined by the amount of lignocellulosic biomass or plant material. Blue-green algae (BGA) equipment and the third and the fourth generations make use of algae of biofuel production to convert lipid into biofuel. While the third generation uses algae directly to produce biofuel, the fourth generation uses metabolically modified algae from oxygenic photosynthetic microorganisms to create artificial carbon reservoirs (Lu et al., 2021). They are also referred to as biofuel that is created both chemically and biologically. Chemical synthesis is used to produce biofuel with the aid of a catalyst, and the influence of several variables, including pH, temperature, and pressure, has proven crucial. Moreover, chemical methods rather than eco-friendly ones are more effective than biological ones in terms of yield. The use of catalysts in chemical processes is preferred over alternative physical procedures because separation is inexpensive and the creation of more specific products. Because they are harder to separate, physical processes usually produce more complex product formations that cost more to process downstream. In biological methods, fungus, bacteria, algae, and halophilic archaea microbially process lignocellulosic biomass. A variety of biocatalysts, also known as enzymes, are used in the production of biofuels in addition to these biological processes (Nanda *et al.,* 2023).

Cellulases, xylanases, and lignolytic enzymes such as laccase, Lytic Polysaccharide Monooxygenase (LPMO), Manganese Peroxidase (MnP), Lignin Peroxidase (LiP), Cellobiose Dehydrogenase (CBDH), and multicopper oxidases are among these enzymes. Furthermore, the enzymatic use of the different biofuel generation techniques is the most environmentally friendly way to get around the numerous challenges of chemical processes. The synthesis of specific products at optimal pressure, temperature, and pH is one benefit of the enzymatic process. As a result, enzymes that are derived from extremophiles have the added advantage of being able to produce a wide range of products in temperatures ranging from 4 to 80 °C and pH values. They are suitable for use in industrial processes because they can also function at higher pressures. Understanding microbial pathways, enzymatic reduction, and their substrate usage strategy is the only way to make biological processes more cost-effective. All biological processes have higher production costs than chemical processes (Callegari and Capodaglio, 2018).

First-Generation Biofuels

At the moment, biogas, ethanol, and biodiesel are the main sources of first-generation biofuels. Biodiesel, which is produced by trans esterifying various vegetable oils and fats, is an alternative biofuel to diesel. However, if its properties are slightly changed, biodiesel might be a better option than diesel. But bioethanol, sometimes known as "flexi fuel," is a better option than gasoline. Additionally, by combining the starch or sugar, bioethanol can be produced from a number of sources. Ethyl butyl ether (ETBE) is made using bioethanol as a feedstock and readily blends with gasoline. Other biofuels, such as biogas and biomethane, are created by anaerobic digestion of household and municipal garbage. The increasing demand for edible oils makes it difficult to use food crops for biorefineries, even though it is easy to produce biodiesel, bioethanol, and biogas from them. The primary barriers to the development of first-generation biofuel are the use of crop pesticides and fertilizers, excessive groundwater consumption, and food as a feedstock (Demirbas, 2011).

Second-Generation Biofuels

Nonfood crops like waste from agriculture (rice straw, wheat straw, sugar cane bagasse, etc.) and biological material from municipal solid waste are used to make second-generation biofuels. The following are the main advantages of 2G bio fuels over the first generation. They do not pose a threat to food supplies their products produce fewer greenhouse gas emissions, and they require less land for raw materials. Nonetheless, the mixed feedstock concept included heterogeneous feed. Higher input costs for process development are also required when operating at a higher technological risk. Plant biomass is composed of 75% polysaccharide, which may be a source of carbon. Advanced biofuels are produced from lignocellulosic biomass through natural gasification or fermentation and hydrolysis. (bioethanol and biobutanol). Miscanthus, switchgrasses, rotating crops (poplar and eucalyptus), and agricultural waste residue are some of the raw materials used to make advanced biofuels. Fischer-Tropsch diesel is made from the glucose residues through the hydrolysis process, and biomass is turned into liquid to completely replace conventional diesel. Advanced bioethanol can be a good substitute for gasoline. In this process, lignocellulosic biomass is transformed into syngas through appropriate gasification. Furthermore, this syngas can be used as a source of liquid hydrocarbons (kerosene, diesel, or bio-SNG) or transformed into methane or dimethyl ether (DME). There are two primary methods for 2G biofuels (Fallde and Eklund, 2015). The initial step is the thermochemical synthesis pathway, that makes use of chemical reformation and thermal degradation at different oxygen concentrations to transform biomass. In the second, biochemical conversion uses biocatalysts or catalysts to convert with the help of bacteria. The main advantage of thermochemical conversion over biochemical conversion is that the entire organic component is converted into biofuel, whereas only the polysaccharide is converted into biofuel in the latter case.

Third-Generation Biofuels

3G biofuel is being developed in the early stages of research using algae. One kind of microalgae and seaweed macroalgae are cyanobacteria, also known as blue-green algae (BGA). The world is home to over 800000 different species of algae. They require very few nutrients to thrive, and they can grow rapidly enough to be collected in a month. Additionally, they can even be profitably produced in wastewater (Ellis *et al.,* 2012). On an area basis, the potential for oil production from algae is 100 times greater than that of canola and soy bean oils (Hu *et al.,* 2008). Algal growth is best suited for temperatures between 20 and 30 °C; below 16 °C, growth is slower, and temperatures over 35 °C are harmful. In microalgae, photosynthesis produces lipid, which can make up depending on the species, 20–80% of the dry weight. However, modifications to the nutritional requirements can change the yield of the lipid, protein, and carbohydrate products (Shen *et al.,* 2009). The leftover carbohydrates and starches are then processed further and may be used to create ethanol. Biodiesel is then made from lipid that has been extracted using various extraction methods. The various extraction techniques used in the lipid extraction process include both chemical and mechanical extractions (Table 2).

Table 2. Methods for lipid extraction from algae (advantages and disadvantages)

Method	Advantages	Disadvantages
Oil expeller	Easy to operate No solvent required	A large biomass size is necessary. Slow functioning. Increased power consumption and issues with scaling up.
Ultrasonication	Shorter extraction duration Minimal solvent needed Higher solvent cell content release	The cost of eliminating solid residue goes up with centrifugation and filtering. Low efficiency, volatile nature, and target chemical.
Microwave	Cost-effective and environmentally beneficial decreased time and solvent usage. A higher yield of extraction	Long extraction time. A large amount of the highly combustible and poisonous solvent is needed. Recovery of solvents requires a lot of energy. High infrastructure and operating costs
Solvent Extraction	Easy and affordable to implement Excellent efficiency, ideal for small-scale	

continued on following page

Table 2. Continued

Method	Advantages	Disadvantages
Supercritical CO2	Time savings, Low solvent toxicity, Improved selectivity and adaptability to temperature and pressure changes. In favor of mass transfer. Extract without a solvent	
Wet extraction	Using less energy to dry biomass Lower usage of solvents	Low-quality lipid extracted

Fourth-Generation Biofuel

Production of the fourth generation of biofuel is presently underway using the latest synthetic biological techniques. The finding has sparked optimism for this generation's photobiological and electrobiological biofuels. The synthetic biology of algae and cyanobacteria uses recombinant deoxyribonucleic acid (DNA) technologies to produce a range of novel, promising strains. This method incorporates new biological components or restructures the biological system to produce biofuel, and it uses new equipment to synthesize the new strain. Photosynthesis is an essential process for the large-scale manufacture of biofuel because it uses energy from the sun to split water molecule into oxygen and hydrogen through a combination of both the I and II photosystems. Additionally, artificial photolysis is the new method for producing biofuel (Gangue *et al.,* 2015). Even CO2 water is a different way to make biofuel using carbon-based solar fuel. Compared to previous generations of biofuels, the resources for fourth-generation energy sources are abundant, affordable, and easily accessible.

Table 3. Comparison of biofuel generations

Generation	Source	Current conditions	Problems
First	Food crop sources Starch and sugar Oil crops	Commercially available. Technically developed	Competition with food supply and land uses Benefit of greenhouse gases are dependent on the feedstock
Second	Lignocellulosic Biomass Agro-waste and energy crop	Advanced status of development and demonstration step	Higher cost, selection cheap, and sustainable raw material Additional cost of pre-treatment. Enzyme cost is higher
Third	Algae	Fast-growing, cultivation land not required, Various potential algae strains are available, "under research and development"	High cost of downstream processing
Fourth (Extension of third generation)	Algae and cyanobacteria	Primary stage of genetic engineering and new recombinant strains development, more promising than 3G	Under research.

MICROORGANISM FOR PRODUCING BIOFUELS

The production of biofuel is still challenging because it is more expensive to produce than the raw material. Microbial action, as opposed to enzyme action, transforms lignocellulosic material into biofuel during the microbial conversions stage of bioprocessing. Researchers are more interested in this method than in the first-generation biofuel production process because of the cost (Ho et al., 2013). According to the most recent bioprocess trend, the microbial route or its mixtures have the potential to produce ethanol with a high yield by primarily using the cellulose mechanism with the pre-treated biomass's other constituents (lignin and hemicellulose). A small amount of ethanol can be produced during the breakdown of pre-treated feedstocks by a variety of aerobic fungi. The electrons generated by the metabolic pathway are moved to the oxygenated chain for oxidative phosphorylation instead of phosphorylation at the substrate level, which is how ethanol is made. The general law of alcohol generation from sugar states that for every mole of hexose sugar, two moles of alcohol are produced. *Saccharomyces cerevisiae* and other yeasts use the process of glycolysis to make alcohol. All industrial processes are conducted at higher pH and temperature ranges to enhance the breakdown of wheat straw, and consortia of thermophiles such as *Halomonas* sp and potent fungal strains such as *Sarocladium strictum* are used appropriately (Jin *et al.,* 2018) (Table 4).

Table 4. Microorganisms and their biofuel yields

Microorganism	Biofuel	Biofuel yield (g/L)	References
Clostridium acetobutylicum	Butanol	3	(Khanna *et al.,* 2011)
Clostridium thermocellum	Isobutanol	5.4	(Lin *et al.,* 2015)
Escherichia coli	Butanol	30	(Shen *et al.,* 2011)
Escherichia coli	Ethanol	25	(Romero-García *et al.,* 2016)
Saccharomyces cerevisiae	Fatty acids	0.38	(Kai *et al.,* 2016)
Saccharomyces cerevisiae	Isoprenoid based biofuel	40	(Westfall *et al.,* 2012)
Pseudomonas putida	Butanol	0.05	(Nielsen *et al.,* 2009)
Cryptococcus sp	Lipids	7.8	(Deeba *et al.,* 2016)
Zymomonas mobilis	2,3 butandiol	10	(Yang *et al.,* 2016)

BIOFUEL TYPES

A vital component of new energy sources are biofuels, that are natural energy sources produced by biological carbon fixation. Therefore, the production of biofuel requires a significant amount of technological research and development (Rydz *et al.,* 2015). Fischer-Tropsch (FT) Fuel,

Algae, Biobutanol, Bioethanol, Biomethanol, Bio-Dimethyl Ether, Biomethane, Biohydrogen, and halophilic lipid-based biofuels must all be appropriately produced from these biomasses.

Gaseous Biofuels

Biological products and residues can be transformed into fuel gases for energy in two ways: mainly; Producer gas can be produced by partially burning dry goods, and biogas can be produced by anaerobic fermentation of wet or semi-wet materials (Budzianowski & Postawa, 2017). Fuel has long been made from these gases. In the most developed countries, running the increasing number of municipal waste treatment plants can be significantly reduced by using biogas from anaerobic fermenters to power stationary engines that produce electricity. Biogas can be used to generate steam in a boiler, power an engine that may or may not be connected to an electric generator, or provide hot water. The main problem with this energy is that only a small percentage of the gas can be stored because gas storage is so costly. As a result, flare out of excess gas is often required. Internal combustion engines may easily employ gaseous fuels. One advantage is that because biofuels mix well with air, they burn more completely than liquid fuels. They also produce less lubricating oil sludge, less contaminating contaminants, no cylinder wall lubrication washdown during engine starting, and less valve burning (Callegari & Capodaglio, 2018).

The digester's and gasifier's working conditions determine the chemical composition of bio gas and generating gas, respectively. The most important component of biogas is methane, which has a heating value of 35-9 MJ/m^3 from an energy perspective. Methane is difficult to liquefy because of its critical liquefaction temperature of 82°C. Others have used liquefied biogas to power tractors in both cases Therefore, using biogas in cars is not cost-effective; its practical use is better suited for stationary motors.

Biogas and Biomethane

A variety of lipid sources, including grease, algae, microorganisms, animal fats, and vegetable oils, are used to make biodiesel, a fatty acid methyl ester. Oil extraction, esterification, transesterification, and purification are the steps in the multi-step process used to create biodiesel. It has become a feasible drop-in biofuel alternative with significant potential to lower greenhouse gas emissions linked to diesel fuel made from fossil fuels. Additionally, biodiesel can be used in diesel engines that are already in use without requiring significant changes (Demirbas, 2011). Before biodiesel can be produced, oil must be extracted from the feedstock source using a number of techniques like mechanical pressing, extraction of solvent, supercritical fluid extraction, ultrasonic extraction, and microwave extraction. When methanol and other acid catalysts are present, these oils are used as feedstock for transesterification, a process that yields biodiesel. Vegetable oils, including sunflower, canola, soybean, corn, grapeseed, cottonseed, palm, and corn oil, are the most frequently utilized raw materials. The second step in the creation of biodiesel, known as transesterification, involves the reaction of an alcohol—typically methanol or ethanol—with oil in the presence of a catalyst. The primary ingredient in biodiesel, fatty acid methyl esters, are created when alcohol and oil combine. The final step in the production process is to remove impurities from the biodiesel. Usually, this procedure involves either water washing or dry washing the biodiesel (Gouda *et al.,* 2024). Unlike hydrolases, which hydrolyze ester bonds, lipases act as catalysts for transesterification. They make it easier for alcohol and lipids to react, producing glycerol and biodiesel. Although they are not as frequently utilized as lipases, other enzymes like cellulases and proteases can also be utilized in the biodiesel production process. Feedstocks containing contaminants such as proteins or cellulosic debris that could obstruct the transesterification process can be cleaned up using these enzymes. Many studies have been conducted on lipases derived from microbiological sources, including bacteria, fungi, and yeast. For instance, lipases from *Pseudomonas cepacia*, *Rhizopus oryzae*, and *Candida antarctica* have demonstrated encouraging stability and activity in the synthesis of biodiesel.

Biogas is a by-product of anaerobic digestion and is a combustible gas produced by microorganisms decomposing organic substrates (Agarwal *et al.*, 2017). It occupies only 0.3% of the renewable fuel market space and has various end-use applications in homes, including cooking, lighting, and space heating. Biogas is primarily used for power generation and is rarely used as car fuel. EU countries, particularly Sweden and Switzerland, are the main producers of biomethane as a transportation fuel. Most digesters use post-treatment bio methanation units for transportation through natural gas pipelines or vehicles. The UK is the largest producer, with 84% of the country's overall biogas production coming from landfills. As landfills decrease, energy production on excess agricultural land will provide a significant portion of these resources (Azad *et al.*, 2015).

One well-known and conventional method is anaerobic digestion for bio converting organic waste & sludge into biogas or biomethane. By decomposing solid residues from fermentation operations and sewage treatment plants, this technique has the ability to both produce biomethane as and utilize the wastes at the same time. Hydrolysis, acidogenesis, acetogenesis, and methanogenesis are the four main processes that make up anaerobic digestion (Pauly & Keegstra, 2008). With a higher calorific value of about 36 MJ/m3, biomethane can take the place of natural gas in both stationary and mobile applications. Because the substrates work together to keep the pH and nitrogen and carbon ratio, which are critical for the synthesis of biomethane, co-digestion of different organic wastes presents a variety of industrial research possibilities in addition to anaerobic digestion. Anaerobic digestion, which occurs without oxygen, uses common methanogenic microbes from the genera *Methanobrevibacter, Methanococcus, Methanogenium, Methanopyrus, Methanosaeta, Methanosarcina, and Methanosphaera.* Anaerobic digestion, particularly the oxidation of volatile fatty acids, depends on syntrophic metabolism, which is mediated by interspecies electron transport. Through interspecies electron transfer, methanogenic and non-methanogenic bacteria exchange the redox mediator that is created when volatile fatty acids undergo biological oxidation. By lowering the partial pressure of hydrogen to less than 10–4 atm, this interspecies hydrogen transfer can promote the emergence of acetogenic processes (Naik *et al.*, 2010). Temperature, the ratio of inoculum to feedstock, and the duration of incubation are some additional experimental variables that have a significant impact on anaerobic digestion and co-digestion.

Syngas

Syngas, also known as synthesis gas, is a mixture of carbon dioxide, carbon monoxide, and hydrogen that is utilized in biomass conversion procedures. It has the ability to transport light molecular weight hydrocarbons as well as remnants of other molecules including CH4, N2, ashes, and tears. Syngas is often kept at the lowest value due to their value being less than other process by-products like biochar and biodiesel (Balat, 2008). Only five percent of the fuel used in the industrial manufacturing of syngas is acceptable for use in the production of important chemicals or fuels due to the intricacy of the process and the need for expensive cleanups. Most fuel used for this purpose consists of Natural gas (22%), Coal (51%), Petroleum wastes (25%), and Petcoke (1%) (El-Malek *et al.,* 2020).

Liquid Biofuel

The two primary types of biofuels utilized in transportation systems worldwide. Biobutanol acts as a substitute for bioethanol due to its superior characteristics (Budzianowski & Postawa, 2017). The manufacturing of biofuels in the EU is influenced by the mixing permitted by each nation, as they are often mixed with fossil fuels.

Biodiesel

Fatty acid methyl ester (FAMEs) from both edible and non-edible oils are combined to create biodiesel that has physical and chemical traits with conventional diesel. Because it emits less carbon dioxide and particles, it is environmentally benign. Edible oils are a food security concern, as non-edible oils require additional processing (Callegari & Capodaglio, 2018). Wasted oils can be used to address disposable oil issues and produce biofuel. Algal biomass offers high production and photosynthesis efficiency, but the main challenge is oil extraction. Proper disposal of oil waste can be cost-effective and environmentally beneficial (Kai et al., 2019).

Bioethanol

The alcoholic fermentation with carbohydrates yields ethanol, a type of biofuel. It is primarily used as an initial-generation fuel in subtropical and tropical regions, with sugarcane being the primary feedstock (Cecconet *et al.,* 2018). It can also be made with lignocellulosic feedstock as a second-generation fuel. Ethanol is also used as a universal ingredient in blended gasoline in various concentrations, such as E15, E85, and BFC. Bioethanol is less polluting than fossil fuels, even though it has a lower energy equivalency. It is renewable, less harmful, and has less harmful byproducts than most alcohol-based fuels. Its partial carbon cycle is due to plants absorbing most of the CO_2 produced from manufacturing and burning, allowing for a partially closed carbon cycle. The use of bioethanol as a replacement for traditional fuels is warranted due to its renewable nature, lower harmful byproducts, and partial carbon cycle (De Melo *et al.,* 2014).

Vehicle emissions can be reduced by using bioethanol, a liquid biofuel with a much greater oxygen concentration of 35%. Bioethanol is commonly blended with gasoline in a variety of ratios for use as a drop-in biofuel in modern motor engines. The efficiency and performance of automobile engines may be enhanced by using bioethanol instead of conventional fuels because of how little carbon it emits. Because bioethanol has a lower volumetric energy density than regular gasoline, cars need a larger volume of it than they do of conventional fuels. Bioethanol can be added as a mixing ingredient to regular liquid gasoline. Through pretreatment, enzymatic hydrolysis, and fermentation, bioethanol is made from a variety of lignocellulosic and sugar-based feedstocks, such as food processing wastes, different energy crops, and crop residues (such as straw, bran, and stalk). Through the simple glycolytic process, a model microbe known as bioethanol can be produced by fermenting starch and hexose carbohydrates, such as glucose, using Baker's yeast (*Saccharomyces cerevisiae*). Food-versus-fuel resulted from these food crops being diverted from consumption to fuel products. First-generation biomasses, such corn, potatoes, and cassava, are suitable feedstocks for fermenting in biorefineries in that generate bioethanol because they are high in starch and/or glucose. However, lignocellulosic or second-generation biomass, like wood and agricultural waste, has emerged as a promising substitute feedstock for the production of bioethanol and other biofuels (Bowyer *et al.,* 2018). However, because lignin prevents enzymes and microorganisms from quickly metabolizing holocellulose (cellulose and hemicellulose) sugars, lignocellulosic biomass presents a number of upstream fermentation problems. While lignin and holocellulose may be separated by pretreatment of biomass, some degradation products, including furfurals, phenols, and carboxylic acids, may also be produced. These substances lower the hydrolysate's pH and stop fermentation bacteria from growing and functioning. Additionally, *S. cerevisiae* lacks a native metabolic pathway for fermenting pentose sugars, which are hemicellulose monomers, that influences how lignocellulosic biomass ferments to produce bioethanol. However, the fermentation of lignin-based products to bioethanol has advanced significantly as a result of continuing investigations in biomass pretreatment techniques, bioprocess technology, and microbial genetic engineering. Using thermophilic bacteria to produce bioethanol is one such method. Microbes that can survive in harsh radiation, osmosis, temperature, pressure, and salt conditions are known as extremophilic bacteria (Shen *et al.,* 2009). With unique enzymes that provide a robust physiological and thermal environment, thermophilic microorganisms offer a range numerous benefits for bioprocessing, including improved reaction kinetics, increased product yields, stability against pollutants and inhibitors, and quicker organic matter breakdown.

The widely used glycolytic fermentation process, which produces ethanol from glucose as a simple sugar. *S. cerevisiae* uses the Embden–Meyerhoff–Parnas glycolytic system, whereas *Zymomonas mobilis* uses the Entner–Doudoroff pathway for glucose metabolism (De Melo *et al.,* 2014). Pseudomonas species commonly use the Entner–Doudoroff path, which is basically an aerobic technique for glucose metabolism. According to theory, for every mole of glucose that is converted to ethanol, the Entner–Doudoroff pathway produces two molecules of Adenosine triphosphate (ATP).

Biobutanol

1-butanol, 2-butanol, iso-butanol, and tert-butanol are the four active butanol isomers. The physicochemical properties of biobutanol show that it is a superior fuel additive, with a higher calorific value of 29 MJ/L than bioethanol (19.6 MJ/L) (Kusuktham & Srinophakun, 2014). Compared to bioethanol, biobutanol is much less volatile, more miscible in gasoline, and much less problematic for engine ignition. Biobutanol's remarkable physicochemical characteristics allow it to be used as a drop-in bio fuel that does not require changes to car engines or as an addition in a variety of fossil fuels, such as gasoline and diesel. Butanol is frequently utilized as a laboratory solution in the chemical, polymers, textile, paint, and cosmetics industries in addition to being used as fuel. A variety of anaerobic bacterial species known as Clostridium are used in acetone–butanol–ethanol (ABE) fermentation, one of the earliest fermentation processes, to physiologically produce biobutanol.

Butanol is a potential green fuel with numerous benefits, particularly for internal combustion engines. Its higher oxygen content makes it easily blendable with gasoline and potentially soluble with diesel, reducing emissions. Biobutanol also has greater evaporation heat that can reduce NOx production during combustion (Fallde & Eklund, 2015). It can be made using fossil fuels or biofuels. However, its main limitation is its low production. N-butanol-powered engine should have lower specific consumption than an ethanol-powered engine due to its higher heating value and energy density. It is less prone to evaporation and has a greater flash point, making it safer to transport or expose to higher temperatures. It is non-corrosive, has greater viscosity and lubricity, and may protect engine components from biobutanol production. Micro-algae is a third-generation energy source with greater potential due to its fast growth rates and carbohydrate content production (Ellis *et al.,* 2012).

APPLICATIONS OF BIOPLASTICS

Agricultural Applications

Bioplastics are utilized in agriculture as mulch films, grow bags, tunnels, pots, seedling trays, pesticide containers, and farm nets due to their biodegradability, durability, protective properties, water resistance, compostability, and other attributes (Santos *et al.,* 2020). Bioplastic makes up 40% of the mulch used in agriculture. Its composition—starch, cellulose, PHA, and PLA—allows soil bacteria to readily break it down, boosting soil fertility and crop productivity. In addition to shielding plants from growth of weeds, insects, and birds, bioplastic mulch preserves the amount of moisture and conformation of the soil. Bioplastics are also used in the manufacturing process of agricultural goods due to their robustness and suppleness. Additionally, bioplastics make other soil polymers that are better suited for seedling bags or pots by speeding up their decomposition. Agricultural nets are commonly made from PHB or bioplastics combined with PLA because of their high tensile strength (Wang et al., 2020).

Industrial Applications

Bioplastics are useful materials used in many different areas for construction, architecture, packaging, electrical and electronics, and others. Bioplastics are used as conductors in electrical and electronics to produce electrochromic devices, diodes, batteries, and fuel cells (Jin *et al.,* 2018). Bioplastics are also used as membranes in sound-transmitting and sound-amplifying equipment, as well as cases for devices like speakers, computer peripherals, and mobile phones. Bioplastics suitable for sensors, solar cells, and newer forms of electronics commonly get reinforcement from carbon nanotubes and cellulose nanofibers. PLA with graphene reinforcement offers wide thermal conductivity, is biodegradable, and shows low deformity. Moreover, bioplastics often find utility in dairy, beverage containers, and packaging products. Low permeability makes them challenging in packaging, and bioplastics are frequently reinforced with other materials, such as films made from thermoplastic starch, cellulose films, clay, and PBAT (Khanna et al., 2017). Reinforced bioplastics are also used in applications across the building industry including doors, window frames, fabrics for buildings, material for earth constructions, and insulation for temporary buildings.

Figure 5. Different applications of bioplastics

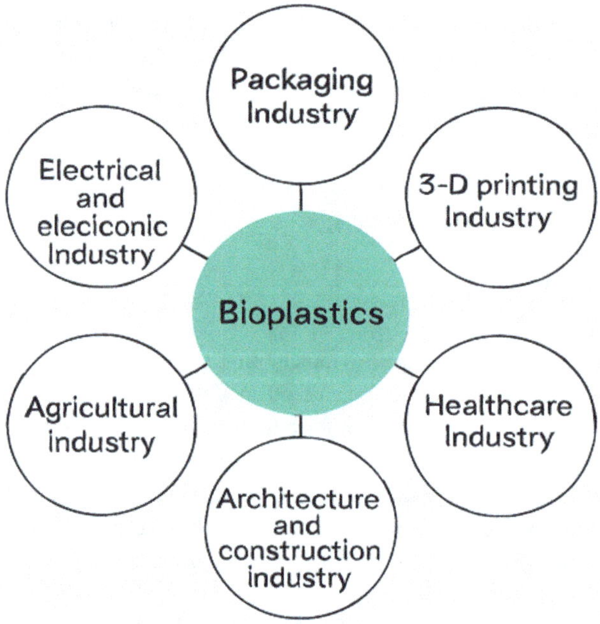

Medical Applications

Because of their non-toxicity, biocompatibility, porosity, and biodegradability, bioplastics are beneficial in a variety of biomedical applications. They are used in drug delivery systems, medical equipment, bone tissue engineering, heart valve replacement, cancer diagnosis, and wound-healing dressings (Garbeva *et al.,* 2018). When combined with PHB, PHBHHx, and hydroxyapatite increase cell proliferation and bone tissue formation. High-antioxidant lignin-reinforced bioplastics protect against oxidative stress and skin radiation, enhancing cartilage tissue growth. Paclitaxel is an anticancer drug, that has been delivered to mice using polyhydroxy octanoate and polyethylene glycol copolymer nanoparticles, reducing colon cancer (Rydz *et al.,* 2015). Biodegradable polymers are used in in vivo implant scaffolds and *in vitro* cell cultures. PLA-PU composites treated with lecithin facilitate sustained hepatocyte growth. PHB film patches enhance blood vessel formation and promote bone production in mice with cranial abnormalities. Bioplastics have drawbacks in biomedicine that accelerate deterioration and lower molecular mass (Rayung *et al.,* 2020). The device design, manufacturing, performance, and polymer chemistry also influence the selection of appropriate polymers for medical applications.

SUSTAINABLE FUTURE OF BIOPLASTIC AND BIOFUEL

In order to reduce environmental pollution, slow down climate change, and promote a resource-efficient, circular economy, bioplastics and biofuels must have a sustainable future. Both of these technologies seek to substitute carbon-emission-free, renewable, and biodegradable energy and materials for those derived from fossil fuels. Bioplastics may lessen dependency on petroleum-based plastics because they are made from natural feedstocks like cellulose, sugarcane, maize starch, or micro algae and have a long environmental half-life. Making them biodegradable under specific conditions can help address one of the most pressing environmental problems: plastic pollution in soils, streams, and oceans. However, biofuels made from biomass sources such as forestry waste, algae, agricultural waste, and even food waste provide a cleaner burning alternative to fossil fuels in industry, transportation, and aviation (Shalaby, 2013). These fuels can contribute to the shift to net-zero energy systems by drastically reducing greenhouse gas emissions. These fuels include advanced drop-in biofuels, bioethanol, and biodiesel. In addition to technological advancement, systemic changes in waste management, production, and consumption are necessary for the integration of bioplastics and biofuels into global economies. Utilizing biomass sources other than food, advanced biotechnological processes such as microbial fermentation, enzymatic conversion, and genetically modified algae allow for increased yields, lower processing costs, and avoidance of conflicts with food production. For instance, a biorefinery model is made possible by the capacity to convert lignocellulosic feedstocks, such as agricultural waste or forestry by-products, into precursors for both biofuels and bioplastics. This enables the production of numerous sustainable products from a single biomass source. This strategy maximizes resource efficiency and reduces waste, which aligns with the circular economy's tenets.

Benefits to the environment go beyond lowering carbon emissions. When combined with sustainable farming methods, biomass generation for bioplastics and biofuels can be planned to repair degraded land, enhance soil health, and support biodiversity. In addition to producing useful products, using waste-derived feedstocks, such as spent cooking oil or organic municipal waste, lowers landfill accumulation and methane emissions (Smuda, 2004). In order to complete the carbon and nutrient cycles, microalgae cultivation can be combined with wastewater treatment and carbon dioxide collection to make the process even more sustainable. To guarantee that bioplastics and biofuels have a truly sustainable future, a few challenges must be overcome. Production scaling up must be accomplished without using excessive amounts of water and land, and life cycle assessments must direct development to guarantee that environmental effects are, in fact, less severe than those of traditional alternatives. To increase acceptance and establish stable markets for these products, policies, incentives, and international cooperation will be crucial. The extent to which bioplastics can minimize pollution will also depend on public awareness and appropriate waste sorting systems. The combination of green chemistry, sustainable manufacturing, and renewable energy systems will make bioplastics and biofuels essential components of a low-carbon economy. They can contribute to the achievement of global climate goals while protecting ecosystems by implementing the principles of the circular economy, cutting waste, and substituting products derived from fossil fuels (Schwaiger *et al.*, 2011). These developments can transition from niche markets to mainstream solutions with sustained research funding, supportive legislation, and industry-community cooperation, clearing the path for a future that is cleaner, more sustainable, and more resilient.

CHALLENGES

A lot of researchers assess sustainability, including biofuels, using life cycle assessment (LCA). Although there is great potential for biomanufacturing biofuels and bioplastics to lessen reliance on fossil fuels, a number of obstacles prevent widespread adoption. The availability and sustainability of feedstocks are a major concern because seasonality, land-use competition, and high logistics costs are common problems for waste biomass, microalgae, and agricultural residues. Technologies for pretreatment and conversion are still inefficient and energy-intensive, and lignocellulosic biomass presents unique challenges because of its resistant structure. Low productivity, product toxicity, and contamination risks at industrial scales are the limitations of enzymatic and microbial fermentation processes. Furthermore, downstream processing is costly and energy-intensive, frequently surpassing production costs, and is used to recover fuels or purify biopolymers, such as polyhydroxyalkanoates (PHA) and polylactic acid (PLA). Another issue is market competitiveness, since bioproducts find it challenging to compete economically due to established petrochemical infrastructure and fluctuating fossil fuel prices. Furthermore, end-of-life management and product performance are important issues. There are concerns regarding the true environmental benefits of bioplastics because many of them lack the mechanical strength, durability, or biodegradability required for widespread use. Inadequate infrastructure for recycling and composting, policy gaps, and low consumer awareness all hinder commercialization. Innovations in metabolic engineering, process intensification, synthetic biology, and circular bioeconomy models are needed to overcome these obstacles. Innovations that can reduce costs and improve sustainability include integrated biorefineries, engineered microbes for increased yields, and more environmentally friendly downstream recovery techniques. These developments have the potential to make biomanufacturing a pillar of a low-carbon and sustainable future when combined with carbon credits, supportive regulations, and investments in waste-to-resource technologies.

CONCLUSION

Bioplastics are being produced from renewable biomass materials, and provide a green substitute for petro-plastics because they are biodegradable, sourced from renewable resources, and have lower carbon content. Poly Hydroxy Alkanoates (PHAs), Poly Lactic Acid (PLA), ulvan, alginate, and carrageenan are some of the bioplastics with varied mechanical, thermal, and biodegradable characteristics applicable to different uses. PHAs are biodegradable replacements for man-made plastics in packaging, agriculture, and pharmaceuticals. PLA that is produced from crops such as corn and sugarcane, has extensive applications in 3D printing and food packaging. Polysaccharides of marine origin, such as ulvan and alginate, present novel routes for biocompatible and fast-degradable bioplastics, especially in food packaging and biomedical applications. Red seaweed-derived carrageenan presents potential in green coatings and films. Sustainability relies on maximizing raw material processing efficiency, energy-efficient manufacturing, and end-of-life treatment by composting or recycling. Bioplastics also have industrial uses in agriculture, packaging, electronics, and the construction industry. Bioplastics are being challenged by cost effectiveness, performance constraints, and industrial scalability.

REFERENCES

Adeniyi, A. G., Ighalo, J. O., & Onifade, D. V. (2018). Biofuels from microalgae biomass: A review of conversion processes and procedures. *Arabian Journal of Chemistry, 15*(6), 103791. DOI: 10.1016/j.arabjc.2022.103791

Agarwal, A. K., Gupta, J. G., & Dhar, A. (2017). Potential and challenges for large-scale application of biodiesel in automotive sector. *Progress in Energy and Combustion Science, 61*, 113–149. DOI: 10.1016/j.pecs.2017.03.002

Ali, I., Ding, W., & Zhang, Z. (2023). Microalgae-based bioplastics: A comprehensive review. *Renewable & Sustainable Energy Reviews, 178*, 113247. DOI: 10.1016/j.rser.2023.113247

Azad, A. K., Rasul, M. G., Khan, M. M. K., Sharma, S. C., & Hazrat, M. A. (2015). Prospect of biofuels as an alternative transport fuel in Australia. *Renewable & Sustainable Energy Reviews, 43*, 331–351. DOI: 10.1016/j.rser.2014.11.047

Balat, M. (2008). Potential importance of hydrogen as a future solution to environmental and transportation problems. *International Journal of Hydrogen Energy, 33*(15), 4013–4029. DOI: 10.1016/j.ijhydene.2008.05.047

Bhatia, S. K., Otari, S. V., Jeon, J. M., & Yang, Y. H. (2019). Biowaste-to-bioplastic (polyhydroxyalkanoates): Conversion technologies, strategies, and challenges. *Bioresource Technology, 298*, 122393. DOI: 10.1016/j.biortech.2019.122393 PMID: 33494006

Bowyer, J., Bratkovich, S., Frank, M., Fernholz, K., & Howe, J. (2018). *Biofuels: A review of the life cycle literature*. Dovetail Partners Inc.

Budzianowski, W. M., & Postawa, K. (2017). Total chain integration of sustainable biogas production. *Renewable Energy, 106*, 41–56. DOI: 10.1016/j.renene.2016.12.073

Callegari, A., & Capodaglio, A. G. (2018). Properties and beneficial uses of (bio)chars, with special attention to products from sewage sludge pyrolysis. *Resources, 7*(1), 20. DOI: 10.3390/resources7010020

Cecconet, D., Molognoni, D., Callegari, A., & Capodaglio, A. G. (2018). Agro-food industry wastewater treatment with microbial fuel cells: Energetic recovery issues. *International Journal of Hydrogen Energy, 43*(1), 500–511. DOI: 10.1016/j.ijhydene.2017.07.231

Chong, J. W. R., Tan, X., Khoo, K. S., Ng, H. S., Jonglertjunya, W., Yew, G. Y., & Show, P. L. (2022). Microalgae-based bioplastics: Future solution towards mitigation of plastic wastes. *Environmental Research, 206*, 112620. DOI: 10.1016/j.envres.2021.112620 PMID: 34968431

Colwill, J. A., Wright, E. I., Rahimifard, S., & Clegg, A. J. (2012). Bio-based plastics in the automotive industry. *Journal of Biobased Materials and Bioenergy, 6*(3), 274–281. DOI: 10.1166/jbmb.2012.1213

Dalton, B., Bhagabati, P., De Micco, J., Padamati, R. B., & O'Connor, K. (2022). A review on biological processes for pharmaceuticals and personal care products removal. *Chemosphere, 286*, 131716. DOI: 10.1016/j.chemosphere.2021.131716

Dang, B. T., Bui, X. T., Tran, D. P., Ngo, H. H., & Nghiem, L. D. (2022). Current application of algae derivatives for bioplastic production: A review. *Bioresource Technology*, *347*, 126698. DOI: 10.1016/j.biortech.2022.126698 PMID: 35026424

De Melo, A. C., de Castro, H. F., & de Moraes, F. F. (2014). Enzymatic synthesis of biodiesel via alcoholysis of palm oil. *Applied Biochemistry and Biotechnology*, *173*(6), 1365–1375. DOI: 10.1007/s12010-014-0934-y

Deeba, F., Pruthi, V., & Negi, Y. S. (2016). Converting paper mill sludge into neutral lipids by oleaginous yeast *Cryptococcus vishniaccii* for biodiesel production. *Bioresource Technology*, *213*, 96–102. DOI: 10.1016/j.biortech.2016.02.105 PMID: 26965670

Demirbas, A. (2011). Competitive liquid biofuels from biomass. *Applied Energy*, *88*(1), 17–28. DOI: 10.1016/j.apenergy.2010.07.016

Di Bartolo, A., Infurna, G., & Dintcheva, N. T. (2021). A review of bioplastics and their adoption in the circular economy. *Polymers*, *13*(8), 1229. DOI: 10.3390/polym13081229 PMID: 33920269

El-Malek, F. A., Khairy, H., Farag, A., & Omar, S. (2020). The sustainability of microbial bioplastics, production and applications. *International Journal of Biological Macromolecules*, *157*, 319–328. DOI: 10.1016/j.ijbiomac.2020.04.076 PMID: 32315677

Ellis, J. T., Hengge, N. N., Sims, R. C., & Miller, C. D. (2012). Acetone, butanol, and ethanol production from wastewater algae. *Bioresource Technology*, *111*, 491–495. DOI: 10.1016/j.biortech.2012.02.002 PMID: 22366611

Fallde, M., & Eklund, M. (2015). Towards a sustainable socio-technical system of biogas for transport: The case of the city of Linköping in Sweden. *Journal of Cleaner Production*, *98*, 17–28. DOI: 10.1016/j.jclepro.2014.08.015

Ganigué, R., Puig, S., Batlle-Vilanova, P., Balaguer, M. D., & Colprim, J. (2015). Microbial electrosynthesis of butyrate from carbon dioxide. *Chemical Communications*, *51*(15), 3235–3238. DOI: 10.1039/C4CC10121A PMID: 25608945

Garbeva, P., Hol, W. H. G., & de Boer, W. (2018). The role of volatile compounds in microbial interactions. *Trends in Microbiology*, *26*(11), 942–953. DOI: 10.1016/j.tim.2018.06.002

Ghobashy, M. M., Elhady, M. A., & El-Sawy, N. M. (2021). Radiation crosslinking of modifying biodegradable plastics for sustainable future: A review. *Journal of Polymer Research*, *28*(10), 389. DOI: 10.1007/s10965-021-02751-3

Gouda, M. K., Swellam, A. E., & Omar, S. H. (2024). Production of biodiesel by enzymatic transesterification [Review]. *Energy Sources. Part A, Recovery, Utilization, and Environmental Effects*, *46*(1), 1–21. DOI: 10.1080/15567036.2023.2283993

Harding, K. G., Dennis, J. S., von Blottnitz, H., & Harrison, S. T. L. (2017). A life-cycle comparison between inorganic and biological catalysis for the production of biodiesel. *Journal of Cleaner Production*, *142*, 3157–3169. DOI: 10.1016/j.jclepro.2016.10.134

Ho, S. H., Huang, S. W., Chen, C. Y., Hasunuma, T., Kondo, A., & Chang, J. S. (2013). Bioethanol production using carbohydrate-rich microalgae biomass as feedstock. *Bioresource Technology, 135*, 191–198. DOI: 10.1016/j.biortech.2012.10.015 PMID: 23116819

Hoang, P. H., Hoang, H. H., & Chung, W. (2022). Extraction and characterization of polyhydroxyalkanoates from microbial biomass. *Journal of Environmental Chemical Engineering, 10*(3), 107419. DOI: 10.1016/j.jece.2022.107419

Hong, M., Chen, E. Y. X., & Chen, X. (2021). Towards truly sustainable polymers: A metal-free recyclable polyester from biorenewable non-strained γ-butyrolactone. *Nature Chemistry, 13*(11), 1043–1049. DOI: 10.1038/s41557-021-00748-5

Hopewell, J., Dvorak, R., & Kosior, E. (2009). Plastics recycling: Challenges and opportunities. *Philosophical Transactions of the Royal Society of London. Series B, Biological Sciences, 364*(1526), 2115–2126. DOI: 10.1098/rstb.2008.0311 PMID: 19528059

Hu, Q., Sommerfeld, M., Jarvis, E., Ghirardi, M., Posewitz, M., Seibert, M., & Darzins, A. (2008). Microalgal triacylglycerols as feedstocks for biofuel production: Perspectives and advances. *The Plant Journal, 54*(4), 621–639. DOI: 10.1111/j.1365-313X.2008.03492.x PMID: 18476868

Jariyasakoolroj, T., Tashiro, K., & Wang, H. (2020). Advanced supramolecular design for direct ink writing of soft materials. *Advanced Materials, 32*(39), 2003760. DOI: 10.1002/adma.202003760

Jayakody, L. N., Ferdouse, J., & Hayashi, K. (2022). Alginate-based composites for packaging applications: A review. *Journal of Polymers and the Environment, 30*(5), 1747–1767. DOI: 10.1007/s10924-021-02315-w

Jin, M., Slininger, P. J., Dien, B. S., Waghmode, S., Moser, B. R., Orjuela, A., & Balan, V. (2018). Microbial lipid-based lignocellulosic biorefinery: Feasibility and challenges. *Trends in Biotechnology, 36*(3), 281–297. DOI: 10.1016/j.tibtech.2017.10.020 PMID: 30278987

Kai, Y., Hasegawa, M., & Ohta, T. (2016). Production of fatty acids in *Saccharomyces cerevisiae*. *Journal of Biotechnology, 222*, 69–77. DOI: 10.1016/j.jbiotec.2016.02.017

Kakadellis, S., & Harris, Z. M. (2020). Don't scrap the waste: The need for broader system boundaries in bioplastic food packaging life-cycle assessment. *The Science of the Total Environment, 727*, 138831. DOI: 10.1016/j.scitotenv.2020.138831

Kanagesan, K., Abdulla, R., & Derman, E. (2022). Ulvan, a bioactive marine polysaccharide as a green ingredient for functional food and pharmaceutical applications. *Molecules (Basel, Switzerland), 27*(20), 7035. DOI: 10.3390/molecules27207035 PMID: 36296626

Kartik, A., Akhil, D., Lakshmi, D., Gopinath, K. P., Arun, J., Sivaramakrishnan, R., & Pugazhendhi, A. (2021). A critical review on production of biopolymers from algae biomass and their applications. *Bioresource Technology, 329*, 124868. DOI: 10.1016/j.biortech.2021.124868 PMID: 33707076

Khanna, S., Goyal, A., & Moholkar, V. S. (2011). Production of n-butanol from biodiesel derived crude glycerol using *Clostridium pasteurianum* immobilized on amberlite. *Fuel, 102*(1), 211–219. DOI: 10.1016/j.fuel.2012.07.011

Kim, J. K., Kim, D. Y., & Lee, N. K. (2020). A review on the properties and applications of carrageenan. *Polymer Korea*, *44*(6), 707–719. DOI: 10.7317/pk.2020.44.6.707

Kusuktham, B., & Srinophakun, P. (2014). Improvement of butanol production from palm empty fruit bunch by *Clostridium beijerinckii*. *Energy Procedia*, *52*, 627–632. DOI: 10.1016/j.egypro.2014.07.118

Lakshmi, D. S., Trivedi, N., & Reddy, C. R. K. (2020). Synthesis and characterization of seaweed cellulose derived carboxymethylcellulose. *Carbohydrate Polymers*, *250*, 116904. DOI: 10.1016/j.carbpol.2020.116904

Lin, P. P., Rabe, K. S., Takasumi, J. L., Kadisch, M., Arnold, F. H., & Liao, J. C. (2015). Isobutanol production at elevated temperatures in thermophilic *Geobacillus thermoglucosidasius*. *Metabolic Engineering*, *24*, 1–8. DOI: 10.1016/j.ymben.2014.03.006 PMID: 24721011

Lu, J., Sheahan, C., & Fu, P. (2021). Metabolic engineering of algae for fourth generation biofuels production. *Energy & Environmental Science*, *4*(7), 2451–2466. DOI: 10.1039/C0EE00593B

Mohammed, A., Rivers, A., Stuckey, D. C., & Ward, K. (2023). Alginate-based bioplastics: A review. *International Journal of Biological Macromolecules*, *233*, 123550. DOI: 10.1016/j.ijbiomac.2023.123550

Naik, S. N., Goud, V. V., Rout, P. K., & Dalai, A. K. (2010). Production of first- and second-generation biofuels: A comprehensive review. *Renewable & Sustainable Energy Reviews*, *14*(2), 578–597. DOI: 10.1016/j.rser.2009.10.003

Nanda, S., Kumar, V., & Vij, R. K. (2023). A review on thermochemical and biochemical conversion of biomass to biofuels. *BioEnergy Research*, *16*(1), 1–26. DOI: 10.1007/s12155-022-10526-x

Nielsen, D. R., Leonard, E., Yoon, S. H., Tseng, H. C., Yuan, C., & Prather, K. L. J. (2009). Engineering alternative butanol production platforms in heterologous bacteria. *Metabolic Engineering*, *11*(4-5), 262–273. DOI: 10.1016/j.ymben.2009.05.003 PMID: 19464384

Pandey, A., Srivastava, S., & Rai, P. (2022). Polyhydroxyalkanoates (PHAs): A review on biosynthesis, properties, and applications. *Bioresource Technology Reports*, *19*, 101163. DOI: 10.1016/j.biteb.2022.101163

Papong, S., Malakul, P., Trungkavashirakun, R., Wenunun, P., Chom-in, T., Nithitanakul, M., & Sarobol, E. (2014). Comparative assessment of the environmental profile of PLA and PET drinking water bottles from a life cycle perspective. *Journal of Cleaner Production*, *65*, 539–550. DOI: 10.1016/j.jclepro.2013.09.030

Pauly, M., & Keegstra, K. (2008). Cell-wall carbohydrates and their modification as a resource for biofuels. *The Plant Journal*, *54*(4), 559–568. DOI: 10.1111/j.1365-313X.2008.03463.x PMID: 18476863

Peng, Y., Wu, P., Schartup, A. T., & Zhang, Y. (2021). Plastic waste release caused by COVID-19 and its fate in the global ocean. *Proceedings of the National Academy of Sciences of the United States of America*, *118*(47), e2111530118. DOI: 10.1073/pnas.2111530118 PMID: 34751160

Rahman, A., & Bhoi, P. R. (2021). An overview of non-biodegradable bioplastics. *Journal of Cleaner Production*, *294*, 126218. DOI: 10.1016/j.jclepro.2021.126218

Ramos, F. D., Delpivo, C., & Borsarelli, C. D. (2019). Polyhydroxyalkanoates (PHAs): Production, applications, and end-of-life strategies. *Biotechnology Advances*, *42*, 107582. DOI: 10.1016/j.biotechadv.2019.107582

Rayung, M., Aung, M. M., Azhar, S. C., & Suait, M. S. (2020). Bio-based polymer electrolytes for electrochemical devices: Insight into the ionic conductivity performance. *Materials (Basel)*, *13*(4), 838. DOI: 10.3390/ma13040838 PMID: 32059600

Razzak, M. T., Darwis, D., & Zainuddin, S. (2017). Irradiation of polyvinyl alcohol and polyvinyl pyrrolidone blended hydrogel for wound dressing. *Radiation Physics and Chemistry*, *140*, 96–100. DOI: 10.1016/j.radphyschem.2017.02.046

Romero-García, J. M., Niño, L., Martínez-Patiño, C., Ruiz, E., Romero, I., & Castro, E. (2016). Bioethanol production from olive tree biomass. *Renewable Energy*, *86*, 1067–1073. DOI: 10.1016/j.renene.2015.09.043

Rosenboom, J. G., Langer, R., & Traverso, G. (2022). Bioplastics for a circular economy. *Nature Reviews. Materials*, *7*(2), 117–137. DOI: 10.1038/s41578-021-00407-8 PMID: 35075395

Rueda, E., García-Galán, M. J., & Ortiz, A. (2023). Life cycle assessment of polyhydroxybutyrate production from *Synechocystis* sp. PCC 6803. *Algal Research*, *69*, 102929. DOI: 10.1016/j.algal.2022.102929

Rydz, J., Sikorska, W., Kyulavska, M., & Christova, D. (2015). Polyester-based (bio)degradable polymers as environmentally friendly materials for sustainable development. *International Journal of Molecular Sciences*, *16*(1), 564–596. DOI: 10.3390/ijms16010564 PMID: 25551604

Santos, A. J., Carvalho, F., Oliveira, C. S., & Fortunato, E. (2020). Bioplastics from agro-waste for food packaging applications. *Food Packaging and Shelf Life*, *25*, 100523. DOI: 10.1016/j.fpsl.2020.100523

Schwaiger, N., Feiner, R., & Wimmer, B. (2011). Bioplastics from renewable resources: The role of life cycle assessment in the development of new products. *The International Journal of Life Cycle Assessment*, *16*(7), 675–676. DOI: 10.1007/s11367-011-0315-5

Shalaby, E. A. (2013). Biofuel: sources, extraction and determination. In Liquid, Gaseous and Solid Biofuels - Conversion Techniques, 18, 451-478. DOI: https://doi.org/DOI: 10.5772/51943

Shen, C. R., Lan, E. I., Dekishima, Y., Baez, A., Cho, K. M., & Liao, J. C. (2011). Driving forces enable high-titer anaerobic 1-butanol synthesis in *Escherichia coli. Applied and Environmental Microbiology*, *77*(9), 2905–2915. DOI: 10.1128/AEM.03003-10 PMID: 21398484

Shen, Y., Yuan, W., Pei, Z., & Mao, E. (2009). Microalgae mass production methods. *Transactions of the ASABE*, *52*(4), 1275–1287. DOI: 10.13031/2013.27771

Smuda, M. (2004). Bioplastics: A growing trend. *Packaging Technology & Science*, *17*(5), 255–261. DOI: 10.1002/pts.663

Sudhakar, M., Priya, M., & Dharani, G. (2024). A review on the environmental impacts of microplastics and its remediation techniques. *Environmental Science and Pollution Research International*, *31*(11), 15927–15951. DOI: 10.1007/s11356-024-32151-1

Vasile, C., Baican, M., & Darie-Ni ă, R. N. (2019). Emerging and advanced technologies in bioplastics. *Journal of Cellular Plastics*, *55*(3), 251–277. DOI: 10.1177/0021955X19833637

Wang, L., Zhang, B., & Xiao, J. (2022). Carrageenan-based films and coatings for food packaging applications: A review. *Trends in Food Science & Technology*, *119*, 257–273. DOI: 10.1016/j.tifs.2021.12.015

Westfall, P. J., Pitera, D. J., Lenihan, J. R., Eng, D., Woolard, F. X., Regentin, R., & Renninger, N. S. (2012). Production of Amorphadiene in yeast, and its conversion to dihydroartemisinic acid, precursor to the antimalarial agent artemisinin. *Proceedings of the National Academy of Sciences of the United States of America*, *109*(3), E111–E118. DOI: 10.1073/pnas.1110740109 PMID: 22247290

Wichard, T., Charrier, B., & Potin, P. (2015). Green algae as model organisms for biological fluid dynamics. *Annual Review of Fluid Mechanics*, *47*, 343–375. DOI: 10.1146/annurev-fluid-010313-141426 PMID: 26594068

Yang, S., Mohagheghi, A., Franden, M. A., Chou, Y. C., Chen, X., & Zhang, M. (2016). Metabolic engineering of *Zymomonas mobilis* for 2,3-butanediol production from lignocellulosic biomass sugars. *Biotechnology for Biofuels*, *9*(1), 1–15. DOI: 10.1186/s13068-016-0606-y PMID: 27594916

Yap, J. X., Chan, Y. H., & Tshai, K. Y. (2023). A review on the degradation of poly(lactic acid) blends. *Polymer Degradation & Stability*, *208*, 110256. DOI: 10.1016/j.polymdegradstab.2023.110256

Chapter 10
Biopharmaceutical Manufacturing:
Challenges and Solutions

Mukul Machhindra Barwant
https://orcid.org/0000-0002-5639-4251
Sanjivani Rural Education Society Sanjivani Arts, Commerce, and Science College, Kopargoan, India

Balwant Singh
https://orcid.org/0000-0002-6224-7194
K.S. Saket PG College, Dr. Ram Manohar Lohia Avadh University, Ayodhya, India

Amir M. Vazirizadeh
Persian Gulf Research and Studies Institute, Fishery and Marine Biology Department, Persian Gulf University, Iran

ABSTRACT

Biopharmaceutical production is an important industry for the production of life-saving biologics such as monoclonal antibodies, recombinant proteins, and vaccines. Nevertheless, the industry is plagued by serious issues of process efficiency, scalability, regulatory compliance, and cost-effectiveness. Bioprocessing technologies such as continuous manufacturing, single-use bioreactors, and automation have changed the face of the industry with their impact on increased flexibility in production and lowering costs. Additionally, incorporating artificial intelligence, process analytical technology (PAT), and digital twin models has streamlined real-time monitoring and predictive maintenance to deliver increased product consistency and regulatory compliance.. On the other hand, sustainable biomanufacturing approaches like use of renewable feedstocks, green bioprocessing, and valorization of wastes are being addressed to reduce environmental footprint.

INTRODUCTION

Biopharmaceuticals, or biologics, are drugs developed from biological material such as tissues, cells, or organisms, and encompass a broad product portfolio including monoclonal antibodies,

DOI: 10.4018/979-8-3373-2873-7.ch010

recombinant proteins, vaccines, and cell or gene therapies (Walsh, 2018). They are complex in both structure and function, distinguishing them significantly from small-molecule drugs. Consequently, their manufacturing processes are highly sophisticated and sensitive to environmental and procedural variations (Rathore & Winkle, 2009). The global biopharmaceutical industry has experienced exponential growth over the last few decades due to advances in molecular biology, recombinant DNA technology, and cell line development (Ecker et al., 2015).

Biomanufacturing forms the cornerstone of the biopharmaceutical sector, utilizing living systems—most notably mammalian cells such as Chinese Hamster Ovary (CHO) cells—to produce high-value therapeutic proteins under strictly regulated conditions. Despite the transformative potential of biopharmaceuticals, the production process is fraught with challenges including high production costs, issues with scalability and reproducibility, regulatory compliance, and the need to meet critical product quality attributes such as purity, potency, and immunogenicity (Huang et al., 2010; Shukla & Thömmes, 2010).

In scaling up from laboratory to commercial production, challenges often arise due to limitations in bioreactor design, suboptimal cell culture conditions, and constraints in downstream processing. Achieving uniform glycosylation profiles, protein folding, and maintaining biological activity adds further complexity to quality control procedures (Liu, 2015). Moreover, biopharmaceutical production must align with stringent regulatory requirements enforced by agencies such as the U.S. Food and Drug Administration (FDA) and the European Medicines Agency (EMA), emphasizing compliance with Good Manufacturing Practices (GMP), Process Analytical Technologies (PAT), and Quality by Design (QbD) principles (FDA, 2004; EMA, 2020).

In recent years, innovative strategies such as single-use bioreactor systems, continuous bioprocessing, and digitalization—integrating automation and artificial intelligence—have begun to transform the landscape of biomanufacturing. These technologies aim to increase efficiency, reduce contamination risk, and facilitate real-time monitoring and control of process parameters (Konstantinov & Cooney, 2015; Zydney, 2016).

This refined understanding of manufacturing challenges and innovations provides the foundation for exploring state-of-the-art solutions. A clear grasp of these evolving trends is critical for optimizing bioprocesses, ensuring regulatory compliance, and enabling the cost-effective and scalable production of safe, high-quality biotherapeutics.

In summary, the background highlights the necessity of advanced strategies to address the multifaceted challenges of biopharmaceutical production and sets the stage for discussing the new technologies and approaches explored in this chapter.

CHALLENGES IN BIOPHARMACEUTICAL MANUFACTURING

Biopharmaceutical production, as significant as its pioneering advances in contemporary medicine, is beset by a myriad of challenges owing to the intrinsic biologic complexity, the vulnerability of living production organisms, and stringent regulatory standards. These challenges pervade the whole pipeline of production—ranging from cell line development and optimization of culture, purification, formulation, to conformance with international quality standards. Figure no 1 represents a schematic overview of the principal challenges encountered in the biopharmaceutical manufacturing process.

Figure 1. Challenges of biopharmaceutical manufacturing

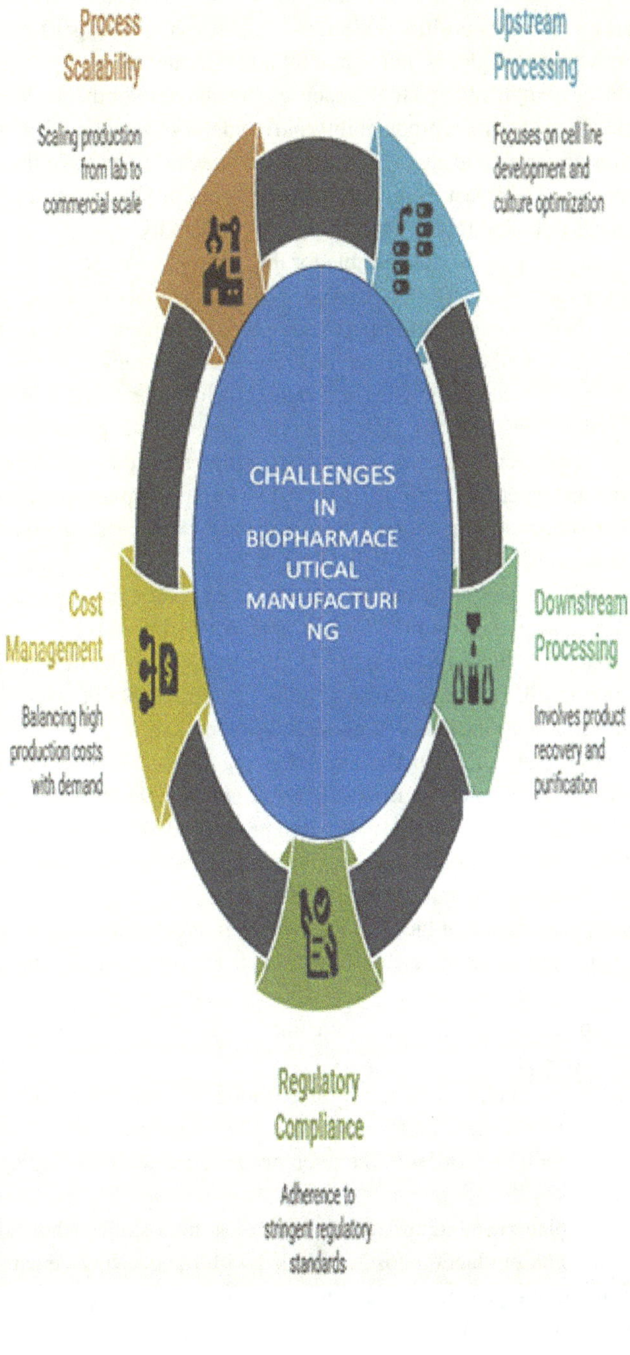

Upstream processing includes the creation of high-productive cell lines and culture condition optimization for the highest possible product expression. A key problem is genetic and phenotypic instability of the recombinant cell lines, which may cause product yield and quality variability with time (Wurm, 2004). In addition, cell lines like Chinese Hamster Ovary (CHO) cells are sensitive to culture medium composition variations, shear stress, and oxygen transfer rates, which can negatively impact protein glycosylation and folding (Gramer, 2014).

A limitation is the complexity and high expense of media development. Chemically defined and serum-free media are ideal for reproducibility and regulatory compliance but involve extensive empirical optimization through testing (Li et al., 2010). Additionally, scale-up from laboratory to industrial bioreactors is subject to limitations concerning mixing, mass transfer, and pH or temperature gradients, which affect cell viability and productivity.

Downstream processing is also responsible for the recovery and purification of the product, which typically forms more than 50% of the overall cost of production (Shukla & Thömmes, 2010). Low product yield, the high burden of impurities, and multi-step chromatographic purification are the key bottlenecks here that can be time- and resource-consuming.

Specifically for monoclonal antibodies and glycoproteins, preserving product integrity and eliminating host cell proteins (HCPs), DNA, and viral impurities is paramount. Glycosylation heterogeneity and the occurrence of process-related impurities make the purification more difficult and impact the product's safety and efficacy (Liu, 2015). Protein aggregation during downstream processing also contributes to immunogenic responses and causes serious concerns for patient safety (Rathore & Kapoor, 2015).

Biopharmaceuticals are highly sensitive to small variations in manufacturing conditions, requiring sophisticated analytical methods for real-time monitoring and control. Nonetheless, the integration of Process Analytical Technology (PAT) and Quality by Design (QbD) strategies in biologics production is still challenging owing to the limited number of fast, non-invasive, and rugged analytical instruments available (Rathore & Winkle, 2009).

Furthermore, developing an exhaustive understanding of critical process parameters (CPPs) and their effects on critical quality attributes (CQAs) is desirable but challenging, especially for new biologics like gene therapies and cell-based products (FDA, 2004). High heterogeneity of biological systems tends to produce process drift and variability in product quality, making regulatory approval and lifecycle management challenging.

Due to the therapeutic nature of biopharmaceuticals, production processes have to adhere to rigorous regulatory guidelines set by agencies like the U.S. Food and Drug Administration (FDA), European Medicines Agency (EMA), and International Council for Harmonisation (ICH). The dynamic and changing nature of regulatory guidelines poses a major challenge to manufacturers aiming for global market access (EMA, 2018).

In addition, proving biosimilarity in the case of biosimilar development is another complicating factor. In contrast to generic small molecules, biosimilars have to be very similar in structure, function, and immunogenicity profiles to the reference product, with demanding comparability studies (Pisal et al., 2010).

Biomanufacturing plants need significant capital outlays, high-skilled labor, and sophisticated quality systems. The high production cost, combined with the growing demand for biologics, puts pressure on improving productivity and minimizing cost of goods sold (COGS) without sacrificing quality (Walsh, 2018).

In addition, process scalability from laboratory to commercial scale is still a challenge because of variations in hydrodynamics, nutrient distribution, and shear forces in large-scale bioreactors. Implementation of continuous manufacturing and single-use technologies is promising but also needs revalidation, retraining, and redesigning of conventional infrastructure (Zydney, 2016).

Table 1. Different types of biopharmaceutical manufacturing and their applications

Type of Biopharmaceutical Manufacturing	Biopharmaceuticals Produced	Applications	References
Mammalian Cell Culture	Monoclonal antibodies, therapeutic proteins	Cancer treatment, autoimmune disorders, hormone therapies, enzyme replacement therapies	Walsh, 2018
Bacterial Fermentation	Insulin, growth factors, vaccines, enzymes	Diabetes management, wound healing, vaccines, metabolic diseases	Adhikari, 2017
Yeast-based Systems	Vaccines, monoclonal antibodies, recombinant proteins	Vaccine production (e.g., hepatitis B), protein therapies, diagnostics	Alper & Stephanopoulos, 2009
Plant-based Systems	Therapeutic proteins, vaccines, enzymes	Production of biopharmaceuticals for rare diseases, therapeutic antibodies	Vojdani & Gerhard, 2019
Insect Cell Expression Systems	Vaccines, biopharmaceuticals, virus-like particles	Vaccine production (e.g., influenza, Zika), gene therapy vectors, diagnostic tools	Choi & Lee, 2013
Cell-Free Protein Synthesis Systems	Peptides, small proteins, enzymes	Rapid protein production for research, diagnostic reagents, small-scale therapeutic proteins	
Hybridoma Technology	Monoclonal antibodies	Diagnostic tests, cancer therapy, autoimmune diseases, immunosuppressive treatments	Köhler & Milstein, 1975
Continuous Bioprocessing	Therapeutic proteins, vaccines, antibodies	High-yield biomanufacturing, reduced production costs, streamlined production for large-scale therapies	Pollard & Woodley, 2007

Upstream Processing Challenges

Upstream processing in biopharmaceutical production is the first part of the production process, which deals with cell line development and cultivation for expression of the target therapeutic protein. It is a vital step because it determines product yield, quality, and reproducibility. Nevertheless, it is also full of pitfalls in terms of biological variability, nutrient handling, and contamination control.

Cell Line Development and Optimization

The choice and design of hardy, high-titer cell lines are essential for the success of upstream processing. Host systems routinely employed include Escherichia coli, yeast (Pichia pastoris, Saccharomyces cerevisiae), and mammalian cells, in particular, Chinese Hamster Ovary (CHO) cells as a result of their capability for complex post-translational processing (Kim et al., 2012).

One of the biggest challenges is genetic stability and stable expression of the therapeutic gene through many passages. Spontaneous mutations, silencing of genes, and clonal heterogeneity can result in reduced productivity or modification of glycosylation patterns (Wurm, 2004). Second, selection of high-producers is time- and material-intensive and usually involves methods such as fluorescence-activated cell sorting (FACS), limiting dilution, or single-cell microscopy (Huang et al., 2010).

Emergent technologies like CRISPR/Cas9 genome editing and omics-based methodologies are increasingly being combined to boost cell line productivity and better forecast cell performance. Yet, such tools need validation and come under regulatory oversight due to the potential for off-target effects and unexpected phenotypic outcomes (Lee et al., 2018).

Media Formulation and Nutrient Supply

Culture medium composition is also a key determinant of cell productivity, growth, and product quality. Media are required to provide not only carbon and nitrogen sources but also vitamins, trace elements, lipids, and growth factors in proper concentrations. The major challenge is to develop chemically defined, serum-free media that allow for high cell density with minimal variability and risk of contamination (Altamirano et al., 2006).

Inadequate media compositions may result in nutrient depletion, metabolite buildup (e.g., lactate, ammonia), and oxidative stress, which negatively impact cell viability and protein expression (Restelli et al., 2006). In addition, nutrient imbalance may change glycosylation patterns and post-translational modifications, which may influence the efficacy and safety of the final product (Kuo et al., 2018).

Dynamic nutrient feeding regimes, including fed-batch and perfusion cultures, are used to ensure the best nutrient levels. However, these require strong monitoring systems and real-time analytical techniques to prevent gradients of nutrients or toxic metabolite buildup (Xie & Wang, 1996).

Contamination Risks and Bioreactor Control

Microbial contamination—specifically by bacteria, fungi, mycoplasma, and viruses—is an ever-present risk in upstream bioprocessing, resulting in batch failure, product loss, and regulatory non-compliance (Langdon et al., 2009). Even residual contamination can elicit immune reactions or shift host cell metabolism, compromising product safety and process economics.

Bioreactor systems, whether stainless steel or single-use, must be kept aseptic under tightly controlled conditions of temperature, pH, dissolved oxygen (DO), and agitation. Changes in these conditions can lead to cellular stress, protein misfolding, or decreased yields (Nienow, 2006). Scale-up from laboratory-scale to production-scale bioreactors also poses other challenges regarding oxygen transfer, mixing homogeneity, and foam control (Borys et al., 2019).

Sophisticated bioreactor control methods combining Process Analytical Technology (PAT), soft sensors, and feedback loops are used more and more to track important process parameters (CPPs) in real time. Their deployment is complicated and requires high process understanding, data integration, and regulatory qualification (Mandenius & Brundin, 2008).

Downstream Processing Challenges

Downstream processing (DSP) comprises the vital steps of protein separation, purification, and formulation following upstream cultivation. It normally represents 60–80% of overall manufacturing costs in biopharmaceutical production due to its complexity, multi-step processes, and rigorous regulatory compliance (Gottschalk, 2017). The major challenges in this phase are how to obtain high purity and recovery of the product with preserved bioactivity and reduced costs.

Protein Purification and Recovery Efficiency

Protein purification is a multi-step process aimed at separating the therapeutic biomolecule from host cell proteins, DNA, endotoxins, viruses, and process-related contaminants. Popular methods include centrifugation, filtration, chromatography (affinity, ion exchange, hydrophobic interaction, size exclusion), and ultrafiltration/diafiltration (Shukla & Thömmes, 2010).

The key challenge is to reconcile purity and yield, particularly for multifaceted biologics such as monoclonal antibodies, fusion proteins, and vaccines. Loss of recovery tends to happen through adsorption onto column matrices, aggregation, or denaturation under extreme processing conditions (Jungbauer, 2013). Moreover, trace impurities or product variants also need to be eliminated to satisfy stringent regulatory requirements for safety, potency, and consistency.

Affinity chromatography, especially with Protein A for monoclonal antibodies, has high selectivity but is high in cost, has low binding capacity, and experiences leaching of the ligand into the product stream (Roque et al., 2004). To overcome this, other ligands, mixed-mode resins, and continuous chromatography systems are being investigated, although their scalability and reproducibility need to be confirmed (Rathore & Rajan, 2008).

In addition, the necessity for product-specific purification approaches enhances process development time and resource usage, since no single purification approach can be utilized across various biologics (Müller-Späth et al., 2008).

High Cost and Time-Intensive Filtration Processes

Filtration is crucial in cell, particulate, and microbial contaminant removal during DSP. Depth filtration is normally employed for harvest clarification, while sterile and virus filtration provide ultimate product protection. Filtration operations tend to be expensive, time-consuming, and fouling-prone, particularly on a large scale (Morales et al., 2008).

High viscosity, host cell protein and DNA presence, and high cell densities all have the potential to lower filter throughput and lifetime substantially, resulting in higher operational costs and downtime (Yigzaw et al., 2006). Virus filtration, a regulatory requirement, further complicates things because it requires the use of costly filters with low capacity and long processing times (Brorson & Xu, 2010).

Disposable filtration systems are offering a substitute for stainless steel configurations, lessening the need for cleaning and contamination danger. They have challenges tied to filter-to-filter performance variability, supply chain reliance, and extractables/leachables of polymeric materials (Jacquemart et al., 2016).

To enhance filtration efficiency and minimize cost, companies are investing in process intensification routes like continuous DSP, pre-flocculation, inline conditioning, and real-time monitoring. Although promising, these technologies need extensive validation, training, and synchronization with quality-by-design (QbD) principles for regulatory qualification (Kelley, 2009).

Regulatory and Quality Control Hurdles

Biopharmaceutical production is tightly controlled to guarantee the safety, effectiveness, and quality of therapeutic goods. In contrast to conventional drugs, biopharmaceuticals are produced from living organisms, which brings with them inherent variability, complexity, and sensitivity to manufacturing conditions. Consequently, sustaining regulatory compliance and product consistency across batches of manufacture continue to be among the most critical challenges in the sector (FDA, 2020; EMA, 2018).

Good Manufacturing Practices (GMP) and Compliance

Good Manufacturing Practices (GMP) are an integral part of regulatory control in the biopharmaceutical industry. Implemented by regulatory agencies like the U.S. Food and Drug Administration (FDA), European Medicines Agency (EMA), and World Health Organization (WHO), GMP regulations confirm products are produced and controlled consistently to the quality standards suited to their intended use (ICH, 2021).

GMP compliance involves an effective quality management system that includes facility design, standard operating procedures (SOPs), training of personnel, documentation, process validation, and change control (FDA, 2020). It is especially demanding to comply with GMP during biopharmaceutical manufacturing owing to the inherent biological variability in raw materials, cell lines, and environmental factors that may impact product quality (Rathore & Winkle, 2009).

In addition, the biomanufacturing industry's globalized character has created intricate supply chains and multi-site manufacturing paradigms. Every production facility needs to ensure GMP compliance, and ensuring practices are harmonized across regions with varying regulatory requirements contributes to the complexity (Kraemer et al., 2011).

Deviation or non-compliance from GMP may result in regulatory warning letters, product recall, and import prohibition, which carry serious financial and reputational implications. To reduce this, firms are increasingly taking risk-based strategies and digital quality management systems to improve real-time monitoring, data integrity, and regulatory traceability (De Felice et al., 2022).

Batch-to-Batch Variability and Product Consistency

Batch-to-batch variability describes unwanted variations in product quality characteristics—e.g., glycosylation profiles, protein structure, or biological function—across different batches. This variability is a major issue in biopharmaceuticals, as slight process changes can result in major differences in safety and efficacy (Gronemeyer et al., 2014).

In contrast to synthetic small molecules, where the final product is chemically defined and reproducible, biopharmaceuticals are extremely sensitive to upstream and downstream condition changes. Cell culture conditions, media formulation, bioreactor conditions, and purification processes can all impact critical quality attributes (CQAs) (Patel et al., 2020).

To address this challenge, producers use Quality by Design (QbD) principles, where product and process understanding is established early in development to determine the design space that will guarantee consistent product quality. QbD also includes process analytical technologies (PAT) for real-time monitoring and control to reduce variability in manufacturing (FDA, 2004).

Even with these advances, complete control over biological systems is still challenging, particularly for new modalities such as gene therapies, biosimilars, and cell-based products. Regulatory agencies now demand rigorous comparability studies in the case of manufacturing changes, such as analytical, non-clinical, and even clinical assessments to confirm consistency (EMA, 2018).

Supply Chain and Scalability Issues

The international biopharmaceutical production environment is critically dependent on a sophisticated, web-like supply chain to provide raw materials, reagents, single-use items, and other key manufacturing inputs in a timely manner. In combination with the scale-up challenges of laboratory to commercial production, these problems can have a dramatic effect on manufacturing timelines, cost-effectiveness, and product availability (Lange et al., 2022).

Raw Material Shortages and Logistics

Raw material scarcity has become a significant constraint in biopharmaceutical manufacturing, particularly brought to the forefront during the COVID-19 pandemic that revealed supply chain vulnerabilities worldwide. Dependence on a few vendors for critical inputs—e.g., cell culture media components, resins, filtration membranes, and single-use systems—can result in major delays and variability (Jacquemart et al., 2016; Pauwels et al., 2021).

Biomanufacturers tend to rely on high-quality, GMP-grade materials, which involve extensive testing, validation, and traceability. Any supply chain or transportation disruption, whether caused by geopolitical tensions, natural disasters, or regulatory controls, can lead to production delays or failure (Fisher et al., 2021). In addition, temperature-sensitive and sterile materials require cold-chain logistics and controlled environments during shipping, contributing to complexity and expense (Shukla et al., 2017).

To address these threats, organizations are embracing dual source approaches, local diversification of suppliers, and just-in-time (JIT) inventory systems. These adjustments call for effective supply chain threat management processes and regulatory adaptability for alternative material verification (Srai & Kumar, 2019).

Scale-up Challenges for Commercial Production

Scaling up biopharmaceutical operations from pilot or laboratory scale to commercial production brings with it specialized technological and operating challenges. With small-molecule drugs, scaling up is frequently linear and can be predicted. Biologics, however, are living organisms with great environmental and mechanical sensitivity (Zydney, 2016).

Important issues to address are sustaining product quality and yield when scale-up to large-scale bioreactors and purification systems. Conditions like oxygen transfer, shear stress, mixing, and heat removal can be substantially different from scale to scale and may influence cell viability, protein expression, and product homogeneity (Farid, 2007; Huang et al., 2010).

Additionally, upstream and downstream operations frequently must be re-optimized to accommodate large volumes. For example, chromatography columns employed in downstream purification can have lower efficiency at scale, necessitating redesign or use of new techniques like continuous or multi-column chromatography (Kelley, 2009).

Moreover, scale-up requires large capital expenditures, facility expansion, and regulatory clearance. The use of single-use technologies, modular bioprocessing units, and digital biomanufacturing platforms is mitigating these hurdles by facilitating flexible and agile scale-up without sacrificing quality (Hickey et al., 2020).

In general, successful scale-up demands thorough knowledge of key process parameters (CPPs) and their connection to key quality attributes (CQAs), backed by strong process analytical technologies (PAT) and quality-by-design (QbD) platforms (FDA, 2004).

In addition to traditional stirred-tank and perfusion bioreactors, emerging systems such as fluidized-bed and photobioreactors are also gaining attention for their utility in continuous and photosynthetic-based biomanufacturing.

TECHNOLOGICAL INNOVATIONS AND EMERGING SOLUTIONS

Technology innovations are transforming the biopharmaceutical manufacturing landscape with revolutionary solutions to surmount long-existing challenges around scalability, efficiency, and regulatory compliance. Among the landmark developments is the implementation of single-use bioreactors (SUBs), which have taken center stage because of their operational flexibility, lower risk of cross-contamination, and lower capital and cleaning costs. SUBs enable fast process development and are especially beneficial for multi-product plants and individualized therapies (Eibl et al., 2010). Additionally, continuous bioprocessing, such as perfusion cultures and combined continuous chromatography, is becoming more prevalent to increase product yield, process reproducibility, and real-time quality control. These continuous systems minimize footprint and energy usage while enhancing manufacturing responsiveness and scalability (Konstantinov & Cooney, 2015).

The embedding of automation and digital technologies in manufacturing processes is one of the key drivers of operational excellence. Automation reduces human error, enhances reproducibility, and allows high-throughput process control. With AI and machine learning algorithms, automation platforms are now able to perform predictive analytics, fault detection early on, and dynamic process optimization. Process Analytical Technology (PAT), which has been supported by regulatory bodies such as the FDA, is an important aspect of this digital revolution. PAT includes real-time measurement and monitoring of critical process parameters and quality attributes by employing sophisticated tools such as spectroscopy, chromatography, and multivariate data analysis, thus assuring consistent product quality and easing compliance with Quality by Design (QbD) paradigms (Rathore & Winkle, 2010; FDA, 2004).

Cell line engineering has also undergone tremendous advancements using the implementation of CRISPR-Cas9 and synthetic biology strategies. CRISPR can be used for precise genome editing, which is used to boost productivity characteristics, stress tolerance, and glycosylation accuracy in production cell lines like Chinese hamster ovary (CHO) and HEK293 cells. This speeds up cell line development (CLD) and diminishes the cost of laborious screening procedures (Ronda et al., 2014). In contrast, synthetic biology makes it possible to design synthetic regulatory devices, biosensors, and metabolic routes to provide tailor-made cell factories that are tailored towards particular therapeutic products (Nielsen & Keasling, 2016).

Emerging digital twin technology is also transforming the industry further by allowing virtual simulation of physical bioprocesses. A digital twin combines sensor data, control system data, and past database data to provide a dynamic, real-time simulation of biomanufacturing operations. The model assists in process development, failure prediction, and real-time decision-making, thus enhancing process robustness and operational efficiency. Combined with Industry 4.0 technologies like the Internet of Things (IoT), cloud computing, and AI, digital twins are leading the way in smart manufacturing strategies, driving innovation, traceability, and regulatory preparedness in biopharmaceutical manufacturing (Verma et al., 2021; Lee et al., 2018).

These technologies together signify a paradigm shift in biopharmaceutical production, opening the way for more nimble, affordable, and scalable production systems to address global healthcare needs with precision and speed. The growing complexity, regulatory rigidity, and cost-intensiveness of biopharmaceutical production have propelled the use of disruptive technologies to enhance efficiency, scalability, and product quality. Technological advances are revolutionizing traditional biomanufacturing paradigms, moving toward automation, digitization, and precision biological engineering (Walsh, 2018; Ghasemi et al., 2021).

Advances in Single-Use Bioreactors and Continuous Processing

Single-use bioreactors (SUBs) have transformed upstream biomanufacturing through flexibility, lower contamination risk, and quicker changeover. Disposable plastic parts-based systems avoid cleaning and sterilization between batches, vastly enhancing plant efficiency (Eibl et al., 2010). SUBs are particularly valuable for multiproduct facilities and clinical-scale manufacturing, where quick turnaround and responsiveness are essential (Langer & Rader, 2014).

Concurrently, continuous bioprocessing—such as perfusion cultures and continuous chromatography—offers a route to enhance yield, consistency, and cost-effectiveness. Continuous operations keep cells in the best growth phases, maximizing volumetric productivity and allowing real-time product monitoring and control (Konstantinov & Cooney, 2015). Hybrid systems combining continuous upstream with batch or semi-continuous downstream processes are now being adopted to transition gradually from conventional batch models.

Automation, AI, and Process Analytical Technology (PAT)

Digitalization and automation play a central role in managing variability and complexity in biomanufacturing. Automated processes minimize the risk of human error, simplify procedures, and enhance reproducibility across different scales of production (Hossain et al., 2023). Integrated with artificial intelligence (AI) and machine learning (ML), manufacturers can currently process large volumes of data to forecast performance patterns, identify anomalies, and refine process parameters in real-time.

Process Analytical Technology (PAT), which the FDA champions, enables real-time monitoring of key quality attributes (CQAs) with tools such as spectroscopy, chromatography, and multivariate analysis. PAT enables feedback control systems that modify process conditions in real time, thereby guaranteeing product quality and regulatory compliance (FDA, 2004; Rathore & Winkle, 2010).

CRISPR and Synthetic Biology for Cell Line Engineering

Recent developments in CRISPR-Cas9 genome editing and synthetic biology have enabled the rational engineering of production cell lines with improved characteristics. CRISPR allows for multiplexed and accurate editing of host genomes—e.g., CHO or HEK293 cells—thus enhancing protein expression, glycosylation consistency, and stress resistance (Ronda et al., 2014).

Synthetic biology also facilitates the design of synthetic promoters, biosynthetic pathways, and regulatory circuits to modulate gene expression and metabolic fluxes in host cells (Nielsen & Keasling, 2016). Such tools enhance cell line development (CLD) by diminishing the requirement for large-scale screening and improving consistency in large-scale production.

In addition, advances in "designer" cell lines with integrated biosensors, knock-in/knock-out, and epigenetic tuning are facilitating next-generation biomanufacturing with enhanced product yield and stability (Wurm, 2013).

Digital Twin Models and Smart Manufacturing

Digital twin technology—virtual representations of physical biomanufacturing systems—facilitates real-time simulation, monitoring, and optimization of process production. Models combine sensor data, PAT tools, and control systems to simulate biological operations, offering predictive understanding of system behavior under different conditions (Verma et al., 2021).

Industry 4.0 technology-enabled smart manufacturing platforms with IoT, cloud computing, and AI enable closed-loop control, preventive maintenance, and continuous improvement of biomanufacturing (Lee et al., 2018). Digital twins also enable quicker process development, risk assessment, and regulatory documentation through data visualizaton and traceability.

Through virtual prototyping of process changes prior to physical execution, digital twins minimize downtime, improve scale-up, and facilitate the shift to continuous and modular manufacturing systems.

SUSTAINABLE AND COST-EFFECTIVE BIOMANUFACTURING STRATEGIES

The increasing need for biopharmaceuticals and cost and environment pressures have caused the industry to move towards developing sustainable and economical manufacturing processes. Green bioprocessing is spearheading this, with the view of reducing biomanufacturing's ecological impacts through the usage of environmentally friendly solvents, low water intake, and green feedstocks. Utilizing plant or microbial biomass-derived feedstocks, including lignocellulosic biomass, algae, and agro-industrial residues, not only diminishes dependence on petroleum-derived substrates but also aligns with the sustainable development goals (Jahangirian et al., 2020). Production based on renewable raw materials, such as glycerol derived from biodiesel or starch hydrolysates derived from agricultural by-products, has shown compatibility with microbial and mammalian expression systems employed in biopharmaceutical manufacturing (Liu et al., 2018).

Waste valorization and circular economy strategies provide further opportunities for sustainable biomanufacturing. Biopharmaceutical production processes create significant amounts of waste in the form of spent media, cellular debris, and single-use items. These wastes can be redirected into bioenergy, biofertilizers, or simply as feedstocks for other biotechnological products by way of valorization. Anaerobic digestion of bioresidues and enzymatic hydrolysis of biomass to recover nutrients represent some of the circular approaches popular in bioprocessing plants (Bhatia et al., 2022). Additionally, developments in synthetic biology and metabolic engineering now facilitate the conversion of biowastes into useful co-products, keeping economic efficiency side by side with sustainability objectives (Choi et al., 2019).

Energy efficiency is another key aspect of sustainable biomanufacturing. Conventional bioprocessing processes, such as sterilization, aeration, and downstream purification, consume high energy. New technologies like membrane-based separation, low-energy freeze-drying, and continuous chromatography systems are being created to minimize energy demands substantially while ensuring product quality (Rathore et al., 2018). The application of process intensification methods, such as integrated and continuous bioprocessing, also helps reduce energy usage and cost of production by eliminating wastage and downtime (Pollard & Woodley, 2007).

Adding life cycle assessment (LCA) and environmental impact modeling helps manufacturers to identify critical areas for environmental improvement over the entire product life cycle, starting from raw material sourcing and ending in product disposal. When combined with digital technologies such as real-time monitoring and predictive analytics, manufacturers are able to dynamically optimize energy and material consumption, improving both ecological and economic performance (Sartorius, 2020). Combined, these sustainable practices not only assist in lowering the carbon footprint but also help ensure regulatory compliance and public acceptance, ultimately pushing the biopharmaceutical sector's shift towards greener and more responsible manufacturing paradigms.

Green Bioprocessing and Renewable Feedstocks

Green bioprocessing is a paradigm change in biopharmaceutical production, with an emphasis on minimizing environmental footprint and enhancing sustainability. This includes the use of environmentally friendly solvents, minimizing water and energy consumption, and using biodegradable or recyclable materials. At the heart of green bioprocessing is the utilization of renewable feedstocks from agricultural wastes, lignocellulosic biomass, algae, or industrial residues. These feedstocks provide sustainable alternatives to petroleum-based substrates and promote the world's shift towards a bio-based economy (Jahangirian et al., 2020).

Microbial and mammalian cell culture systems have been shown compatible with renewable feedstocks like glycerol from biodiesel production and hydrolysates of starchy or cellulosic biomass (Liu et al., 2018). Such replacement not only decreases raw material costs but also saves the carbon impact of conventional inputs. Moreover, advances in metabolic engineering have made possible the construction of engineered strains that can metabolize efficiently complex feedstocks, making green biomanufacturing more feasible.

Waste Valorization and Circular Economy Approaches

During biopharmaceutical manufacturing, large volumes of waste are produced, such as spent media, cell debris, and single-use plastic items. Waste valorization practices, consistent with circular economy values, seek to convert these by-products into valuable resources. For instance, anaerobic digestion can transform organic bioprocess waste into biogas for energy recovery, while enzymatic treatments can recover nutrients for recycle into media formulations (Bhatia et al., 2022).

Synthetic biology and metabolic engineering provide means to produce waste as desired co-products like biosurfactants, bioplastics, or secondary metabolites, thereby establishing closed-loop manufacturing systems (Choi et al., 2019). These circular methodologies assist in the reduction of environmental impact, decrease waste disposal expenditure, and enhance the economic value of biomanufacturing operations.

Energy-Efficient Biomanufacturing Practices

Energy usage is one of the major contributors to both the environmental and economic impact of biopharmaceutical plants. Large energy sinks are sterilization, temperature maintenance, aeration, and downstream process operations such as chromatography and drying. Energy-efficient technologies have been developed in recent years to bridge these challenges. For example, membrane filtration and low-energy lyophilization techniques have been used to replace traditional energy-consuming separation and drying techniques (Rathore et al., 2018).

Process intensification by sustained bioprocessing, such as perfusion culture and integrated purification systems, has also been established to enhance energy efficiency by saving batch downtime and optimizing equipment use (Pollard & Woodley, 2007). Also, energy monitoring and real-time analysis with the help of digital platforms enable dynamic process adjustments with minimal unnecessary consumption of energy, thereby increasing the operational sustainability (Sartorius, 2020).

CONCLUSION

The landscape of biopharmaceutical manufacturing is facing crucial change spurred on by the demand for advanced therapeutics and the imperative for sustainability. With the industry expanding, meeting the challenges that are part of biopharmaceutical manufacturing—varying from upstream processing, downstream purification, regulatory approval, to scalability—is still imperative. Advances in biomanufacturing technologies, including single-use technologies, continuous processing, and advanced automation, are already mitigating many of these challenges. Implementation of such technologies, aside from boosting productivity and quality, also cuts cost and the negative effect on the environment. Furthermore, emerging biomanufacturing strategies emphasizing sustainability, like green bioprocessing, waste valorization, and energy-efficient methods, hold promising potential for reducing the environmental impact of biopharmaceutical manufacturing. The use of renewable feedstocks, recycling of waste streams, and circular economy concepts is at the core of the vision of a more sustainable biopharmaceutical industry. Also, the use of advanced technologies such as artificial intelligence, CRISPR, and process analytical technologies (PAT) is poised to further enhance process efficiency, minimize variability, and facilitate real-time monitoring of biomanufacturing processes. While these improvements have been made, there are still large barriers that are mainly issues of regulatory complexity, batch-to-batch consistency, and new technology scalability. Ongoing coordination among academia, industry, and regulatory agencies will be essential to address these challenges. New biomanufacturing materials and methods must also comply with regulatory requirements while not compromising product quality or patient safety. Ultimately, the future of biopharmaceutical production will be based on the integration of innovative technology and sustainable processes. Through a solution that addresses economic and environmental issues, the industry can fulfill increasing demand for biologics and ensure sustainable long-term biopharmaceutical production. The ongoing emphasis on research and development, together with the implementation of best practices and innovative technologies, will be central to the future of biopharmaceutical manufacturing, allowing the industry to address global healthcare needs effectively and sustainably.

These transformative trends—including modular design, automation, and the drive for scalable, sustainable solutions—will be instrumental in shaping a resilient and forward-looking biomanufacturing ecosystem.

REFERENCES

Adhikari, M. (2017). Recent advances in bacterial fermentation for the production of therapeutic proteins. *Biotechnology Advances*, *35*(3), 391–403.

Alper, H. S., & Stephanopoulos, G. (2009). Engineering yeasts for biofuels production: From strains to systems. *Bioresource Technology*, *100*(4), 2335–2341.

Altamirano, C., Paredes, C., Cairó, J. J., & Gòdia, F. (2006). Improvement of CHO cell culture medium formulation: Simultaneous substitution of glucose and glutamine. *Biotechnology Progress*, *22*(3), 609–617. PMID: 16739940

Bhatia, S. K., Kim, J. H., Song, H. S., Jeon, J. M., Kim, Y. G., & Yang, Y. H. (2022). Waste to bioenergy: A sustainable approach for production of biohydrogen using organic waste. *Bioresource Technology*, *344*, 126203.

Borys, M. C., Linzer, D. I. H., & Papoutsakis, E. T. (2019). Culture of CHO cells for recombinant protein production. In Smith, E. (Ed.), *Biopharmaceutical Production Technology* (Vol. 1, pp. 41–82). Wiley-VCH.

Brorson, K. A., & Xu, Y. (2010). Virus filtration of biotechnology products. *Biotechnology and Bioengineering*, *106*(2), 203–212. PMID: 20178120

Choi, S. Y., Song, C. W., Shin, J. H., & Lee, S. Y. (2019). Biorefineries for the production of top building block chemicals and their derivatives. *Metabolic Engineering*, *28*, 223–239. PMID: 25576747

Choi, Y. J., & Lee, S. Y. (2013). Insect cell culture and its application in biopharmaceutical production. *Biotechnology Advances*, *31*(6), 996–1008.

De Felice, F., Petrillo, A., Cioffi, R., & Calabrese, M. (2022). Digital transformation and regulatory compliance in biopharmaceutical manufacturing: A framework proposal. *Technovation*, *117*, 102526.

Ecker, D. M., Jones, S. D., & Levine, H. L. (2015). The therapeutic monoclonal antibody market. *mAbs*, *7*(1), 9–14. PMID: 25529996

Eibl, R., Kaiser, S., Lombriser, R., & Eibl, D. (2010). Disposable bioreactors: The current state-of-the-art and recommended applications in biotechnology. *Applied Microbiology and Biotechnology*, *86*(1), 41–49. DOI: 10.1007/s00253-009-2420-4 PMID: 20094714

EMA. (2018). *Guideline on the requirements for quality documentation concerning biological investigational medicinal products in clinical trials*. European Medicines Agency. https://www.ema.europa.eu

Farid, S. S. (2007). Process economics of industrial monoclonal antibody manufacture. *Journal of Chromatography. B, Analytical Technologies in the Biomedical and Life Sciences*, *848*(1), 8–18. PMID: 16899415

FDA. (2004). *Guidance for Industry: PAT — A Framework for Innovative Pharmaceutical Development, Manufacturing, and Quality Assurance*. U.S. Food and Drug Administration. https://www.fda.gov

FDA. (2020). *Guidance for Industry: CGMP for Phase 1 Investigational Drugs*. U.S. Food and Drug Administration. https://www.fda.gov

Fisher, A. C., Franco, R. D., & Ho, C. (2021). Biomanufacturing in the age of COVID-19: Advances and challenges in vaccine production. *Trends in Biotechnology*, *39*(11), 1164–1176.

Ghasemi, M., Kanani, M., & Rahimnejad, M. (2021). Recent advances in biopharmaceuticals production with flexible and smart manufacturing systems. *Biotechnology Letters*, *43*(3), 519–532.

Gottschalk, U. (2017). *Process scale purification of antibodies*. CRC Press.

Gramer, M. J. (2014). Product quality considerations for mammalian cell culture process development and manufacturing. *Advances in Biochemical Engineering/Biotechnology*, *139*, 123–166. PMID: 23748351

Gronemeyer, P., Ditz, R., & Strube, J. (2014). Trends in upstream and downstream process development for antibody manufacturing. *Bioengineering (Basel, Switzerland)*, *1*(4), 188–212. PMID: 28955024

Hickey, J. M., Santiago, M. G., & Carlson, E. D. (2020). Flexible biomanufacturing: Industry perspectives on single-use technologies and facility design. *Biotechnology Advances*, *44*, 107608.

Hossain, M. M., Kabir, M. H., & Kim, J. H. (2023). Application of AI in biomanufacturing: Challenges and future prospects. *Computers in Biology and Medicine*, *155*, 106554.

Huang, Y. M., Hu, W., Rustandi, E., Chang, K., Yusuf-Makagiansar, H., & Ryll, T. (2010). Maximizing productivity of CHO cell culture using chemically defined media in fed-batch culture. *Biotechnology Progress*, *26*(5), 1400–1410. PMID: 20945494

Huang, Y. M., Hu, W., Rustandi, E., Chang, K., Yusuf-Makagiansar, H., & Ryll, T. (2010). Maximizing productivity of CHO cell-based fed-batch culture using chemically defined media in stirred-tank bioreactors. *Biotechnology and Bioengineering*, *106*(4), 804–814. PMID: 21404255

Huang, Y. M., Hu, W., Rustandi, E., Chang, K., Yusuf-Makagiansar, H., & Ryll, T. (2010). Maximizing productivity of CHO cell-based fed-batch culture using chemically defined media in stirred-tank bioreactors. *Biotechnology and Bioengineering*, *105*(5), 1002–1015. PMID: 19882695

ICH. (2021). *ICH Q12: Technical and Regulatory Considerations for Pharmaceutical Product Lifecycle Management*. International Council for Harmonisation. https://www.ich.org

Jacquemart, R., Lin, Y. H., & Kamen, A. A. (2016). Biomanufacturing of viral vectors: Industrial challenges and opportunities. *Biotechnology Journal*, *11*(4), 473–484. PMID: 26632496

Jacquemart, R., Lin, Y. H., Stern, B., Azouz, A., & Kamen, A. (2016). Manufacturing of adenovirus vectors: Part I. Upstream processes. *Pharmaceutical Bioprocessing*, *4*(3), 183–197.

Jahangirian, H., Lemraski, E. G., Webster, T. J., Rafiee-Moghaddam, R., & Abdollahi, Y. (2020). A review of environmentally friendly synthesis of pharmaceuticals using biocatalysis and green chemistry principles. *Biotechnology Advances*, *38*, 107322.

Jungbauer, A. (2013). Product purification: Protein A chromatography. In Harnisch, J. P. (Ed.), *Biopharmaceutical Manufacturing* (pp. 151–176). Wiley.

Kelley, B. (2009). Industrialization of mAb production technology: The bioprocessing industry at a crossroads. *mAbs*, *1*(5), 443–452. PMID: 20065641

Kim, J. Y., Kim, Y. G., & Lee, G. M. (2012). CHO cells in biotechnology for production of recombinant proteins: Current state and further potential. *Applied Microbiology and Biotechnology*, *93*(3), 917–930. PMID: 22159888

Köhler, G., & Milstein, C. (1975). Continuous cultures of fused cells secreting antibody of predefined specificity. *Nature*, *256*(5517), 495–497. PMID: 1172191

Konstantinov, K. B., & Cooney, C. L. (2015). White paper on continuous bioprocessing. *May 20, 2015*. American Institute of Chemical Engineers (AIChE). https://www.aiche.org

Konstantinov, K. B., & Cooney, C. L. (2015). White paper on continuous bioprocessing. *Journal of Pharmaceutical Sciences*, *104*(3), 813–820. DOI: 10.1002/jps.24252

Kraemer, M., Reed, J., & Tobin, S. (2011). Global regulatory challenges in biopharmaceutical manufacturing. *Pharmaceutical Technology Europe*, *23*(4), 42–47.

Kuo, C. C., Lin, Y. T., & Liu, C. H. (2018). Glycosylation of therapeutic proteins in mammalian cells. *Current Opinion in Chemical Engineering*, *22*, 1–7.

Langdon, S. P., Wyld, D., & Reeves, J. R. (2009). Contamination in cell culture: Risks and preventive measures. *Methods in Molecular Biology (Clifton, N.J.)*, *946*, 15–28.

Lange, I., Kourentzi, K., & Willson, R. C. (2022). Supply chain resilience in the biopharmaceutical industry. *Biotechnology Journal*, *17*(7), 2100425.

Langer, E. S., & Rader, R. A. (2014). Single-use bioprocessing: A technology that is revolutionizing the biomanufacturing industry. *BioProcess International*, *12*(6), 24–30.

Lee, J., Bagheri, B., & Kao, H. A. (2018). A cyber-physical systems architecture for Industry 4.0-based manufacturing systems. *Manufacturing Letters*, *3*, 18–23.

Lee, J. S., Kallehauge, T. B., Pedersen, L. E., & Kildegaard, H. F. (2018). Site-specific genome engineering for high-level protein production in CHO cells. *Biotechnology Journal*, *13*(3), 1700645.

Li, F., Vijayasankaran, N., Shen, A., Kiss, R., & Amanullah, A. (2010). Cell culture processes for monoclonal antibody production. *mAbs*, *2*(5), 466–479. PMID: 20622510

Liu, H. (2015). Impact of glycosylation on the efficacy and safety of monoclonal antibodies. *mAbs*, *7*(2), 256–263.

Liu, L., Li, Y., Li, S., Du, G., & Chen, J. (2018). Renewable bio-resources: A review on microbial production of platform chemicals. *Biotechnology Advances*, *36*(6), 1423–1440.

Mandenius, C. F., & Brundin, A. (2008). Bioprocess optimization using design-of-experiments methodology. *Biotechnology Progress*, *24*(6), 1191–1203. PMID: 19194932

Morales, M., Ma, J., Al-Rub, K. A., & Scheper, T. (2008). Challenges in downstream processing: From clarification to purification. *Biotechnology Journal*, *3*(3), 327–337.

Müller-Späth, T., Morbidelli, M., & Hubbuch, J. (2008). Purification of therapeutic proteins using simulated moving bed chromatography. *Journal of Chromatography. A*, *1171*(1-2), 46–58.

Nielsen, J., & Keasling, J. D. (2016). Engineering cellular metabolism. *Cell*, *164*(6), 1185–1197. PMID: 26967285

Nienow, A. W. (2006). Reactor engineering in large scale animal cell culture. *Cytotechnology*, *50*(1), 9–33. PMID: 19003068

Patel, S. K. S., Choi, S. H., & Kang, Y. C. (2020). Recent developments in process analytical technologies (PATs) for biopharmaceutical production. *Biotechnology Journal*, *15*(5), 1900569.

Pauwels, E., Breuer, L., & Lander, B. (2021). The pandemic and the global biopharmaceutical supply chain. *Nature Biotechnology*, *39*(7), 749–752.

Pisal, D. S., Kosloski, M. P., & Balu-Iyer, S. V. (2010). Delivery of therapeutic proteins. *Journal of Pharmaceutical Sciences*, *99*(6), 2557–2575. PMID: 20049941

Pollard, D., & Woodley, J. M. (2007). Biocatalysis for pharmaceutical intermediates: The future is now. *Trends in Biotechnology*, *25*(2), 66–73. PMID: 17184862

Pollard, D. J., & Woodley, J. M. (2007). Biocatalysis for pharmaceutical intermediates: The future is now. *Trends in Biotechnology*, *25*(2), 66–73. PMID: 17184862

Rathore, A. S., Agarwal, H., & Sharma, A. (2018). Energy-efficient and sustainable bioprocessing strategies. *Current Opinion in Chemical Engineering*, *22*, 42–48.

Rathore, A. S., & Kapoor, G. (2015). Analytical characterization of protein aggregates. *Biopharm International*, *28*(5), 28–34.

Rathore, A. S., & Rajan, R. S. (2008). Current perspectives on validation of protein purification processes. *Biotechnology Progress*, *24*(5), 1090–1098. PMID: 19194918

Rathore, A. S., & Winkle, H. (2009). Quality by design for biopharmaceuticals. *Nature Biotechnology*, *27*(1), 26–34. PMID: 19131992

Rathore, A. S., & Winkle, H. (2010). Quality by design for biopharmaceuticals. *Nature Biotechnology*, *28*(9), 831–835. PMID: 19131992

Restelli, V., Wang, M. D., Huzel, N., & Butler, M. (2006). The effect of enhanced oxygenation on the metabolic profile and productivity of recombinant CHO cells. *Biotechnology and Bioengineering*, *94*(4), 679–687. DOI: 10.1002/bit.20899

Ronda, C., Pedersen, L. E., Hansen, H. G., Kallehauge, T. B., Betenbaugh, M. J., & Kildegaard, H. F. (2014). Accelerating genome editing in CHO cells using CRISPR Cas9 and CRISPy, a web-based target finding tool. *Biotechnology and Bioengineering, 111*(8), 1604–1616. PMID: 24827782

Roque, A. C. A., Lowe, C. R., & Taipa, M. A. (2004). Antibodies and genetically engineered related molecules: Production and purification. *Biotechnology Progress, 20*(3), 639–654. PMID: 15176864

Sartorius. (2020). *Sustainable Biomanufacturing: Environmental Footprint Assessment of Bioprocesses.* White Paper. Retrieved from https://www.sartorius.com

Shukla, A. A., & Thömmes, J. (2010). Recent advances in large-scale production of monoclonal antibodies and related proteins. *Trends in Biotechnology, 28*(5), 253–261. PMID: 20304511

Shukla, A. A., Wolfe, L. S., Mostafa, S. S., & Norman, C. (2017). Evolving trends in biopharmaceutical process development and manufacturing. *Bioengineering & Translational Medicine, 2*(1), 58–69. DOI: 10.1002/btm2.10049 PMID: 29313024

Srai, J. S., & Kumar, M. (2019). Supply network configuration for distributed manufacturing: Case studies in the biopharmaceutical industry. *International Journal of Production Research, 57*(8), 2436–2453.

Verma, D., Sharma, R., & Sharma, A. (2021). Digital twins in biopharmaceutical manufacturing: A transformative approach for smart production. *Biotechnology Advances, 49*, 107764.

Vojdani, F., & Gerhard, L. (2019). Plant-based expression systems for biopharmaceuticals: Developments and challenges. *Frontiers in Plant Science, 10*, 1276.

Walsh, G. (2018). Biopharmaceutical benchmarks 2018. *Nature Biotechnology, 36*(12), 1136–1145. PMID: 30520869

Walsh, G. (2018). *Biopharmaceuticals: Biochemistry and Biotechnology*. Wiley-Blackwell.

Wurm, F. M. (2004). Production of recombinant protein therapeutics in cultivated mammalian cells. *Nature Biotechnology, 22*(11), 1393–1398. PMID: 15529164

Wurm, F. M. (2013). CHO quasispecies—Implications for manufacturing processes. *Processes (Basel, Switzerland), 1*(3), 296–311.

Xie, L., & Wang, D. I. C. (1996). High cell density and high monoclonal antibody production through medium design and rational feeding in a fed-batch culture of hybridoma cells. *Biotechnology and Bioengineering, 51*(6), 725–729. PMID: 18629840

Yigzaw, Y., Piper, R., Tran, M., & Shukla, A. A. (2006). Exploiting the adsorptive properties of depth filters for host cell protein removal during monoclonal antibody purification processes. *Biotechnology Progress, 22*(1), 288–296. PMID: 16454522

Zydney, A. L. (2016). Continuous downstream processing for high value biological products: A review. *Biotechnology and Bioengineering, 113*(3), 465–475. PMID: 26153056

Chapter 11
Sustainable Biomanufacturing:
Green Technologies for Environmental and Economic Benefits

Muhammad Anas
https://orcid.org/0000-0001-5127-8043
Selçuk University, Turkey

Waseem Ahmed Khattak
Quaid-i-Azam University, Islamabad, Pakistan

Erdogan E. Hakki
Selçuk University, Turkey

Javed Iqbal
https://orcid.org/0000-0002-9032-2622
Bacha Khan University, Pakistan

Banzeer Ahsan Abbasi
https://orcid.org/0000-0003-3036-4481
Rawalpindi Women University, Pakistan

Ghulam Murtaza
Yunnan University, Kunming, China

ABSTRACT

This chapter comprehensively explores the principles, technologies, applications, economic considerations and future directions of green biomanufacturing. It covers biological production platforms, waste valorization, sustainable materials, regulatory dynamics, analyze core principles; waste minimization, energy efficiency & lifecycle assessment. Evaluating enabling technologies; microbial fermentation, enzyme catalysis, synthetic biology, plant/algae-based systems. It reviews industrial applications in pharmaceuticals, biofuels, biomaterials, waste management and explore economic viability, policy incentives and challenges in scalability. The study finds that green biomanufacturing offers significant environmental and economic benefits, including reduced emissions, enhanced resource efficiency and new value chains from waste streams. Future research should focus on optimizing process control through AI, next-gen bioreactors, expanding public-private partnerships for scale-up infrastructure and harmonizing global regulatory frameworks.

DOI: 10.4018/979-8-3373-2873-7.ch011

INTRODUCTION

Definition and Scope of Sustainable Biomanufacturing

Sustainability in Biomanufacturing is the use of biological systems or organisms (including cells, enzymes, and tissues) to produce a broad range of products for human use (Zhang et al., 2017). Sustainable biomanufacturing is significantly different than traditional manufacturing which is heavily dependent on fossil sources of energy and leaves behind significant amounts of environmental pollutants, and instead is focused on use of renewable feedstocks, energy efficient process configurations, and zero/low waste production in confluence with circular economy philosophies. This strategy involves biotechnology, engineering, and sustainability science to reshape the way materials are made, from feedstock choice and bioengineered strain construction to bioreactor engineering and waste utilization (Aggarwal et al., 2024). Sustainable biomanufacturing is a far-reaching area that encompasses both energy and healthcare, as well as agriculture and consumer goods sectors. It includes new science, like metabolic engineering and synthetic biology, as well as green chemistry and resource recovery technologies, and it puts industries on a path from extraction to regenerative production (Lozano et al., 2018). Being a discipline which combines various fields like science, technology and economics, it is not only addressing technical and scientific challenges, but also has regulatory, social and economic dimensions and is an essential part of the world-wide bioeconomy (Anas et al., 2025, Haris et al., 2023).

Importance of Green Technologies in Industrial Bioprocessing

Green technologies are at the heart of sustainable biomanufacturing practices, the adoption of which would allow industries to lower their environmental footprint, while enhancing efficiency and product quality (Shokoohi & Attar, 2024a). These technologies are intended to lower energy demand, obviate usage of harmful chemicals, and employ resources more efficiently across the bioprocessing value chain. For example, we can observe highly selective low-energy enzyme-based catalysis in the context of pharmaceutical or textile production, and continuous fermentation systems lead to both the reduction of resources use and enhanced yields compared to the batch processing. Bio-based solvents, energy-saving bioreactors, and closed-loop water systems are also examples of how green technologies make for cleaner industries(Osman et al., 2024, Ahmad et al., 2022). Furthermore, waste valorization approaches, e.g., turning lignocellulosic biomass into high-value bio-products or capturing and utilizing CO_2 emission, improve environmental and economic performance(Ahmed et al., 2021). The use of these emerging technologies not only tackles climate and pollution challenges but also enables companies to meet more stringent environmental regulations and build consumer confidence by creating a sustainable brand. This demonstrates that such green technologies are not only compliance tools but strategic enablers for innovation and competitiveness in the bio-based economy(Ladu & Quitzow, 2017, Abbasi et al., 2020).

Economic and Environmental Drivers for Sustainable Practices

The shift to sustainable biomanufacturing is driven by both economic and environmental imperatives. Economically, increasing costs of fossil fuels, consumer demand for green products, and the increasing global demand for bio-based products are forcing industries to go -"green"(Yang et al., 2021, Abbasi et al., 2019). Long-term in-service cost can be reduced by sustainable manufacturing approaches, such as energy saving techniques, minimizing waste and benefits from green financing and incentive, e.g. carbon credit and sustainability linked loan. In environmental terms, the growing problems of climate change, loss of biodiversity and pollution have given further emphasis to the need for cleaner production systems. Biomanufacturing provides a means to mitigate these issues through lower carbon emissions, reduced material usage, and circular economy(Clomburg et al., 2017a; Leong et al., 2021). Regulatory impact is also a major driver as the global ecosystem of governments and international institutions are responsive with reinforced environmental standards and incentives to adopt eco-innovation(Achmad et al., 2023). Furthermore, eco-friendly activities also improve brand image, supply chain stability and help develop new sectors in the green market. These economic and environmental drivers combine to make a compelling argument for a shift away from traditional, extractive models toward more sustainable, regenerative models of biomanufacturing.

PRINCIPLES OF GREEN BIOMANUFACTURING

Green biomanufacturing denotes sustainable design and operation of biological production systems that are both economically affordable and environmentally benign(A. Ali et al., 2024). It puts materials and energy to responsible use to prevent waste, environmental pollution, and ecological degradation. Unlike classic manufacturing, which is generally linear in nature - extract, manufacture, use and discard - green biomanufacturing aims to develop circular systems, in which natural resources are regenerated, and long-term ecological balance is maintained. The underlying principles of green biomanufacturing largely originate from sustainability science and industrial ecology and can be simplified into a few fundamental ideas, (Clomburg et al., 2017b). This chapter considers three critical principles driving most modern green biomanufacturing technologies: (1) minimizing waste by leveraging circular economy approaches, (2) energy efficiency and adoption of renewable energy sources, and (3) biodegradability and the use of life cycle assessments (LCA) to direct environmental decision-making.

Waste Reduction and Circular Economy Approaches

Waste reduction is one of the key features of green biomanufacturing and it is in direct accordance with the objectives of the circular economy. Linear industrial models often lead to large piles of waste, a lot of which constitutes toxic, non-reusable waste, or waste that can only be dumped in seas or river rocks or can simply be trashed. Green biomanufacturing, on the other hand, used systems approach to eliminate the waste by designing the product and optimizing the process, and to make use of the by-products(Rangel et al., 2020). Waste reduction is one of the most important methods and is accomplished through biomass valorization, a process in which agricultural residues, food waste and other nonutilized organic sources are converted into valuable products that include biofuels, bioplastics and fine specialty chemicals. As an example, lignocellulosic biomass such as crop residues and byproducts of the forestry industry can be converted into fermentable sugars and then processed into bio-based ethanol to displace production from petroleum-based fuels as well as limit agricultural waste. Industrial symbiosis is another vital waste reducing practice wherein the waste byproducts of one biomanufacturing site is used as a feedstock of another(Rangel et al., 2020). This model has been realized in eco-industrial parks, namely within the Kalundborg in Denmark, where several industries are using steam, water and organic waste in a co-dependent manner. These collaborations help realize increased material efficiency and decreased emissions and waste emissions generally. Furthermore, biological and enzymatic processes are utilized to transform the low-value or polluting waste into valuable products. For instance, some bacterial strains have the ability to use crude glycerol as carbon source for the synthesis of value-added products such as 1,3-propanediol or biopolymers(Garlapati et al., 2016). Process intensification is the other driving motivation for waste minimization in green biomanufacturing, which utilizes processes that feature fewer unit operations, input of energy and raw materials. By integrating processes or by replacing currently batch-wise working equipment with continuous systems many industries can greatly reduce their adverse environmental impact. Moreover, process integration approaches such as recycle of process water, recovery of solvents, and direct on-site treatment of effluent water have been developed to reduce the amount of waste emissions. Novel technologies, such as membrane filtration, anaerobic digestion, and bio-electrochemical systems are, increasingly being utilized for the treatment of wastewater and production of valuable nutrients or energy(Madondo et al., 2023). In a circular economy, products are also designed for end-of-life. Bioengineered products such as bioplastics are now also designed to be recyclable, compostable, or biodegradable. These systems make it possible for them to re-enter a production cycle via mechanical recycling, biodegradation or incineration with energy recovery. To summarize, green biomanufacturing encompasses waste minimization, resource efficiency and closed loop systems, and accordingly, it represents the practicization of circular economy in the bioeconomy(Halim-Lim et al., 2025).

Energy Efficiency and Renewable Energy Integration

The second fundamental principle of green biomanufacturing refers to energy efficiency and the use of renewable forms of energy. Industrial process energy represents one of the largest sources of greenhouse gas (GHG) emissions and climate change(Worrell et al., 2018). In conventional manufacturing, these processes typically run on fossil fuels, which use up natural resources and release carbon dioxide and other emissions. Green biomanufacturing aims at making biomanufacturing far less energy-intensive than it currently is, by streamlining process designs, by capturing waste heat, and by using low-carbon or carbon-neutral energy sources(Kurt et al., 2023). The first step towards energy efficiency is energy-intelligent process design. This also involves the choice of biological systems being conducted on the ambient temperature scales, making the heating or cooling process less frequent. Enzyme-facilitated reactions, for example, can occur at modest temperatures and pressure, unlike chemical catalysts that necessitate harsh conditions(Armstrong, 1987). Likewise, if thermochemical synthesis routes are compared to the energy consuming microbial fermentation processes. Efforts towards developing microbial strains with increased substrate uptake rates or product yields, also lead to lower energy use per unit of product.

Even more energy-efficient bioreactor concepts are under development. Technologies like airlift bioreactors, membrane bioreactors and photo bioreactors are customized for the product pathway and the microbe demand, which reduce mix or aeration which requires large energy input. What's more, process control systems employing real-time sensors and by process learning algorithms can automatically adjust operating settings, such as pH, temperature, and nutrient feed rates, in real time to effectively keeps the system optimized. By minimizing transients and operating steadily, such systems avoid waste of energy. The use of renewable energy sources within biomanufacturer also further establish an important strategy. Power Towards sustainability. Buildings can be powered with photovoltaics, wind turbines, and biomass generated power yielding near zero carbon emissions. Anaerobic digesters, for example, turn organic waste into biogas, which can be burned to produce power or heat for fermentation tanks and distillation columns. That negates that amount of fossil fuel used and provides a second income in energy production. Algae-based biomanufacturing, phototrophic cultivation as applied in the production of algae uses sunlight as the main input of energy for biomass formation, which constitutes a direct replacement of inputs of fossil origin for renewable ones(Mahmood et al., 2023).

An additional enabling trend is the link of CCU with biomanufacturing. In such a model, CO_2 from energy generation or industrial activities is trapped and put into microbial systems that can transform it into useful products, such as organic acids, alcohols, or polymers. The Lanza Tech example of circular carbon economy technologies is an example of one such process, where renewable power and CO_2 feedstocks are combined into a single pathway. Government and institutional backing also helps to push energy efficiency and renewables use. Price supports energy, incentives for carbon pricing, and tax policy encourage industries to transform and invest in clean energy technology. In addition, green designations and environmental data frameworks, like the ISO 50001 energy management system, drive organizations to track and make reductions in their energy consumption on an ongoing basis(Marimon & Casadesús, 2017). Finally, there are other reasons to integrate energy efficiency and renewable energy into biomanufacturing, such as decreasing the environmental footprint of this industry and increasing its economic competitiveness by minimizing the amount of fossil fuel it requires and lowering the exposure to fluctuating costs of those fuels. These strategies will be crucial to secure the long-term sustainability of the bioeconomy as global demand for energy rises and climate targets tighten(Gawel et al., 2019).

Biodegradability and Lifecycle Assessment (LCA)

The green biomanufacturing foundations pave the path for a sustainable future industry that wed technology to the environment. Waste minimization under circular economy means materials and energy are reused, recycled or recovered, rather than being lost by waste. Energy saving and renewable energy sources could radically reduce the carbon footprint of production processes and the need for finite fossil resources. Lastly, through an emphasis on biodegradability and a detailed life-cycle analysis, green biomanufacturing minimizes its environmental impacts throughout the value chain(S. S. Ali et al., 2022). Taken together, these principles allow industries to meet changing environmental requirements, while also becoming more sustainable and more marketable, and yet more socially responsible. As the world goes to decarbonization and circularity, these principles are paramount to the development and success of the bio-based economy (Figure 1).

Figure 1. Strategies for promoting sustainable product development, including waste minimization, energy conservation, use of biodegradable materials, and life cycle assessment. These practices aim to reduce environmental impacts by incorporating circular economy principles, renewable energy sources, and comprehensive evaluation throughout the value chain

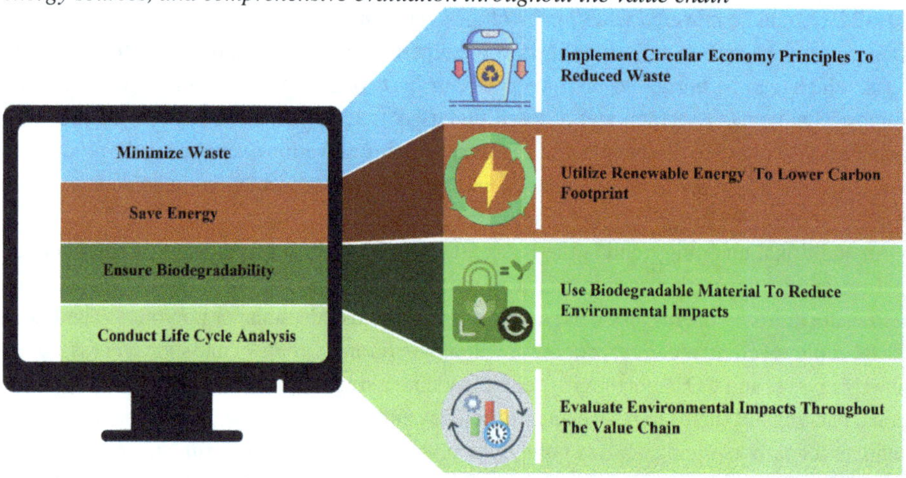

KEY GREEN TECHNOLOGIES IN BIOMANUFACTURING

Green biomanufacturing is at the confluence of environmental sustainability and industrial biotechnology(Shokoohi & Attar, 2024b). The goal of this property is to generate products (including biofuels, bioplastics, pharmaceuticals, and chemicals) in ways that have low ecological footprints and be as efficient as possible. This can be accomplished by incorporating advanced, sustainable technologies based on biological organisms. These technologies have been identified as the most disruptive: microbial and cell-free fermentation, enzymatic biocatalysis, photosynthesis- and plant-based bioproduction, and synthetic biology(Singla, 2020). Collectively, they constitute the bedrock of modern green biomanufacturing with disparate yet complementary routes toward cleaner, safer and more efficient industrial processes

Microbial Fermentation Technology

Microbial fermentation is one of the most established and versatile green technologies in biomanufacturing, utilizing microorganisms such as bacteria, fungi, and yeast to convert renewable feedstocks into bio-based products. Traditional fermentation has long been used in food and beverages, but modern industrial applications extend to antibiotics, vaccines, amino acids, vitamins, enzymes, organic acids, and biofuels (Liao et al., 2016). In recent years, microbial fermentation has been harnessed for the production of biodegradable plastics, such as polylactic acid (PLA) and polyhydroxyalkanoates (PHA), which provide sustainable alternatives to petroleum-derived plastics (Chen & Jiang, 2018). Operating under mild temperature and pH conditions, fermentation processes reduce energy demand and minimize hazardous byproducts, aligning with green chemistry principles (Choi et al., 2020). Additionally, metabolic engineering has enhanced microbial strains for improved stress tolerance and substrate utilization, further increasing process efficiency (Lee et al., 2019). Importantly, fermentation can valorize agricultural residues and lignocellulosic biomass, contributing to circular economy models that transform waste streams into valuable resources (Li et al., 2022). Thus, microbial fermentation remains a cornerstone of green biomanufacturing, combining eco-efficiency, renewability, and industrial scalability.

Metabolic Engineering and Synthetic Biology

Metabolic engineering and synthetic biology represent cutting-edge approaches that enable the rational redesign of microbial metabolism for the efficient production of pharmaceuticals, fuels, and fine chemicals. Unlike traditional fermentation, which relies on the natural metabolic state of microorganisms, metabolic engineering employs genetic modifications such as CRISPR/Cas9 editing, gene knockouts, and pathway optimization to redirect cellular fluxes toward target metabolites (Nielsen & Keasling, 2016). Synthetic biology extends this concept further by introducing standardized biological parts, modular circuits, and de novo pathway construction to build synthetic cell factories (Way et al., 2014). Applications range from microbial synthesis of amino acids (e.g., lysine, glutamate) and vitamins, to high-value pharmaceuticals such as artemisinin and insulin (Keasling, 2017). These technologies also enable sustainable production of biofuels, bioplastics, and natural pigments (Silverman & Karim, 2020). Importantly, metabolic engineering and synthetic biology contribute to green manufacturing by improving yields, reducing toxic byproducts, and enabling the use of renewable carbon sources such as glucose, glycerol, and CO_2 (Zhou et al., 2021). The integration of computational tools, high-throughput screening, and machine learning has accelerated the design–build–test–learn cycle, bringing microbial engineering closer to industrial deployment (Carbonell et al., 2018). Collectively, these technologies provide precision, scalability, and sustainability, making them essential drivers of the bioeconomy.

Cell-Free Biomanufacturing

Cell-free biomanufacturing is an emerging technology that eliminates the constraints of living cells by using cell extracts or purified enzymes to perform biosynthetic reactions in vitro. Unlike microbial fermentation or metabolic engineering, which are limited by cell viability and regulation, cell-free systems allow full control over reaction conditions, enabling higher yields, rapid prototyping, and tolerance to toxic intermediates (Swartz, 2012). These systems are particularly suited for testing synthetic pathways, producing pharmaceuticals, and generating proteins that are otherwise unstable or toxic to host cells (Silverman et al., 2020). One notable example is the on-demand production of vaccines and therapeutic proteins, which has demonstrated significant potential for deployment in remote or resource-limited settings (Hodgman & Jewett, 2012). Cell-free systems also enable multi-enzyme cascade reactions, reducing solvent use and intermediate purification steps, thereby saving time and resources (Kay & Jewett, 2015). Advances in enzyme stabilization, energy regeneration systems, and cell-free extract preparation have made these approaches increasingly scalable for industrial applications (Karim & Jewett, 2016). From a green chemistry standpoint, cell-free biomanufacturing is resource-efficient, requiring less energy, water, and nutrients than traditional cell-based processes while generating fewer byproducts.

This positions it as a complementary technology to microbial fermentation and biocatalysis, accelerating the transition toward sustainable industrial biotechnology.

Enzyme-Based Biocatalysis for Sustainable Synthesis

Biocatalysis with enzymes is another important green technology in biomanufacturing, providing an environmentally friendly alternative to conventional chemical catalysts. Enzymes are nature's catalysts exquisitely specific, efficient and biodegradable(Buller et al., 2023). They have gained immense application in industries owing to their capability of catalysing a wide range of reactions under Eco compatible conditions. Enzymes, in contrast to typical catalysts which often work at high temperature, high pressure, and in toxic solvents, work well at the mild temperature and pH that typify water and thus reduce the energy demand and chemical hazards associated with the process. Enzyme catalysis Reaction selectivity is one of the most important benefits of enzyme catalysis. The regioselectivity, chemo selectivity, and stereoselectivity of enzymes is particularly important in the synthesis of drugs, where impurities in a product cannot be tolerated. Such selectivity diminishes reliance on elaborate separation protocols, limits the production of side-products, and enhances overall product yield. Enzymes such as lipases, transaminases, and oxidoreductases are, e.g., widely applied in active pharmaceutical ingredient (API) synthesis, flavor, fragrances, and fine chemicals production(Meghwanshi et al., 2020). Enzymes also can facilitate cascade reactions, where multistep enzymatic transformations take place in the same reactor with no intermediate purification. This lowers use of solvent, process time, and waste. Biocatalysis can usually be fitted into current manufacturing facilities and is a readily adoptable component of greener manufacturing processes for companies wanting to minimize their impact(Sheldon & Brady, 2022). In addition, protein engineering and directed evolution have considerably broadened the potential of enzymes by increasing their stability, activity, and substrate specificity. Enzyme immobilization to enable their re-use through multiple reaction cycles further improves the cost effectiveness and environmental friendliness of the enzymes. From the environmental point of view, the enzyme-mediated biocatalysis follows the green chemistry concepts such as atom economy, little or no derivation and renewable feedstock. Enzymes also help to substitute hazardous substances in bleaching, desizing, cleaning etc processes in industries, such as textile, paper, detergent etc. For example, the textile industry employs cellulases and amylases which eliminates starches while promoting the manufacture of higher-quality fabrics but without using harmful chemicals. The enzyme-based biocatalysis represents the essence of the guiding principles for green biomanufacturing: efficiency, specificity, and environmental friendliness. On-going developments in enzyme engineering and reductions in costs may lead to an increasing application of biocatalysis in many other industrial areas(Wu et al., 2021). Enzyme-based biocatalysis has become a cornerstone of green biomanufacturing, offering high selectivity, efficiency, and environmental compatibility compared to conventional chemical catalysts (Table 1)

Table 1. Real-time examples of enzyme-based biocatalysis: applications, performance techniques, and outcomes

Enzyme	Application	Performance Technique	Results	Reference
Lipase (*Candida antarctica*)	Synthesis of chiral intermediates for pharmaceuticals	Immobilization on silica, protein engineering	High enantioselectivity, >95% yield	Meghwanshi et al. (2020)
Transaminase	Production of optically pure amines for drug synthesis	Directed evolution for substrate specificity	Production of enantiopure amines with >98% ee	Sheldon & Brady (2022)
Oxidoreductase (Alcohol dehydrogenase)	Conversion of alcohols to aldehydes/ketones in fine chemicals	Cofactor recycling systems (NADH/NADPH)	Selective oxidation under mild conditions	Wu et al. (2021)
Cellulase	Textile biopolishing, paper pulping	Immobilization, synergistic enzyme cocktails	Eco-friendly textile finishing, reduced chemical usage	Buller et al. (2023)
Amylase	Starch hydrolysis in food and textile industries	Thermostabilization by protein engineering	Efficient starch hydrolysis, energy saving	Wu et al. (2021)

Algae and Plant-Based Bioproduction

Algae and plants present bioproduction systems promising for the sustainable production of fuels, chemicals, nutraceuticals, and high-value biomolecules using sunlight, CO_2, and water as nutrients and biosynthesis driving force(Yadav et al., 2021). These photosynthetic biomanufacturing systems have excellent prospects about the decarbonization of economies and resource regeneration. microalgae are highly efficient in converting solar energy into biomass and can, therefore, be grown on non-arable lands using wastewater or brackish water and do not displace food crops and freshwater resources. The microalgae *Chlorella, Spirulina*, and *Nannochloropsis* produce lipids as feedstock for biodiesel, proteins as animal feeds, pigments, for example, astaxanthin, and premium human nutrition, for example, antioxidants such as omega-3 fatty acids. microalgae are also highly effective as carbon dioxide capture and bioremediation options due to their rapid growth and high nutrient acquisition efficiency. They can be cultivated on a large scale in either open pond systems or closed, artificially lighted photobioreactors with minimum inputs compared to outputs. Cultivation of algae with other industrial processes such as aeration of flue gases for carbon dioxide could lead to near-zero emissions and enable circular industrial ecology(Paul *et al.*, 2021). Similarly, plant-based compact biomanufacturing, known as molecular farming, employs genetically modified crops such as tobacco or plant cell systems to create more complex proteins, enzymes, and secondary metabolites. These methods are particularly promising for the very low-cost production of therapeutic proteins such as antibodies, vaccines, and enzymes. For instance, growing tobacco plants modified to produce monoclonal antibodies was instrumental in the production of ZMapp, an experimental treatment for the Ebola virus. The risks of infection with human pathogens are significantly lower with plant-based transient expression systems. They are also much faster and simple to scale up than traditional fermentation-based systems (Figure 2). Finally, environmentally friendly and relatively easily biodegradable and low toxicity to humans and the environment products are obtained from algae and plants. Plant biomass can be converted into bioenergy, and algae can be composted after harvesting, making these systems almost perfectly circular in the biorefinery model. While there are still challenges, especially regarding photosynthesis efficiency optimization, genetic engineering complexity and costs scale, the advances in synthetic biology and controlled environment farming are addressing those and many other issues. Thus, biosynthetic products from algae and plant-based systems have enormous potential as sustainable carbon-negative biomanufacturing options, which bode well for achieving global climate and resource recovery goals (Khalid *et al.,* 2020).

Figure 2. Unlock the potential of algal and plant-based bioproduction by harnessing sustainable resources, carbon capture, and circular economy benefits while proactively addressing photo-synthetic efficiency, genetic complexity, and scaling hurdles

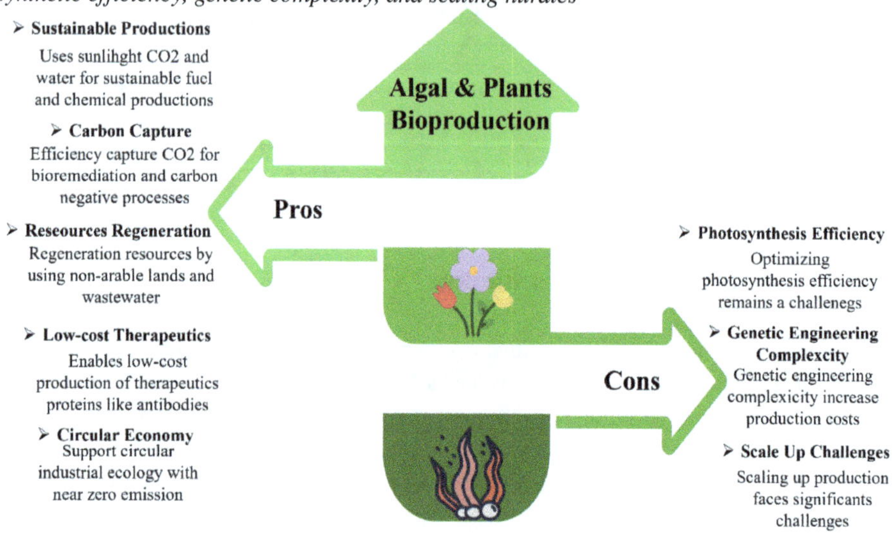

Synthetic Biology for Eco-Friendly Process Optimization

Synthetic biology represents a paradigm shift in green biomanufacturing, enabling the rational engineering of biological systems for improved sustainability and efficiency of production. It is more than simple genetic engineering since it places a range of these standard parts together, can create entirely new pathways and custom microbes for various applications. Using synthetic biology, we can now program cells to convert renewable feedstocks such as agricultural waste, CO 2 or even plastics into desirable products, with high specificity and low waste. Metabolic pathway optimization is the most influential contribution of synthetic biology toward sustainability(Agapakis et al., 2012). Synthetic pathways, a bypass for flow of cellular metabolism to the desired merchandise can be generated, with high productivity and yield. For instance, engineered design of *Escherichia coli* and yeast strains has been accomplished to produce chemicals such as isobutanol, artemisinin and lactic acid with industrial application. Often these alien producers grow faster than the native producers, are more tolerant to toxic intermediates or resources efficient. Synthetic biology enables the development of biosensor designs and dynamic control devices. By wiring genetic circuits to environmental sensors (e.g., pH, oxygen and metabolite concentration), microorganisms as production systems can behave in an auto-regulatory manner, tuning their response to maximize yields and minimizing the need for energy and resources. This leads to self-optimizing bioprocesses with less intervention and less process variability and regularity. Why not create enzyme cascades that use substrates and cofactors later oxidized to fluorescent or luminescent molecules? And synthetic biology outside the cell, where synthetic pathways run extracellularly, enables rapid prototyping and safer production, particularly in pharma. Synthetic biology for eco-friendly process optimization also involves the reduction in toxic intermediates and solvents, construction of microbial consortia for complex transformations and utilization of minimal genome strains to alleviate metabolic load and waste generation(Qumsani, 2024). To this end E. coli have been engineered which have been crippled in terms of non-essential genes so that more of the cellular resources are channelled into product formation. Furthermore, CRISPR and genome-scale metabolic modeling have greatly increased the speed and accuracy of strain design, rendering synthetic biology an indispensable tool in green manufacturing(Zeng et al., 2022). Synthetic biology can also promote life cycle thinking by enabling design-for-degradation or the design of products that are engineered to degrade safely after use or design-for-reuse, which allows for the reutilization of microbes or enzymes across production batches. These concepts improve circularity and bring synthetic biology in line with green chemistry and sustainability. However, ethical, regulatory and biosafety challenges need to be overcome for responsible application in the future. Nevertheless, synthetic biology has the unique power to transform biomanufacturing into a cleaner, smarter, and more sustainable industry, providing scalable solutions to some of the biggest environmental problems facing the planet.

INDUSTRIAL APPLICATIONS

The industrial importance of green biomanufacturing has seen a considerable increase over the last 10 years due to advances in biotechnology, synthetic biology, green chemistry, and a market demand shift toward sustainability. This green biomanufacturing technology is no long be limited to the lab or the pilot plant but had been widespread across various segments of the world economy, for this can provide us with a green and sustainable alternative economically compared to the traditional manufacture. In sectors that historically have leaned on fossils, biomanufacturing is under exploration or being applied for its capacity to lower emissions, reduce energy use and supply products that are biodegradable or renewable such as: QUICKLY biomanufacturing is being applied in sectors that in the past have leaned heavily on fossils because of its ability to cut emissions, lower energy use and supply products that are biodegradable or are renewable. This chapter presents major industrial applications across four important sectors, including (1) pharmaceutical and nutraceutical development, (2) biofuels and renewable chemicals, (3) sustainable packaging and bio-based materials, and (4) waste valorization with byproduct utilization. These applications also show economic viability of green biomanufacturing in each of these regions and how biomanufacturing contributes to global sustainability efforts(Shokoohi & Attar, 2024c).

Pharmaceutical and Nutraceutical Production

Pharmaceutical and nutraceutical industries is one of the major transformative agents of green biomanufacturing where biotechnology-based strategies have been used for the development of efficient, safe, and environmentally friendly manufacturing systems(Süntar et al., 2021). Classical drug synthesis often includes complicated multi-step chemical routes which need intense energy and toxic solvents and heavy metal catalysts. Biomanufacturing, on the other hand, uses microbial and enzymatic systems for making active pharmaceutical ingredients (APIs), vaccines and health supplements, under gentle and environmentally friendly conditions. The transition has diminished not only the environmental footprint, but reaction selectivity, product yield and process safety. One of the milestones is microbial production of artemisinin, a key anti-malarial drug. Derived from the plant sweet wormwood (Artemisia annua), extraction of artemisinin is season-sensitive, land-demanding and not reliably efficient. By way of synthetic biology, they converted Saccharomyces cerevisiae to produce the artemisinin precursor artemisinin acid at scale in a fermentable process. Developed and widely licensed to Sanofi in collaboration with PATH and Amyris, this technology represented a significant advancement in bio-based pharmaceutical production, providing an economical and consistent process with a low environmental burden.

Recombinant DNA technology has also turned around vaccine and insulin manufacture. Instead of isolating insulin from animal pancreases, contemporary green biomanufacturing relies on genetically modified strains of *E. coli* or yeast to ferment human insulin a method that is both more ethical and scalable, and more resource-efficient. What's more, companies including Medicago and Greenovation Biotech are using plant-based expression systems that is, growing genetically altered tobacco or moss to make vaccines and monoclonal antibodies, which need far less water, energy and infrastructure than mammalian cell cultures(Jadhav & Khare, 2024). Within the nutraceutical industry, biomanufacturing is producing omega-3 fatty acids, antioxidants such as astaxanthin, and amino acids, such as L-glutamine, which are crucial for the health and wellness sectors. The microalgae, including *Schizochytrium and Haematococcus* species, are grown in tailored bioreactors to produce these substances in an economically viable and environmentally friendly manner, and avoid the need to use marine resources from which fish oil is extracted. In a world of increasing consumer preference for clean label, plant-based, and environmentally friendly products, green biomanufacturing is ready to drive the pharmaceutical and nutraceutical supply chain of the future.

Biofuels and Renewable Chemicals

Biofuels and renewable chemicals are among the first, and most huge, utilizations of green biomanufacturing. With the world being challenged by decreasing dependence on fossil fuel and reduced CO2 emission, bio-based energy from bioethanol, biodiesel and biogas have been highlighted significantly. Depending on the nature of the bioethanol there are a number of methods to reduce carbon emissions: when sugars extracted from corn, sugar cane or lignocellulose are fermented by micro-organisms, ethanol is created; this can be mixed with petrol to make it a lower-emission fuel. For example, Brazil has been a world leader in sugarcane ethanol for decades and produces almost the entirety of the energy it needs for transportation(Vandenberghe et al., 2022). The enzymatic hydrolysis and Consolidated Bioprocessing (CBP) have made the second-generation biofuels more attractive, using non-food feed stocks such as agriculture or forestry waste(Olguin-Maciel et al., 2020). Other companies, such as POET-DSM and Novozymes, have created "one-stop shop" platforms (referred to as "integrated") that do both breakdown cellulose into fermentable sugars and fermentation of those sugars into ethanol with the help of engineered microbes in the mix, which allows for the sidestepping of the tail-chewing over competition with global food supply chains. Aside from fuels, renewable chemicals made through green biomanufacturing are replacing petrochemicals used in plastics, coatings, solvents and industrial intermediates. For example, succinic acid, and intermediate platform chemical for biodegradable polymers can be generated by Actinobacillus succinogenes or engineered E. coli strains. Polylactic acid (PLA), which is produced by microbial fermentation of glucose to lactic acid, can also be used as a form of bioplastic. Leading the charge to build a scalable plant for making biopolymers are global firms such as NatureWorks and Total Corbion. Another success story is in synthetic biology for drop in fuels and specialty chemicals. For example, LanzaTech's gas fermentation platform uses (acetogenic) bacterial strains to turn industrial waste gases (CO, CO_2) into ethanol and other high-value chemicals. Their pilot plants in China and Belgium are a proof of concept that green biomanufacturing can be grafted to heavy industry, doing while so not only reducing harmful emissions, but also creating economic value(Pesch, 2023). These latest advances demonstrate that green biomanufacturing is both an environmental and economic solution in driving the transition toward green, sustainable, and low-carbon energy and materials economy.

Sustainable Packaging and Biomaterials

The packaging and materials industries are at a turning point with increased awareness about plastics pollution, government regulations to ban single use of plastics, and consumer demand for biodegradable options(Barone et al., 2025). In this transition, green biomanufacturing becomes a crucial enabler as it provides us with bio-based, compostable and renewable material alternatives to petrol-based products. These eco-friendly biomaterials have multiple uses across the packaging, construction, textiles and electronics sectors, and are both versatile and environmentally friendly. One leading synthesized biomaterial is polylactic acid (PLA), a biodegradable thermoplastic produced by fermenting plant sugars. Today, PLA is commonly found in food packaging, disposable cutlery, and is even used as a 3D printing material! It decomposes into water and CO2 in an industrial compost under the ecological chain of life and production. Another prominent example of a bioplastic is polyhydroxyalkanoates (PHAs), Young et al., 2016, obtained intracellularly from bacteria such as, Cupriavidus necator, under environmentally stressful conditions due to high carbon availability. PHAs are completely biodegradable also in terrestrial and marine environments, and this is very important for packaging applications because in this case the risk of dispersion in ecosystems is not negligible(Meereboer et al., 2020).

Apart from plastics, the trend of green biomanufacturing can help to develop 'mycelium packaging', as this uses the root systems of fungi to generate artificial foam — and thus, a Styrofoam alternative. Start-ups like Ecovative have brought these products to market for consumer electronics and protective packaging for fragile vehicles. Lastly other biopolymers such as nanocellulose (derived from plant biomass) are being used in coatings, film and biodegradable composites for packaging and structural applications. A significant example is Danone's introduction of plant-based PET bottles with the MEG component sourced through biomanufacturing from "green" feedstocks. Although it still depends on petrochemical TPA feedstock, such partial bio-based packaging substantially reduces the product's carbon footprint, providing an example of how legacy materials may become greener as a result of bio-based inputs. The dye, adhesive and coating are integrated, reflecting the broadening of the green biomanufacturing domain of green materials. Based on natural sources, such as lignin or microbial pigments, these bioproducts substitute petroleum or even hazardous compounds(Philippini et al., 2020). With the introduction of extended producer responsibility (EPR) laws and more stringent environmental requirements across the globe, sustainable biomaterials for packaging applications have evolved from simply an option for ethical consideration, to a mandated and economic necessity.

Waste Valorization and Byproduct Utilization

The conversion of waste to value is one of the most attractive advantages of green biomanufacturing. The valorization of waste is the reclamation of waste materials that have value for reuse, recycling or recovery into products or materials of value. This is at the core of circular economy logic, which tackles environmental pollution and resource scarcity simultaneously, by closing material cycles and preventing landfilling or incineration. The valorization of glycerol, a byproduct of biodiesel generation, is a case in point. Crude glycerol is hard to get rid of - it's full of impurities - but it's full of carbon and hydrogen. This waste stream, when processed with engineered species (such as *Klebsiella or Clostridium*), can synthesize desirable compounds such as 1,3-propanediol, succinic acid, or biosurfactants. This process saves biodiesel plants in waste management fees, and generates value-added markets from byproducts (carbon dioxide and protein meal). Another appropriate substrate for biomanufacturing valorization is the food waste and agricultural residues. Anaerobic digestion of food waste generates biogas, and, for some forms of digestate, valuable biofertilizer(Sharma et al., 2023). Organic acids, enzymes or bioethanol production comes from fruit peel or dairy waste fermentation. More and more startups and research institutions are turning to urban waste-to-biofactory models where even their neighborhood waste streams are used to produce goods that can value from smart city and zero-waste programs.

Another potential is the brewery and distillery industry, with its significant amounts of spent grain and yeast. Spent-grain fiber and protein content can be significantly targeted via enzymatic treatment into a variety of feed products, biodegradable films, or even into bioplastics(Karlsen & Skov, 2022). Spent yeast biomass as well can be converted to nutraceuticals or bio-flavor. For example, green biomanufacturing is being considered by AB InBev and other multinational beverages producers to be included in the supply chain to enhance waste management and sustainability profiles. In the textile industry, cotton and synthetic fiber waste blends are being enzymatically treated to recover cellulose or polyester for reuse, which has big potential in reducing the massive landfill tip-fee of this industry. (Kumar & Verma, 2024). Taking a different perspective of waste one in which it is seen not as an end waste stream but as feedstock the use of waste to make materials and products opens new value chains, mitigates environmental degradation and harmonizes industries with the objectives of the circular economy. These developments don't just reduce cost and cut carbon; they also create new markets for bio-based products once thrown out with the trash.

ECONOMIC AND REGULATORY CONSIDERATIONS

Green manufacturing transitions from a niche to mainstream industrial practice, its economic reality and regulatory placement have gained concomitant importance. The case for environmentally sound and ethical manufacturing is clear, but the pace and extent of uptake of such green technologies are shaped by economic and policy contexts, which impact strategies (when, how and where) that industries pursue. Cost and risk considerations, but often more specifically ROI, competitive market positioning become critical drivers of the ERO. But it is public policy and regulatory incentives that are equally important in the acceleration, or set back, of greener biomanufacturing methods. Specifically, the chapter discusses the economics behind green biomanufacturing from the perspective of cost-benefit analysis, compares global and national policies created to drive sustainable practice at every level of green manufacturing, and presents key barriers that must be surmounted to achieve success in terms of scale-up of green technologies from pilot to commercial scale

Cost-Benefit Analysis of Green Biomanufacturing

Green biomanufacturing, once increasingly encouraged due to its environmental benefits, needs to be economically powerful enough to be adopted by the whole industry. A clear cost/benefit analysis is therefore necessary to determine the trade-offs, the payback, and the economic sustainability of these new technologies versus traditional manufacturing processes. Typical green biomanufacturing costs are related to research and development (R&D), CAPEX on new or retrofit facilities or infrastructure, feedstock (especially if advanced or engineered organisms are employed), along with OPEX covering maintenance, energy, labor, and compliance costs. Nonetheless, the long-term operational savings and the various environmental and market-related advantages can often justify these up-front investments. Resource efficiency is one of the most important economic benefits of green biomanufacturing. In many cases, these processes need less water, less toxic solvents and less energy than chemical syntheses. This reduces both ongoing utility bills, as well as expenses associated with waste treatment, emission control and hazardous material disposal. Furthermore, the potential to work with renewable or waste feed-stocks including agricultural residues, glycerol, and carbonaceous flue gases results in a lower input cost and new revenue sources through waste spinalization(Manara & Zabaniotou, 2016).

Market differentiation is another important economic factor. Consumers, investors, regulators all want a more environmental products Companies that can churn our products via 'green bio-manufacturing' can charge a premium, develop deeper brand loyalty and limit potential liabilities. The increasing demand for certified biodegradability, non-toxic and carbon neutral products provides a case for investment in sustainability. For instance, bioplastics such as PLA and PHA are likely to command a premium over traditional plastics because they are environmentally sound, especially in markets that are mandated or have implemented bans on conventional plastics(K-ourmentza et al., 2020). Passing over the direct financial return, the indirect and immeasurable return is huge. These range from improved employee engagement, stronger community relations, futureproofing against stricter regulations, and access to green financing or sustainability-linked loans. A powerful cost-benefit criterion is not merely based on profit and loss calculations, but also on life cycle costs, internalization of environmental externalities, and the congruence with long-term goals. The economic viability of green biomanufacturing is however subject dependent. For low-resource or developing countries, the high initial investment of capital, as well as a lack of infrastructure, may prevent widespread use without policy backing or external funding. Accordingly, economic analysis should be localized to the sector, the geography and the technology, and would consider the cost for short term and the longer term ("cost horizons").

Policy Frameworks and Incentives for Sustainable Practices

Green biomanufacturing is strongly facilitated by policy frames and government incentives(Love et al., 2025). Because systemic changes are needed for the transition from fossil to bio-based industries, public intervention may be called for to compensate for market failures, to provide financial support, and to establish sustainability criteria. Governments worldwide are beginning to perceive the potential of the bioeconomy as strategic and are designing legislation to stimulate research, commercialization, and adoption of green biomanufacturing technologies. At an international level, the likes of the Paris Climate Accord and the United Nations Sustainable Development Goals (SDGs) offer top-down goals to encourage countries to decarbonize their industries. Several countries have in turn formulated their own national bioeconomy strategies. For example, the European Union: created the EU Bioeconomy Strategy and Green Deal, promoting sustainable use of biomass, eco-innovations, and the biorefineries creation(Woźniak et al., 2021). Money from programs such as Horizon Europe and the European Innovation Council are made available for biomanufacturing projects relating to climate action and resource efficiency. Such bioenergy, carbon capture, and rural biomanufacturing infrastructure is provided for in the US by the Inflation Reduction Act (IRA) and Farm Bill. Federal grants and tax incentives also are available for biobased innovations from agencies such as the Department of Energy (DOE), National Science Foundation (NSF), and Department of Agriculture (USDA). State-based programs including California's Low Carbon Fuel Standard (LCFS) and New York's Green Bank also encourage investment in sustainable technology .Incentives play a crucial role in promoting the adoption of green biomanufacturing by creating favorable economic conditions that encourage sustainable practices. Governments and regulatory bodies often provide tax credits to companies that utilize renewable feedstocks or produce biodegradable goods, thereby reducing production costs and stimulating eco-friendly innovation. Similarly, feed-in tariffs and subsidies for bioenergy production make renewable energy more financially attractive compared to fossil fuels. Carbon pricing and cap-and-trade schemes further enhance the competitiveness of green alternatives by internalizing the environmental costs of conventional manufacturing. Additionally, loan guarantees and venture funding serve as vital financial instruments to support bio-based startups, helping them overcome high initial capital requirements. At the policy level, green procurement programs strengthen market demand by prioritizing biomanufactured goods in public sector purchasing. Collectively, these incentives not only accelerate industrial transition toward greener technologies but also ensure long-term sustainability and competitiveness in biomanufacturing.

Additionally, regulatory harmonization and standardization are essential. Certification systems like ISO 14001 (Environmental Management Systems)(Massoud et al., 2010), USDA Certified Biobased Product Label, and Ecolabel EU help define quality and sustainability benchmarks, providing credibility and market access for green products(Rossi et al., 2024). Without these standards, industries may face barriers in international trade or consumer trust. However, policy effectiveness depends on proper implementation, enforcement, and integration across sectors. Fragmented or inconsistent policies can undermine investor confidence and delay technological diffusion. Therefore, governments must coordinate regulatory instruments, remove contradictory subsidies (e.g., for fossil fuels), and ensure long-term stability to foster green industrial transformation.

Challenges in Scaling Up Green Technologies

Challenges and opportunities for scaling of green biomanufacturing processes While there is great potential and ongoing progress in development of green biomanufacturing technologies, scaling technologies from lab or bench scale to full scale industrial operations remains a significant limitation. Numerous green technologies have proven to be extremely efficient and beneficial for the environment at the small scale; however, they are faced with technical, financial and logistical challenges when scaled up to production levels(Song et al., 2019). These are fundamental challenges that need to be solved in general for large scale deployment. One of the most challenging issues is the complexity of the process. Biomanufacturing is comprised of living organisms or highly intricate biochemical dynamics reacting to temperature, pH, oxygen and other environmental factors(Wang et al., 2024). These operations require high-degree process control, in-line monitoring, advanced real-time measurement and good bioreactor up/downstream integration. Small impurities can be responsible for reducing yield, contamination or complete batch loss. Because of these complexities, scaling up is riskier and more expensive than traditional chemical manufacturing. Another obstacle is capital intensity. These costs can be in the hundreds of millions of dollars for large-scale fermentation infrastructure, bioreactor systems, purification units and biomass preprocessing. GREEN REFINERIES Unlike mature petrochemical refineries, green biomanufacturing facilities do not have established supply chains and will have to construct logistics of feedstock collection, preprocessing and storage. In addition to high upfront costs (which can, however, vary wildly depending on the resource to be developed) the economy of returns is also often cited as a discouraging factor to take the plunge. Public funding and VC investments have done much to get there, but scaling up over time often requires the backing of dedicated capital and alliances with big industry players.

Variability of feedstock and supply chain constraints are furthermore challenging(Yue et al., 2014). The composition, source and quality of agricultural waste residues, algae or waste are different during the season, geography and its method of processing(Koul et al., 2022). This variability also influences processing uniformity and the quality of processed materials, necessitating adaptable systems along with advanced pretreatment techniques. Additionally, biomass logistics could be costly, including transportation, drying, and storage, especially in remote and less developed areas. Regulatory and permitting obstacles can also slow or complicate scale-up. Large-scale biomanufacturing operations may require environmental-impact studies, water-use permits, emissions-control technology, and biosafety approval just to get through the front doors of a processing plant. These legislative requirements, while vital, increase deployment time and cost. In addition, absence of policies related to synthetic biology or GMOs in some countries has also limited commercialization(Anyshchenko & Yarnold, 2021).

Another underappreciated problem is workforce constraints. Biomanufacturing facilities require expert staff in molecular biology, process engineering, data science and environmental management(Shokoohi & Attar, 2024d). There are also few regions with training programs or a talent pool that could fuel mass biomanufacturing. This disparity can delay the time to deployment and add to the operational risk. Finally, there is the question of market acceptance and consumer education. Even with environmentally responsible products, consumers might think twice about switching to new bio-based substitutes that they are not familiar with to because their performance and price seem different from what they are used to. That's especially crucial in some markets--like packaging, food, and pharmaceuticals--where trust and compliance are critical. A multi-faceted approach is required to address these scale-up challenges. Risk sharing and infrastructure sharing can be realized by means of public-private partnerships, long-term financing instruments, innovation hubs, and integrated bioclusters(Srivastav et al., 2024). R&D is crucial and should be continued not only for discovery, but for scale-up technologies (modular bioreactors, advanced fermentation systems, automation tools). Flexible feedstock-agnostic platforms can also help mitigate the variation in raw materials. Finally, the clarity of regulations, public education and the development of talents are part of an effective scaling strategy.

FUTURE TRENDS AND INNOVATIONS

Due to increasing global challenges for sustainability and the transition of industrial processes towards low-carbon, resource-efficient production, green biomanufacturing is expected to play a central role as a driver of the bioeconomy. The future of this industry will be redefined by next-level technology and further integration of digital with bio and systems engineering. Especially in green biomanufacturing, we are in the business of leveraging intelligent, real-time, analytics, precision engineering to develop smarter, scalable, and more adaptable bioprocesses. Historical trends suggest that AI (artificial intelligence), advanced reactor design, and market globalization will be prominent elements of the next generation of green biomanufacturing. In this chapter, the authors provide a perspective of the innovation landscape by considering three main areas: The application of AI and machine learning for the optimization of bioprocessing processes(Khanal et al., 2023). The introduction of next-generation bioreactors and continuous manufacturing systems. The anticipated worldwide expansion and market development of green biomanufacturing in the future (Figure 3).

Figure 3. Integration of AI-driven optimization, advanced bioreactors, and global expansion drives the transition from unsustainable, high-carbon bioprocesses toward a low-carbon, efficient, and sustainable bioeconomy

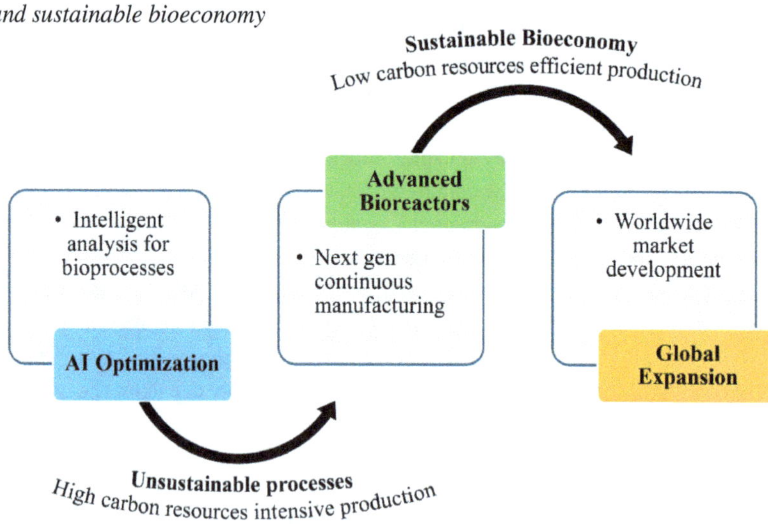

AI and Machine Learning for Process Optimization

AI and ML are going to revolutionize green biomanufacturing by boosting precision, flexibility and predictability in the value chain. Conventional biomanufacturing operations often use fixed recipes, empirical trial and error optimization, and static control systems. AI-enabled systems can, on the other hand, process massive volumes of process data in real-time, find hidden patterns, and continuously repattern parameters for optimal yield, minimal waste, and maximum energy efficiency. Perhaps the greatest benefit that AI can provide to biomanufacturing is in process modeling and optimization. Algorithms from machine learning can be trained on past and present data sets to forecast the favorable conditions for growth of microorganisms, enzyme activities, or metabolite production. This ability is particularly important in industrial high-throughput fermentation systems where dozens of variables including temperature, pH, substrate concentration, oxygen content level and agitation interact in multivariate nonlinear would. AI-based tools like neural networks, decision trees and reinforcement learning algorithms will be better able to pinpoint optimal operating regimes more quickly and accurately than conventional design-of-experiment (DoE) approaches.

AI is also revolutionizing metabolic engineering and strain design. Methods such as deep learning and genetic algorithms have the potential to help researchers identify targets of gene editing, predict pathway bottlenecks, and forecast nonspecific effects. Platforms like Google DeepMind's AlphaFold, which predicts the folding of proteins with uncanny alacrity, are already hastening the discovery and engineering of enzymes for bio-catalysis and synthetic pathways. Together with omics (genomics, transcriptomics, proteomics) data, the AI can be used to generate the digital twins of microbial systems that can be in silico simulated and optimized prior to being tested in the lab scale. In downstream processes, AI also improves predictive maintenance, failure detection, and quality management. Through image recognition systems based on computer vision, contamination factor or abnormal cell morphology can be identified in bioreactors. Anomaly detection applications can be used to identify potential process abnormalities or unconventional equipment conditions, such as vibrations, energy used and flow rates. Finally, AI can aid in supply chain optimization, predicting biomass feedstock availability, energy use, such as transportation energy, or logistics needs due to weather trends, demand patterns, or geopolitical tensions. Examples of AI in action include Siemens' real-time bioprocess monitoring solution "BioPAT" suite and Ginkgo Bioworks' use of ML algorithms in an organism design automation platform. With costs of hardware dropping and computational resources becoming more available, these tools will be used by smaller and mid-size biotech companies as well. AI in the future is expected to be developed into autonomous biomanufacturing, where self-learning algorithms adapt production with input from a user being minimal.

Next-Gen Bioreactors and Continuous Manufacturing

The physical platform of biomanufacturing is changing quickly in response to the needs for greater throughput, more cost-effective production and environmentally friendly operations. Conventional good-old batch bioreactors, undoubtedly robust work horses, however, suffer from the capability as well as in the process stability and time to-market. The emerging development of next-generation bioreactors and the shift towards continuous processing also offers an attractive alternative, resulting in process control in real-time, modular scalability, and much lower footprint and environmental impact. The continuous biomanufacturing process includes continuous upstream and downstream processes such that feed is introduced and product is withdrawn continuously. This contrasts with the batch manufacturing systems where there is set-up time and set-down time associated with every production run, resulting in downtime and reduced productivity. Continuous systems result in higher volumetric productivity, smaller footprint, and tighter process control due to keeping cells or enzymes in their optimal operating conditions. They are particularly suited for high value products like pharmaceuticals, where quality and cleanliness are essential. E.g., advances in perfusion bioreactors, that constantly remove waste and resupply nutrients, have enabled extended viability of cells. So do membrane bioreactors, which separate cells with selective membranes, and allow metabolites to pass by, resulting in the enhancement of product yield but not biomass. Lab on-a-chip systems, microfluidic bioreactors, are a convenient mean for high throughput screening of very small volumes and low consumption of reagents, nearly no waste disposal. These systems are ideal for strain screening, enzyme kinetics and precision fermentation research. The transition to next-gen bioreactors is furthermore in line with the tenets of Industry 4.0, i.e., smart manufacturing, where sensors, data analytics, and cyber-physical systems play a predominant role (33–36). Nowadays, there are bioreactors possessing real-time sensors for pH, dissolved oxygen (DO), biomass density, and metabolite content, and their sensed information are widely input into AI in real-time control. This digital integration adds not just consistency of product, but also regulatory compliance with a traceable and auditable process history.

Modular bioreactor designs, meanwhile, also help the sustainability case by allowing scaling out (adding more units) rather than up (increasing the tank size), which means that they are more suited to localized production or distributed models. Such flexibility is especially advantageous when manufacturing vaccines or specialty chemicals in emerging areas, remote regions, or in emergency response situations, for example, pandemic emergencies. The development of these next-gen systems is being spearheaded by companies such as Cytiva, Sartorius and GE Healthcare. Pfizer has developed a COVID-19 mRNA vaccine with continuous manufacturing processes, illustrating that these processes can be scaled up and employed under accelerated schedules. We anticipate that the future for green biomanufacturing will involve broad dissemination of these systems in which automation, robotics, and AI are integrated to provide the intelligent, sustainable and agile manufacturing systems of the future, enabled on a culture vessel platform.

Global Adoption and Market Growth Projections

Green biomanufacturing is being implemented worldwide at an increasing rate due to the urgency of environmental issues, the potential of new economic opportunities, and supportive policy instruments. With climate change mitigation, resource efficiency and waste reduction taking top priority across countries and industries, green biomanufacturing is a solution that can solve many challenges at once. If current market trends and forecasts are to be believed, growth in all four of the primary areas of the bioeconomy biofuels, bioplastics, bio-based chemicals, pharmaceuticals and other bioactive products and intellectual property will take the bioeconomy to a future of multitrillion-dollar prosperity. GLOBAL BOMANUFACTURING MARKETS Source: Recent market intelligence reports suggests that the biomanufacturing market will hit more than USD1.4 trillion by 2030, in a CAGR across the period of 2023 and 2030 of over 9%. The bioplastics sector alone is projected to exceed USD 65bn by 2028, driven by prohibitions on single-use plastics and consumer appetite for environmentally friendly packaging. The biofuel industry, especially 2nd generation ethanol and biodiesel, is growing as governments set blending targets along with investments in the industrial rural bio-refinery plant. Brazil, India and US are increasingly adopting ethanol blending program, thus driving the market for the scalable biomanufacturing systems.

In pharmaceutical field, local manufacturing, rapid vaccine production, and resiliency of supply chain are encouraging implementation of green biomanufacturing. The rise of personalized medicine and biologics is also driving the need for flexible biomanufacturing that is dispersed and available in Asia-Pacific and Africa. The nutraceutical market comprising bio-based vitamins, probiotics, and functional foods is also up and coming at more than 7% globally as such concerns for health and sustainability come under focus. From a geographic standpoint, North America and Europe dominate in biomanufacturing capacities and R&D. Nevertheless, the Asia-Pacific region is experiencing fastest growth, supported by government regulations, awareness of the environment and investment in bioeconomy projects. On the one hand, the China's "Made in China 2025" plan and India's "National Bio-Energy Mission" are representative of state-led initiatives in green manufacturing sector. Some African countries have also started to invest in bio-based industrial parks, in particular Kenya, Nigeria and South Africa.

The expansion of green biomass production is inseparable from the development of supportive ecosystems (e.g. policy, joint R&D between academia and industry, and infrastructure). Innovation clusters such as BioVale (UK), Biobased Delta (Netherlands), and AgriBio (Australia) are provided as examples of the way in which regional ecosystems can facilitate the adoption of an industrial cluster through integrated networks of producers, researchers, and industry policy makers. But the path to widespread use is not without roadblocks. BARRIERS: Issues including cost competition, perceptions of the public, infrastructure deficiencies and intellectual property (IP) need to be overcome for an inclusive and sustainable expansion to take place. Establishing technology, funding and know how transfer to developing countries will be required to a truly global green biomanufacturing implementation. In the future, the macro-infrastructure for growth will be things like continued investment in synthetic biology and AI, greater access to green finance, alignment of international standards for bio-based products, and tighter global collaboration in climate and sustainability goals. With this growing interest from countries on bio-based economies, green biomanufacturing will be the key in shaping a sustainable, inclusive and socially/environmentally sustainable global future industrial society.

CONCLUSION

Sustainable biomanufacturing is key to a paradigm change in how society conceives of industrial production, from fossil based, linear to bio-based, circular, and environmentally sustainable. In summary, across the various dimensions covered in this chapter it has become clear that green biomanufacturing is more than just a potential remedy for ecological and climate challenges; it is an enabler of innovation, economic development, and industrial durability. At its core, the basic tenets of green biomanufacturing sense waste elimination, energy conservation, and life-cycle perspective—reframe industrial efficiency by bringing biological production in concert with the objectives of sustainability. The realization of those principles is linked to state-of-the-art technologies such as microbial fermentation, enzyme bio-catalysis, synthetic biology, or photosynthetic systems including algae and plants. They also make it possible to produce pharmaceuticals, fuels, chemicals, biomaterials and food ingredients in a sustainable manner, with less reliance on non-renewable inputs and fewer adverse environmental impacts. The industrial applications and case studies that are reported—from artemisinin biosynthesis to biodegradable plastics and to CO2-derived ethanol— show that green biomanufacturing is no longer a dream of the future but a reality that is implementable at scale. Waste valorization approaches are also more applied recycling strategies towards cyclic economy that helps transform waste into value added resources along with demonstrating a higher level of economic sustainability. The economics and regulatory dynamics of this shift are both a testament to its potential and a mirror of its hurdles. However, with financial barriers still manifesting in initial capital outlay and infrastructure scale-up challenges, cost-benefit analyses usually highlight long-term operational savings, as well as enhanced brand positioning and risk reduction. Roebuck adds: "With governments at all levels implementing policy, tax rebate incentives, environmentally friendly finance, and global sustainability goals, adoption is on the rise in every region and from every industry." In the future, advancements such as AI-enabled process optimization, next-gen bioreactors, and continuous manufacturing will drive the industry forward and its production processes smarter, more sustainable, and more flexible. Market trends and forecasts agree on the solid, global growth in bioplastics, biofuels and green chemicals, with yet another evidence of future demand momentum. It is discussing what a green biomanufacturing would look like, and not 'just' technically as an evolutionary development, but that concept should begin to define our conception of how to shape a resilient, low carbon and sustainable industrial future. Through interdisciplinary thinking, supportive policy and ongoing innovation, it has the power to revolutionize production on a global level – in the best interests of both individuals and the environment.

REFERENCES

Abbasi, B. A., Iqbal, J., Kiran, F., Ahmad, R., Kanwal, S., Munir, A., & Mahmood, T. (2020). Green formulation and chemical characterizations of Rhamnella gilgitica aqueous leaves extract conjugated NiONPs and their multiple therapeutic properties. *Journal of Molecular Structure*, *1218*, 128490.

Abbasi, B. A., Iqbal, J., Mahmood, T., Qyyum, A., & Kanwal, S. (2019). Biofabrication of iron oxide nanoparticles by leaf extract of Rhamnus virgata: Characterization and evaluation of cytotoxic, antimicrobial and antioxidant potentials. *Applied Organometallic Chemistry*, *33*(7), e4947.

Achmad, G. N., Yudaruddin, R., Nugroho, B. A., Fitrian, Z., Suharsono, S., Adi, A. S., Hafsari, P., & Fitriansyah, F. (2023). Government support, eco-regulation and eco-innovation adoption in SMEs: The mediating role of eco-environmental. *Journal of Open Innovation*, *9*(4), 100158.

Agapakis, C. M., Boyle, P. M., & Silver, P. A. (2012). Natural strategies for the spatial optimization of metabolism in synthetic biology. *Nature Chemical Biology*, *8*(6), 527–535. PMID: 22596204

Aggarwal, N., Pham, H. L., Ranjan, B., Saini, M., Liang, Y., Hossain, G. S., Ling, H., Foo, J. L., & Chang, M. W. (2024). Microbial engineering strategies to utilize waste feedstock for sustainable bioproduction. *Nature Reviews Bioengineering*, *2*(2), 155–174.

Ahmad, M., Ali, A., Ullah, Z., Sher, H., Dai, D. Q., Ali, M., & Ali, I. (2022). Biosynthesized silver nanoparticles using Polygonatum geminiflorum efficiently control fusarium wilt disease of tomato. *Frontiers in Bioengineering and Biotechnology*, *10*, 988607. PMID: 36159677

Ahmed, I., Zia, M. A., Afzal, H., Ahmed, S., Ahmad, M., Akram, Z., Sher, F., & Iqbal, H. M. (2021). Socio-economic and environmental impacts of biomass valorisation: A strategic drive for sustainable bioeconomy. *Sustainability*, *13*(8), 4200.

. Ali, A., Usman, M., Jayamani, E., Soon, K., & bin Ab Wahab, M. K. (2024). Sustainable Biomanufacturing. In *Biomedical Implants* (pp. 195–217). CRC Press.

Ali, S. S., Elsamahy, T., Abdelkarim, E. A., Al-Tohamy, R., Kornaros, M., Ruiz, H. A., Zhao, T., Li, F., & Sun, J. (2022). Biowastes for biodegradable bioplastics production and end-of-life scenarios in circular bioeconomy and biorefinery concept. *Bioresource Technology*, *363*, 127869. PMID: 36064080

Anas, M.. (2025). Mitigating heavy metal pollution in agriculture: A multi-omics and nanotechnology approach to safeguard global wheat production. *Journal of Hazardous Materials Advances*, *17*, 100584. https://doi.org/https://doi.org/10.1016/j.hazadv.2024.100584

Anyshchenko, A., & Yarnold, J. (2021). From 'mad cow' crisis to synthetic biology: Challenges to EU regulation of GMOs beyond the European context. *International Environmental Agreement: Politics, Law and Economics*, *21*(3), 391–404.

Armstrong, R. N. (1987). Enzyme-catalyzed detoxication reactions: Mechanisms and stereochemistr. *Critical Reviews in Biochemistry*, *22*(1), 39–88. PMID: 3115676

Barone, A. S., Maragoni-Santos, C., de Farias, P. M., Cortat, C. M. G., Maniglia, B. C., Ongaratto, R. S., Ferreira, S., & Fai, A. E. C. (2025). Rethinking single-use plastics: Innovations, polices, consumer awareness and market shaping biodegradable solutions in the food packaging industry. *Trends in Food Science & Technology*, •••, 104906.

Buller, A. R., Brinkmann-Chen, S., Garcia-Borràs, M., Houk, K. N., & Arnold, F. H. (2023). Enzyme engineering and biocatalysis for green chemistry. *Nature Reviews. Chemistry*, *7*(1), 45–60. DOI: 10.1038/s41570-022-00440-8 PMID: 38123688

Buller, R., Lutz, S., Kazlauskas, R., Snajdrova, R., Moore, J., & Bornscheuer, U. (2023). From nature to industry: Harnessing enzymes for biocatalysis. *Science*, *382*(6673), eadh8615. PMID: 37995253

Carbonell, P., Jervis, A. J., Robinson, C. J., Yan, C., Dunstan, M., & Swainston, N. (2018). An automated Design–Build–Test–Learn pipeline for enhanced microbial production of fine chemicals. *Communications Biology*, *1*(1), 66. DOI: 10.1038/s42003-018-0076-9 PMID: 30271948

Chen, G. Q., & Jiang, X. R. (2018). Engineering microorganisms for improving polyhydroxyalkanoate biosynthesis. *Current Opinion in Biotechnology*, *53*, 20–25. DOI: 10.1016/j.copbio.2017.11.003 PMID: 29169056

Choi, K. R., Jang, W. D., Yang, D., Cho, J. S., Park, D., & Lee, S. Y. (2020). Systems metabolic engineering strategies: Integrating systems and synthetic biology with metabolic engineering. *Trends in Biotechnology*, *38*(7), 760–772. DOI: 10.1016/j.tibtech.2019.12.015 PMID: 30737009

Clomburg, J. M., Crumbley, A. M., & Gonzalez, R. (2017a). Industrial biomanufacturing: The future of chemical production. *Science*, *355*(6320), aag0804. PMID: 28059717

Clomburg, J. M., Crumbley, A. M., & Gonzalez, R. (2017b). Industrial biomanufacturing: The future of chemical production. *Science*, *355*(6320), aag0804. PMID: 28059717

Garlapati, V. K., Shankar, U., & Budhiraja, A. (2016). Bioconversion technologies of crude glycerol to value added industrial products. *Biotechnology Reports (Amsterdam, Netherlands)*, *9*, 9–14. PMID: 28352587

Gawel, E., Pannicke, N., & Hagemann, N. (2019). A path transition towards a bioeconomy—The crucial role of sustainability. *Sustainability*, *11*(11), 3005.

Halim-Lim, S. A., Jamaludin, A. A., Islam, A. T., Weerabahu, S., & Priyono, A. (2025). Unlocking potential for a circular bioeconomy transition through digital innovation, lean manufacturing and green practices: A review. *Management of Environmental Quality*, *36*(1), 130–154.

Haris, M., Fatima, N., Iqbal, J., Chalgham, W., Mumtaz, A. S., El-Sheikh, M. A., & Tavafoghi, M. (2023). Oscillatoria limnetica mediated green synthesis of iron oxide (Fe2O3) nanoparticles and their diverse in vitro bioactivities. *Molecules (Basel, Switzerland)*, *28*(5), 2091. PMID: 36903337

Hodgman, C. E., & Jewett, M. C. (2012). Cell-free synthetic biology: Thinking outside the cell. *Metabolic Engineering*, *14*(3), 261–269. DOI: 10.1016/j.ymben.2011.09.002 PMID: 21946161

Jadhav, R. R., & Khare, D. (2024). Green biotherapeutics: Overcoming challenges in plant-based expression platforms. *Plant Biotechnology Reports, 18*(4), 465–486.

Karim, A. S., & Jewett, M. C. (2016). A cell-free framework for rapid biosynthetic pathway prototyping and enzyme discovery. *Metabolic Engineering, 36*, 116–126. DOI: 10.1016/j.ymben.2016.03.002 PMID: 26996382

Karlsen, F., & Skov, P. V. (2022). Review–Potentials and limitations of utilising brewer's spent grain as a protein source in aquaculture feeds. *Journal of Cleaner Production, 357*, 131986.

Kay, J. E., & Jewett, M. C. (2015). Lysate of engineered Escherichia coli supports high-level conversion of glucose to 2,3-butanediol. *Metabolic Engineering, 30*, 190–200. DOI: 10.1016/j.ymben.2015.06.004 PMID: 26428449

Keasling, J. D. (2017). Synthetic biology and the development of tools for metabolic engineering. *Metabolic Engineering, 44*, 177–185. DOI: 10.1016/j.ymben.2017.10.004 PMID: 22314049

Khalid, M., De la ROsa, D., & Fikre, B. (2020). *Enhancing environmental sustainability in slow fashion apparel industry: Risk identification and supply chain mapping of bio-based polymer fibers.*

Khanal, S. K., Tarafdar, A., & You, S. (2023). Artificial intelligence and machine learning for smart bioprocesses. *Bioresource Technology, 375*, 128826. PMID: 36871700

Koul, B., Yakoob, M., & Shah, M. P. (2022). Agricultural waste management strategies for environmental sustainability. *Environmental Research, 206*, 112285. PMID: 34710442

Kourmentza, K., Kachrimanidou, V., Psaki, O., Pateraki, C., Ladakis, D., & Koutinas, A. (2020). Competitive advantage and market introduction of PHA polymers and potential use of PHA monomers. In *The Handbook of Polyhydroxyalkanoates* (pp. 167–202). CRC Press.

Kumar, V., & Verma, P. (2024). Microbial valorization of kraft black liquor for production of platform chemicals, biofuels, and value-added products: A critical review. *Journal of Environmental Management, 366*, 121631. PMID: 38986370

Kurt, E., Qin, J., Williams, A., Zhao, Y., & Xie, D. (2023). Perspectives for Using CO2 as a Feedstock for Biomanufacturing of Fuels and Chemicals. *Bioengineering (Basel, Switzerland), 10*(12), 1357. PMID: 38135948

Ladu, L., & Quitzow, R. (2017). Bio-based economy: Policy framework and foresight thinking. *Food Waste Reduction and Valorisation: Sustainability Assessment and Policy Analysis*, 167–195.

Lee, S. Y., Kim, H. U., Chae, T. U., Cho, J. S., Kim, J. W., & Shin, J. H. (2019). A comprehensive metabolic map for production of bio-based chemicals. *Nature Catalysis, 2*(1), 18–33. DOI: 10.1038/s41929-018-0212-4

Leong, H. Y., Chang, C.-K., Khoo, K. S., Chew, K. W., Chia, S. R., Lim, J. W., Chang, J.-S., & Show, P. L. (2021). Waste biorefinery towards a sustainable circular bioeconomy: A solution to global issues. *Biotechnology for Biofuels, 14*, 1–15. PMID: 33827663

Li, Z., Zhang, W., & Wang, Y. (2022). Valorization of lignocellulosic biomass into value-added products via microbial fermentation. *Bioresource Technology*, *363*, 127975. DOI: 10.1016/j.biortech.2022.127975

Liao, J. C., Mi, L., Pontrelli, S., & Luo, S. (2016). Fuelling the future: Microbial engineering for the production of sustainable biofuels. *Nature Reviews. Microbiology*, *14*(5), 288–304. DOI: 10.1038/nrmicro.2016.32 PMID: 27026253

Love, J. C., Reynolds, E. B., Goldston, D., & Frye, H. E. (2025). Biomanufacturing in the US: A MIT. *Policy Brief.*

Lozano, F. J., Lozano, R., Freire, P., Jiménez-Gonzalez, C., Sakao, T., Ortiz, M. G., Trianni, A., Carpenter, A., & Viveros, T. (2018). New perspectives for green and sustainable chemistry and engineering: Approaches from sustainable resource and energy use, management, and transformation. *Journal of Cleaner Production*, *172*, 227–232.

Madondo, N. I., Rathilal, S., Bakare, B. F., & Tetteh, E. K. (2023). Application of bioelectrochemical systems and anaerobic additives in wastewater treatment: A conceptual review. *International Journal of Molecular Sciences*, *24*(5), 4753. PMID: 36902185

Mahmood, T., Hussain, N., Shahbaz, A., Mulla, S. I., Iqbal, H. M., & Bilal, M. (2023). Sustainable production of biofuels from the algae-derived biomass. *Bioprocess and Biosystems Engineering*, *46*(8), 1077–1097. PMID: 36331626

Manara, P., & Zabaniotou, A. (2016). Co-valorization of crude glycerol waste streams with conventional and/or renewable fuels for power generation and industrial symbiosis perspectives. *Waste and Biomass Valorization*, *7*, 135–150.

Marimon, F., & Casadesús, M. (2017). Reasons to adopt ISO 50001 energy management system. *Sustainability*, *9*(10), 1740.

Massoud, M. A., Fayad, R., Kamleh, R., & El-Fadel, M. (2010). *Environmental management system (ISO 14001) certification in developing countries: Challenges and implementation strategies.*

Meereboer, K. W., Misra, M., & Mohanty, A. K. (2020). Review of recent advances in the biodegradability of polyhydroxyalkanoate (PHA) bioplastics and their composites. *Green Chemistry*, *22*(17), 5519–5558.

Meghwanshi, G. K., Kaur, N., Verma, S., Dabi, N. K., Vashishtha, A., Charan, P., Purohit, P., Bhandari, H., Bhojak, N., & Kumar, R. (2020). Enzymes for pharmaceutical and therapeutic applications. *Biotechnology and Applied Biochemistry*, *67*(4), 586–601. PMID: 32248597

Meghwanshi, G. K., Kaur, N., Verma, S., Gupta, N., Kumar, R., & Prakash, V. (2020). Enzymes for pharmaceutical and therapeutic applications. *Biotechnology Reports (Amsterdam, Netherlands)*, *25*, e00427. DOI: 10.1016/j.btre.2020.e00427 PMID: 32248597

Nielsen, J., & Keasling, J. D. (2016). Engineering cellular metabolism. *Cell*, *164*(6), 1185–1197. DOI: 10.1016/j.cell.2016.02.004 PMID: 26967285

Olguin-Maciel, E., Singh, A., Chable-Villacis, R., Tapia-Tussell, R., & Ruiz, H. A. (2020). Consolidated bioprocessing, an innovative strategy towards sustainability for biofuels production from crop residues: An overview. *Agronomy (Basel), 10*(11), 1834.

Osman, A. I., Chen, Z., Elgarahy, A. M., Farghali, M., Mohamed, I. M., Priya, A., Hawash, H. B., & Yap, P. (2024). Membrane technology for energy saving: Principles, techniques, applications, challenges, and prospects. *Advanced Energy and Sustainability Research*, *5*(5), 2400011.

Paul, S., Bera, S., Dasgupta, R., Mondal, S., & Roy, S. (2021). Review on the recent structural advances in open and closed systems for carbon capture through algae. *Energy Nexus*, *4*, 100032.

Pesch, H. (2023). *Exploring the use of plant factories for the production of biomass for the biorefining industry*.

Philippini, R. R., Martiniano, S. E., Ingle, A. P., Franco Marcelino, P. R., Silva, G. M., Barbosa, F. G., Dos Santos, J. C., & da Silva, S. S. (2020). Agroindustrial byproducts for the generation of biobased products: Alternatives for sustainable biorefineries. *Frontiers in Energy Research*, *8*, 152.

Qumsani, A. T. (2024). The contribution of microorganisms to sustainable development: Towards a green future through synthetic biology and systems biology. *Journal of Umm Al-Qura University for Applied Sciences*, 1–17.

Rangel, A. E., Gómez Ramírez, J. M., & Gonzalez Barrios, A. F. (2020). From industrial by-products to value-added compounds: The design of efficient microbial cell factories by coupling systems metabolic engineering and bioprocesses. *Biofuels, Bioproducts & Biorefining*, *14*(6), 1228–1238.

Rossi, C., Shen, L., Junginger, M., & Wicke, B. (2024). Sustainability certification of bio-based products: Systematic literature review of socio-economic impacts along the supply chain. *Journal of Cleaner Production*, •••, 143079.

Sharma, P., Bano, A., Verma, K., Yadav, M., Varjani, S., Singh, S. P., & Tong, Y. W. (2023). Food waste digestate as biofertilizer and their direct applications in agriculture. *Bioresource Technology Reports*, *23*, 101515.

Sheldon, R. A., & Brady, D. (2022). Green chemistry, biocatalysis, and the chemical industry of the future. *ChemSusChem*, *15*(9), e202102628. PMID: 35026060

Sheldon, R. A., & Brady, D. (2022). The limits to biocatalysis: Pushing the envelope. *Chemical Science (Cambridge)*, *13*(12), 3232–3245. DOI: 10.1039/D1SC05620A

Shokoohi, M., & Attar, T. (2024a). Biomanufacturing for a sustainable future: Unleashing the potential of biotechnology in pharmaceutical raw material production. [IJHES]. *International Journal of New Findings in Health and Educational Sciences*, *2*(2), 142–153.

Shokoohi, M., & Attar, T. (2024b). Biomanufacturing for a sustainable future: Unleashing the potential of biotechnology in pharmaceutical raw material production. [IJHES]. *International Journal of New Findings in Health and Educational Sciences*, *2*(2), 142–153.

Shokoohi, M., & Attar, T. (2024c). Biomanufacturing for a sustainable future: Unleashing the potential of biotechnology in pharmaceutical raw material production. [IJHES]. *International Journal of New Findings in Health and Educational Sciences, 2*(2), 142–153.

Shokoohi, M., & Attar, T. (2024d). Biomanufacturing for a sustainable future: Unleashing the potential of biotechnology in pharmaceutical raw material production. [IJHES]. *International Journal of New Findings in Health and Educational Sciences, 2*(2), 142–153.

Silverman, A. D., & Karim, A. S. (2020). Cell-free gene expression: An expanded repertoire of applications. *Nature Reviews. Genetics, 21*(3), 151–170. DOI: 10.1038/s41576-019-0185-8 PMID: 31780816

Silverman, A. D., Karim, A. S., & Jewett, M. C. (2020). Cell-free gene expression: An expanded repertoire of applications. *Nature Reviews. Genetics, 21*(3), 151–170. DOI: 10.1038/s41576-019-0185-8 PMID: 31780816

Singla, P. (2020). Plant synthetic biology: A paradigm shift targeting stress mitigation, reduction of ecological footprints and sustainable transformation in agriculture. *Plant Stress Biology: Strategies and Trends*, 435–489.

Song, M., Fisher, R., & Kwoh, Y. (2019). Technological challenges of green innovation and sustainable resource management with large scale data. *Technological Forecasting and Social Change, 144*, 361–368.

Srivastav, A. K., Das, P., & Srivastava, A. K. (2024). Future Trends, Innovations, and Global Collaboration. In *Biotech and IoT: An Introduction Using Cloud-Driven Labs* (pp. 309–398). Springer.

Süntar, I., Çetinkaya, S., Haydaroğlu, Ü. S., & Habtemariam, S. (2021). Bioproduction process of natural products and biopharmaceuticals: Biotechnological aspects. *Biotechnology Advances, 50*, 107768. PMID: 33974980

Swartz, J. R. (2012). Transforming biochemical engineering with cell-free biology. *AIChE Journal. American Institute of Chemical Engineers, 58*(1), 5–13. DOI: 10.1002/aic.13701

Vandenberghe, L., Valladares-Diestra, K., Bittencourt, G. A., Torres, L. Z., Vieira, S., Karp, S. G., Sydney, E., de Carvalho, J. C., Soccol, V. T., & Soccol, C. R. (2022). Beyond sugar and ethanol: The future of sugarcane biorefineries in Brazil. *Renewable & Sustainable Energy Reviews, 167*, 112721.

Wang, G., Mohsin, A., Chu, J., Zhuang, Y., & Zhang, S. (2024). Advances and prospects for advanced biomanufacturing. *Scale-up and Chemical Process for Microbial Production of Plant-Derived Bioactive Compounds*, 1–16.

Way, J. C., Collins, J. J., Keasling, J. D., & Silver, P. A. (2014). Integrating biological redesign: Where synthetic biology came from and where it needs to go. *Cell, 157*(1), 151–161. DOI: 10.1016/j.cell.2014.02.039 PMID: 24679533

Worrell, E., Bernstein, L., Roy, J., Price, L., & Harnisch, J. (2018). Industrial energy efficiency and climate change mitigation. In *Renewable energy* (p. Vol1_548-Vol1_568). Routledge.

Woźniak, E., Tyczewska, A., & Twardowski, T. (2021). Bioeconomy development factors in the European Union and Poland. *New Biotechnology*, *60*, 2–8. PMID: 32835869

Wu, S., Snajdrova, R., Moore, J. C., Baldenius, K., & Bornscheuer, U. T. (2021). Biocatalysis: Enzymatic synthesis for industrial applications. *Angewandte Chemie International Edition*, *60*(1), 88–119. PMID: 32558088

Wu, S., Snajdrova, R., Moore, J. C., Baldenius, K., & Bornscheuer, U. T. (2021). Biocatalysis: Enzymatic synthesis for industrial applications. *Angewandte Chemie International Edition*, *60*(1), 88–119. DOI: 10.1002/anie.202006648 PMID: 32558088

Yadav, D. K., Singh, A., Agrawal, V., & Yadav, N. (2021). Algal Biomass: A Natural Resource of High-Value Biomolecules. *Bioprospecting of Plant Biodiversity for Industrial Molecules*, 303–334.

Yang, L., Wang, X.-C., Dai, M., Chen, B., Qiao, Y., Deng, H., Zhang, D., Zhang, Y., de Almeida, C. M. V. B., & Chiu, A. S. (2021). Shifting from fossil-based economy to bio-based economy: Status quo, challenges, and prospects. *Energy*, *228*, 120533.

Yue, D., You, F., & Snyder, S. W. (2014). Biomass-to-bioenergy and biofuel supply chain optimization: Overview, key issues and challenges. *Computers & Chemical Engineering*, *66*, 36–56.

Zeng, Y., Hong, Y., Azi, F., Liu, Y., Chen, Y., Guo, C., Lin, D., Wu, Z., Chen, W., & Xu, P. (2022). Advanced genome-editing technologies enable rapid and large-scale generation of genetic variants for strain engineering and synthetic biology. *Current Opinion in Microbiology*, *69*, 102175. PMID: 35809388

Zhang, Y.-H. P., Sun, J., & Ma, Y. (2017). Biomanufacturing: History and perspective. *Journal of Industrial Microbiology & Biotechnology*, *44*(4–5), 773–784. PMID: 27837351

Zhou, S., Zhuang, Y., & Li, Y. (2021). Engineering microbial cell factories for sustainable production of chemicals. *Biotechnology Advances*, *51*, 107733. DOI: 10.1016/j.biotechadv.2021.107733

Chapter 12
Biomanufacturing for Environmental Sustainability and Remediation

Rajan Kumar Singh
https://orcid.org/0009-0003-9010-4072
Parul Institute of Technology, Parul University, India

Shourya Bodla
https://orcid.org/0009-0003-8393-3112
Parul Institute of Technology, Parul University, India

Nethikunta Aashrith Patel
Parul Institute of Technology, Parul University, India

Samhita Kumar Polavarapu
Parul Institute of Technology, Parul University, India

Bollapu Rohini Reddy
Parul Institute of Technology, Parul University, India

Soham Trivedi
Parul Institute of Technology, Parul University, India

Vivek Kumar
Center of Microbiome Research, Microbiomes Institute, University of Southern Florida, USA

ABSTRACT

Rising global demand for waste-to-wealth generation has caught a lot of attention towards the biological remediation methods with human interventions to enhance capabilities to detoxify pollutants. This comprehensive book chapter aims to focus on the different biomanufacturing strategies and their roles in bioremediation processes. Metabolic engineering and synthetic biology leverage the production of enhanced biosystems. This chapter highlights various applications of biomanufacturing in the fields of pollution control and waste treatment. Engineered proteins and microbes are developed to degrade plastic waste and accompany a bioleaching process for extracting heavy metals from e-waste and also bioelectricity generation. Specific microbes are studied which can enhance the absorption of heavy metals such as Pseudomonas fluorescens

DOI: 10.4018/979-8-3373-2873-7.ch012

and Bacillus subtilis. The circular economy strategies like reuse, reduce, and recycle, enhances economic, social, and environmental balance by increasing resource efficiency and providing long-term sustainability without any environmental effects.

INTRODUCTION

Role of Biomanufacturing in Environmental Sustainability

Biomanufacturing is a process which is used to produce biomolecules that can be used in various fields like agriculture, material, energy and pharmaceuticals by using biological systems which are metabolically and genetically enhanced to produce desired products (Zhang et al., 2017). There are various biological systems used in this process such as microorganisms, enzymes, plants or animal cells. Biomanufacturing plays a pivotal role in maintaining environmental sustainability as it utilizes naturally occurring and renewable biological systems unlike traditional manufacturing that relies on fossil fuels and also generates significant waste (Oluyemi et al., 2024). It is already performed by everyone in their daily routine and has been started for many years like preparation of curd, cheese, soy sauce, wine, bread etc, all these come under biomanufacturing as naturally occurring microbes are used in these processes. Also, the production of various primary metabolites (ethanol, acetone, butanol), secondary metabolites (Penicillin, streptomycin) and biomolecules such as proteins and enzymes.

Examples of modern biomanufacturing technologies include mammalian cell culture systems, enzymatic biocatalysis, and microbial fermentation. These systems have been enhanced by advancements in metabolic engineering and synthetic biology, enabling them to create biofuels, bioplastics, and specialized chemicals in an efficient manner (Bhatia et al., 2024). The use of fossil fuels has been greatly reduced because of biotechnology advancements that have made it possible for organisms like Saccharomyces cerevisiae and E. coli that were created using a systems biology approach to convert industrial wastes or agricultural waste into products with additional value. Biodegradable and less polluting than traditional plastics, bioplastics such as polylactic acid (PLA) and polyhydroxyalkanoates (PHAs) are made via microbial synthesis. Through the production of valuable goods from food, agricultural, and industrial waste, biomanufacturing also helps to increase the value of waste. Significant ecological benefits can be obtained from biomanufacturing. It frequently uses less water and energy, produces gentler pollution discharges, and uses waste-based or renewable materials, all of which reduce carbon emissions. Additionally, biological systems frequently generate less hazardous waste that functions in an environmentally beneficial way. Biomanufacturing has drawbacks. These include problems with scalability, irregular biomass supply, increased production costs, and regulatory obstacles pertaining to genetically modified organisms. But because of developments in synthetic biology, metabolic engineering, and artificial intelligence, biomanufacturing is becoming more and more feasible on an industrial scale while also increasing yields and reducing prices (Nielsen & Keasling, 2016).

Applications of Biomanufacturing in the Pollution Control and Waste Management

Bio-manufactured products are inherently sustainable and cost effective due to easy availability which are used for various applications like Synthetic Biosystems, Microbial detoxification, Anaerobic Digesters and Composting Systems, Bioelectricity Generation, Phyto-remediation.

Synthetic Biosystems

Global metrics of e-waste deposition shows there is a significant increase in non-degradable plastic waste accumulation in landfills and ocean bodies. The projections show that there will be a significant increase by 70 metric tonnes till 2030. The major disposal regions include landfills and waste scraps (Forti et al., 2020). E-waste contains different mixtures of composite materials mainly consisting heavy metals (lead, cadmium, mercury, nickel and copper) and plastic composites (poly-aromatic hydrocarbons, polystyrene, acrylonitrile butadiene styrene, polycarbonate). These compositions make e-waste difficult for degradation (Tsydenova & Bengtsson, 2011). Traditional methods of e-waste disposal make it difficult for recycling and it causes biomagnification of toxic metals. There are yet established procedures to recycle the metals from e-waste, but the plastic recycling methods are limited due to complex chemical composition and expensive methods. So alternative biological methods have been experimented synthetically by engineering protein structure and modifying enzyme's catalytic binding sites can improve plastic degradation (Austin et al., 2018). Some microbes are also bioengineered to secrete these recombinant enzymes to degrade heterogenous plastic composites (Jaiswal et al., 2020). Heavy metals from e-waste deposits can be extracted by the method of bioleaching by using acidophilic bacteria (Pant et al., 2012). Bioengineered microbes have improved metal tolerance and metal degradation capabilities, and are used for mineralization of gold in oceanic bodies, making them more efficient and cost effective. The major application of these microbes is in the solubilization of gold (Johnston et al., 2013).

Microbial Detoxification

Rapid development, urbanization and exponential increase in population has caused a rise in pollution levels (Sharma et al., 2022). There are physicochemical methods that are being employed to control pollution and waste disposal. But due to the associated problems that arise due to these methods, biological measures are being explored which can be self-sustaining and safe to use (Mishra et al., 2021). Biological methods of detoxification include usage of wild type or engineered microbes that are obtained from water bodies. Some wild type microbes are genetically modified to specifically remove toxic metals and chemicals from waste to make them less harmful and exposed to the environment. These microbes are extensively studied for their potential for human diseases (Bala et al., 2022). Microbial detoxification strategies include mineralization and bioremediation. Removing heavy metals from toxic industrial effluents has been a difficult task that involves usage of chemical reactions. Replacing the traditional methods of microbes such as *Pseudomonas fluorescens*, *P. aeruginosa*, *Lysinibacillus sphaericus* and *Cladosporium sp.* are used to remove metals like iron, cobalt, zinc, copper etc (Paranthaman & Karthikeya, 2015; Mohammadian et al., 2015; Peña-Montenegro et al., 2015). Some organisms of *Streptomyces* sp. are used to decontaminate petroleum soil and degrade hydrocarbons. BL-27 strain of *Bacillus subtilis* can degrade crude oil in 5 days (Wang et al., 2019).

Plastic waste disposed of into the environment are harmful as they decompose slowly releasing toxic chemicals into water bodies. These chemicals include PET, Polystyrene, LDPE, HDPE, Polyvinylchloride (PVC) and polyethylene. Though microbes such as *Pseudomonas fluorescens, Bacillus siamensis* and *Aspergillus flavus* degrade plastic in more than 50 days they are more reliable for safe and faster degradation than traditional methods (Elahi et al., 2021; Maroof et al., 2021; Taghavi et al., 2021).

Anaerobic Digesters and Composting Systems

A number of studies have looked into how different types of bioplastics break down under anaerobic conditions, mainly focusing on PHAs, PLA, starch-based materials like Mater-Bi, and others. There are multiple temperature conditions for the degradation process with mesophilic conditions (30–38 °C), thermophilic (52–58 °C) (Appels et al., 2011). These plastics are tested in various forms-powder, film, granules, and even real-world items like cups or plates-and results showed big differences depending on the material, how it was treated beforehand, and how the tests were done. PHAs and TPS came out as the most easily degradable, often producing good amounts of methane, which means they could be useful for energy recovery (Benn & Zitomer, 2018). But some plastics like PBAT, PBS, and a few PLA blends don't really break down much, even when tested at higher temperatures. A few types of plastics are pre-treated—like heated up or treated with chemicals—before digestion. While a lot of studies used tools like SEM or FTIR to check how much the materials had degraded, not many actually looked into what microbes were responsible. From what we know, it's mostly anaerobic bacteria and methanogens doing the work. So, while anaerobic digestion looks like a good option for certain bioplastics when the conditions are right, others still need intensive research-either in how they're made or how they're processed-to really make them work for this kind of waste treatment (Falzarano et al., 2023).

Composting is a natural process in which organisms and microbes present in soil use the organic matter from dead leaves, animal waste and manure. These organisms convert the organic compounds into humic substances that are further used by plants (Ingrao et al., 2017). Use of compostable plastic material for packaging has gained importance due to the emergence of the replacement of traditional plastics derived from petroleum sources which causes pollution and release toxins upon degradation. Bio-based plastic composts have been developed to imitate the properties of the domestic plastic properties and applications. Depending on the material there are many types of composting systems such as drum reactors, row composting and table composting. The efficiency of the composting method depends on the method and characteristic of the material (Dilkes-Hoffman et al., 2019).

Bioelectricity Generation

Globally the increasing demand for electric supply and rapid multiplication of electric grid lines led to the increased focus on renewable energy such as wind, solar and tidal energy. Traditional fuel such as coal and oil is still being used to balance the requirements. Though there are renewable sources of energy, biological sources are being explored to replace the requirement of heavy machinery and costly equipment (Al-Yasiri, 2021). To eliminate the requirement of fossil fuels like petroleum and gasoline, biofuels like methane and ethane are produced by anaerobic digesters and conversion tanks which convert organic waste into methane and other products. These also constitute the renewable sources of electricity generation (Kabeyi & Olanrewaju, 2022). There is another biological system available that can convert biological energy into electric energy called Microbial Fuel Cell.

Microbial Fuel Cells are the example of Bioelectricity where the bacterial present in the fuel cell uses the organic matter for metabolism to generate electrons which are transferred to the electrodes of the cell. These MFC (Microbial Fuel Cells) are installed in the sewage treatment plants to harness the electric power generated by them due to their accelerated metabolism and methane produced after the digestion is used as biogas (Hoang et al., 2022).

Phytoremediation

Recent advancements in green technology for waste treatment and pollution control led to the usage of a safest alternative 'Phytoremediation'. Hydrocarbon removal from effluent deposits and landfills can be performed using mycoremediation and phytoremediation. There are different plant species that can absorb and stabilize the pollutants. For example, sunflowers and willows can detoxify lead and arsenic from contaminated soil. With recent advancements in genetic engineering and recombinant DNA technology there are modified plants that can be grown specific for contaminant removal from polluted lands (Ahmad et al., 2024).

Components like heavy metals present in the effluents can be reused after they are taken up by the plants. The biomass formed can also be used as a feedstock and can be used as a fuel too. Biofuel producing plants are grown in petroleum contaminated regions where these plants use the hydrocarbons and for biofuel that can be refined **(Wijekoon et al., 2025).**

Objectives and Scope of the Chapter

This chapter aims to explore different methods of biomanufacturing that will be needed for environmental remediation and identifying green technologies that can be viable for this process. The chapter also provides a brief scope for further research and application that need to be developed to create a far more reliable alternative for waste treatment and toxin removal. It also discusses the major aspects of biomanufacturing practices and the methodologies that can be sustainable for the future.

SCIENTIFIC & TECHNICAL FOUNDATIONS FOR SUSTAINABLE BIOMANUFACTURING PRACTICES

Environmental-friendly, responsible production of materials, chemicals and energy will be niches for biomanufacturing from bio-based feedstocks, among other emerging production-platform protocols (Ali et al., 2024). The establishment of a series of bioprocesses for several types of commercial products has provided a secure platform for further expansion into the industrial sector. Biomanufacturing is an emergent field that needs to have access to the most recent and advanced bioprocess technologies, since it is used already for more and more applications, including agro-products, food fermentations, diagnostics, bioremediation, biofuels, biotherapeutics and other sustainable environmental solutions (Pandey et al., 2024). Thus, this integration seeks to move from a fossil-based economy to a bio-based economy through integrations. Microorganisms, when genetically engineered, can create new products at a more effective rate. The fact that life-cycle assessments for carbon footprints and integrative options show that micro-integration is an option for lessening the environmental impact of bioproducts when compared to micro-refineries means the goal is to re-establish levels of environmental impact, economic viability, and socio-ethical responsibility (Benavides et al., 2024). Therefore, integration with green chemistry, enzyme technology, and microbial engineering hopes to promote more sustainable and effective industrial applications and processes. Bio-fabrication as it currently exists is a cumbersome process and energy intensive. Something must be adjusted to promise that these sustainable efforts do not cause further harm to the planet when such thoughts are brought to large-scale production.

Energy consumption remains a major concern in large-scale biomanufacturing, energy generation, lab use, factory output and pollution. Yet, energy generation and consumption can be avoided through computational prediction strategies which ease processes, make them more targeted and less energy dependent. Encouraging such sustainable bio-fabrication factors would better align this process with circular economic factors (Filippi et al., 2025). The more and more sustained bio-fabrication would otherwise become a sustainable platform the easier it would be to produce these value-added items from chemicals to compostable fabrics, as generated bioproducts or things made from bio-reagents would be the equivalent to things that could not be made from renewable or fossil resources. Although the process for batch and fed-batch exists in the current industry, interest is rapidly increasing in Continuous Biomanufacturing (CBM), nominally to reduce capital and operational costs. Transition to the continuous mode of operation is expected to improve productivity and reduce environmental pollution, which may affect sustainability targets. This shift is considered to be pivotal, making CBM (Continuous Biomanufacturing) a potential key technology towards a sustainable bioeconomy. In other words, sustainable biomanufacturing approaches like biotechnology allow using renewables to produce products and efficient processes such as CBM (Continuous Biomanufacturing) with reduced environmental effects (Del Hierro et al., 2024). The products from biopharmaceutical production are of high value for human health. A majority, however, express a strong desire to reduce its environmental impact using science-based strategies for environmental burden reduction and development of rational solutions. The latter is achieved by developing new sustainability programs, certifications, initiatives, and in-service training and the promotion of sustainability in publications, foundation donations, and consortia sponsorship.

In addition, it is processes and facility suite designs that experienced architectural and process design sponsors can employ to drive reductions, in an economical manner, of many categories of environmental stress, while also satisfying the applicable expectations of the client, society, and legislation (Whitford et al., 2022).

Use of Renewable sources and Waste-derived Feedstocks for Biomanufacturing

Biomanufacturing techniques make use of renewable and waste-based feedstocks such as animal waste, food processing by-products, lignocellulosic biomass, municipal solid wastes, and green waste. Such operations decrease the processing time and the energetic expenses, and enhance the product quality and the product yield (Narisetty et al., 2023). The electro-catalysed CO2 reduction reaction can also be carried out to convert the CO2 into feedstocks. This may serve to highlight the significance of green hydrogen at cheaper rates that can not only boost the efficiency, but also the scalability of biomanufacturing processes (Ma et al., 2022). Industrial by-products and municipal solid wastes can be used as raw materials for the production of biofuels, biochemicals and other bioproducts via anoxic fermentation. They can be converted into biohydrogen and biopolymers to minimize the environmental impact and encourage the use of green and low-carbon resources in the green economy model (S et al., 2018). Methanol, formate, acetate can be further processed in engineered microbial strains to generate various platform chemicals and food additives that contributes to diminish the reliance on the fossil resources while reducing the carbon footprint and circular economy and environmental-friendly (Zhang et al., 2022). Agriculturally derived biowastes can be processed and transformed into a variety of materials that can be subsequently used for additive manufacturing processes (Rahman et al., 2023). Different ways exist for the use of agro-wastes such as animal waste, agro- industrial waste, crop residues, and fruit and vegetable waste in value added products. These techniques are burning, gasification, pyrolysis, fermentation, transesterification and anaerobic digestion (Yaashikaa et al., 2022). Agricultural-related wastes give rise to a lot of quantity of lignocellulosic biomass as the abundant renewable resource material for wide application of bioproducts (Mujtaba et al., 2023). Sustainability goals pervade the industry and are nudging it from fossil fuels as a finite resource to biotechnology. It is known to convert renewable feedstocks such as glucose to chemicals, the major next step is in the use of waste feedstocks. Synthetic microorganisms that can convert various C-rich polymeric waste materials, such as lignocellulosic and plastic waste, to value-added chemicals are engineered. This unexploited potential underpins the circular bioeconomy, prevents land-use conflicts with food and is in line with circular economy aspects (Pitzalis & Sadler, 2025; Serna Loaiza et al., 2019; Sebastián Serna Loaiza et al., 2022; Willett & Hajduk, 2024).

Circular Economy in terms of SDG (Sustainable Development Goals) and Resource Efficiency

The circular economy concept or strategy of supply chain enhancement or management enhances the economic, social, and environmental balance by improving the efficiency of resources and supporting sustainable developmental goals (Gao et al., 2024). Strategies like reuse, reduce and recycle promote sustainable designing which in-turn helps circular economy in decoupling the economic growth from environmental harm by which it fosters long-term in terms of sustainability by extending the life cycles, directly providing support to the global resources (Rodriguez et al., 2019) (Figure 1). Digital technologies and closed-loop systems help the circular economy help in promoting waste minimization and resource optimization providing a helping-hand towards innovation and economic growth despite obstacles or challenges like costs and resistance from the organization (Balaji et al., 2025). SDGs (Sustainable Development Goals) like SDG6(clean water), SDG8 (economic growth), SDG11 (sustainable cities), SDG12 (responsible consumption) and SDG13 (climate action) go for a balanced and systematic approach to ensure that the strategies of circular economy get a boost-up from environmental, economic and social dimensions without any challenges or obstacles (Dong et al., 2021; Sorooshian, 2024). Some more SDGs (Sustainable Development Goals) like SDG15 protect the terrestrial ecosystems through the help of biological practices such as composting and biomimicry. The integration of the circular economy by policy reduces the industrial dependence on finite resources (Valverde & Avilés-Palacios, 2021).

Figure 1. Illustration representing the stages of the circular economy process starting from production and distribution to the re-use of the raw material and energy for domestic and commercial purposes

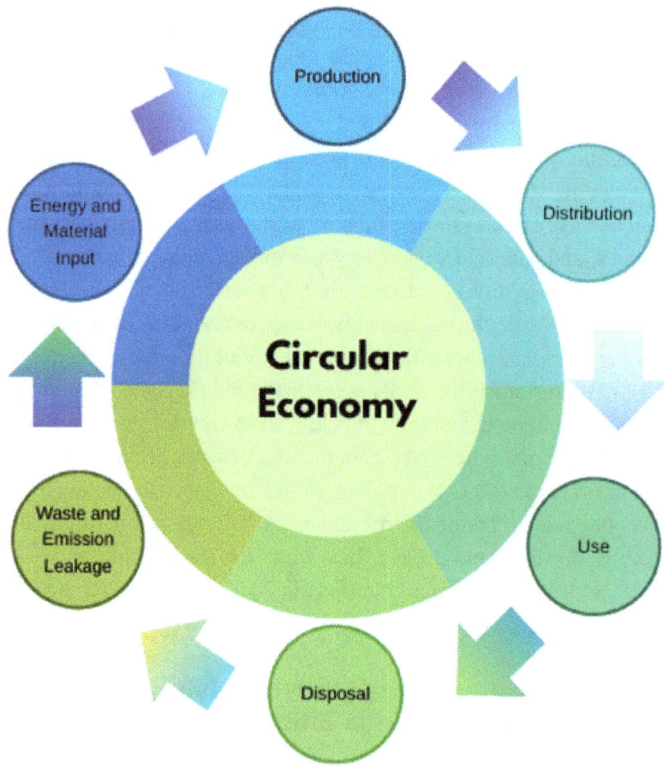

Industrial Waste Valorization

Artificial waste valorization is the prime mover in promoting indirect frugality policy and sustainable development objectives through the upgrading of colourful artificial residues and by-products into value-added chemicals, energy, and products and thus maximizing coffers' utilization and minimizing environmental goods. Being a more global artificial enterprise, the subsequent rise in the product of wastes i.e., from husbandry, food processing, manufacturing, mining, and energy product calls for new forms of disposing of wastes other than traditional jilting and incineration. Such traditional steps take into consideration a significant contribution to hothouse gas emigrations, land loss, and recoverable coffers loss, thereby propounding the need for resource valorization and recovery processes (Cichoski et al., 2024).

Valorization is a new concept in which waste is converted to a resource using a wide variety of technological routes. Organic artificial wastes, especially agrarian and food processing wastes, are of particular interest due to their water and nutrient values and amenability for processes like anaerobic digestion, turmoil, composting, and bioactive motes recovery. Anaerobic digestion allows biodegradable organic waste to be converted into biogas and dig estate, the latter of which is further used as a biofertilizer, hence allowing for energy production as well as agricultural output. Strains like Saccharomyces cerevisiae and Lactobacillus spp. Utilized in microbial unrest to produce industrially significant chemicals such as bioethanol, lactic acid, and acetic acid, instead of cleaner substitutes to the fossil fuel commodities (Beleno & Ramos, 2024). Either, bioactive composite recovery of food process by-products — e.g., polyphenols, carotenoids, and healthy fibre — is an unstated line of interest that has emerged with focus, particularly in the nutraceutical, pharmaceutical, and floral diligence, wherein substrates including fruit peel, seeds, and coffee refuse yield high functional biomolecule and antioxidant recoveries. Lignocellulosic biomass, which is one of the major by-products of agriculture and forestry with cellulose, hemicellulose, and lignin, is also a top choice for valorization. These are convertible through pyrolysis, hydrothermal liquefaction, and gamification thermochemical conversion processes and enzymatic hydrolysis and turmoil biochemical conversion processes. These pathways yield biofuels like bioethanol, biobutanol, and biodiesel, and platform chemicals like levelling acid and culture, which can be the bioplastic precursors, detergents, and resins. Organic waste valorization has been of great interest, but inorganic artificial remainders — typically more difficult to valorize — are no longer being added to indirect frugality strategies. Wastes like bauxite refinery red sludge, coal cover ash of coal combustion, sword sediment, and mining wastes are natural accoutrements to be used as building material as cementitious accoutrements, summations, or as drug for geopolymers. They not only redirect these wastes away from tips but also reduce the use of raw materials and lower the carbon footprint of cement and concrete products (Xian et al., 2023). Furthermore, new recovery technologies such as hydrometallurgy and hydrometallurgy are used to recover precious essences such as lithium, cobalt (Okolie et al., 2023) (Figure 2).

Figure 2. Flowchart depicting key valorization routes for organic, lignocellulosic, and inorganic waste in sustainable waste management and circular economies

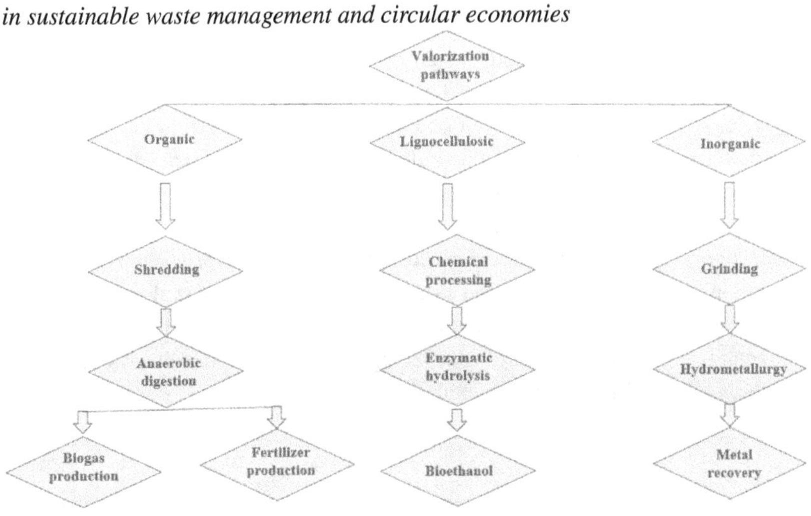

Organic waste is processed via anaerobic digestion to produce biogas and fertilizer. Lignocellulosic biomass undergoes chemical processing and enzymatic hydrolysis to yield bioethanol. Inorganic waste is treated through grinding and hydrometallurgy for metal recovery.

Nickel and Rare-Earth Metal Extraction from Electronic Waste and Artificial Waste

Similar recovered essence is critical to electronics, renewable energy technology, and electric vehicle batteries and therefore aligning waste valorization conditioning with decarbonization and overall sustainability targets (Castro-Criado et al., 2023). The revenue-generating ideas of waste valorization are unwanted in that they give room for thrift to offset the cost of waste disposal, create new sources of income, and enhance their sustainability profile. Anaerobic digestion stores, for example, yield not only renewable energy but also biofertilizers, which may be sold and hence offer multi-stream income potential. Aside from this, possible recovery of bioactive emulsion and biopolymer from agro-industry waste have by implication high-value application opportunities such as food, health, and packaging (Arvelli et al., 2025). However, the transition to widespread valorization of waste is not trouble-free. Sophisticated walls such as artificial waste aqueducts' heterogeneity make process scaling and optimization difficult, and financial walls such as excessive capital expenditure and limited access to funds make abandonment of such technologies by specifically small and medium-sized enterprises (SMEs) unsuitable. Policy and legislation trials such as variable waste bracket, nonsupervisory penalization of valorised goods, ban on transboundary waste transport, etc. also limit the advancement of waste valorization conditioning (Mishra et al., 2022). In an attempt to combat such hindrances, policy interventions such as subventions, exemption of duty, extended patron responsibility (EPR) schemes, and decompression of legal fabrics are no longer being advocated and proposed across the world. One of the more consolidated strategies in play is integrated biorefineries, whereby a variety of aqueducts of wastes are combined into pools to make several products within a span covering energies and chemicals to accessories. Such plants are the indirect frugality morality for ensuring maximal input-oriented effectiveness, product variety, and minimum production of wastes. Emerging technologies such as microwave oven-assisted pyrolysis, supercritical CO_2 birth, and machine literacy-driven waste sorting technologies are increasing process dexterity, scalability, and economically viable feasibility (Bano et al., 2025). Brazilian and Mexican nation-level case studies are representative of environment-specific valorization models that leverage available domestic coffers and sustain indigenous sustainability conditions. Brazil, for instance, is turning fruit and vegetable wastes into animal feed and functional foods, while Mexico is investing in recycling technology to make essence out of synthetic sludge and electronic waste to power its shift towards renewable energy and reduced foreign raw material dependence (Cecilia et al., 2019). These community-scale enterprises are examples of bottom-up valorization strategies for having great ability to contribute significantly to public and transnational sustainability efforts. Public education systems, transnational partnership, and public-private partnerships further propel invention, technology transfer, and structure capacity for waste valorization. Full life cycle examinations (Lucas) and techno-economic analyses (Teas) also badly require evaluation to determine actual ecological and rewarding advantages of valorization pathways, environmentally sustainable as well as sellable (Dhiman et al., 2025).

BIOREMEDIATION AND PHYTOREMEDIATION AS BIOMANUFACTURING TOOLS FOR SUSTAINABILITY

Bio-manufacturing is the use of living systems to create products with low environmental impact. As bioremediation and phytoremediation technologies become prevalent, to meet challenges in the area of pollution, they provide eco-friend technology to remove pollutants like plastics, organic waste, heavy metals (Ali et al., 2019). These strategies take advantage of microbial ability and plants to degrade, transform or sequester contaminants, and are scalable, cost effective (Ahmad et al., 2014). This chapter highlights microbe and biodegradation methods for bioremediation processes, biodegradation approaches to waste management, and phytoremediation technologies for heavy metal detoxification, incorporating new industry dynamics and developments to demonstrate their role in eco-efficient bio-manufacturing (Anjum et al., 2012).

Microbial Approaches for Bioremediation

Microorganisms are used for the decomposition or transformation of environmental pollutants into non-toxic compounds and such process is known as bio-remediation. These are survival genes of *Pseudomonas sps, Rhodococcus, Mycobacterium sps.,* and *Bacillus sps.* microbes which have been chosen for their metabolic plasticity and ability to withstand adverse conditions (Azubuike et al., 2016). They are also able to decompose hydrocarbons, pesticides and industrial solvents, and are thus essential for environmental purification. The efficacy depends on the appropriate choice of the microbial strains and the environmental (Bhattacharyya et al., 2021).

Mechanisms of Microbial Bioremediation

Microbial bioremediation includes many ideas depending on individual pollutants and site characteristics (Tomczyk et al., 2023):

- **Bioaugmentation:** Addition of specific populations of microbes to help in the degradation of pollutants. For instance, *Pseudomonas putida* breaks down aromatic hydrocarbons found in oil-contaminated soils.
- **Biostimulation:** The addition of nutrients, such as nitrogen or phosphorus, to promote the growth of indigenous microbial group involved in clean-up of petroleum products.
- **Biosparging:** The process of bubbling air through groundwater to stimulate aerobic biodegradation of volatile organic compounds (VOCs) like benzene (Das & Dash, 2014).
- **Bioventing:** The process of inducing air flow through unsaturated soil to stimulate microbial respiration competent cells effective for petroleum hydrocarbons.
- **Composting:** Blending of secondary-contaminated soil and organic matter, for example, agriculture waste, so that to accelerate microbial degradation (Gadd, 2010).

Recent Advancements in Microbial Bioremediation

Designing of microbial bioremediation systems require several strategies which accompany the production of advanced methodologies such as:

- **Synthetic Biology:** Engineered microbes (Singh et al., 2011) with expanded degradation pathways could provide alternative strategies for bioremediation, pollutants like polychlorinated biphenyls (PCBs) can be managed, Eg. modified *Escherichia coli* degrades polyethylene terephthalate (PET) plastics.
- **Metagenomics**: DNA sequencing reveals new species from weird fumaroles which creates greater diversity in the bioremediation tool kit.
- **Bio electrochemical Systems**: Microorganisms cooperating with electrodes, as in microbial fuel cells (Microbial Fuel Cells) enables simultaneous wastewater treatment and power generation (Glick, 2010).

Biodegradation of Plastics, Industrial and Organic Waste

A massive disposal table of plastics and organic waste Plenty of environmental issues resulted from the accumulation of plastics and organic waste adding to landfill overflow and emissions. Biodegradation through microbial digestors. For those products, it provides a circular solution, converting waste into biogas, compost and monomers. This section presents an overview of digestor types, mechanisms, and industrial developments for digestors (Priya et al., 2022).

Types of Digestors

Digesters are managed in a manner adapted to the types of waste to be treated. The following table summarizes their characteristics:

- **Anaerobic Digestors:** Bacteria that thrive without oxygen break down organic waste in the absence of oxygen through the process of anaerobic digestion applications, resulting in energy, biogas, and digestate production for energy and agricultural uses (Khan et al., 2018).
- **Aerobic Composting:** Conditions with high oxygen content encourage microbes that convert waste into stable Arena: The name for the area where a particular operation takes place compost, we're decreasing your volume and making a soil amendment (Lovley, 2006).
- **Enzymatic Digestors:** Catabolism of bioplastic polymers by enzymes, such as hydrolases and oxidoreductases to monomers, or metabolized to CO2 and water. Enzymes like cutinases cleave polymer chains to oligomers, which can be further metabolized by microorganisms to form CO2, water, and biomass, thereby accomplishing the biodegradation cycle (Sharma et al., 2018) (Figure 3).

Figure 3. Breakdown of bioplastic polymers by enzymes (such as hydrolases and oxidoreductases) into monomers

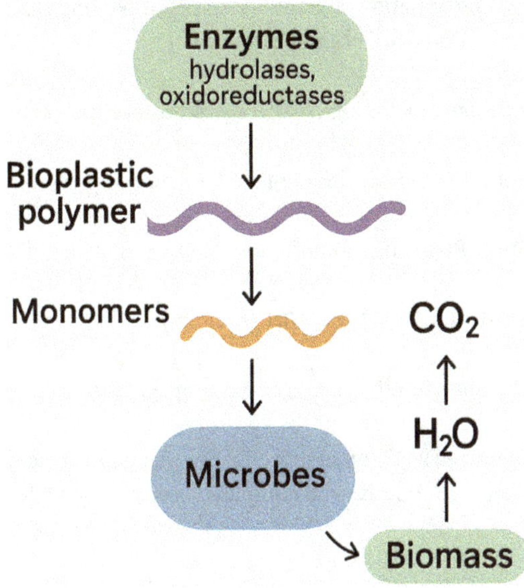

The microbial metabolism converts these monomers into CO_2, H_2O, and biomass, completing the biodegradation cycle and contributing to a sustainable bioplastic life cycle.

Industry Innovations

Production of biologically sustainable products require innovations in the industrial scale manufacturing design and planning. These products thereby meet the standards of the domestic usage and industrial design.

- **Starch Derived Bioplastics:** Processed from potato skins and remnants of banana are biodegradable and are used in packaging.
- **Advanced Sorting:** Composting facilities logically use near-infrared spectroscopy to separate bioplastics, improving degradation efficiency.
- **Processed biogas plants:** Modern plants process mixed waste streams, which can convert 60–70% of the pollutants contained in the mixed waste organic trash into biogas for fuel.

Bioremediation and Phytoremediation to Detoxify Heavy Metals Obtained from Different Industries

Heavy metals (Megharaj et al., 2011) released by human industrial or agricultural activities are persistent and toxic.

Phytoremediation Techniques

Phytoremediation is a remediation strategy based on employing plants to remove, stabilize, or transform heavy metals (Pilon-Smits, 2005).

- **Phytoextraction:** Plants including *Brassica juncea* take metals up into shoots which are then harvested.
- **Phytostabilization:** Metals are immobilized in roots by plants that include *Vetiveria zizanioides.*
- **Phytovolatilization:** Plants like *Populus spp.* convert metals into volatile forms

Plant Growth-Promoting Rhizobacteria (PGPR)

Bacteria such as Bacillus subtilis increase the crop growth and metal uptake (Reddy & Cameselle, 2009).

Mycorrhizae: Fungus such as Glomus spp. enhance metal uptake and plant tolerance. Green Belts: Metal plants collect around industrial complexes and passively detoxify (Tiquia-Arashiro & Rodrigues, 2016).

Table 1. Overview of key microbial strains and algal species involved in the bioremediation of toxic heavy metals such as cadmium, lead, mercury, and uranium

S.no	Pollutant	Microorganism	Functions and Affects on Heavy Metals	References
1	Cadmium	*Bacillus cereus* HQ-1	Biosorption via cell wall; Langmuir isotherm model	**(Hu et al., 2007)**
2	Lead	*Bacillus cereus* SEM-15	Adsorption via IAA secretion & Phosphate solubilization	**(Li et al., 2023)**
3	Mercury	*Pseudomonas aeruginosa*	This strain can absorb ~180 mg Hg/g for the toxin removal	**(Tang et al., 2024)**
4	Chromium	*Aspergillus flavus* and *A. fumigatus* (fungi)	They remove >70 % Cr (VI) via surface binding to the metal ion.	**(Tarfeen et al., 2022)**
5	Copper	*Cystoseira crinitophylla* algae	It adsorbs 160 mg Cu/g of copper waste.	**(Tarfeen et al., 2022)**
6	Zinc	*Rhodobacter capsulatus*	164 mg Zn/g uptake through the cell wall.	**(Tang et al.,2024)**
7	Arsenic	*Halomonas sp*	Oxidizes arsenite [As^{3+}] to less toxic forms to for safer disposal.	**(Qattan, 2025)**
8	Iron	*Geobacter sulfurreducens*	Reduces ferric (oxy)hydroxides (e.g., hematite nanoparticles, 10–50 nm) under varied pH and hydrogen conditions	**(Yan et al., 2008)**
9	Uranium	*Stenotrophomonas sp.*	Achieves ~98% U removal from mining wastewater (47 mg/L) in 72 h; ~1,199 mg U/g biomass in alginate-embedded systems	**(Sánchez-Castro et al., 2021)**
10	Nickel	*Lysinibacillus sp.*	Cell wall functional groups (carboxyl, hydroxyl, amino) bind Ni; both live and dead biomass effective in effluent treatment.	**(Prithviraj et al., 2014)**

SUSTAINABLE PRODUCT DEVELOPMENT THROUGH GREEN BIOMANUFACTURING

Biodegradable Bioplastics for Sustainable Packaging

Conventional plastics have been used extensively since the 1940s to replace goods made of paper, glass, and metal because of their affordability, versatility, and desired qualities (Thakur et al., 2018). Later on, these plastics are being used everywhere for example they are used in clothing, packaging, food services, agriculture, consumer electronics, automotive, consumer goods, building and construction. Among all of these nowadays plastics are mostly used in food packaging, that is approximately about 40% (Narancic et al., 2020). Every year 300 million tons of plastic is generated but only small amounts are recycled, the remaining is all waste and is dumped into the water bodies which takes millennia to decompose. They also contribute to microplastic pollution and greenhouse gas emissions that have a negative effect on ecosystems and human health (Fredi & Dorigato, 2021; Gurunathan et al., 2025). Twelve million tons of plastic enter the ocean annually. Of these, 1.75 tonnes come directly from the shipping and fishing sectors, while 9.5 million tonnes make their way to the ocean via land (Khalid et al., 2022). So, these plastics are harmful for the environment as they are non-biodegradable and get accumulated on land and in the marine ecosystem (Kirar et al., 2024), they should be replaced by a healthy option which can be bioplastics.

Bioplastics are prepared from various sources like rice straw, wood pulp, cereals etc. The rice straw is a huge waste and it increases soil fertility but also produces disease causing organisms. Also, it is not easily degradable. It is reported that most of the farmers in North India are burning rice straw which is causing environmental pollution as it leads to greenhouse gas emission (Gadde et al., 2009). Therefore, instead of burning the rice straw they can be used in the preparation of bioplastic packaging materials. It is observed that there is steady increase in the use of bioplastic for food packaging, when 65% of bioplastic produced in 2018 is used in it (D'Almeida & de Albuquerque, 2024). The cellulose in the rice straw and also the chitosan from the shrimp shells can be used in this bioplastic packaging material. The bioplastics have a different characteristic depending on the composition of the ratio of chitosan and cellulose such as (chitosan: cellulose) 3:10, 4:10, 5:10. Various characteristics such as density, tensile strength, water absorption, modulus of elasticity, and elongation at break are calculated (Sain, 2020). The bioplastic's density determines how well it shields packaged goods from the elements. Greater air and moisture resistance can be achieved by using higher density bioplastics, which could increase the products' shelf life (Pratiwi et al., 2017). Water absorption is significant because it can impact the mechanical characteristics and rate of bioplastic breakdown. In particular, high-water absorption in starch-based bioplastics can cause swelling, deterioration, and even hydrolysis (material breakdown). A material's tensile strength tells how much stress it can bear before breaking. A bioplastic with a higher tensile strength may withstand greater weight and stress during handling, storage, and transit without rupturing or shattering. The stiffness or resistance to deformation under stress is measured by modulus of elasticity. Certain packing applications that call for stiffness may benefit from a stiffer material, which is indicated by a higher modulus of elasticity. Tensile strength and it are strongly related. The amount of strain a material can withstand before breaking is measured by its elongation at break. For flexibility and impact resistance, this is crucial. For packaging that must endure impacts, a higher elongation at break indicates that the material may bend more before breaking.

Among the ratios mentioned above, the one having the high chitosan (5:10) has a higher density than the other two. The ratio 4:10 has a high tensile strength, modulus of elasticity, and elongation at break and the one with less chitosan has the high-water absorption which is an essential property for the bioplastic to degrade (Sain, 2020).

Bio-Filter for Pollution Control and Abetment

To control the rising pollution in different forms that affect all life forms which has created a global crisis of critical climate change and threat to human health; United Nations has formed 17 "The Sustainable Development Goals" (Carlsen & Bruggemann, 2022). Water is most abundantly found on earth where only 3 percent water is portable and the remaining counterpart to be in salty water in oceans. Disposal of waste and effluents from domestic households to industries has created accumulation of harmful toxic waste into water bodies. It is estimated that around 2 billion people use the contaminated water which causes cancers and many chronic disorders. This has created a requirement for a filter that can absorb, detoxify, precipitate and coagulate the entry of wastes into water bodies (Kumar et al., 2011). Biofilters are generally containers that are packed with biofilm with microbes growing actively and constantly feeding on the organic substrates. These biofilters need to possess some key features which makes them suitable for industrial effluent treatment. They are (Andres et al., 2006):

- Size and porosity of the packing bed.
- Enriching nutrient supply for high metabolic activity.
- Heterogenous mixture of microbes for multiple toxin removal.
- Mechanical stability of the packing bed.

Biofilters are made including these mentioned characteristics using agricultural wastes and animal husbandry by products. Different compositions of elements can be used for the biofilter packaging which includes ceramic, porcelite and perlite (Sakuma et al.,2006). Biofiltration also depends on some associated parameters such as Moisture level, Substrate composition, Optimum temperature and packaging composition and type of microbes (Pachaiappan et al.,2022). The biomanufacturing steps that are followed during the product of biofilters are:

1. Microbial species selection and genetic modification: Identifying and genetically enhancing microbes which can have high tolerance to high pollutant-degrading capabilities.
2. Base media preparation: Developing porous, durable, and bio-compatible support materials that allow microbial growth and stability.
3. Immobilization: Microbes are immobilized on the media either naturally by biofilm development or by synthetic means like encapsulation.
4. Assembly: The filter media loaded with microbes is assembled into filter units and tested under controlled environmental conditions to ensure microbial activity is stable and effective.
5. Scaling and customization: Biomanufacturing allows scalable production and modification of biological processes—ranging from household units to industrial-scale (Le Borgne & Baquerizo (2019).

Biofilters also possess some critical challenges that can affect their applications in various waste treatments which are coagulation and formation of flocks by the microbes during their growth which hampers the filtration process, sometimes microbes present in the biofilm can produce inhibitory compounds in reaction to toxic compounds which terminates the filtration and finally the denitrification of rice straws takes prolonged period due to the release of carbon at a faster rate (Zhao et al., 2020).

Sustainable Biofuel Production

Diminishing fossil fuel reserves, rising pollution and global warming has led to the production of sustainable and renewable biofuels through microbial metabolic mechanisms. This has promising positive impacts on environment and carbon footprint (Herdlevær & Barth., 2024). Production of biofuels from organic wastes of industrial processes like paper pulp mills involves certain chemical reactions like hydrolysis, acidogenesis, acetogenesis and methanogenesis. These processes produce methane as a primary product and a mixture of other gases which includes ammonia, carbon dioxide and nitrogen. Bacteria utilize these reactions to convert organic waste to other desired products (Chan-Yam et al., 2022). Other useful byproducts that are produced through anaerobic digestion of organic waste are biohydrogen, ethanol and biodiesel. Though these products are produced after anaerobic digestion their amount and quality depend on the type of raw material and environmental conditions (Kumar et al., 2025). Based on the type of raw materials used in the production of biofuels; they are classified into 4 generations (Figure 4):

Figure 4. Pictographically representation of the 4 generations of Biofuels which are produced with specific raw materials and associated products after biological manufacturing methods

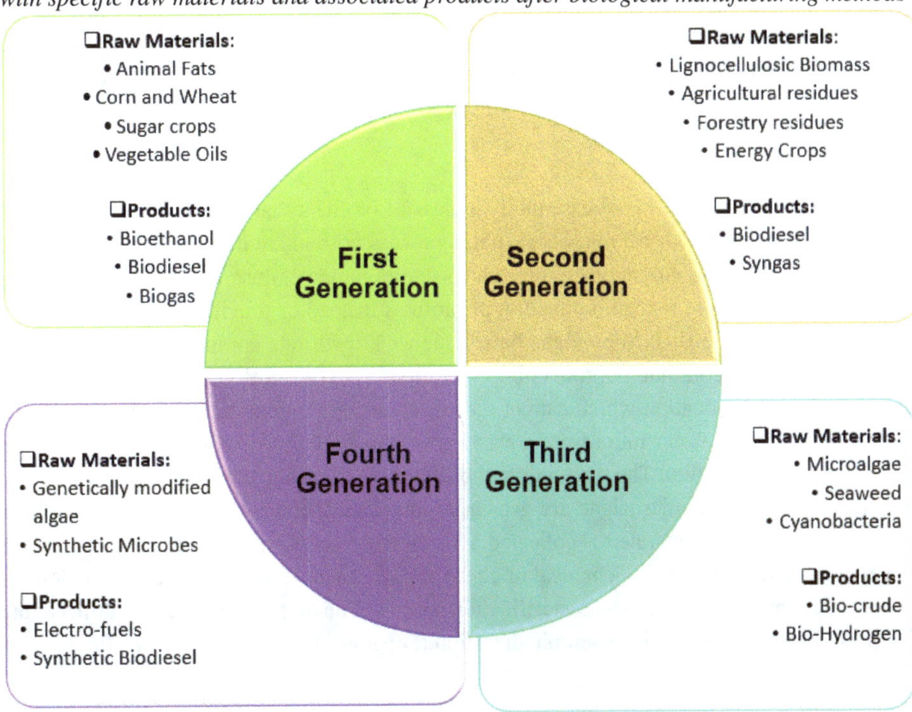

First Generation Biofuels

First generation biofuels are derived from edible parts of the plants which primarily contain starch, fatty acids and oils. Plants that produce an abundance of these biomolecules are sugar-cane, corn and beet roots. Biofuels such as biodiesel and ethanol are produced by processing the edible feedstocks. The biomanufacturing steps involve feedstock cultivation, harvesting & extraction, Conversion and Purification & distillation (Naik et al., 2010). Conversion of sugar/starch/oil crops into ethanol and biodiesel employs the usage of fermentation process using yeast and bacteria. Commercial biofuel producing crops require expensive pesticides, herbicides and also require large land requirements. Due to this economic feasibility of first-generation biofuels are not a cost-effective alternative for fossil fuels. Usage of edible crops for biofuel production also raises concerns over food security (Hirani et al., 2018).

Second Generation Biofuels

Second generation biofuels are produced from the non-edible parts of plants and animals. The major raw material that is used for their production is lignocellulose which is majorly present in vegetable and agricultural residues (Sims et al., 2010). Processing of these lignocellulosic biomass produces ethanol and alcohol. Lignin is most abundantly found in agricultural plant waste which replaces the regular disposal and pollution (Godbolea et al., 2018). The manufacturing of these biofuels involves steps such as pretreatment, enzyme hydrolysis, fermentation and purification. Pretreatment includes the chemical breakdown of lignocellulose. After the primary treatment enzyme hydrolysis uses cellulose and hemicellulose to produce sugars. These sugars are converted into ethanol and methane which are used as biofuels and biogas. This process is cost effective and contributes to environmental remediation as agricultural wastes are used as raw material for the conversion. Genetically modified microbes are used for fermentation of feedstock which enhances the product quality and reduces the byproduct inhibition (Naik et al., 2010).

Third Generation Biofuels

Third generation biofuels are essentially a class of biofuels that are produced from micro algae and other photosynthetic microbes. In this process normal environmental conditions are utilized which helps autotropic algae to produce starch, lignocellulose and fatty acids. This is then used as a substitute for the production of biofuels instead of providing additional energy sources (Dutta et al., 2014). Microalgae have a higher growth rate compared to other sources which helps for the continuous production of biofuel. They do not require sophisticated lab equipment for multiplication which caught recent researchers' attention (Kumar et al., 2018). Microalgae grow at a faster rate in waste water and sewage deposits which contributes to the environmental remediation. The production of biofuels via microalgae follows 2 phases: Firstly, Biological phase where microalgae are grown in ponds and photobioreactors which use light and CO_2. The biomass generated is collected and filtered. Secondly, the chemical phase where the cells are disrupted using mechanical or chemical treatment. Lipids extracted from biomass are converted into biodiesel by transesterification process. The by-products are then utilized into bioethanol and biogas through anaerobic digestion (Dragone et al., 2010).

Fourth Generation Biofuels

In recent years a new class of biofuel has been established which utilizes genetically altered microbes such as cyanobacteria, algae and fungi as feedstock. These microbes are engineered to tolerate toxic chemicals and inhibitory compounds. They are also modified to express their entire potential of converting substrates (Abdullah et al., 2019). Biomanufacturing of 4th generation biofuels include strategies of metabolic engineering and CRISPR-based gene editing. These GMOs are cultivated in bioreactors with an optimized fermentation with maximum yield. Some systems integrate carbon capture where cyanobacteria absorb CO2 during fuel synthesis. Post fermentation separation technologies such as solvent extraction and distillation are used for the purification of the biofuel produced (Love, 2022). The by-products produced from this process are used as raw materials in the waste valorization. Overall analysis of 4th generation biofuels is a promising alternative for biofuel production with minimal land usage and zero carbon footprint which is potent to replace the entire fossil fuels. Currently research is being undergone to fully utilize microbial effectiveness for biofuel production (Joshi & Mishra 2022).

ECONOMICAL AND SOCIAL IMPACT

The traditional methods are not cost efficient and non-prominent when efficiency is provided as an importance. The use of micro-organisms for the removal of pollutants in the environment is an inexpensive and eco-friendly approach of bioremediation of environment contaminated with toxic chemicals (Liu et al., 2019). Noticeable limitations, uncertainties and lack of genericity of efficacy and long-term environmental effects are concluded based on the past to present subsequent research studies, signalling that equity and cost-efficiency reviews are needed to reduce the limitations that characterize the literature. The necessity of physical and chemical modifications to achieve better performance is highlighted and the possibility of finding synergy between other types of remediation is discussed. Altogether, these advances are imperative to construct durable, sustainable biochar-based solutions in support of its commercialisation for massive environmental remediation (Masud et al., 2023). Biomanufacturing offers a green alternative to replace fossil feedstocks with valorization of agricultural and forest residues to biofuels and biochemicals. Problems of the complicated structure of lignocellulose and high costs of the conventional pretreatment techniques and exogenous hydrolase supplement are still unsolved. Future research will aim to couple enzyme production, hydrolysis, and fermentation in a single and less expensive process. The engineering of microbial co-culturing systems are considered as a very promising approach to counter metabolic burdens that lead to functional specialisation, and to improve the efficiency and stability of bioconversion towards a fossil-free future (Liu et al., 2021). Challenges associated with it are over-coming the complicated variability of feed stock, capital, and processing costs.

Overall, clear, comparable life-cycle assessments are necessary to inform research and policy toward a sustainable, fossil-free future (Benavides et al., 2024). There are problems to be solved in this field, including issues relating to product titre, product yield, and product productivity, for example. A key issue to be considered is the influence of the life span and aging of microorganisms on cell viability, process performance, and production longevity in industrial fermentation (Yang et al., 2023).

Economic Challenges & Regulatory Issues

Biomanufacturing for green principles is confronted with economical barriers, especially the high cost of scaling up to be remained competitive in the market. Presently, it is challenging to have clear and accepted guidelines and the standard criteria for combined TEA and LCA methods. These challenges result in poor predictability of impacts and process optimisation, which in turn risk the commercial success of bio-based innovations (Meramo et al., 2022). Some important concerns remain with respect to regulation of genetically modified organisms (GMOs) which can have concerns over biosafety and pathogenicity. Water, Existence and characterization of CRISPR/Cas systems in thermophilic bacteria and at the eukaryotic-microbial interface (Sharma et al., 2024). Key issues include possible transfer of genes to other microbes by horizontal gene transfer and the general impact on ecosystem flexibilities. The lack of adherence to appropriate bio-based plastic waste handling practices results in compromised environmental remediation. Inconsistent labelling and the absence of harmonized sustainability assessment methods result in 'greenwashing' and a general lack of transparency, for which dedicated regulatory frameworks and clearer guidelines are needed to deliver real environmental benefits and improve investors' confidence (de Souza et al., 2024). Microalgae are necessary for an environmentally friendly practice by helping to clean wastewater, capture carbon and make bioplastics – all essential for a circular economy. Their large-scale commercialization is hindered by the high costs associated with biomass production. Economically, the cost of CO2 capture by means of microalgae is much higher than chemical methods.

In addition, the industry faces regulatory barriers, including novel food authorisations and standardisation, as well as low public acceptability and investor scepticism (Tang et al., 2025). The bio-pharmaceutical manufacturing industry is also taking the reins on working to minimize its' environmental footprint through science and sensible design processes. It is essential that experienced architectural and process design sponsors in materials, processes, and suite designs to enable cost-effective reduction of several categories of environmental stress. Moreover, the design work is critical to meeting all appropriate regulatory requirements (Whitford et al., 2022). Single-use equipment provides environmental benefits by saving natural resources, particularly water and energy. It is related to cleaning operations. Furthermore, the addition of regulatory problems is most important. This is because of Good Manufacturing Practice, as well as the adoption of Quality by Design. These are essential for product quality and process integrity (Lalor et al., 2019). To solve these problems, people ask the government to create a simpler and perhaps separate regulation system for bio-based products. Also, there must be increased public spending on infrastructure and market incentives for greater competitiveness and acceleration of sustainable development (Attal-Juncqua et al., 2024). Tackling these challenges will require improved enforcement mechanisms, a convergence of international policies, and heightened investment in green chemistry and sustainable practices (Jairoun et al., 2025).

Challenges for Industrial Adoption

Economic Barriers

While biomanufacturing technologies hold promise for enhancing environmental sustainability, economic limitations present considerable obstacles. The development and installation of specialized bioreactors and biorefineries required for bioprocessing require significant capital inputs. Like conventional chemical factories, biomanufacturing facilities also have upfront fixed expenses. The initial setup costs are further increased by the fact that biomanufacturing facilities, in contrast to conventional chemical plants, need more controlled conditions and advanced biogenic maintenance equipment (Meyer et al., 2017).

Furthermore, when comparing the return on investment (ROI) of sustainable chemical alternative processes to that of sustainable biomanufacturing R&D, the former is always lengthier. Private financiers and corporations seeking faster financial returns are put off by these lengthier timeframes to realize rewards. Another difficulty is competing with economically motivated froths from less expensive fossil fuel products in addition to non-competitively priced bio-fuel substitutes that are characterized by biological marketing. One reason why stakeholders are reluctant to adopt these systems is the perceived financial risk involved in investing in unproven technologies that are defined by unique market constructs (Emadian et al., 2017).

Technical and Scale-Up Limitations

Scaling up biomanufacturing methods from laboratory to industry is a difficult undertaking that is frequently highly expensive and associated with challenges. When biomanufacturing processes are expanded from a highly controlled laboratory setting with access to cutting-edge technologies to the real world, they face operational, contamination, and environmental unpredictability. The stability, effectiveness, yield, and operational costs of the bioprocess are impacted by the sensitivity of critical bioremediation and biosynthetic microorganisms or enzymes to pH, temperature, and pollution load (Wang et al., 2020). The unpredictability of feedstock is another significant obstacle. Agricultural or industrial waste resources are frequently used in sustainable bioprocesses; however, the components of these resources vary depending on the source, time of year, or processing technique. Standardization and scale-up are complicated by these disparities, which necessitate regular adjustments to bioprocessing parameters (Giacomucci et al., 2020).

Regulatory and Quality-Assurance Constraints

Biomanufacturing processes, particularly those that use genetically modified organisms (GMOs), are subject to a stringent and intricate regulatory framework. The approval process is unduly drawn out when using modified microbes or new enzymes in open systems because they require thorough biosafety assessments of the altered microbe (Chomac-Pierzecka, 2025). Different countries' regulatory rules make it more difficult to coordinate internationally and transfer technology. The scalability and commercial viability of biomanufacturing technologies are undermined by the absence of harmonization of international standards. Furthermore, there are no consistent standards for assessing the efficacy and security of bio-based remediation treatments. Because of inconsistent quality control and monitoring practices, stakeholders are unable to evaluate the efficacy and compliance of various products, resulting in regulatory fragmentation. The market opportunity is impacted by this regulatory uncertainty, which also deters potential investors. (Lee et al., 2019).

Supply-Chain & Infrastructure Gaps

The current industrial infrastructure in many areas is not built to support large-scale biomanufacturing and bioprocessing plants. The lack of bioprocessing facilities in developing nations limits the adoption of sustainable technology. Regarding the logistics of moving and storing biologically active materials, biomanufacturing likewise has particular needs. In order to sustain activity, active microbial cultures, enzymes, and biomass need cold chain logistics and environmental control, which raises operating costs. Operational adoption is significantly hampered by the absence of established supply chains for acquiring and delivering feedstock and final products (Vučurović, 2024). In addition, downstream processing technologies for bioproduct separation, purification, and packaging are still in their infancy and cannot match the scalability and efficiency of chemical processes (Xiao et al., 2024).

Social Acceptance & Skill-Gaps

Public perception and social acceptance remain major obstacles for the biomanufacturing sector, particularly when it comes to genetically modified technologies. Concerns about biosafety, ecological balance, and ethics have led to a great deal of opposition and mistrust towards the use of modified microbes. Furthermore, practitioners' and regulators' understanding of biomanufacturing limitations and capacities is conspicuously lacking. There is now a shortage of qualified experts in the field, particularly those with training in microbiology, biochemistry, synthetic biology, and data science (Xu & Wang, 2015). The lack of integrated biomanufacturing process frameworks in training and education programs is impeding the development and uptake of these technologies (Zhang et al., 2025).

Future Prospects for Sustainable Biomanufacturing

Advanced Strain & Enzyme Engineering

Emergence of technologies like synthetic biology and genetic engineering are enhancing sustainable biomanufacturing. Genome editing techniques such as CRISPR allow shedding to be tailored towards degrading pollutants or synthesizing biopolymers. These engineered microbes improved efficiency, resistance to environmental changes, and enhanced metabolic capabilities (Bell et al., 2024). Other methods such as directed evolution and protein engineering have boosted enzyme efficiency under industrial conditions. These reductions make processes more biological in nature and environmentally friendly. Another development is the formation of microbial consortia toward complex wastes for bioprocessing which aids in increasing the scope and efficiency of bioremediation (Costa et al., 2021).

Smart Bioreactors & AI-Driven Control

Merging biomanufacturing infrastructure with digital tools gives rise to smart and responsive bioprocessing. For instance, modern bioreactors have real time sensors that measure the level of pH, oxygen, temperature, pollutant level, etc. This information is integrated through machine learning to adjust working conditions to enhance output and minimize resource usage. AI-powered control systems can anticipate and implement real-time corrective actions for any deviations from processes, thereby minimizing downtime and waste. Such innovation is expected to enhance the reliability, scalability, and economic efficiency of biomanufacturing (Silva et al., 2024).

Circular-Economy Integration

The concept of digital twins, which refers to the virtual replicas of physical bioprocessing systems, enables the simulation and optimization of various processes which helps in reducing the cost and time of industrial implementation.

Sustainable biomanufacturing is a key pillar of the circular economy revolving around waste mitigation and resource swapping, where agricultural by-products, food waste, and municipal sludge serve as raw materials for biofuels, bioplastics, high-value enzymes, and other biochemicals. Such as the reduced costs and environmental impact related to waste disposal. This method cuts down the ecological impact associated with waste disposal and economically benefits resource recovery. Another potential application is carbon capture and utilization (CCU) using engineered autotrophs or photosynthetic organisms which turn CO2 emissions into valuable products like organic acids or bio-based polymers. Such systems are designed to accomplish both pollution control and sustainable production for climate change reduction strategies (Liang et al., 2020).

Policy Incentives & Market Mechanisms

Policies and financial support are necessary to encourage sustainable biomanufacturing. They are providing green technologies funding, tax breaks, and subsidies. Regulatory sandboxes permit the controlled application of new biotechnologies, expediting their clinical utilization while balancing biosafety. In addition, carbon credits and sustainability-linked bonds also offer new revenue opportunities for companies that reduce emissions and restore the environment. Cross-border agreements and harmonized regulations are essential to facilitate international collaboration and investment. Providing supportive and efficient regulatory pathways will foster investor confidence and speed up industrial adoption (Chen & Jiang, 2018).

Collaborative Innovation Ecosystems

The future of biomanufacturing rests on collaborative innovation ecosystems integrating civil society, government, industry, and academia. A combination of sectors in public-private partnerships can more efficiently develop and deploy technologies by blending their resources, infrastructure, and expertise. Startups, researchers, and other individuals in low-resourced settings are now able to contribute to the field due to unrestricted access to genetic tools, process designs, and strain libraries made available through bio foundries and open-source platforms. In addition to interdisciplinary research initiatives, international consortia are also enabling innovation that make biomanufacturing solutions contextually relevant and globally scalable. These collaboration frameworks are critical for effectively tackling multifaceted environmental issues alongside realizing the full potential of sustainable biomanufacturing (Shahab et al., 2025).

CONCLUSION

As industrial processes increase and environmental pollution rises, the need for safe, efficient, and sustainable alternatives to conventional remediation methods has increased. The areas of application of biologically mediated technologies range from hydrocarbon and heavy metal degradation to plastic wastes recycling to renewable resources, which are essential for next-generation environmental and industrial technologies. The metabolic capabilities of various fungal and bacterial organisms have turned microbial bioremediation into one of the most innovative techniques. Microorganisms such as Pseudomonas, Bacillus, Mycobacterium, and Streptomyces have adept abilities to hydrolyse solvents, pesticides, and even resistant plastics. Under different environmental conditions, these microbes' abilities are enhanced through bioaugmentation, biostimulation, and bio-sparging. Furthermore, recently emerged synthetic biology is providing new opportunities for more targeted tolerance and specificity genetic engineering of microbes. Today, with the aid of CRISPR-Cas9 and metabolic pathway design, more efficient engineered strains than those found in nature are being developed for the digestion of recalcitrant pollutants such as polychlorinated biphenyls (PCBs) and polyethylene terephthalate (PET).

Purification of the contaminated site by soil and water phytoremediation in the microcosm model is environmentally and economically appealing and has been widely adopted today. Some plants including Vetiveria zizanioides, Populus spp., & Brassica juncea are reported for the bio-extraction of heavy metals like cadmium, arsenic, lead and chromium. They have the ability to detoxify these metals via phytoextraction, Phyto stabilization and even phytovolatilization. Mycorrhizal fungi and PGPRs, which secrete phytohormones and work synchronously with plants provide an advantage. These symbiotic systems increase the metabolomic response of the plant to environmental stress and contribute to the nutrients uptake and efficient utilization. Recent advances in plant biotechnology, have resulted in the development of a new class of genetically engineered plants for rural as well as urban areas which can take up high concentration of pollutants, open up the possibilities to phytoremediate the area of contamination. Biomanufacturing is important for sustainable development because of its' ability to convert waste into useful products. Anaerobic digestion, aerobic composting, and enzymatic digestion can produce biogas, compost, and bio-fertilizers, from surplus agricultural products, food wastes, and even plastics like biodegradable plastics. Hydrolases and cutinases have been exploited to degrade PLA and starch-based plastics as a renewable alternative to petroleum-based materials. MFCs (Microbial Fuel Cells) are categorized as Benign Systems as they have the capability to produce electricity with waste treatment within the presence of microbes. These strategies conform to the UN Sustainable Development. These are in accordance with the following United Nations Sustainable Development Goals (SDG 6: Clean Water, SDG 12: Responsible Consumption, and SDG 13: Climate) Nevertheless, there are issues including (1) high startup cost, (2) no infrastructure, (3) outdated legislation and (4) low public interest hampering it from widespread application. These issues are not likely to be solved by any one industry in particular, but will only be effectively addressed through industry collaboration, innovative regulations and fiscals, public education, and technological literacy. Thus, this chapter provides a comprehensive and detailed overview of the current biomanufacturing techniques and advancements in the field on engineering and technology. It also emphasizes the role of sustainable goals which contribute to the development of novel and ecofriendly products. It also provides a future scope in understanding better alternatives for traditional manufacturing methods.

ACKNOWLEDGEMENTS

The authors are highly obliged to Parul Institute of Technology, Parul University, Vadodara, Gujarat, India, for allowing them to carry out this work. The authors are also thankful to Er. Ayush Madan, Department of Biotechnology, School of Research & Technology, People's University, Bhanpur, Bhopal, Madhya Pradesh 462037, India for his constant help and support while preparation of this book chapter.

REFERENCES

Abdullah, B., Muhammad, S. A. F. A. S., Shokravi, Z., Ismail, S., Kassim, K. A., Mahmood, A. N., & Aziz, M. M. A. (2019). Fourth generation biofuel: A review on risks and mitigation strategies. *Renewable & Sustainable Energy Reviews, 107*, 37–50. DOI: 10.1016/j.rser.2019.02.018

Ahmad, J., Marsidi, N., Sheikh Abdullah, S. R., Hasan, H. A., Othman, A. R., Ismail, N., & Kurniawan, S. B. (2024). Integrating phytoremediation and mycoremediation with biosurfactant-producing fungi for hydrocarbon removal and the potential production of secondary resources. *Chemosphere, 349*, 140881. DOI: 10.1016/j.chemosphere.2023.140881 PMID: 38048826

Ahmad, M., Rajapaksha, A. U., Lim, J. E., Zhang, M., Bolan, N., Mohan, D., Vithanage, M., Lee, S. S., & Ok, Y. S. (2014). Biochar as a sorbent for contaminant management in soil and water: A review. *Chemosphere, 99*, 19–33. DOI: 10.1016/j.chemosphere.2013.10.071 PMID: 24289982

Al-Yasiri, A. J. (2021). Global Energy Demand For Different Energy Sources: Current Status and Future Prospects. *Akkad Journal Of Contemporary Economic Studies, 1*(4), 186–196. DOI: 10.55202/ajces.v1i4.96

Ali, A., Usman, M., Jayamani, E., Soon, K., & bin Ab Wahab, M. K. (2024). Sustainable Biomanufacturing. In Biomedical Implants (pp. 195-217). CRC Press. https://doi.org/DOI: 10.1201/9781003375098-12

Ali, H., Khan, E., & Ilahi, I. (2019). Environmental chemistry and ecotoxicology of hazardous heavy metals: Environmental persistence, toxicity, and bioaccumulation. *Journal of Chemistry, 6730305*. Advance online publication. DOI: 10.1155/2019/6730305

Andres, Y., Dumont, E., Le Cloirec, P., & Ramirez-Lopez, E. (2006). Wood bark as packing material in a biofilter used for air treatment. *Environmental Technology, 27*(12), 1297–1301. DOI: 10.1080/09593332708618747 PMID: 17285934

Anjum, N. A., Ahmad, I., & Duarte, A. C. (Eds.). (2012). *The plant family Brassicaceae: Contribution towards phytoremediation*. Springer., https://www.researchgate.net/publication/230729665_The_Plant_Family_Brassicaceae_Contribution_Towards_Phytoremediation

Appels, L., Lauwers, J., Degrève, J., Helsen, L., Lievens, B., Willems, K., & Dewil, R. (2011). Anaerobic digestion in global bio-energy production: Potential and research challenges. *Renewable & Sustainable Energy Reviews, 15*(9), 4295–4301. DOI: 10.1016/j.rser.2011.07.121

Arvelli, S., Jia, L., Zhang, M., & Zhao, J. (2025). Review of Advanced Technologies and Circular Pathways for Food Waste Valorization. *Journal of Agricultural and Food Chemistry, 73*(26), 16085–16108. DOI: 10.1021/acs.jafc.5c03394 PMID: 40549968

Attal-Juncqua, A., Getz, J., Morhard, R., & Gronvall, G. K. (2024). Integrating safety, security, sustainability, and social responsibility principles into the U.S. bioeconomy. *MSphere, 9*(5), e0008424. DOI: 10.1128/msphere.00084-24 PMID: 38687115

Austin, H. P., Allen, M. D., Donohoe, B. S., Rorrer, N. A., Kearns, F. L., Silveira, R. L., Pollard, B. C., Dominick, G., Duman, R., El Omari, K., Mykhaylyk, V., Wagner, A., Michener, W. E., Amore, A., Skaf, M. S., Crowley, M. F., Thorne, A. W., Johnson, C. W., Woodcock, H. L., & Beckham, G. T. (2018). Characterization and engineering of a plastic-degrading aromatic polyesterase. *Proceedings of the National Academy of Sciences of the United States of America, 115*(19), E4350–E4357. DOI: 10.1073/pnas.1718804115 PMID: 29666242

Azubuike, C. C., Chikere, C. B., & Okpokwasili, G. C. (2016). Bioremediation techniques-classification based on site of application: Principles, advantages, limitations and prospects. *World Journal of Microbiology & Biotechnology, 32*(11), 180. DOI: 10.1007/s11274-016-2137-x PMID: 27638318

Bala, S., Garg, D., Thirumalesh, B. V., Sharma, M., Sridhar, K., Inbaraj, B. S., & Tripathi, M. (2022). Recent Strategies for Bioremediation of Emerging Pollutants: A Review for a Green and Sustainable Environment. *Toxics, 10*(8), 484. DOI: 10.3390/toxics10080484 PMID: 36006163

Balaji, S. G., Penubaka, K. K. R., Kumar, M., Goel, P., Jadhav, A. B., & Mohakud, S. (2025). Circular economy strategies for resource efficiency and sustainable development in manufacturing industries. *Journal of Neonatal Surgery, 14*(13s). https://www.researchgate.net/publication/390598115

Bano, S., Singh, K., Chaudhary, A., & Chandra, R. (2025). Innovative methods for the valorisation of solid wastes from sugar mill and refineries for sustainable development: A review. *Cleaner Waste Systems, 10*, 100230. DOI: 10.1016/j.clwas.2025.100230

Beleno, M. T., & Ramos, R. T. (2024). Agro-industrial waste valorization: An environmental improvement strategy. In Agro-industrial environmental improvement models [Chapter]. Autonomous University of Baja California. https://doi.org/DOI: 10.13140/RG.2.2.27769.28005

Bell, E. L., Hutton, A. E., Burke, A. J., O'Connell, A., Barry, A., O'Reilly, E., & Green, A. P. (2024). Strategies for designing biocatalysts with new functions. *Chemical Society Reviews, 53*(6), 2851–2862. DOI: 10.1039/d3cs00972f PMID: 38353665

Benavides, P. T., Balchandani, S., & Gracida-Alvarez, U. R. (2024). Environmental analysis of biotechnologies for biofuels, bioplastics, and bioproducts: A greenhouse gas (GHG) emissions review. *Biotechnology for the Environment, 1*(1), 10. DOI: 10.1186/s44314-024-00010-5

Benn, N., & Zitomer, D. (2018). Pretreatment and anaerobic co-digestion of selected PHB and PLA bioplastics. *Frontiers in Environmental Science, 5*, 93. DOI: 10.3389/fenvs.2017.00093

Bhatia, S. K., Bhatia, S., Inda-Webb, M. E., Kourmentza, K., Moon, T. S., Singh, V., & Zhao, J. (2024). Biotechnology for sustainable materials: Innovating today for a greener tomorrow. *Biotechnology for Sustainable Materials*, *1*(1), 3. DOI: 10.3390/su16198515

Bhattacharyya, P., Roychoudhury, N., & Banerjee, S. (2021). Bioremediation of heavy metals using microbial consortia: Recent trends and applications. *Environmental Technology & Innovation*, *24*, 101893. DOI: 10.1007/978-981-16-0602-1_12

Carlsen, L., & Bruggemann, R. (2022). The 17 United Nations' sustainable development goals: A status by 2020. *International Journal of Sustainable Development and World Ecology*, *29*(3), 219–229. https://ui.adsabs.harvard.edu/link_gateway/2022IJSDW.29.219C/doi:10.1080/13504509.2021.1948456

Castro-Criado, D., Rivera-Flores, O., Abdullah, J. A. A., Castro-Osorto, E., Alonso-González, M., Ramos-Casco, L., Perez-Puyana, V. M., Sánchez-Barahona, M., Sánchez-Cid, P., Jiménez-Rosado, M., & Romero, A. (2023). Valorization of Honduran Agro-Food Waste to Produce Bioplastics. *Polymers*, *15*(12), 2625. DOI: 10.3390/polym15122625 PMID: 37376271

Cecilia, J. A., García-Sancho, C., Maireles-Torres, P., & Luque, R. (2019). Industrial food waste valorization: A general overview. In Bastidas-Oyanedel, J.-R., & Schmidt, J. E. (Eds.), *Biorefinery* (pp. 253–272). Springer., DOI: 10.1007/978-3-030-10961-5_11

Chan-Yam, K., Meyer, T., Scott, J. A., & Basiliko, N. (2022). Methane production potential of pulp mill sludges: Microbial community and substrate constraints. *FEMS Microbiology Letters*, *368*(21-24), fnab161. Advance online publication. DOI: 10.1093/femsle/fnab161 PMID: 34994385

Chen, G. Q., & Jiang, X. R. (2018). Engineering microorganisms for improving polyhydroxyalkanoate biosynthesis. *Current Opinion in Biotechnology*, *53*, 20–25. DOI: 10.1016/j.copbio.2017.10.008 PMID: 29169056

Chomać-Pierzecka, E. (2025). Innovation as an Attribute of the Sustainable Development of Pharmaceutical Companies. *Sustainability*, *17*(6), 2417. DOI: 10.3390/su17062417

Cichoski, T., Calian, M., Dias, F. T., Valente, R. C., & Guerra, J. B. S. O. A. (2024). Industrial waste valorization: Contributions to achieving the SDGs in Brazil. Case Study for the Multistakeholder Forum on Science, Technology and Innovation for the SDGs. http://dx.doi.org/DOI: 10.13140/RG.2.2.27769.28005

Costa, R., Conceição, M. M., da Silva, A. R., & Conceição, J. T. P. (2021). Marketing verde–A importância do consumo sustentável para as empresas. Research. *Social Development*, *10*(7), e26310716812–e26310716812. DOI: 10.33448/rsd-v10i7.16812

D'Almeida, A. P., & de Albuquerque, T. L. (2024). Innovations in Food Packaging: From Bio-Based Materials to Smart Packaging Systems. *Processes (Basel, Switzerland)*, *12*(10), 2085. DOI: 10.3390/pr12102085

Das, S., & Dash, H. R. (2014). Microbial bioremediation: A potential tool for restoration of contaminated areas. *Environmental Science and Pollution Research International*, *21*(17), 10255–10272. DOI: 10.1007/978-981-16-0602-1_17 de Souza, N. R. D., Groenestege, M., Spekreijse, J., Ribeiro, C., Matos, C. T., Pizzol, M., & Cherubini, F. (2024). Challenges and opportunities toward a sustainable bio-based chemical sector in Europe. *Wiley Interdisciplinary Reviews. Energy and Environment, 13*(5), e534. DOI: 10.1002/wene.534

Del Hierro, A. G., Moreno-Cid, J. A., & Casey, E. (2024). Continuous biomanufacturing for sustainable bioeconomy applications. *EFB Bioeconomy Journal, 4*, 100071. DOI: 10.1016/j.bioeco.2024.100071

Dhiman, P., Aggarwal, S., & Sethi, M. (2025). Technological innovations in food waste valorisation. *Discover Sustainability, 6*, 45. DOI: 10.1007/s43621-025-01073-4

Dilkes-Hoffman, L. S., Pratt, S., Lant, P. A., & Laycock, B. (2019). The role of biodegradable plastic in solving plastic solid waste accumulation. In *Plastics to energy* (pp. 469–505). William Andrew Publishing., DOI: 10.1016/b978-0-12-813140-4.00019-4

Dong, L., Liu, Z., & Bian, Y. (2021). Match circular economy and urban sustainability: Re-investigating circular economy under sustainable development goals (SDGs). *Circular Economy and Sustainability, 1*, 243–256. DOI: 10.1007/s43615-021-00021-2

Dragone, G., Fernandes, B., Vicente, A. A., & Teixeira, J. A. (2010). Third generation biofuels from microalgae. In Méndez-Vilas, A. (Ed.), *Current research, technology and education topics in applied microbiology and microbial biotechnology* (pp. 1355–1366). FORMATEX., https://www.researchgate.net/publication/236006059_Third_generation_biofuels_from_microalgae

Dutta, K., Daverey, A., & Lin, J. G. (2014). Evolution retrospective for alternative fuels: First to fourth generation. *Renewable Energy, 69*, 114–122. DOI: 10.1016/j.renene.2014.02.044

Elahi, A., Bukhari, D. A., Shamim, S., & Rehman, A. (2021). Plastics degradation by microbes: A sustainable approach. *Journal of King Saud University. Science, 33*(6), 101538. DOI: 10.1016/j.jksus.2021.101538

Emadian, S. M., Onay, T. T., & Demirel, B. (2017). Biodegradation of bioplastics in natural environments. Waste management, 59, 526-536. https://doi.org/DOI: 10.1016/j.wasman.2016.10.006

Falzarano, M., Polettini, A., Pomi, R., Rossi, A., & Zonfa, T. (2023). Anaerobic Biodegradability of Commercial Bioplastic Products: Systematic Bibliographic Analysis and Critical Assessment of the Latest Advances. *Materials (Basel, Switzerland), 16*(6), 2216. DOI: 10.3390/ma16062216 PMID: 36984096

Filippi, M., Mekkattu, M., & Katzschmann, R. K. (2025). Sustainable biofabrication: From bioprinting to AI-driven predictive methods. *Trends in Biotechnology, 43*(2), 290–303. DOI: 10.1016/j.tibtech.2024.07.002 PMID: 39069377

Forti, V., Balde, C. P., Kuehr, R., & Bel, G. (2020). The Global E-waste Monitor 2020: Quantities, flows and the circular economy potential. https://ewastemonitor.info/wp-content/uploads/2020/11/GEM_2020_def_july1_low.pdf

Fredi, G., & Dorigato, A. (2021). Recycling of bioplastic waste: A review. *Advanced Industrial and Engineering Polymer Research, 4*(3), 159–177. DOI: 10.1016/j.aiepr.2021.06.006

Gadd, G. M. (2010). Metals, minerals and microbes: Geomicrobiology and bioremediation. *Microbiology (Reading, England)*, *156*(Pt 3), 609–643. DOI: 10.1099/mic.0.037143-0 PMID: 20019082

Gadde, B., Bonnet, S., Menke, C., & Garivait, S. (2009). Air pollutant emissions from rice straw open field burning in India, Thailand and the Philippines. *Environmental Pollution*, *157*(5), 1554–1558. DOI: 10.1016/j.envpol.2009.01.004 PMID: 19201513

Gao, J. Q., Li, D., & Qiao, G. H. (2024). Circular economy strategies in supply chains: Enhancing resource efficiency and sustainable development goals. *Environmental Science and Pollution Research International*, *31*(7), 8751–8767. DOI: 10.1007/s11356-023-31551-z PMID: 38180660

Giacomucci, L., Raddadi, N., Soccio, M., Lotti, N., & Fava, F. (2020). Biodegradation of polyvinyl chloride plastic films by enriched anaerobic marine consortia. *Marine Environmental Research*, *158*, 104949. DOI: 10.1016/j.marenvres.2020.104949 PMID: 32217303

Glick, B. R. (2010). Using soil bacteria to facilitate phytoremediation. *Biotechnology Advances*, *28*(3), 367–374. DOI: 10.1016/j.biotechadv.2010.02.001 PMID: 20149857

Godbolea, A., Awate, S., Varadana, O. N., & Suresha, S. (2018). Biomass to Biofuel: A Review of Technologies of Production and Future Prospects. *International Journal of Engineering Research & Technology (Ahmedabad)*, *7*, 24–32. DOI: 10.17577/IJERTV7IS040017

Gurunathan, M. K., Navasingh, R. J. H., Selvam, J. D. R., & Čep, R. (2025). Development and characterization of starch bioplastics as a sustainable alternative for packaging. *Scientific Reports*, *15*(1), 15264. DOI: 10.1038/s41598-025-00221-0 PMID: 40312412

Herdlevær, K. M., & Barth, T. (2024). Optimizing formic acid-assisted Co-HTL of digested sewage sludge and lignocellulosic waste for enhanced bio-crude yield and energy recovery. *Energies*, *17*(1), 258. DOI: 10.3390/en17010258

Hirani, A. H., Javed, N., Asif, M., Basu, S. K., & Kumar, A. (2018). A review on first-and second-generation biofuel productions. Biofuels: greenhouse gas mitigation and global warming: next generation biofuels and role of biotechnology, 141-154. http://dx.doi.org/DOI: 10.1007/978-81-322-3763-1_8

Hoang, A. T., Nižetić, S., Ng, K. H., Papadopoulos, A. M., Le, A. T., Kumar, S., Hadiyanto, H., & Pham, V. V. (2022). Microbial fuel cells for bioelectricity production from waste as sustainable prospect of future energy sector. *Chemosphere*, *287*(Pt 3), 132285. DOI: 10.1016/j.chemosphere.2021.132285 PMID: 34563769

Hu, Q., Qi, H., Bai, Z., Dou, M., Zeng, J., Zhang, F., & Zhang, H. (2007). Biosorption of cadmium by a Cd 2+-hyperresistant Bacillus cereus strain HQ-1 newly isolated from a lead and zinc mine. *World Journal of Microbiology & Biotechnology*, *23*, 971–976. DOI: 10.1007/s11274-006-9322-2

Ingrao, C., Gigli, M., & Siracusa, V. (2017). An attributional Life Cycle Assessment application experience to highlight environmental hotspots in the production of foamy polylactic acid trays for fresh-food packaging usage. *Journal of Cleaner Production*, *150*, 93–103. DOI: 10.1016/j.jclepro.2017.03.007

Jairoun, A. A., Al-Hemyari, S. S., Shahwan, M., Alkhoujah, S., El-Dahiyat, F., Jaber, A. A. S., & Zyoud, S. H. (2025). Towards eco-friendly pharmaceuticals: Regulatory and policy approaches for sustainable medicines use. *Exploratory Research in Clinical and Social Pharmacy, 17*, 100576. DOI: 10.1016/j.rcsop.2025.100576 PMID: 40026320

Jaiswal, S., Sharma, B., & Shukla, P. (2020). Integrated approaches in microbial degradation of plastics. *Environmental Technology & Innovation, 17*, 100567. DOI: 10.1016/j.eti.2019.100567

Johnston, C. W., Wyatt, M. A., Li, X., Ibrahim, A., Shuster, J., Southam, G., & Magarvey, N. A. (2013). Gold biomineralization by a metallophore from a gold-associated microbe. *Nature Chemical Biology, 9*(4), 241–243. DOI: 10.1038/nchembio.1179 PMID: 23377039

Joshi, S., & Mishra, S. (2022). Recent advances in biofuel production through metabolic engineering. *Bioresource Technology, 352*, 127037. DOI: 10.1016/j.biortech.2022.127037 PMID: 35318143

Kabeyi, M. J. B., & Olanrewaju, O. A. (2022). Technologies for biogas to electricity conversion. *Energy Reports, 8*, 774–786. DOI: 10.1016/j.egyr.2022.11.007

Khalid, M. Y., Arif, Z. U., Ahmed, W., & Arshad, H. (2022). Recent trends in recycling and reusing techniques of different plastic polymers and their composite materials. *Sustainable Materials and Technologies, 31*, e00382. DOI: 10.1016/j.susmat.2021.e00382

Khan, M. I., Shin, J. H., & Kim, J. D. (2018). The promising future of microalgae: Current status, challenges, and optimization of a sustainable and renewable industry for biofuels, feed, and other products. *Microbial Cell Factories, 17*(1), 36. DOI: 10.1186/s12934-018-0879-x PMID: 29506528

Kirar, S., Mohne, D., Singh, M., Sagar, V., Bhise, A., Goswami, S., & Bhaumik, J. (2024). Eco-friendly lignin nanocomposite films as advanced UV protective and antimicrobial sustainable packaging materials. *Sustainable Materials and Technologies, 40*, e00864. DOI: 10.1016/j.susmat.2024.e00864

Kumar, T. P., Rahul, M., & Chandrajit, B. (2011). Biofiltration of volatile organic compounds (VOCs): an overview. Res J Chem Sci, 2231, 606X. https://isca.me/rjcs/Archives/vol1/I8/ISCA-RJCS-2011-174-15.pdf

Kumar, V., Nanda, M., Joshi, H. C., Singh, A., Sharma, S., & Verma, M. (2018). Production of biodiesel and bioethanol using algal biomass harvested from fresh water river. *Renewable Energy, 116*, 606–612. DOI: 10.1016/j.renene.2017.10.016

Kumar, V., Verma, P., de Freitas, F. A., Srivastava, P. K., Vashishth, A., & Américo-Pinheiro, J. H. P. (2025). A critical review on biofuels generation from pulp-paper mill sludge with emphasis on pretreatment methods: Renewable energy for environmental sustainability. *BMC Environmental Science, 2*(1), 2. DOI: 10.1186/s44329-024-00016-0

Lalor, F., Fitzpatrick, J., Sage, C., & Byrne, E. (2019). Sustainability in the biopharmaceutical industry: Seeking a holistic perspective. *Biotechnology Advances, 37*(5), 698–707. DOI: 10.1016/j.biotechadv.2019.03.015 PMID: 30922993

Le Borgne, S., & Baquerizo, G. (2019). Microbial Ecology of Biofiltration Units Used for the Desulfurization of Biogas. *ChemEngineering, 3*(3), 72. DOI: 10.3390/chemengineering3030072

Lee, S. Y., Kim, H. U., & Chae, T. U. (2019). A comprehensive metabolic map for production of bio-based chemicals. *Nature Catalysis*, *2*(1), 18–33. DOI: 10.1038/s41929-018-0212-4

Li, Q., Zhang, W., Liao, S., Xing, D., Xiao, Y., Zhou, D., & Yang, Q. (2023). Mechanism of lead adsorption by a Bacillus cereus strain with indole-3-acetic acid secretion and inorganic phosphorus dissolution functions. *BMC Microbiology*, *23*(1), 57. DOI: 10.1186/s12866-023-02795-z PMID: 36869296

Liang, B., Zhao, Y., & Yang, J. (2020). Recent Advances in Developing Artificial Autotrophic Microorganism for Reinforcing CO2 Fixation. *Frontiers in Microbiology*, *11*, 592631. DOI: 10.3389/fmicb.2020.592631 PMID: 33240247

Liu, L., Bilal, M., Duan, X., & Iqbal, H. M. N. (2019). Mitigation of environmental pollution by genetically engineered bacteria - Current challenges and future perspectives. *The Science of the Total Environment*, *667*, 444–454. DOI: 10.1016/j.scitotenv.2019.02.390 PMID: 30833243

Liu, Y., Tang, Y., Gao, H., Zhang, W., Jiang, Y., Xin, F., & Jiang, M. (2021). Challenges and Future Perspectives of Promising Biotechnologies for Lignocellulosic Biorefinery. *Molecules (Basel, Switzerland)*, *26*(17), 5411. DOI: 10.3390/molecules26175411 PMID: 34500844

Love, J. (2022). Microbial pathways for advanced biofuel production. *Biochemical Society Transactions*, *50*(2), 987–1001. DOI: 10.1042/BST20210764 PMID: 35411379

Lovley, D. R. (2006). Bug juice: Harvesting electricity with microorganisms. *Nature Reviews. Microbiology*, *4*(7), 497–508. DOI: 10.1038/nrmicro1442 PMID: 16778836

Ma, X., Liang, H., Panda, S., Fung, V. K. Y., Zhou, J. F. J., & Zhou, K. (2022). C2 feedstock-based biomanufacturing of value-added chemicals. *Current Opinion in Biotechnology*, *73*, 240–245. DOI: 10.1016/j.copbio.2021.08.017 PMID: 34536659

Maroof, L., Khan, I., Yoo, H. S., Kim, S., Park, H. T., Ahmad, B., & Azam, S. (2021). Identification and characterization of low density polyethylene-degrading bacteria isolated from soils of waste disposal sites. *Environmental Engineering Research*, *26*(3). Advance online publication. DOI: 10.4491/eer.2020.167

Masud, M. A. A., Shin, W. S., Sarker, A., Septian, A., Das, K., Deepo, D. M., Iqbal, M. A., Islam, A. R. M. T., & Malafaia, G. (2023). A critical review of sustainable application of biochar for green remediation: Research uncertainty and future directions. *The Science of the Total Environment*, *904*, 166813. DOI: 10.1016/j.scitotenv.2023.166813 PMID: 37683867

Megharaj, M., Ramakrishnan, B., Venkateswarlu, K., Sethunathan, N., & Naidu, R. (2011). Bioremediation approaches for organic pollutants: A critical perspective. *Environment International*, *37*(8), 1362–1375. DOI: 10.1016/j.envint.2011.06.003 PMID: 21722961

Meramo, S., Fantke, P., & Sukumara, S. (2022). Advances and opportunities in integrating economic and environmental performance of renewable products. *Biotechnology for Biofuels*, *15*, 144. DOI: 10.1186/s13068-022-02239-2 PMID: 36550529

Meyer, H. P., Minas, W., & Schmidhalter, D. (2017). Industrial-scale fermentation. Industrial biotechnology: products and processes, 1-53. http://dx.doi.org/DOI: 10.1002/9783527807833.ch1

Mishra, B., Mohanta, Y. K., Reddy, C. N., Reddy, S. D. M., Mandal, S. K., Yadavalli, R., & Sarma, H. (2023). Valorization of agro-industrial biowaste to biomaterials: An innovative circular bioeconomy approach. *Circular Economy*, *2*, 100050. DOI: 10.1016/j.cec.2023.100050

Mishra, B., Varjani, S., Kumar, G., Awasthi, M. K., Awasthi, S. K., Sindhu, R., & Zhang, Z. (2021). Microbial approaches for remediation of pollutants: Innovations, future outlook, and challenges. *Energy & Environment*, *32*(6), 1029–1058. DOI: 10.1177/0958305X19896781

Mohammadian Fazli, M., Soleimani, N., Mehrasbi, M., Darabian, S., Mohammadi, J., & Ramazani, A. (2015). Highly cadmium tolerant fungi: Their tolerance and removal potential. *Journal of Environmental Health Science & Engineering*, *13*, 19. DOI: 10.1186/s40201-015-0176-0 PMID: 25806110

Mujtaba, M., Fernandes Fraceto, L., Fazeli, M., Mukherjee, S., Savassa, S. M., Araujo de Medeiros, G., do Espírito Santo Pereira, A., Mancini, S. D., Lipponen, J., & Vilaplana, F. (2023). Lignocellulosic biomass from agricultural waste to the circular economy: A review with focus on biofuels, biocomposites and bioplastics. *Journal of Cleaner Production*, *402*, 136815. Advance online publication. DOI: 10.1016/j.jclepro.2023.136815

Naik, S. N., Goud, V. V., Rout, P. K., & Dalai, A. K. (2010). Production of first and second generation biofuels: A comprehensive review. *Renewable & Sustainable Energy Reviews*, *14*(2), 578–597. DOI: 10.1016/j.rser.2009.10.003

Narancic, T., Cerrone, F., Beagan, N., & O'Connor, K. E. (2020). Recent advances in bioplastics: Application and biodegradation. *Polymers*, *12*(4), 920. DOI: 10.3390/polym12040920 PMID: 32326661

Narisetty, V. R. R., Maitra, S., Tarafdar, A., Alphy, M. P., Kumar, A. N., Madhavan, A., Sirohi, R., Awasthi, M. K., Sindhu, R., Varjani, S., & Binod, P. (2023). Waste-Derived Fuels and Renewable Chemicals for Bioeconomy Promotion: A Sustainable Approach. *BioEnergy Research*, *16*(1), 16–32. DOI: 10.1007/s12155-022-10428-y PMID: 35350609

Nielsen, J., & Keasling, J. D. (2016). Engineering Cellular Metabolism. *Cell*, *164*(6), 1185–1197. DOI: 10.1016/j.cell.2016.02.004 PMID: 26967285

Okolie, O., Kumar, A., Edwards, C., Lawton, L. A., Oke, A., McDonald, S., Thakur, V. K., & Njuguna, J. (2023). Bio-Based Sustainable Polymers and Materials: From Processing to Biodegradation. *Journal of Composites Science*, *7*(6), 213. DOI: 10.3390/jcs7060213

Oluyemi, G. F., Afolabi, R. O., Zamora, S. C., Li, Y., & McElroy, D. (2024). Environmental Impact Assessment of a Plant Cell-Based Bio-Manufacturing Process for Producing Plant Natural Product Ingredients. *Sustainability*, *16*(19), 8515. DOI: 10.3390/su16198515

Pachaiappan, R., Cornejo-Ponce, L., Rajendran, R., Manavalan, K., Femilaa Rajan, V., & Awad, F. (2022). A review on biofiltration techniques: Recent advancements in the removal of volatile organic compounds and heavy metals in the treatment of polluted water. *Bioengineered*, *13*(4), 8432–8477. DOI: 10.1080/21655979.2022.2050538 PMID: 35260028

Pandey, K., Pandey, M., Kumar, V., Aggarwal, U., & Singhal, B. (2024). Bioprocessing 4.0 in biomanufacturing: Paving the way for sustainable bioeconomy. *Systems Microbiology and Biomanufacturing, 4*(2), 407–424. DOI: 10.1007/s43393-023-00206-y

Pant, D., Joshi, D., Upreti, M. K., & Kotnala, R. K. (2012). Chemical and biological extraction of metals present in E waste: A hybrid technology. *Waste Management (New York, N.Y.), 32*(5), 979–990. DOI: 10.1016/j.wasman.2011.12.002 PMID: 22217552

Paranthaman, S. R., & Karthikeyan, B. (2015). Bioremediation of heavy metal in paper mill effluent using Pseudomonas spp. *International Journal of Microbiology, 1*(1), 1–5. https://microbiozjournals.com/abstract-bioremediation-of-heavy-metal-in-paper-mill-effluent-using-pseudomonas-spp/

Peña-Montenegro, T. D., Lozano, L., & Dussán, J. (2015). Genome sequence and description of the mosquitocidal and heavy metal tolerant strain Lysinibacillus sphaericus CBAM5. *Standards in Genomic Sciences, 10*, 2. DOI: 10.1186/1944-3277-10-2 PMID: 25685257

Pilon-Smits, E. (2005). Phytoremediation. *Annual Review of Plant Biology, 56*, 15–39. DOI: 10.1146/annurev.arplant.56.032604.144214 PMID: 15862088

Pitzalis, M. F., & Sadler, J. C. (2025). Chemical bio-manufacture from diverse C-rich waste polymeric feedstocks using engineered microorganisms. *RSC Sustainability, 3*(4), 1672–1684. DOI: 10.1039/D5SU00013K

Pratiwi, R., Rahayu, D., & Barliana, M. I. (2017). Characterization of Bioplastic from Rice Straw Cellulose. *Research Journal of Pharmaceutical, Biological and Chemical Sciences, 8*, 217–221. https://www.rjpbcs.com/pdf/2017_8(1S)/[32].pdf

Prithviraj, D., Deboleena, K., Neelu, N., Noor, N., Aminur, R., Balasaheb, K., & Abul, M. (2014). Biosorption of nickel by Lysinibacillus sp. BA2 native to bauxite mine. *Ecotoxicology and Environmental Safety, 107*, 260–268. DOI: 10.1016/j.ecoenv.2014.06.009 PMID: 25011123

Priya, A. K., Jalil, A. A., Vadivel, S., Dutta, K., Rajendran, S., Fujii, M., & Soto-Moscoso, M. (2022). Heavy metal remediation from wastewater using microalgae: Recent advances and future trends. *Chemosphere, 305*, 135375. DOI: 10.1016/j.chemosphere.2022.135375 PMID: 35738200

Qattan, S. Y. (2025). Harnessing bacterial consortia for effective bioremediation: Targeted removal of heavy metals, hydrocarbons, and persistent pollutants. *Environmental Sciences Europe, 37*(1), 1–35. DOI: 10.1186/s12302-025-01103-y

Rahman, A. M., Rahman, T. T., Pei, Z., Ufodike, C. O., Lee, J., & Elwany, A. (2023). Additive Manufacturing Using Agriculturally Derived Biowastes: A Systematic Literature Review. *Bioengineering (Basel, Switzerland), 10*(7), 845. DOI: 10.3390/bioengineering10070845 PMID: 37508872

Reddy, K. R., & Cameselle, C. (2009). *Electrochemical remediation technologies for polluted soils, sediments and groundwater*. John Wiley & Sons., DOI: 10.1002/9780470523650

Rodríguez, J., Rubio, L., Celemín, M., & Alonso-Almeida, M. (2019). Analysis of the relations between circular economy and sustainable development goals. *International Journal of Sustainable Development and World Ecology*, *26*(1), 1–13. DOI: 10.1080/13504509.2019.1666754

Sain, M. (2020). Production of bioplastics and sustainable packaging materials from rice straw to eradicate stubble burning: A Mini-Review. *Environment Conservation Journal*, *21*(3), 1–5. DOI: 10.36953/ECJ.2020.21301

Sakuma, T., Hattori, T., & Deshusses, M. A. (2006). Comparison of different packing materials for the biofiltration of air toxics. Journal of the Air & Waste Management Association (1995), 56(11), 1567–1575. https://doi.org/DOI: 10.1080/10473289.2006.10464564

Sánchez-Castro, I., Martínez-Rodríguez, P., Abad, M. M., Descostes, M., & Merroun, M. L. (2021). Uranium removal from complex mining waters by alginate beads doped with cells of Stenotrophomonas sp. Br8: Novel perspectives for metal bioremediation. *Journal of Environmental Management*, *296*, 113411. DOI: 10.1016/j.jenvman.2021.113411 PMID: 34351286

Šašinková, D., Serbruyns, L., & Julinová, M., FayyazBakhsh, A., De Wilde, B., & Koutný, M. (2022). Evaluation of the biodegradation of polymeric materials in the freshwater environment—An attempt to prolong and accelerate the biodegradation experiment. *Polymer Degradation & Stability*, *203*, 110085. DOI: 10.1016/j.polymdegradstab.2022.110085

Sebastián Serna Loaiza, Miltner, A., & Miltner, M. (2022). Microbial utilization of next generation feedstocks for biomanufacturing. *Frontiers in Bioengineering and Biotechnology*, *10*, 874612. Advance online publication. DOI: 10.3389/fbioe.2022.874612 PMID: 35480982

Serna Loaiza, S., Miltner, A., Miltner, M., & Friedl, A. (2019). A review on the feedstocks for the sustainable production of bioactive compounds in biorefineries. *Sustainability*, *11*(23), 6765. DOI: 10.3390/su11236765

Shahab, M. A., Destro, F., & Braatz, R. D. (2025). Digital twins in biopharmaceutical manufacturing: Review & human-machine collaborative intelligence. arXiv. http://dx.doi.org//arXiv .2504.00286DOI: 10.48550

Sharma, B., Dangi, A. K., & Shukla, P. (2018). Contemporary enzyme based technologies for bioremediation: A review. *Journal of Environmental Management*, *210*, 10–22. DOI: 10.1016/j.jenvman.2017.12.075 PMID: 29329004

Sharma, P., Bano, A., Singh, S. P., Dubey, N. K., Chandra, R., & Iqbal, H. (2022). Recent advancements in microbial-assisted remediation strategies for toxic contaminants. *Cleaner Chemical Engineering*, *2*, 100020. DOI: 10.1016/j.clce.2022.100020

Sharma, S., Pathania, S., Bhagta, S., Kaushal, N., Bhardwaj, S., Bhatia, R. K., & Walia, A. (2024). Microbial remediation of polluted environment by using recombinant E. coli: A review. *Biotechnology for the Environment*, *1*(1), 8. DOI: 10.1186/s44314-024-00008-z

Silva, A. P. S. e, Araújo, N. M. da F. T. de S., Oliveira, M. D. S. de, Chagas, S. C. S., Marques, F. R. V., Britto, L. P. da S., … Nascimento, A. V. S. do. (2024). Industry 4.0 and Biotechnology: Strategies For Innovation snd Sustainability. Revista De Gestão - RGSA, 18(10), e08998. https://doi.org/DOI: 10.24857/rgsa.v18n10-094

Sims, R. E., Mabee, W., Saddler, J. N., & Taylor, M. (2010). An overview of second generation biofuel technologies. *Bioresource Technology*, *101*(6), 1570–1580. DOI: 10.1016/j.biortech.2009.11.046 PMID: 19963372

Singh, J. S., Abhilash, P. C., Singh, H. B., Singh, R. P., & Singh, D. P. (2011). Genetically engineered bacteria: An emerging tool for environmental remediation and future research perspectives. *Gene*, *480*(1-2), 1–9. DOI: 10.1016/j.gene.2011.03.001 PMID: 21402131

Sorooshian, S. (2024). The sustainable development goals of the United Nations: A comparative midterm research review. *Journal of Cleaner Production, 142272*. Advance online publication. DOI: 10.1016/j.jclepro.2024.142272

Taghavi, N., Singhal, N., Zhuang, W. Q., & Baroutian, S. (2021). Degradation of plastic waste using stimulated and naturally occurring microbial strains. *Chemosphere*, *263*, 127975. DOI: 10.1016/j.chemosphere.2020.127975 PMID: 32828061

Tang, D. Y. Y., Ooi, C., & Show, P. L. (2025). Blue bioeconomy and biotechnology: Towards a sustainably growing microalgae industry. *Blue Biotechnology*, *2*, 13. DOI: 10.1186/s44315-025-00036-8

Tang, H., Xiang, G., Xiao, W., Yang, Z., & Zhao, B. (2024). Microbial mediated remediation of heavy metals toxicity: Mechanisms and future prospects. *Frontiers in Plant Science*, *15*, 1420408. DOI: 10.3389/fpls.2024.1420408 PMID: 39100088

Tarfeen, N., Nisa, K. U., Hamid, B., Bashir, Z., Yatoo, A. M., Dar, M. A., Mohiddin, F. A., Amin, Z., Ahmad, R. A., & Sayyed, R. Z. (2022). Microbial Remediation: A Promising Tool for Reclamation of Contaminated Sites with Special Emphasis on Heavy Metal and Pesticide Pollution: A Review. *Processes (Basel, Switzerland)*, *10*(7), 1358. DOI: 10.3390/pr10071358

Thakur, S., Chaudhary, J., Sharma, B., Verma, A., Tamulevicius, S., & Thakur, V. K. (2018). Sustainability of bioplastics: Opportunities and challenges. *Current Opinion in Green and Sustainable Chemistry*, *13*, 68–75. DOI: 10.1016/j.cogsc.2018.04.013

Tiquia-Arashiro, S. M., & Rodrigues, D. F. (2016). *Bioremediation and biotechnology: Sustainable approaches to pollution degradation*. Springer International Publishing., DOI: 10.1007/978-3-030-35691-0

Tomczyk, P., Wdowczyk, A., Wiatkowska, B., & Szymańska-Pulikowska, A. (2023). Assessment of heavy metal contamination of agricultural soils in Poland using contamination indicators. *Ecological Indicators*, *156*, 111161. DOI: 10.1016/j.ecolind.2023.111161

Tsydenova, O., & Bengtsson, M. (2011). Chemical hazards associated with treatment of waste electrical and electronic equipment. *Waste Management (New York, N.Y.)*, *31*(1), 45–58. DOI: 10.1016/j.wasman.2010.08.014 PMID: 20869229

Valverde, J. M., & Avilés-Palacios, C. (2021). Circular economy as a catalyst for progress towards the sustainable development goals: A positive relationship between two self-sufficient variables. *Sustainability*, *13*(22), 12652. DOI: 10.3390/su132212652

Vučurović, D., Bajić, B., Trivunović, Z., Dodić, J., Zeljko, M., Jevtić-Mučibabić, R., & Dodić, S. (2024). Biotechnological Utilization of Agro-Industrial Residues and By-Products—Sustainable Production of Biosurfactants. *Foods*, *13*(5), 711. DOI: 10.3390/foods13050711 PMID: 38472824

Wang, B., Wang, Z., Chen, T., & Zhao, X. (2020). Development of Novel Bioreactor Control Systems Based on Smart Sensors and Actuators. *Frontiers in Bioengineering and Biotechnology*, *8*, 7. DOI: 10.3389/fbioe.2020.00007 PMID: 32117906

Wang, D., Lin, J., Lin, J., Wang, W., & Li, S. (2019). Biodegradation of Petroleum Hydrocarbons by Bacillus subtilis BL-27, a Strain with Weak Hydrophobicity. *Molecules (Basel, Switzerland)*, *24*(17), 3021. DOI: 10.3390/molecules24173021 PMID: 31438460

Whitford, B., Jones, D., & Kinnane, S. (2022). Biomanufacturing design: Reducing the environmental burden. *Current Opinion in Biotechnology*, *76*, 102717. DOI: 10.1016/j.copbio.2022.102717 PMID: 35439701

Wijekoon, W., Priyashantha, H., Gajanayake, P., Manage, P., Liyanage, C., Jayarathna, S., & Kumarasinghe, U. (2025). Review and prospects of phytoremediation: Harnessing biofuel-producing plants for environmental remediation. *Sustainability*, *17*(3), 822. DOI: 10.3390/su17030822

Willett, A., & Hajduk, M. (2024). Perspectives for using CO_2 as a feedstock for biomanufacturing. *Bioengineering (Basel, Switzerland)*, *10*(12), 1357. Advance online publication. DOI: 10.3390/bioengineering10121357 PMID: 38135948

Xian, Z. N., Yin, C. F., Zheng, L., Zhou, N. Y., & Xu, Y. (2023). Biodegradation of additive-free polypropylene by bacterial consortia enriched from the ocean and from the gut of Tenebrio molitor larvae. *The Science of the Total Environment*, *892*, 164721. DOI: 10.1016/j.scitotenv.2023.164721 PMID: 37301383

Xiao, X., Cheng, Y., & Zhang, Y. (2024). Sustainable Innovation in the Biopharmaceutical Industry: An Analysis of the Impact of Policy Configuration. *Sustainability*, *16*(6), 2339. DOI: 10.3390/su16062339

Xu, D., & Wang, J. (2015). Strategic emerging industries in China: Literature review and research prospect. *American Journal of Industrial and Business Management*, *5*(07), 486. DOI: 10.4236/ajibm.2015.57049

Yaashikaa, P. R., Senthil Kumar, P., & Varjani, S. (2022). Valorization of agro-industrial wastes for biorefinery process and circular bioeconomy: A critical review. *Bioresource Technology*, *343*, 126126. DOI: 10.1016/j.biortech.2021.126126 PMID: 34673193

Yan, B., Wrenn, B. A., Basak, S., Biswas, P., & Giammar, D. E. (2008). Microbial reduction of Fe(III) in hematite nanoparticles by Geobacter sulfurreducens. *Environmental Science & Technology*, *42*(17), 6526–6531. DOI: 10.1021/es800620f PMID: 18800525

Yang, S.-T., Wang, G., & Qin, Z. (2023). A perspective in future biomanufacturing: Challenges in industrial fermentation—understanding and controlling microbial lifespan and aging. *Synthetic Biology and Engineering*, *1*(3), 10019. DOI: 10.35534/sbe.2023.10019

Zhang, C., Ottenheim, C., Weingarten, M., & Ji, L. (2022). Microbial Utilization of Next-Generation Feedstocks for the Biomanufacturing of Value-Added Chemicals and Food Ingredients. *Frontiers in Bioengineering and Biotechnology*, *10*, 874612. DOI: 10.3389/fbioe.2022.874612 PMID: 35480982

Zhang, X., Luo, W., & Xiang, D. (2025). Strategic emerging industries and innovation: Evidence from China. *International Review of Economics & Finance*, *98*, 103858. DOI: 10.1016/j.iref.2025.103858

Zhang, Y. P., Sun, J., & Ma, Y. (2017). Biomanufacturing: History and perspective. *Journal of Industrial Microbiology & Biotechnology*, *44*(4-5), 773–784. DOI: 10.1007/s10295-016-1863 -2 PMID: 27837351

Zhao, Y., Wang, H., Dong, W., Chang, Y., Yan, G., Chu, Z., & Li, C. (2020). Nitrogen removal and microbial community for the treatment of rural domestic sewage with low C/N ratio by A/O biofilter with Arundo donax as carbon source and filter media. *Journal of Water Process Engineering*, *37*, 101509. DOI: 10.1016/j.jwpe.2020.101509

Chapter 13
Regulatory Framework and Quality Assurance in Biomanufacturing:
Ensuring Quality Compliance and Biosafety

Waseem Ahmed Khattak
Quaid-i-Azam University, Islamabad, Pakistan

Muhammad Anas
https://orcid.org/0000-0001-5127-8043
Selçuk University, Turkey

Erdogan E. Hakki
Selçuk University, Turkey

Javed Iqbal
https://orcid.org/0000-0002-9032-2622
Department of Botany, Bacha Khan University, Pakistan

Banzeer Ahsan Abbasi
https://orcid.org/0000-0003-3036-4481
Rawalpindi Women University, Pakistan

Rashid Iqbal
The Islamia University of Bahawalpur, Pakistan

ABSTRACT

This chapter explores the comprehensive regulatory landscape and quality assurance principles governing biomanufacturing, emphasizing the intersection of compliance, biosafety and innovation. It is inherently complex due to its reliance on living systems and biologically derived products, requires stringent oversight to ensure product consistency, patient safety and therapeutic efficacy. The chapter outline global regulatory frameworks and regulatory pathways for biopharmaceutical approval. It also highlights the growing emphasis on risk management and biosafety, addressing risk assessment methodologies, biosafety level classifications and containment strategies for handling GMOs. The roles of internal audits, external inspections, and continuous improvement initiatives are presented as essential tools for sustaining compliance and operational excellence. Through a multidisciplinary lens, the chapter provides insights into how regulatory science is adapting to meet demands of the increasingly complex biologics while fostering innovation and safeguarding public health.

DOI: 10.4018/979-8-3373-2873-7.ch013

INTRODUCTION

Regulatory Landscape and the Imperative of Quality and Biosafety in Bioprocessing

The biomanufacturing sector, which is an anchor for the biotechnological industry, has transformed from an art-based fermentation processes to precision-engineered and highly regulated manufacturing processes of complex biologics, cell therapies and gene-based products. Biomanufacturing operates in a manner that is distinct from conventional manufacturing due to constraints established by living systems, process variation, and the sensitivity of biological products to environmental conditions. These considerations require a strict and coordinated regulatory framework to guarantee safety efficacy and quality of products throughout widely different geographical areas.

The Emergence and Structuring of the Global Regulatory Framework

The landscape of biomanufacturing regulations "serve as the scenery" within which major national (and international) regulatory entities have worked. In the US, the Food and Drug Administration (FDA) has a significant oversight in the development and marketing of biologics and is responsible for the Biologics License Application (BLA) and compliance with current Good Manufacturing Practices (cGMP) that are codified in 21 CFR Parts 210 and 211. Concurrently, the European Medicines Agency (EMA) grants marketing authorization for biologics to all EU member states via the centralized procedure, predominantly based on International Council for Harmonization (ICH) guidelines. ICH guidelines in particular ICH Q5A--Q11 provide fundamental requirements in viral safety, stability studies, process validation and quality risk management (ICH Q9). It is through their transposition into regional law, that global harmonization is achieved albeit with through different actions. The World Health Organization (WHO) has also now facilitated this process by generating biosimilar guidelines that are being used more and more when approving products in emerging markets (Sahoo et al., 2009; Raybould & Pillai, 2023). The PIC/S (the Pharmaceutical Inspection Co-operation Scheme) and the Cartagena Protocol on Biosafety are further mechanisms for global governance of biological risks and transboundary movement of GMOs that contribute to integrating national biosafety into regulatory practice (Figure 1) (Singh et al., 2024). Whilst significant progress has been made in harmonizing requirements, divergent regulatory requirements, in particular cell and live cell based and GE products, still represent a challenge for multinational biopharmaceutical companies. New modalities (e.g., CRISPR-based therapeutics and microbiome interventions) have been brought into focus on recent years, and regulators have turned more towards adaptive oversight approaches including early engagement, conditional approvals, and real-world evidence (Fisher et al., 2019).

Figure 1. Evolution of biomanufacturing regulation

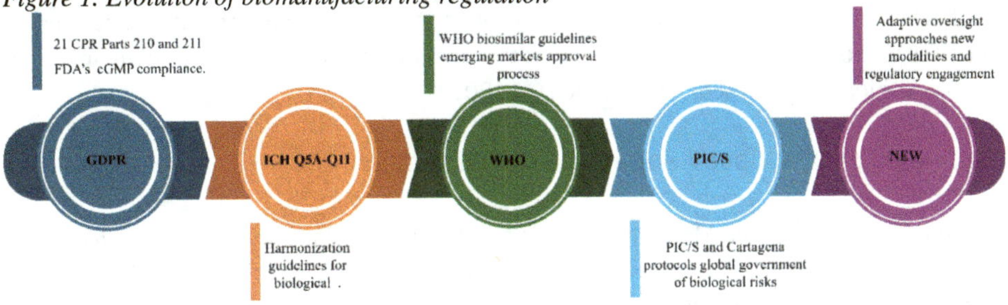

Quality Paradigms in Bioprocess Development: From QbT to QbDD

Quality of biologics in the past was enforced by Quality by Testing (QbT), which simply means that batch was required to be released based on product assays. This method frequently missed "hidden" defects resulting from process variance. The FDA's initiative of Pharmaceutical cGMPs for the 21st Century in 2004 accelerated the shift to Quality by Design (QbD), a strategy that focuses on the design and control of manufacturing processes to achieve a predetermined quality. In QbD, process understanding is achieved through multivariate statistical methods and risk assessment, resulting in the definition Critical Quality Attributes (CQAs), Critical Process Parameters (CPPs), and a Design Space adjustable in real time without regulatory approval (ICH Q8–Q11). The QbD concept has now developed. Quality by Digital Design (QbDD) applies mechanistic and knowledge-driven models for bioprocesses to do digital simulation, optimization and control before the actual real-life process. This approach saves experimental effort for DoE experiments and shortens the time2market (von Stosch et al., 2021). The more frequent use of Process Analytical Technologies (PAT) and Digital Twins also support Real-Time Release Testing (RTRT), where during-processing measurements certify quality and reduce the dependence on end-point testing (Cordiner et al., 2024).

Biosafety: A Core Element of Biomanufacturing Governance

It relates to the safe containment, control, and reduction of potential hazards that may occur in biomanufacturing. With the emergence of high-risk vectors, such as viral-based gene therapies and microbial hosts carrying antibiotic resistance genes, regulatory bodies like the EMA and the FDA require a tiered level of biosafety (BSL) for containment. As noted by Hundleby & Sack (2018) These hazard characterization frames provided by the Recombinant DNA Advisory Committee (RAC) and the OECD Consensus Documents are important for assessing risks of expression systems, host strains and genetically modified agents. Moreover, biosafety is not limited to a lab scale. Implement it in upstream and downstream processes with strong inactivation processes, viral filters and cleaning operations that have been proved. The BMBL manual and EU Directive 2000/54/EC defined details for workplace and environmental safety concepts also highlighting integration of the biosafety in quality assurance system of the laboratories (Raybould and Pillai, 2023). The COVID-19 pandemic underscored the vulnerability inherent to biomanufacturing supply chains and cross-contamination or biosecurity lapses. In the face of this challenge has arisen the concept of Cyber biosecurity, involving the application of cybersecurity practices to bioprocess control systems to protect against intentional attacks or non-authorized access on bioproduction settings (Mantle et al., 2019).

Technological Disruption and Regulatory Evolution

Bioprocessing 4.0 The Merging of Industry 4.0 into Biomanufacturing has regulatory Requirements Evolving. The advancement of technologies such as AI, IoT, cloud computing and augmented reality (AR) allows predictive maintenance, remote real-time monitoring and automated sampling, which can lead to higher process robustness and avoid human errors. Although AIDCs and digital infrastructures offer promise, regulatory systems have incomplete provisions for platform validation standards (Cordiner et al., 2024). The ISPE initiatives Pharma 4.0 aim at closing this gap by describing integrated model systems in which the PAT, MES and ERP are inter-connected through a single data backbone. This enables assured data integrity in a plug-and-play manner consistent with the ALCOA+ notions and leads to a unified control concept (von Stosch et al., 2021). ICH Q13 now has also incorporated explicit support for continuous manufacturing in the regulations, further endorsing the regulatory push towards more flexible production systems able to rapidly adjust to fluctuations in demand without risk to quality or safety. These trends have led to regulatory realignments, with groups like the FDA, EMA, and Health Canada instituting innovation branches such as FDA's CBER Advanced Technologies Program to streamline review pathways for digital biomanufacturing technologies (Fisher et al., 2019).

Globalization and the Need for Regulatory Convergence

Between extremes: the recognition of regional manufacturing the global nature of biopharmaceutical manufacturing has advantages and drawbacks. Reconciliation of conflicting national laws is still one of the most pressing issues, especially in countries where regulatory systems are still developing. Bodies like APEC, AMA, and BRICS as a more recent regulatorily have the goal of bridging the gap between the disparities with mutual recognition of one another´s standards and investment with media, literature, information, and infrastructure. However, there are still inconsistencies in the enforcement of GMP, in the expectation for data integrity and in the biosafety regulations often requiring product specific bridging studies (Sahoo et al., 2009). We are moving towards regulatory convergence and not strict harmonization. That way, scientific principles will become aligned, and we will be able to trust in international guidelines, while maintaining national autonomy. It supports the efficient global distribution, helps to avoid redundant testing, and places the product sooner in the hands of those in need. Mechanisms such as the WHO Collaborative Registration Procedure have shown effective to accelerate vaccine and biologic access in low- and middle-income countries (LMICs) building on existing stringent regulatory authority (SRA) review.

Global Regulatory Authorities in Biomanufacturing

Global control of biomanufacturing products is a patchwork of agencies and harmonization initiatives, all of which are key in safeguarding the safety, efficacy, and quality of bioproducts, especially complex treatmentssuch as monoclonal antibodies, biosimilars, vaccines, and advanced therapies. A good understanding of the region-specific (or global) regulatory bodies such as US FDA, EMA, ICH, World Health Organization (WHO), and country-specific regulators such as Japanese PMDA, Australian TGA, and Indian CDSCO is an important requirement for any entity involved in global biopharma.

U.S. Food and Drug Administration (FDA)

FDA Regulation of Biologics including Vaccines, Cell Therapies and Gene Therapies Biologics products are regulated by the U.S. Food and Drug Administration (FDA), under the Center for Biologics Evaluation and Research (CBER). Appropriate GxP regulations such as those found in 21 CFR Parts 210, 211, and 600–680, which encompass current Good Manufacturing Practices (cGMP) and specific biologics regulations, are required by the FDA. Market approval is granted (by the BLA (Biologics License Application) process) following a demonstration of detailed data on characterization, manufacturing, and clinical effectiveness (Cauchon et al., 2019). Today, the FDA has been the greatest promoter of flexible regulatory mechanisms such as Breakthrough Therapy Designation, Fast Track, and Accelerated Approval in the name of getting innovative biotherapeutics to patients. Furthermore, the FDA actively endorses PAT- and QbD-based frameworks, which focus on strengthened process monitoring and real-time quality control in capillary (Sharma et al., 2022).

European Medicines Agency (EMA)

The EMA is tasked with the scientific assessment of medicines in the European Union. Biologics are assessed through the centralized procedure, which grants access to the market throughout the European Union (EU) by means of a single procedure. All assessments of potency are led by the Committee for Medicinal Products for Human Use (CHMP) and the Biologics Working Party (BWP) for quality and biosafety (Rahalkar et al., 2021). As the first regulatory agency to release a guideline on the approval of biosimilars in 2005 and establish a regulatory pathway, the EMA has served as a model for many biosimilar guidelines issued by various regulatory authorities. This guidance provides recommendations for comparability studies for analytical, nonclinical and clinical studies. EMA implements ICH guidelines and has been very active in the international regulatory harmonization (Rahalkar et al., 2021).

ICH Guidelines (International Council for Harmonization)

The ICH serves as a model to harmonize regulatory requirements worldwide. It is composed of regulatory and industry members from the U.S., EU, Japan, and, as of recently, observers including India and China. ICH guidance guidelines including Q5A–Q11 are of particular importance to biomanufacturing. These guidelines include, but are not limited to, guidance for viral safety evaluation (Q5A), comparability of biotechnological products (Q5E), process validation (Q8–Q11), and quality risk management (Q9). ICH Q12 (Technical and Regulatory Considerations for Pharmaceutical Product Lifecycle Management) and the released for comment draft ICH Q13 on continuous manufacturing are of particular interest to contemporary biomanufacturing facilities. These guidelines encourage post-approval flexibility and efficient lifecycle management something essential in a fast-paced world of biopharma (Geigert, 2023).

WHO Guidelines and Standards

Global production of vaccines The WHO sets international standards and guidelines, for vaccine production and biosimilars, that are highly recommended by regulatory agencies of low- and middle-income countries. The WHO guidelines focused on global access to health, uniformity and safety. On the other hand, for biosimilars, the WHO SBP guidelines (2022 revision) recommend a stepwise route to confirm bio similarity with the generation of strong comparability. WHO also undertakes regulatory capacity building through joint registration systems and prequalification arrangements, especially in Africa, Latin America, and South-East Asia (Rahalkar et al., 2021).

CASE STUDIES

Case Study 1: Microbial Fermentation for Insulin Production

Recombinant DNA technology has enabled large-scale production of **human insulin** using microbial hosts. *Escherichia coli* was the first organism employed in 1982 to produce recombinant human insulin ("Humulin"), approved by the **FDA**, marking a breakthrough in biomanufacturing. Today, both *E. coli* and *Saccharomyces cerevisiae* remain central to cost-effective insulin production, ensuring global supply for diabetes patients. This success exemplifies how microbial fermentation bridges theoretical biotechnology and real-world therapeutics (Walsh & Walsh, 2022).

Case Study 2: Enzyme-Based Technology in Dairy Industry

The application of lactase enzyme (β-galactosidase) in dairy processing is a well-established industrial success. Lactase breaks down lactose into glucose and galactose, enabling the production of lactose-free milk and dairy products. Companies such as DSM and Novozymes have developed robust enzyme formulations now widely used in Europe and North America. This case highlights how enzyme-based biomanufacturing aligns with consumer health needs and adds economic value through product diversification (Jothyswarupha et al., 2025).

Case Study 3: Algae-Based Bioproducts for Nutraceuticals & Biofuels

Microalgae such as *Chlorella vulgaris* and *Spirulina platensis* have gained global recognition as sources of proteins, antioxidants, and biofuels. For instance, Algenol Biotech LLC developed a process using algae to produce ethanol directly from CO_2 and sunlight, while Cyanotech Corporation commercialized *Spirulina*-based nutraceuticals for human health. These examples demonstrate how algae biomanufacturing supports SDG-12 (Responsible Production & Consumption) and SDG-13 (Climate Action) by offering sustainable alternatives to petrochemicals and synthetic supplements. (Sarma et al., 2021)

Country-Specific Regulatory Agencies

PMDA (Pharmaceuticals and Medical Devices Agency, Japan)

PMDA, which is a part of Japan's Ministry of Health, Labor and Welfare (MHLW), evaluates pharmaceuticals, biologics, etc. Japan follows ICH guidelines and has strict post-marketing surveillance. The (Japanese New Drug Application J-NDA) akin to the U.S. BLA process, incorporates lifecycle management evaluations, and extensive consultation periods with manufacturers.

TGA (Therapeutic Goods Act, Australia)

Australia TGA follows the concepts based on ICH and WHO. It provides assessment of the biologicals via the Biologicals Model by dividing autologous from allogeneic therapies. The TGA participates in PIC/S (Pharmaceutical Inspection Co-operation Scheme) and also pursues reliance-based approvals with organizations such as the EMA and FDA. The TGA has also created transparent guidelines for advanced therapies and regenerative medicine products (Ali and Nollet, 2024).

CDSCO (Central Drugs Standard Control Organization, India)

India's DSCO, which falls within Ministry of Health and Family Welfare, is the country's rubber-stamp authority for approving drugs, including biologics and similar biologics. The Biosimilar Guidelines (2012; updated in 2016 and 2019) are modelled on WHO and EMA guidelines but reflect local needs, such as having the option for a local clinical study unless there is a waiver. The RCGM (Review Committee on Genetic Manipulation) and DBT (Department of Biotechnology) are equally involved actively in biosafety evaluations and preclinical development supervision (Rahalkar et al., 2021; Sangavi, 2023). However, CDSCO has a type II (abridged) and a type III (full) review dependent on whether the product is already approved in the reference market like EMA, USFDA etc. India has adopted a more reliance-based approach, especially for biologics related to COVID-19, for which approval may be given based on the foreign regulatory authorities' data under emergency use (Rahalkar et al., 2021).

Lessons from Comparison, Enhancements to Harmonization

On review of the regulatory environment in these emerging markets in BRICS-TM countries, we find that a move towards harmonization with ICH and WHO principles is slowly moving forth, even though a fair degree of heterogeneity still exists. For example, ANVISA in Brazil and SAHPRA in South Africa follow EMA requirements while MoH in Russia and COFEPRIS in Mexico adopt heterogeneity on biosimilar requirements, including reference biologic acquisition and bridging studies. Agencies employ various health technology assessment models for regulatory review (Type I Verification, Type II Abridged, Type III Full), with a different level of data evaluation and time to market. Type III reviews are the most prevalent while type II reviews are burdensome emerging regulators such as TITCK (Turkey) and CDSCO (India) are relying more and more on type II reviews with the assistance of regulatory files from established regulatory peers (Rahalkar et al., 2021). International platforms, such as the International Pharmaceutical Regulators Programme (IPRP) and the WHO's Collaborative Registration Procedure (CRP), are increasingly contributing to developing regulatory convergence. Such systems seek to minimize duplication, enable efficient files review and increase access to biotherapeutics in resource-limited areas.

Regulatory Pathways for Biopharmaceuticals

The global regulatory approval process for biopharmaceuticals follows a rigorous, multi-phase structure encompassing investigational stages, clinical evaluations, and market authorization strategies, all tailored to safeguard human health while facilitating innovation. The complexity of biologic entities such as monoclonal antibodies, gene therapies, and cell-based products necessitates harmonized yet region-specific regulatory pathways. These regulatory frameworks are influenced by national health authorities and international councils like the U.S. Food and Drug Administration (FDA), European Medicines Agency (EMA), Japan's PMDA, and others, which align with the standards established by the International Council for Harmonization (ICH).

INVESTIGATIONAL NEW DRUG (IND) APPLICATION – UNITED STATES (FDA)

On the U.S. side, it is mandatory to obtain an IND any novel biopharmaceutical product prior to human clinical trials. Under 21 CFR Part 312, the IND is not a request for marketing, but a statutory reservation of right to cross state lines with an investigational article, and its position is to be orally transmitted if requested by the same recipient (Jain, 2016). An IND consists of Preclinical Studies (Toxicity, Pharmacokinetics) Results. Postulated therapy for human testing (Phases I–III). Manufacturing and CMC Data. IRB approvals This is a human subjects' case report, and thus, there are no IRB requirements or approvals. Credentials of investigators and risk–benefit assessment. IND Categories There are five IND categories: Commercial INDs (submitted for market approval by pharmaceuticals sponsors). Non-commercial INDs, such as Investigator INDs, Emergency Use INDs, or Treatment INDs for compassionate or investigational uses (FDA, 2023). A pre-IND meeting with FDA is often recommended to gain consensus on study design, safety data, and regulatory requirements. The FDA has 30 days after the IND is submitted to object to it, if not the clinical trials can begin.

BIOLOGICS LICENSE APPLICATION (BLA)

After Phase I-III trials are completed successfully on an approved IND, the sponsor files a Biologics License Application (BLA). The BLA is authorized and described by CBER [Center for Biologics Evaluation and Research] in 21 CFR 600–680, the regulations that pertain to biological products. Detailed clinical trial results, Manufacturing consistency and compliance with GMP, Labeling information, REMS, Facility inspection data (Jain, 2016; Cosenza, 2021). It is the Center for Biologics Evaluation and Research (CBER) that manages the BLA procedure. The FDA assesses. Whether the product is safe and effective for the purpose for which it is labelled. Whether the labeling is accurate. Whether the product quality Reliable material: The products manufactured with high quality material, never deteriorate over time is reliable. Fast Track, Priority Review, Accelerated Approval, and Breakthrough Designation are the most common pathways through which products for the treatment of unmet medical needs or for life-threatening conditions are designed (Figure 2) (FDA, 2023; Rahalkar et al., 2018).

Figure 2. Biological license applications process

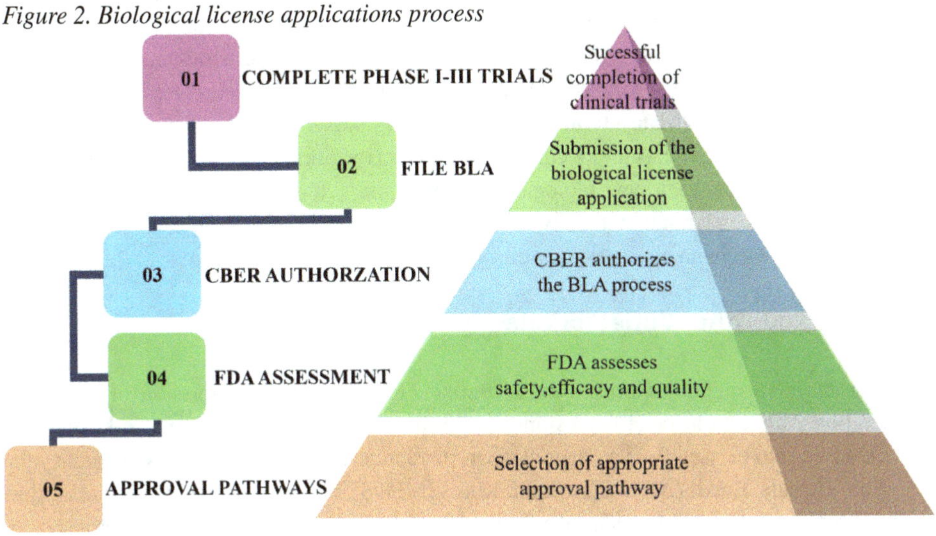

MARKETING AUTHORIZATION IN THE EUROPEAN UNION (EMA)

The EMA oversees biologics and biopharmaceuticals within the European Union (EU) through four primary approval frameworks: Centralized Procedure (CP) required advanced therapy medicinal products, orphan drugs and biopharmaceuticals recombinant. Decentralized Procedure (DCP) to be applied when the product has not received an authorization in any EU Member State. Mutual Recognition Procedure (MRP) where the medicine is already authorized in one Member State. Procedure (NP) for local authorization (Jain, 2016; EMA, 2022). The version that is centralized requires a CHMP review and usually ends in 210 days, disregarding sponsor responses clock-stops.

Japan: PMDA and the J-NDA Pathway

Japan's Pharmaceuticals and Medical Devices Agency (PMDA) regulates biologics under the Pharmaceutical and Medical Device Act (PMD Act). The pathway includes Submission of a Clinical Trial Notification (CTN) before starting trials. Rigorous pre- and post-market surveillance. Marketing Authorization via Japanese New Drug Application (J-NDA), requiring comprehensive clinical data, CMC, and risk assessment documentation. Japan participates in ICH and often aligns with U.S. and EU regulations. For advanced biologics like gene or cell therapies, PMDA has introduced an adaptive approval pathway to accelerate time-to-market with conditional approvals (Joga et al., 2024).

India: CDSCO and Emerging Markets

India's Central Drugs Standard Control Organization (CDSCO) oversees biopharmaceutical approvals in conjunction with the Department of Biotechnology (DBT) and the Review Committee on Genetic Manipulation (RCGM). For biologics, the key submissions are: Clinical Trial Application under Schedule Y of the Drugs and Cosmetics Act. A Biologics Dossier (often CTD format). Local clinical trial data is typically required unless waived through reliance on established markets (e.g., USFDA, EMA) under certain conditions (Rahalkar et al., 2021; Sangavi, 2023). India distinguishes between new biologics and biosimilars, the latter requiring head-to-head comparison studies and immunogenicity data. The Indian model increasingly leverages abridged (Type II) review mechanisms, especially during public health emergencies.

Australia and Other Jurisdictions

Australia's Therapeutic Goods Administration (TGA) requires submission of a Product Registration Application for biologics under its Biologicals Regulatory Framework. Products are classified into classes (I–IV) depending on manipulation levels and donor–recipient relationships. Canada, Brazil (ANVISA), South Korea (MFDS), and other emerging markets follow ICH-aligned procedures with localized adjustments in data requirements, reference comparators, and language formats (Rahalkar et al., 2018; Sharma et al., 2025)

Good Manufacturing Practices (GMP)

GMP Principles and Classification

Good Manufacturing Practices (GMP) is an internationally recognized regulatory method that guarantees pharmaceutical products have been made according to a system, designed to control the quality of products intended for human use. In its most broadly conceived form, the basic tenets of GMP, which are codified broadly in regulatory guidelines such as FDA 21 CFR Parts 210 and 211, ICH Q7, WHO GMP, and PIC/S, revolve around five P's: (1) people, (2) premises, (3) processes, (4) products, and (5) procedures. These are also risk-based and focus on avoiding contamination, mix-ups, non-conformance with guidelines and errors. Systems of such kind (GMP) categorize production premises and kinds of product with regard to risk for the patient and complexity of the production process. Where sterile biopharmaceutical production is concerned, for example, more rigor is needed than for non-sterile processes and production must meet standards according to cleanroom classifications such as ISO 5–8 or EU GMP Grades A–D. These classes detail the environmental controls, that is, limits for particles and microorganisms, gowning, and airflow direction. Each shares similarities with operating areas (background areas (Grade D), preparation areas (Grade C) and aseptic filling zones (Grade A)

FACILITY DESIGN AND ENVIRONMENTAL MONITORING

The design of such facilities is paramount to the avoidance of cross-contamination and for process integrity. The construction of a GMP compliant biomanufacturing plant is necessary for unidirectional personnel and material flows, easy to clean surfaces and pressure differential to minimize contamination. Design must allow for separation of product types and activities (weighing, compounding, filling) and contain pass-throughs for material and waste transfer. Heating, ventilation and air conditioning (HVAC) systems also play crucial role in cleanroom standards, and these systems must be validated to assert compliance with such standards in terms of air change rates, pressure cascades and HEPA filtration efficiencies. EM is a 24/7/365 GMP requirement, especially in aseptic processing areas. This includes active air sampling, settle plates, surface swabs and personnel monitoring to identify microbial or particulate contamination. EM plans should include critical areas, sampling frequency, testing procedures, and alert/action limits. Any such divergences must be subjected to in-depth probe and corrective action planning. Increasingly, also real-time monitoring systems with data integrity compliance (21 CFR part 11) are being applied in ATMP manufacturing sites (Figure 3).

Figure 3. Ensuring GMP compliance in biomanufacturing

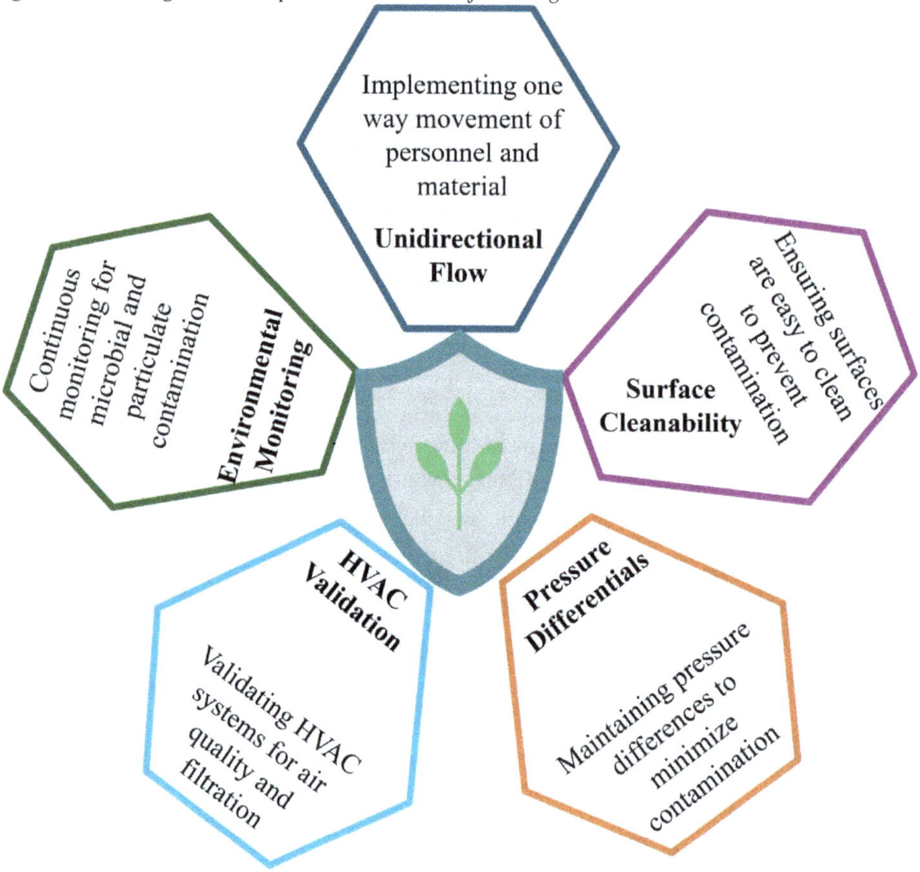

DOCUMENTATION AND RECORD-KEEPING REQUIREMENTS

Good documentation practices are the key of GMP compliance. The sentiment "if it's not written down it didn't happen" emphasizes the need for contemporaneous, well-documented and trackable records. SOP, MBR, logbooks, deviation report, validation protocol and training records are some of the documentations which come in the list of GMP documentation. Each of these documents should be reviewed and approved by QA, should be version-controlled, should be kept for a certain period and should not be altered or accessed by unauthorized persons. Electronic documentation systems (e.g., eQMS or MES platforms) must comply with 21 CFR Part 11 or EU Annex 11, ensuring features such as audit trails, electronic signatures, and secure access. The concept of data integrity is encapsulated in the ALCOA+ principles: Attributable, Legible, Contemporaneous, Original, Accurate, plus Complete, Consistent, Enduring, and Available. Additionally, validation documentation is required for all processes and equipment used in production. This includes Installation Qualification (IQ), Operational Qualification (OQ), and Performance Qualification (PQ). GMP documentation that already exist include preventive maintenance, balances calibration logs cleaning validation, and environmental monitoring data for the internal audit and/or regulatory request for an inspection to take place.

Quality Assurance (QA) and Quality Control (QC)

In biomanufacturing, Quality Assurance (QA) and Quality Control (QC) are fundamental components of a pharmaceutical quality system which serve to ensure the safety, efficacy, and consistency of biopharmaceutical products. Related QA and QC are related but different functions. QA is procedure and definition driven and covers all control of processes or techniques through quality system or control of process activities to ensure that a product sees the quality requirements. It is used to validate the completeness of the processes, documentation, and system as the regulatory bodies would expect. On the other hand, QC is 'real' product focused and consists of activities and techniques that not only validate and control the quality by means analytical testing and inspection of the product (Montgomery, 2006; Christiansen, 2020).

ROLES AND RESPONSIBILITIES OF QA AND QC TEAMS

The QA team is responsible for setting up and maintaining quality systems that ensure compliance to cGMP, SOPs, training programs, deviation, and change control systems. QA is also responsible for administering documentation control, conducting audits, and approving the release of products based on batch records, deviations, and CAPA (Corrective and Preventive Actions). Quality Functions also overlap with regulatory affairs involving pre-inspection coordination and submission audit readiness, with greater incorporation of Quality Risk Management (QRM) concepts and ICH Q10 systems. Besides, QC teams, on the other hand, which focus on testing all raw materials, intermediate products and end products through an analytical process. They carry out bioassays, sterility checks, endotoxin tests, potency assays, stability and so forth, in accordance with validated methodologies and quality specifications. QC is also used in environmental monitoring, utility operation testing (e.g., water-for-injection, cleanroom air), and sample retention (Dwivedi, 2006).

STANDARD OPERATING PROCEDURES (SOPS)

Both QA and QC systems are based around the SOP system, which provides procedures for all biomanufacturing, including documentation, sampling, testing, deviation reporting, and batch review. They standardize the way things are done throughout the organization and achieve reproducible and regulatory compliance. They are author ed and revise d, approved and periodically update d by QA and should be strictly followed for all staff. Violation of SOPs is a regulatory offence and can lead to FDA 483 citations or warning letters (Haider and Asif, 2016). SOPs need to have versioning, be securely housed with readily available access for audits/inspections. All electronic SOP systems should be 21 CFR Part 11 compliant–i.e. capable of secure digital signatures and audit trail.

IN-PROCESS AND FINAL PRODUCT TESTING

QC labs conduct in process and final product testing's to maintain quality throughout the production process. In-process tests such as pH, osmolality, cell viability, bioburden, and identity are key for real-time process control and can be integrated in accordance with PAT (Process Analytical Technology) concepts proposed by regulatory agencies. Final product testing consists of thorough examination of character, purity, strength, sterility and safety parameters. The tests should be validated according to ICH Q2 (R1) specifications, and the pre-set acceptance criteria should be met before the release of the product. Batch release is conducted by QA upon review of all relevant documentation, including but not limited to, batch manufacturing records (BMR), QC test results, and deviation reports. All out of specification (OOS)/out of trend (OOT) results have to be fully investigated, documented and resolved before release. The stability of the product is also tested in accordance with ICH Q1A(R2) for shelf life and storage conditions (Nanov et al., 2024)

VALIDATION AND QUALIFICATION PROCESSES

QC and QA have at their heart validation and qualification. Validation Documentation by which the process, the method or the system is established and the terms for a process, method or system to be considered acceptable is determined. It includes process validation, analytical method validation, cleaning validation and computer system validation. The FDA and ICH Q8–Q11 have recommended life cycle approaches for process validation with three stages: (1) process design, (2) process qualification, and (3) continued process verification (CPV) (Pazhayattil et al., 2023). These steps are intended to be performed in a way to recognize and control critical quality attributes (CQAs) and critical process parameters (CPPs). Qualification refers to procedures that establish that the equipment and systems function properly, from a design, installation and operation perspective (divided into DQ, IQ, OQ, PQ). Equipment used in QC testing is required to be qualified for the regulated testing before its use, such as including HPLC, spectrophotometer, and incubator (Montgomery, 2006). These systems are operated with rigorous calibration and maintenance standard operating procedures (SOPs) to provide accurate and reliable data.

DATA INTEGRITY AND ELECTRONIC SYSTEMS

Modern Current QA/QC systems are primarily based on data quality and electronic records. FDA's 21 CFR Part 11 and EU's Annex 11 states that systems are to provide for electronic records to be: attributable, legible, contemporaneous, original, and accurate (ALCOA + guidelines). Sample tracking, deviation handling, CAPA workflows, and audit trails are handled by LIMS (Laboratory Information Management Systems) and QMS (Quality Management Systems). Enterprise batch records (EBRs) provide the means to assure compliance with automated checks and live deviation alerts reducible by the device. Moreover, document management systems (DMS) are essential for maintaining the controlled documents, change requests, version history, and approvals. In today legislative setup the validation of these computerized systems (Computer System Validation- CSV) owe to be conducted to guarantee data correctness as well as security.

REGULATORY OVERSIGHT AND INSPECTIONS

QA and QC departments need to be "ready for inspection". Quality systems will be compared to cGMP to assure compliance with relevant standards during regulatory inspection from agencies like U.S. FDA, EMA, and WHO. Analysis will also concentrate on data integrity, deviations, CAPA effectiveness and traceability of both raw materials and batches of product. The audit also looks at how QA exercises control over CMOs, APIs supplier and outsourced testing laboratories. Lapses in QA oversight have resulted in past product recalls and enforcement, further highlighting the importance of a strong quality system.

Risk Management and Biosafety

Risk Assessment Methodologies

In biomanufacturing, risk assessment focuses on the correct detection, characterization and control of hazards related to biological materials. Bio-risk associated in the handling of infectious diseases, toxins, genetically modified organisms (GMOs) and other biological materials of concern It is very necessary to address biosafety and biosecurity risks that arise out of pathogens, toxins, other dangerous microorganisms and materials (Kaur & Chugh, 2021). To address these threats, institutions implement structured risk assessment processes that are based on international guidelines and frameworks like the World Health Organization (WHO) Laboratory Biosafety Manual (WHO, 2004), ISO 35001:2019, the NIH Guidelines (NIH, 2019), etc. Bio risk assessment is the central element in bio risk management and is a process that according to ISO 35001 refers to the combination of the likelihood of occurrence, and the severity of harm, resulting from an adverse event concerning a biological agent. The evaluation often occurs tier-based: hazard identification, hazard characterization, exposure assessment, and risk characterization. Each of these steps needs information about the pathogenicity of the organism, route of transmission, infectious dose, environmental survival, and susceptibility of the population. The WHO and CDC endorse a risk-based categorization of agents in four risk groups (RGs) of increasing categories of disease and efficacy of treatment or containment. RG1 indicates low risk, and RG4 is used for agents like *Ebola virus* which produce severe disease and for which few effective prophylaxis or therapy is available (WHO, 2004). Risk assessment techniques help determine the level of containment, the type of PPE, emergency procedures, and training necessary. Beeckman and Rüdelsheim (2020) reported that the activity-based approach should take account of not just the intrinsic properties of biological agents, but also the procedures performed and the exposure routes. This is consistent with "... as low as reasonably achievable ..." principle, whereby biosafety risks are reduced and eliminated by practical measures. Health risk assessments should also include consideration of site-specific items including containment designs; operational aspects of different container systems; HVAC contracting integrity; direction of airflow; and decontamination (Carpenter, 2018). Further regulations, including the European Union Directive 2000/54/EC on work-related biological agents and the United States (U.S.) Occupational Safety and Health Administration (OSHA) Bloodborne Pathogens Standard (29 CFR 1910.1030), demand documented evaluations, to be readily available for review during audits and inspections institutions (Mitchell et al., 2019).

BIOSAFETY LEVELS (BSLS) AND CONTAINMENT STRATEGIES

Containment is the cornerstone of biosafety and is implemented through a combination of laboratory practices, safety equipment, and facility design, collectively known as biosafety levels (BSLs). There are four recognized BSLs, each with defined criteria established by organizations such as the CDC and WHO. BSL-1 facilities handle agents not known to cause disease in healthy humans and require minimal containment, such as handwashing and decontamination of surfaces (Gupta & Zahir, 2020). BSL-2 applies to moderate-risk agents (e.g., *Salmonella* spp., adenoviruses) and mandates access restrictions, use of biosafety cabinets (BSCs), and specific waste decontamination procedures (Pasrija & Kumari, 2025).

BSL-3 is designated for airborne pathogens like *Mycobacterium tuberculosis*. These labs necessitate controlled access, negative air pressure, HEPA filtration, and sealed penetrations (Suganthi et al., 2023).

BSL-4 is the highest containment level, used for agents like *Marburg* virus, where no known treatments exist. Facilities require full-body, air-supplied positive-pressure suits, airlocks, chemical showers, and dedicated exhaust systems (CDC, 2009) (Figure 4) (Diederich, 2025).

Figure 4. Biosafety levels in biomanufacturing

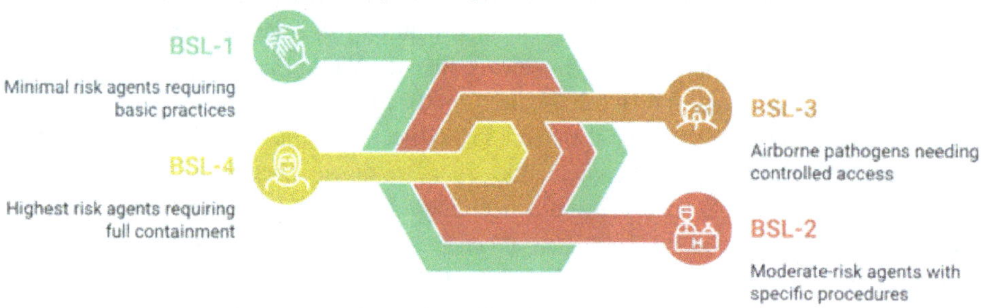
BSL-1
Minimal risk agents requiring basic practices
BSL-4
Highest risk agents requiring full containment
BSL-3
Airborne pathogens needing controlled access
BSL-2
Moderate-risk agents with specific procedures

In biomanufacturing, especially in the production of vaccines or therapeutic proteins using viral vectors, BSL-2 and BSL-3 practices are common. Selection of BSL depends not only on the organism but also on its manipulation in culture volumes, aerosol generation potential, and genetic modification status. The NIH guidelines for recombinant DNA research provide specific criteria for scaling up containment, stressing the role of physical containment (P1–P4) and biological containment such as auxotroph or suicide genes in GMOs (NIH, 2019). The design and operation of containment systems are further dictated by international standards such as ISO 14644 for cleanroom classification and Good Manufacturing Practice (GMP) regulations, which require unidirectional airflow, pressure differentials, and validated decontamination systems for critical environments. Environmental and personnel monitoring are essential to assess the integrity of containment during operations. According to the Canadian Biosafety Handbook (2015), containment failure scenarios must be routinely modelled and mitigated using validated protocols.

HANDLING OF GENETICALLY MODIFIED ORGANISMS (GMOS)

The intentional use of GMOs during biomanufacturing raises unique biosafety and regulatory concerns. GMO management includes organisms that altered through recombinant DNA technology, synthetic biology; and CRISPR/Cas-mediated gene editing (Li et al., 2022). Their biosafety is evaluated based on gene insert structure, gene expression, host-vector system, and possible environmental stability. The use of GMOs is, in many jurisdictions, controlled by contained use legislation, including for example European Directive 2009/41/EC which requires prior authorization and risk classification of work with GMOs, and that containment and emergency plans are provided. According to Gupta et al. (2014), regulations are much different from area to area but mostly based on comparative risk analysis like comparisons of modified organisms with their wildtype isogenies. Primary risk issues associated with GMOs include horizontal gene transfer, allergenic responses – environmental spread, and unintended genetic impacts. These challenges are overcome by tight containment methods through the usage of genetic safety measures such as kill-switches, auxotroph or conditional gene expression systems. The Cartagena Protocol also includes an international framework for biosafety from the transboundary movement of Living Modified Organisms (LMOs) calling for the documentation of identity, handling, and safe use (SCBD, 2000). Risk assessment for GMOs also applies to the downstream. For example, in fermentation with GMO hosts, biomass and effluents need to be decontaminated by an approved process such as heat inactivation or chemical disinfection before disposal (DiGiandomenico et al., 2020). The management of bioburden should protect against accidental release and conform to local environmental and occupational regulations for both upstream and downstream processes. The GMO facilities have to have GMO-specific SOPs in place, and manage genetically characterized cell banks, as well as to carry out environmental monitoring in the production areas (Whomsley et al., 2021). Staff should be subjected to an intensive training on processing, emergency response and containment methods. Also, the ability to be inspection ready to the satisfaction of regulatory oversight (e.g. USDA-APHIS, EFSA, or the national biosafety committees) (Rowe et al., 2012).

INTEGRATION OF RISK MANAGEMENT AND BIOSAFETY IN REGULATORY FRAMEWORKS

A well-designed biosafety system in biomanufacturing is the infusing of risk management into the quality systems. This should consist of the introduction of the ISO 35001:2019 Bio risk Management Standard for a more systematic way to recognize, assess and manage biohazards. This standard fosters a safety culture through leadership commitment, work force involvement, and process safety technology as well as communication, and incident investigation (Callihan et al., 2021). The WHO and FAO are just two of the national and international bodies involved in global biosafety governance, the Biological Weapons Convention (BWC) being another example. BWC neither permits proliferation nor stockpiling of bioweapons, Biotechnology facilities attribute duties of preventing misuse of dual-use research (BWC, 1972). In addition, the Nagoya Protocol introduces the principle of traceability and the obligation to ensure the equitable sharing of benefits in the utilization of genetic resources as part of the regulatory framework of biosafety along with bioethical obligations (SCBD, 2011). This process of biosafety should also encompass the development of incident preparedness and response system. Facilities are to develop emergency plans for containing spills, reporting exposures and taking corrective actions if there is an accidental release. Lessons from previous outbreaks, such as laboratory-acquired SARS infections, have demonstrated the importance of global surveillance and standardization. As Beeckman and Rüdelsheim (2020) note, whereas biosafety is intended to prevent accidental exposure, biosecurity concerns deliberate misuse – theft, for example, or sabotage – whether it is part of a weapons-related activity. A complete risk management system will address them both, most particularly when it comes to valuable biological materials (VBMs such as recombinant cell lines, pathogens, and expression systems). The safe, ethical operation of biomanufacturing facilities includes risk management and biosafety (Shokoohi & Attar, 2024). Using carefully developed methodologies of risk assessment, categorization into biosafety levels and containment measures are the institutions can prevent the risk caused by pathogenic and genetically modified organisms. Guidelines for the practice of these procedures are well harmonized at an international level (by global organizations/authorities such as WHO, ISO, NIH, and the Cartagena Protocol). With the rapid development of biotechnology, especially in the areas of synthetic biology and genome editing, biosafety regulations and risk control will require further improvement to protect workers, the public and environment (Sun et al., 2022).

Audits, Inspections, and Compliance

Valid audit and inspection tools are crucial for regulatory compliance and plant integrity in biomanufacturing facilities. About Paragon Gene Therapy We develop and manufacture viral vectors, including lentivirus and adeno-associated virus (AAV) vectors, for gene or cell therapies and other applications; and to develop next-generation technologies, including novel production systems and techniques that can deliver higher yields of high-quality materials in a significantly simplified process that is cost-effective with faster turnaround (Bulcha et al., 2021). Regulatory requirements from bodies such as the FDA, EMA and WHO necessitate a strong internal and external audit framework as part the QMS for pharmaceutical industry (Lengare et al., 2024).

Internal and External Audits

Internal audits are the proactive quality surveillance mechanisms. They're scheduled events done by an organization's Quality Assurance (QA) team to ensure that activities are in accord with Good Manufacturing Practices (GMP), company procedures, and regulatory requirements. They wish to review details (by type of audit) with respect to such items as documentation, equipment qualification, validation documentation, adherence to SOPs and compliance with training requirements (Singh et al., 2024). The focus is on the recognition of non-conformities and the generation of correct measures in terms of corrections and corrective actions (CAPA) prior regulatory inspections. External audits, on the other hand, are performed by regulators or by independent certifiers. These can include supplier audits, CMO assessments and mock pre-approval inspections (Medina, 2016). Agencies can also request for-cause inspections in response to complaints, deviations or whistleblower reports regarding product. External audits require extensive documentation trails to ensure audit readiness reports, risk assessments, deviation logs, and CAPA results can be provided. To facilitate each audit type, entities devise audit schedules, audit readiness plans, and mechanisms to track audit findings (Pinto, 2024). Contemporary audit procedures are adopting digital and risk based auditing frameworks. Audit trail analysis, automated audit management systems, and ISO 19011-compliant processes help organizations implement more effective internal audit systems while promoting transparency and responsibility. "Pharmaceutical companies that have structured internal audit cycles meeting the ICH Q10 (Pharmaceutical Quality Systems) requirements have better regulatory preparedness as well as operational robustness" (Tawade and Pandya, 2023)

REGULATORY INSPECTIONS AND RESPONSES

These are official reviews by the government of the entity to ensure it meets both the legal and GMP obligations. The FDA's inspection approach, for example, is based on 21 CFR Part 211 (for finished pharmaceuticals) and Part 600-680 (for biologics). Such audit often would involve the review of the batch production records, raw material control, environmental monitoring data as well as quality control test report (Christiansen, 2020). In addition, the integrity of electronic systems is considered under 21 CFR Part 11 by inspectors. There are four phases of the inspection cycle: pre-inspection preparedness or readiness, on-site activities, response readiness, and follow-up. Inspectors record observations in Form FDA 483 (Baratta et al., 2024). If not resolved, such observations may prompt warning letters, import alerts, consent decrees, or product recall. FDA 483 responses are required within 15 days and include information related to root cause analysis, corrective actions, and implementation timeframes (ul Alam, 2024). GMP is, of course, a big part of what the EMA inspects under the EudraLex Volume 4 Annexes for the EU as well as at non-EU facilities exporting into Europe. WHO prequalification audits are a requirement for vaccine manufacturers seeking to supply the UN procurement agencies. Responses to such inspections may involve CAPA plans which are checked for closure at subsequent inspections or remote assessments. To reduce this risk, companies have Inspection Ready Programs (IRPs) which consist of, simulation audits, document control systems, and response SOPs (Gee, 2021). Christiansen (2020) states that proactively planning, establishing strong documentation control and maintaining cross-functional coordination are necessary for handling regulatory scrutiny and maintaining ongoing market access.

Compliance Metrics and Continuous Improvement

Tracking performance data gives actionable information on how well the quality system is working and is a vital aspect of--and it is critical to--continuous improvement efforts. Examples of KCI include trends in audit findings; Cycle-times for CAPAs;Rates of recurrence for deviations; Back log in change control; Defect frequency for product and training compliance scores. The U.S. FDA has advocated the use of Quality Metrics Programs to support proactive quality monitoring and anticipate potential drug shortages based on GMP violations (Aglave et al., 2024). Within biomanufacturing, a relentless improvement philosophy is frequently based on Six Sigma, Total Quality Management (TQM) and Lean Manufacturing strategies. These methodologies use the quantitative analysis of compliance data to improve processes and control outcomes with less variance and improved quality of the product. As reported in Lengare et al. (2024), application of artificial intelligence to quality surveillance (e.g., predictive analysis of trends in deviation or real-time process control), which sparked a drastic change in the management of compliance.

Application of benchmarking metrics through manufacturing sites, suppliers and partners to drive a culture of quality excellence (Alsharari & Aljohani, 2024). For example, proof of the effectiveness of measures applied for CAPA is measured longitudinally, by assessing whether the implemented actions effectively control the root causes. Management's quarterly or annual reviews of quality metrics further help ensure that high level executives are kept informed and stay committed to regulatory compliance and business integrity (Pazhayattil & Sharma, 2025). The WHO also urges to establish the QRM programs as part of the QMS which is based on ICH Q9. Those systems evaluate the risk of compliance from product impact, process complexity and history of deviations that can help to prioritize improvement projects. In addition, scorecards and dashboards are becoming common instruments for monitoring audit results and CAPA effectiveness on-line these days (O'Donnell & Kartoglu, 2024).

Ongoing compliance also includes training of employees, governing changes through change controls, and a vendor qualification program. Any modification to process, equipment or ingredient should be compared for regulatory impact and validated with concurrent SOPs (Roy et al., 2025). Lurie was referring to the impact of quality culture on the sustainability of compliance, and the importance today of holding leaders accountable which is now seen as a regulatory expectation. Audits, inspections, and compliance programs form the backbone of the biomanufacturing industry's commitment to manufacturing safe and effective biologics (Srivastav & Das, 2025). Internal and external audits provide surveillance for operational discipline and vulnerabilities. Regulatory inspections confirm this adherence and maintain industry standards. To be competitive, let alone compliant, companies need to use data-based compliance metrics and commit to continuous improvement. The advancement of technology trends and digital solutions, predictive analytics and a harmonized approach to global standards will continue to influence the way audits and inspections are handled and how compliance is maintained (Odetunde et al., 2022).

Regulatory Trends and Innovations

Role of Digital Technologies in Regulatory Compliance

Biomanufacturing's digital transformation is changing how companies achieve and maintain compliance. The incorporation of artificial intelligence (AI), machine learning (ML), digital twins and cloud-based platforms into manufacturing and quality systems has brought to them real-time tracking, predictive analytics, anywhere decision-making which fits in well with emerging regulatory expectations **(Ajayi, 2025)**. Regulatory bodies like the FDA and the EMA are increasingly adopting these approaches as part of their larger digital health and quality maturity model programs. Now, modern electronic batch record (EBR) systems, integrated with laboratory information management systems (LIMS), provide complete lot traceability and audit-readiness to enable your company to remain in compliance with 21 CFR Part 11 and EU Annex 11 regulations for electronic records and signatures. such as a reduction in dependence on paper records and improved data integrity an oft-cited regulatory violation **(Famili & Cleary, 2022).** Also, digital tools support continuous process verification (CPV) and proactive quality management along product lifecycles (Schmitt et al. With increasing frequency, digital twins, i.e., virtual image of physical processes, are employed for in silico validation and process optimization. They find its utility because it can effectively mimic process behavior, optimize the range of parameters and can also be applied for QbD approach. AI and digital twins have found favor in nascent regulation of personalized medicine and ATMPs, where time to iterate, customize, and evolve is crucial (Nargund et al., 2024). Cloud platforms are also now being used for submission to regulatory agencies and audit readiness. All documentation needs to be in one place and ready for regulatory submission through digital repositories – which also cuts time into submission and increases transparency. Tools such as blockchain are also being tested to help establish better traceability and validation of source materials, and this is especially important in cell therapy manufacturing where donor traceability is **essential (Aguilar-Gallardo & Bonora-Centelles, 2023).**

Evolving Regulations for Cell and Gene Therapies

The regulatory environment for cell and gene therapies (CGTs) is in a state of flux to respond to the intricacies of these emerging modalities. Unlike conventional small molecules, CGTs are highly individualized, biologically variable therapies, and are typically produced in small lots, requiring a dynamic though robust regulatory paradigm. In the United States, these products are regulated by the FDA-CBER through systems like 21 CFR Parts 1271 (Human Cells, Tissues, and Cellular and Tissue-Based Products – HCT/Ps) and 351/361 pathways, based on their level of risk (Sawarkar & Bapat, 2022). FDA's RMAT designation expedites review for CGTs meeting criteria, including unmet need. In Europe, CGTs are regulated by the European Medicines Agency (EMA) under the Committee for Advanced Therapies (CAT) and legislation for advanced therapy medicinal products (ATMP), which includes gene therapy medicinal products (GTMP), somatic cell therapy products (sCTMP), and tissue engineered products (TEP) (Salazar-Fontana, 2022). There is need for centralized marketing authorization, which entails the review of the Committee for Advanced Therapies (CAT) (Zia et al., 2024). PMDA (Japan), Health Canada and TGA (Australia) all use similar structures; however, harmonization is not yet achieved. Key regulatory issues are limited to the absence of standardized potency assays, process consistency (85) and long-term safety data (particularly for integrating vectors such as lentiviruses or adeno-associated viruses (AAV) (85)). There is now a regulatory demand for comprehensive comparability studies post process modifications (EMA, 2022), and a growing interest in these being conducted in real time using advanced analytics (Escandell et al., 2022). Moreover, post-market monitoring for CGTs frequently incorporates long-term follow-up (LTFU) over 15 years, especially for gene therapies with genome integration. Innovative platforms by organizations, such as the FDA's Project Optimus and Project Front Runner, also aim to be reimagining endpoints and trial design for ATMPs compatible with their mode of action **(Dahiya et al., 2025).**

QUALITY BY DESIGN (QBD) AND PROCESS ANALYTICAL TECHNOLOGY (PAT)

QbD and PAT are core elements of regulatory innovation in bioprocessing. These approaches move quality assurance away from end-product testing and towards process control and understanding, as highlighted in the ICH guidelines Q8–Q11. QbD consists in establishing a Quality Target Product Profile (QTPP) and identifying Critical Quality Attributes (CQAs), Critical Process Parameters (CPPs), and a design space within which product may be manufactured without having an impact on quality (Duarte et al., 2025). This organized guidance improves process windiness, regulatory independence, and product lifecycle administration. Regulatory authorities have been advocating for the implementation of QbD as part of the ICH Q12 documents on LCM (da Silva et al., 2024). QbD is also supported by PAT which allows for the real-time monitoring and controlling of the CPPs. Tools like near infrared (NIR) and Raman spectroscopy, as well as on-line HPLC allow manufacturers to follow processes such as pH, levels of metabolites, cell density, or concentration of proteins during production. These devices are linked to feedback control loops that provide consistently high-quality products without having to monitor this batch-wise (Gyorgypal et al., 2022). In monoclonal antibody (mAb) production, for example, PAT provides for real-time monitoring of glycosylation profile and thereby controls batch-to-batch homogeneity. For gene therapy, PAT enables testing for vector integrity, analysis for impurities, and DNA/RNA ratio determination. The FDA's PAT Framework incentivizes the use of these technologies by easing up regulatory constrictions by easing up regulatory restrictions i.e. reduced validation overheads, flexible post-approval change processes (Schmitt et al., 2019). Among the recent advancements is the introduction of model predictive control (MPC) systems that use mathematical models of the bioprocess to detect incipient deviations and actuate pre-emptive changes. Acceptance of such models by the regulators will be based on validation, transparency and reproducibility of the models as an empirical relation. Both the EMA and FDA have released guidance for model-based control submissions as part of QbD dossiers. In particular, the application of QbD and PAT is crucial in continuous biomanufacturing, because classic batch release processes are inadequate. PAT operates in real-time and RTRT is employed to keep the stock lower, to be reactive and to not to allow delay in product quality (Wasalathanthri et al., 2020).

Regulatory drivers and biomanufacturing innovations are converging with a deep undercurrent of the industry's push towards predictive, data-rich, and adaptive quality systems. By using digital technology compliance, traceability and efficiency is increased, which is in line with the advancing wishes, of the regulators (Tounekti et al., 2025). With cell and gene therapies, stakeholders around the world are adapting frameworks to accommodate the development of such complex and high-impact modalities without compromising patient safety. Quality by Design and Process Analytical Technology are based on that evolution and will lead to a science-based culture of process understanding and improvement. These new technologies make regulatory compliance easier, improve product quality, speed time to market and in the long run advance global harmonization in biopharmaceutical development (de Matas et al., 2016).

CONCLUSION

The regulatory landscape for biomanufacturing has developed into a complex, internationally linked, integrated network for the harmonization of quality, safety, and efficacy for the multitude of modalities and geographies. Biomanufacturing is rooted in living systems and biological variability, presenting challenges not encountered in conventional pharmaceutical manufacturing. Thus, well regulated governance is required, including implementation of strict GMPs (Good Manufacturing Practices), QA (Quality assurance) systems, and international guidelines adherence. During this chapter, we have emphasized the need for regulatory mechanisms that are globally synchronized but locally flexible. The FDA, EMA, PMDA, WHO and similar agencies are key in establishing standards and furthering harmonization efforts. But the arrival of new types of treatments such as cell and gene therapies has challenged our traditional regulatory frameworks. These treatments, which are necessarily complex and frequently individualized, require adaptive regulatory pathways, risk-based supervisions, and post-market monitoring that can stretch years beyond launching a product. The regulation of its systems for these therapies is a testament to its commitment to balance safety with innovation. Central in current biomanufacturing discussions is the transition from reactive to proactive quality assurance. The inclusion of QbD, PAT, and real-time monitoring devices represents a turning point in the understanding and appropriate use of quality. This shift from Quality by Testing to Quality by Design not only enhances the knowledge of processes but also enables manufacturers to more effectively react to process variability. Furthermore, digital technologies such as electronic batch records, digital twins and AI-driven analytics enable higher data integrity, faster decision-making and enhanced compliance. Biosafety continues to be a cornerstone in regulatory oversight considering increasing reliance on GMOs and FACPs as well as biohazards for production. The risk assessments, biosafety levels (BLs) and containment measures need to be appropriately followed to safeguard the staff and the environment. Harmonized biosafety standards and use of bio risk management systems promote safe handling and containment at all levels and settings. And lastly, it is continual improvement, coming from internal audits, regulatory inspections and key performance measures -that is the one thing that supports good compliance. A culture of quality, supported by clear documentation, skilled staff, and top-down support, is also key to long-term success in biomanufacturing. The future of the industry will increasingly hinge not only on its ability to integrate science, technology and regulation into smooth, efficient systems that simply get things done while meeting compliance levels but also pre-empting the unmet needs of a swiftly changing therapeutic world.

REFERENCES

Aglave, G., Yerram, S., Patnam, J. D., Ajmal, C., Nizam, V. M., Joga, R., Raghuvanshi, R. S., & Srivastava, S. (2024). Proactive Approaches to cGMP Compliance: Insights and Key Takeaways from USFDA Warning Letters to Pharmaceutical Industries Between 2019 and 2024. *Journal of Pharmaceutical Innovation*, *19*(4), 49.

Aguilar-Gallardo, C., & Bonora-Centelles, A. (2023). Blockchain technology for advanced therapy medicinal products: Applications in tracking, data sharing, and supply chain automation. *Journal of Pharmaceutical and Biopharmaceutical Research*, *5*(2), 430–443.

Ajayi, R. (2025). Integrating IoT and cloud computing for continuous process optimization in real-time systems. *Int J Res Publ Rev*, *6*(1), 2540–2558.

Ali, F., & Nollet, L. M. L. (2024). *Global Regulations of Medicinal, Pharmaceutical, and Food Products*. Springer.

Alsharari, N. M., & Aljohani, M. S. (2024). The benchmarking implementation and management control process as influenced by interplay of environmental and cultural factors: Institutional and contingency perspectives. *Benchmarking*, *31*(9), 3327–3348.

Baratta, M., Jian, W., Hengel, S., Kaur, S., Cunliffe, J., Boer, J., Hughes, N., Kar, S., Kellie, J., & Kim, Y. J. (2024). 2023 White Paper on Recent Issues in Bioanalysis: Deuterated Drugs; LNP; Tumor/FFPE Biopsy; Targeted Proteomics; Small Molecule Covalent Inhibitors; Chiral Bioanalysis; Remote Regulatory Assessments; Sample Reconciliation/Chain of Custody (PART 1A–Recommendations on Mass Spectrometry, Chromatography, Sample Preparation Latest Developments, Challenges, and Solutions and BMV/Regulated Bioanalysis PART 1B-Regulatory Agencies' Inputs on Regulated Bioanalysis/BMV, Biomarkers/IVD/CDx/BAV, Immunogenicity, Gene & Cell Therapy and Vaccine). *Bioanalysis*, *16*(9), 307–364. PMID: 38913185

Beeckman, D. S. A., & Rüdelsheim, P. (2020). Biosafety and biosecurity in containment: A regulatory overview. *Frontiers in Bioengineering and Biotechnology*, *8*, 650. DOI: 10.3389/fbioe.2020.00650 PMID: 32719780

Biological Weapons Convention (BWC). (1972). *Convention on the Prohibition of the Development, Production and Stockpiling of Biological and Toxin Weapons*. https://www.un.org/disarmament/biological-weapons/

Bulcha, J. T., Wang, Y., Ma, H., Tai, P. W., & Gao, G. (2021). Viral vector platforms within the gene therapy landscape. *Signal Transduction and Targeted Therapy*, *6*(1), 53. PMID: 33558455

Callihan, D. R., Downing, M., Meyer, E., Ochoa, L. A., Petuch, B., Tranchell, P., & White, D. (2021). Considerations for laboratory biosafety and biosecurity during the coronavirus disease 2019 pandemic: applying the ISO 35001: 2019 standard and high-reliability organizations principles. *Applied Biosafety : Journal of the American Biological Safety Association*, *26*(3), 113–122. PMID: 36035545

Carpenter, C. B. (2018). Safety considerations for working with animal models involving human health hazards. *Animal Models and Experimental Medicine*, *1*(2), 91–99. PMID: 30891553

Cauchon, N. S., Oghamian, S., & Hassanpour, S.. (2019). Innovation in Chemistry, Manufacturing, and Controls—A Regulatory Perspective from Industry. *Journal of Pharmaceutical Sciences*, *108*(1), 1–12. https://www.sciencedirect.com/science/article/pii/S0022354919300929 PMID: 30794794

CDC. (2009). *Biosafety in Microbiological and Biomedical Laboratories* (5th ed.). https://www.cdc.gov/labs/BMBL.html

Christiansen, G. D. (2020). *Quality Control and Quality Assurance Issues in Biopharmaceutical Processing*. Taylor and Francis., DOI: 10.1201/9781003055297-3

Christiansen, G. D. (2020). *Quality Control and Quality Assurance Issues in Biopharmaceutical Processing*. CRC Press., DOI: 10.1201/9781003055297-3

Christiansen, G. D. (2020). Quality control and quality assurance issues in biopharmaceutical processing. In *Biotechnology* (pp. 33–71). CRC Press.

Cordiner, J. L., Kis, Z., Moghadam, P. Z., & Isoko, K. (2024). Bioprocessing 4.0: A Pragmatic Review and Future Perspectives. *Digital Discovery*, *3*, 1662–1681. DOI: 10.1039/d4dd00127c

Cosenza, M. E. (2021). *Global Regulatory Expectations and Interactions*. In *Translational Medicine* (pp. 103–122). CRC Press.

da Silva, F. V. S., Murtagh, J., & Mu'azzam, K. (2024). *A roadmap for model-based bioprocess development. Biotechnology Advances*. https://www.sciencedirect.com/science/article/pii/S0734975024000727

Dahiya, A., Singh, K., & Ashish, A., Nipun, Bhadyaria, A., Thakur, S., Kumar, M., Das Gupta, G., Das Kurmi, B., & Pal, R. R. (2025). Global harmonization in advanced therapeutics: Balancing innovation, safety, and access. *Personalized Medicine*, •••, 1–11. PMID: 40277251

de Matas, M., De Beer, T., Folestad, S., Ketolainen, J., Lindén, H., Lopes, J. A., Oostra, W., Weimer, M., Öhrngren, P., & Rantanen, J. (2016). Strategic framework for education and training in Quality by Design (QbD) and process analytical technology (PAT). *European Journal of Pharmaceutical Sciences*, *90*, 2–7. PMID: 27112991

Diederich, S. (2025). *Biosafety Level 4 (BSL4)–Virus research at the highest level of biosafety and biosecurity* (Vol. 122). Academic Press.

DiGiandomenico, K., Dunn, E., Sadowski, C., Godwin, S., Keeler, M., Preston, F., Niven, P., Ramsey, P., & Hay, H. (2020). Environmental health and biosafety risk assessment guidance for commercial-scale cell and gene therapy manufacturing. *Applied Biosafety : Journal of the American Biological Safety Association*, *25*(4), 201–213. PMID: 36032393

Duarte, J. G., Duarte, M. G., Piedade, A. P., & Mascarenhas-Melo, F. (2025). Rethinking Pharmaceutical Industry with Quality by Design: Application in Research, Development, Manufacturing, and Quality Assurance. *The AAPS Journal*, *27*(4), 96. PMID: 40389714

Dwivedi, C. M. (2006). Validation of Cell Culture-Based Processes. In *Cell Culture Technology for Pharmaceutical and Cell-Based Therapies*. Taylor and Francis.

EMA. (2022). *Marketing Authorisation Procedures in the EU.* European Medicines Agency. https://www.ema.europa.eu

Escandell, J. M., Pais, D. A., Carvalho, S. B., & Vincent, K. (2022). *Leveraging rAAV bioprocess understanding and next generation bioanalytics development. Trends in Biotechnology.* https://www.sciencedirect.com/science/article/pii/S0958166921002421

Famili, P., & Cleary, S. (2022). Laboratory Information Management System (LIMS) and Electronic Data. *Analytical Testing for the Pharmaceutical GMP Laboratory*, 345-373.

FDA. (2021). *Guidance for Industry: Quality Metrics Reporting Program.* https://www.fda.gov/media/90320/download

FDA. (2023). *FDA Guidance for Industry: Expedited Programs for Serious Conditions – Drugs and Biologics.* https://www.fda.gov/media/86377/download

Fisher, A. C., Kamga, M. H., Agarabi, C., & Brorson, K. (2019). Integrated Continuous Biomanufacturing. *Trends in Biotechnology*, *37*(8), 802–815. DOI: 10.1016/j.tibtech.2019.01.013

Gee, A. P. (2021). Development and Maintenance of a Quality Program. In *Cell Therapy: cGMP Facilities and Manufacturing* (pp. 195–208). Springer.

Geigert, J. (2023). *Regulatory Pathways Impacting Biopharmaceuticals.* In *The Challenge of CMC Regulatory Compliance* (pp. 35–56). Springer. Link

Gupta, A., & Zahir, F. (2020). Biosafety Issues for Scientists and Laboratory Workers. In *Introduction to Occupational Health Hazards* (pp. 114–157). Bentham Science Publishers.

Gupta, K., Karihaloo, J. L., & Khetarpal, R. K. (2014). *Biosafety regulations for GM crops in Asia-Pacific.* Asia-Pacific Association of Agricultural Research Institutions.

Gyorgypal, A., Yang, O., & Chopda, V. (2022). *Recent advances in integrated process analytical techniques and control strategies for monoclonal antibody biomanufacturing. Journal of Chemical Technology and Biotechnology.* https://www.researchgate.net/publication/351056378

Haider, S. I., & Asif, S. E. (2016). *Quality Control Training Manual: Comprehensive Training Guide for API, Finished Pharmaceutical and Biotechnologies Laboratories.* CRC Press.

Hundleby, P. A. C., & Sack, M. (2018). Biosafety, Risk Assessment and Regulation of Molecular Farming. In *Plant Biotechnology and Emerging Areas.* Wiley., DOI: 10.1002/9781118801512.ch13

ICH Q9. (2023). *Quality Risk Management.* International Council for Harmonisation. https://www.ich.org/page/quality-guidelines

Jain, S. (2016). Regulatory Requirements for New Drug Approval in Different Countries: An Overview. [Link to PDF]. *World Journal of Pharmaceutical Research*, *5*(6), 786–816.

Joga, R., Srivastava, S., & Nagpal, K. (2024). Regulatory Landscape and Challenges in CAR-T Cell Therapy Development in the US, EU, Japan, and India. *European Journal of Pharmaceutical Sciences, 2024.* Advance online publication. DOI: 10.1016/j.ejps.2024.106557

Jothyswarupha, K., Venkataraman, S., Rajendran, D. S., Shri, S. S., Sivaprakasam, S., Yamini, T., Karthik, P., & Kumar, V. V. (2025). Immobilized enzymes: Exploring its potential in food industry applications. *Food Science and Biotechnology, 34*(7), 1533–1555. PMID: 40129709

Kaur, P., & Chugh, A. (2021). Challenges in governance of Synthetic Biology: Biorisk assessment. *Asian Biotechnology and Development Review, 23*(3).

Lengare, R. R., Arjun, Y. N., & Bais, S. K. (2024). A Review on Quality Control and Quality Assurance in Pharmaceuticals. [PDF Link]. *International Journal of Pharmacy and Herbal Technology, 2*(4), 2507–2520.

Li, W., Huang, C., & Chen, J. (2022). The application of CRISPR/Cas mediated gene editing in synthetic biology: Challenges and optimizations. *Frontiers in Bioengineering and Biotechnology, 10*, 890155. PMID: 36091445

Mantle, J. L., Rammohan, J., & Romantseva, E. F.. (2019). Cyberbiosecurity for Biopharmaceutical Products. *Frontiers in Bioengineering and Biotechnology, 7*, 116. DOI: 10.3389/fbioe.2019.00116 PMID: 31214582

Medina, C. (2016). A cGMP Risk Assessment and Management Strategy: Guidelines for the Pre-Approval Inspection. In *Preparing for FDA Pre-Approval Inspections* (pp. 107–147). CRC Press.

Mitchell, A. H., Pannell, M. A., Arbury, S., Thomas, R., & Hodgson, M. J. (2019). Bloodborne pathogens standard enforcement at the occupational safety and health administration: The first twenty-five years. *New Solutions, 29*(2), 172–185. PMID: 30917759

. Montgomery, S. A. (2006). *Operations and Quality Systems: Building in Success.* BioProcess International, Supplement, March 2006. Link to Full Text PDF

Nanov, M., Despotovska, S., Mitrovska, G., Koceva, V. D., & Acevska, J. (2024). Advantages of trend analysis in stability studies for prediction of potential OOS result within estimated shelflife of medicinal product. *Macedonian Pharmaceutical Bulletin/Makedonsko Farmacevtski Bilten, 70*(1).

Nargund, S., Mauch, K., & Esswein, S. (2024). *Biopharma 4.0: Digital technologies driving smart manufacturing. Springer.* https://link.springer.com/chapter/10.1007/978-3-031-45669-5_11

NIH. (2019). *Guidelines for Research Involving Recombinant or Synthetic Nucleic Acid Molecules.* https://osp.od.nih.gov/biotechnology/nih-guidelines/

O'Donnell, K., & Kartoglu, U. (2024). QRM, Knowledge Management, and the Importance of ICH Q9 (R1).

Odetunde, A., Adekunle, B. I., & Ogeawuchi, J. C. (2022). Using Predictive Analytics and Automation Tools for Real-Time Regulatory Reporting and Compliance Monitoring. *Int. J. Multidiscip. Res. Growth Eval, 3*(2), 650–661.

Pasrija, R., & Kumari, D. (2025). Introduction to BSL-2 Facilities. In *Protocols for Studying Pathogenic Fungi* (pp. 1-25). Springer.

Pazhayattil, A. B., & Sharma, S. (2025). Post-RCA Impact Assessment, CAPA, and Effectiveness Checks. In *Pharmaceutical Manufacturing Deviation and Failure Investigations: Principles, Practices, and Case Studies* (pp. 77-91). Springer.

Pazhayattil, A. B., Sharma, S., Philip, J. P., Gischewski-Silva, M., & Ingram, M. (2023). Qualification, Continued Process Verification, and Lifecycle Management. In *Technology Transfer: Drug Product Manufacturing Process* (pp. 97-117). Springer.

Pinto, A. R. O. (2024). *A Framework for Leveraging IT Audit Using Artificial Intelligence*. Universidade NOVA de Lisboa.

Rahalkar, H., Cetintas, H. C., & Salek, S. (2018). Quality, non-clinical and clinical considerations for biosimilar monoclonal antibody development: EU, WHO, USA, Canada, and BRICS-TM regulatory guidelines. *Frontiers in Pharmacology*, *9*, 1079. DOI: 10.3389/fphar.2018.01079 PMID: 30364154

Rahalkar, H., Sheppard, A., Santos, G. M. L., Dasgupta, C., Perez-Tapia, S. M., Lopez-Morales, C. A., & Salek, S. (2021). Current Regulatory Requirements for Biosimilars in Six Member Countries of BRICS-TM: Challenges and Opportunities. *Frontiers in Medicine*, *8*, 726660. DOI: 10.3389/fmed.2021.726660 PMID: 34568384

Raybould, A., & Pillai, S. P. (2023). Insights in Biosafety and Biosecurity: Current Challenges and Future Perspectives. *Frontiers in Bioengineering and Biotechnology*, *11*, 1118506. DOI: 10.3389/fbioe.2022.1118506 PMID: 36714616

Rowe, J. D., Amijee, F., Brody, S. D., Wandrey, G. G., & Dreyer, C. C. (2012). The globalization of agricultural biotechnology: implications for regulatory compliance, stewardship and stakeholder engagement. In *Regulation of Agricultural Biotechnology: The United States and Canada* (pp. 335-375). Springer.

Roy, S., Mandal, B., & Das, B. K. (2025). Quality Assurance in Laboratory Practices and Equipment Maintenance: Ensuring Precision, Reliability, and Compliance. In *Laboratory Techniques for Fish Disease Diagnosis* (pp. 79-103). Springer.

Sahoo, N., Choudhury, K., & Manchikanti, P. (2009). Manufacturing of Biodrugs: Need for Harmonization in Regulatory Standards. *BioDrugs*, *23*(1), 1–9. DOI: 10.2165/11317110-000000000-00000 PMID: 19697964

Salazar-Fontana, L. I. (2022). A regulatory risk-based approach to ATMP/CGT development: Integrating scientific challenges with current regulatory expectations. *Frontiers in Medicine*, *9*, 855100. PMID: 35646952

Sangavi, C. (2023). *Regulatory Requirements for the New Drug Approval Process in Different Countries*. International Journal Of Drug Regulatory Affairs. https://www.researchgate.net/publication/372914168

Sangavi, C. (2023). *Regulatory Requirements for the New Drug Approval Process in Different Countries*. International Journal of Drug Regulatory Affairs. ResearchGate.

Sarma, S., Sharma, S., Rudakiya, D., Upadhyay, J., Rathod, V., Patel, A., & Narra, M. (2021). Valorization of microalgae biomass into bioproducts promoting circular bioeconomy: a holistic approach of bioremediation and biorefinery. *3 Biotech, 11*(8), 378.

Sawarkar, S., & Bapat, A. (2022). Global Regulatory Frameworks and Quality Standards for Stem Cells Therapy and Regenerative Medicines. In *Stem Cell Production: Processes, Practices and Regulations* (pp. 69-111). Springer.

SCBD. (2000). *Cartagena Protocol on Biosafety to the Convention on Biological Diversity.* https://bch.cbd.int/protocol

SCBD. (2011). *Nagoya Protocol on Access and Benefit-Sharing*. https://www.cbd.int/abs/

Schmitt, R. H., Ochs, J., & Moutsatsou, P. (2019). Automation in cell and gene therapy manufacturing: From past to future. *Biotechnology Letters, 41*(10), 1179–1190. https://link.springer.com/article/10.1007/s10529-019-02732-z PMID: 31541330

Sharma, S., Monga, A., Jamwal, P., & Kaur, A. (2025). Biosimilars: A Critical Review of Development, Regulatory Landscape, and Clinical Implications. *AAPS PharmSciTech.* Advance online publication. DOI: 10.1208/s12249-025-03038-2 PMID: 39870890

Sharma, S., Rabbani, S. A., & Sharma, R. (2022). *Regulatory Affairs in the Pharmaceutical Industry*. Elsevier. https://www.sciencedirect.com/science/article/pii/B9780128222119000058

Shokoohi, M., & Attar, T. (2024). Biomanufacturing for a sustainable future: Unleashing the potential of biotechnology in pharmaceutical raw material production. [IJHES]. *International Journal of New Findings in Health and Educational Sciences*, 2(2), 142–153.

Singh, P., Shukla, S., & Misra, G. (2024). Good Manufacturing Practices in Quality Control. In *Quality Control and Regulatory Aspects for Biologicals* (pp. 100–118). CRC Press.

Srivastav, A. K., & Das, P. (2025). *Artificial Intelligence in the Production of Biotherapeutics: Principles, Practices and Standards.* CRC Press.

Suganthi, P., Usharani, B., Venkateswari, R., & Muthuraj, M. (2023). Biosafety Practices in Mycobacteriology Laboratory. *Research Advances in Microbiology and Biotechnology, 3*(3), 1–39.

Sun, T., Song, J., Wang, M., Zhao, C., & Zhang, W. (2022). Challenges and recent progress in the governance of biosecurity risks in the era of synthetic biology. *Journal of Biosafety and Biosecurity, 4*(1), 59–67. PMID: 35005525

Tawade, M., & Pandya, S. (2023). *Optimizing Pharmaceutical Quality Audits: Enhancing Compliance and Performance through Best Practices*. ResearchGate.

Tounekti, O., Prior, S., Wassmer, S., Xu, J., Wong, A., Fang, X., Sonderegger, I., Smeraglia, J., Huleatt, J., & Loo, L. (2025). 2024 White Paper on Recent Issues in Bioanalysis: Evolution of Immunogenicity Assessment beyond ADA/NAb; Regulated Genomic/NGS Assays; Hypersensitivity Reactions; Minimum Noise Reduction; False Positive Range; Modernized Vaccine Approaches; NAb/TAb Correlation (PART 3A–Recommendations on Advanced Strategies for Molecular Assays and Immunogenicity of Gene Therapy, Cell Therapy, Vaccine; Biotherapeutics Immunogenicity Assessment & Clinical Relevance PART 3B–Regulatory Agencies' Input on Immunogenicity/Technologies of Biotherapeutics, Gene, Cell & Vaccine Therapies). *Bioanalysis, 17*(3), 105–149. PMID: 39862111

Alam, A. M. (2024). Analyzing FDA form 483 data of 2023: Identifying trends and areas of concern in regulatory compliance. *Journal of Pharmaceutical and Biological Sciences, 12*(1), 3-7.

von Stosch, M., Oliveira, R., & Peres, J. (2021). Digital Twins in Bioprocessing: Applications and Challenges. *Current Opinion in Chemical Engineering, 34*, 100735. DOI: 10.1016/j.coche.2021.100735

Walsh, G., & Walsh, E. (2022). Biopharmaceutical benchmarks 2022. *Nature Biotechnology, 40*(12), 1722–1760. PMID: 36471135

Wasalathanthri, D. P., Rehmann, M. S., Song, Y., Gu, Y., Mi, L., Shao, C., Chemmalil, L., Lee, J., Ghose, S., & Borys, M. C. (2020). Technology outlook for real-time quality attribute and process parameter monitoring in biopharmaceutical development—A review. *Biotechnology and Bioengineering, 117*(10), 3182–3198. PMID: 32946122

WHO. (2004). *Laboratory Biosafety Manual* (3rd ed.). https://www.who.int/publications/i/item/9241546506

Whomsley, R., Palmi Reig, V., & Hidalgo-Simon, A. (2021). Environmental risk assessment of advanced therapies containing genetically modified organisms in the EU. *British Journal of Clinical Pharmacology, 87*(6), 2450–2458. PMID: 33600022

Zia, S., Paris, F., & Alviano, F. (2024). *Emerging technologies for quality control of cell-based ATMPs. Journal of Pharmaceutical and Biomedical Analysis.* https://www.sciencedirect.com/science/article/pii/S073170852400222X

Chapter 14
Biomanufacturing Challenges in Developing Economies

Oyindamola John Samson
https://orcid.org/0000-0003-0404-7634
Olabisi Onabanjo University, Nigeria

Jamiu Oluwatosin Adeyemi
Olabisi Onabanjo University, Nigeria

Kashish Saxena
University of York, UK

Ismail Babatunde Onajobi
Olabisi Onabanjo University, Nigeria

ABSTRACT

Biomanufacturing, the application of biological systems for producing bio-based products, holds significant potential for industrial growth, economic development, and sustainability. However, developing economies face multiple challenges that hinder its progress. Key constraints include limited access to advanced bioprocessing technologies, inadequate infrastructure, and insufficient research funding. Additionally, regulatory bottlenecks, weak policy frameworks, and a lack of skilled workforce further impede the sector's expansion. The high cost of raw materials and dependence on imported biotechnological inputs exacerbate financial burdens on local industries. Moreover, inconsistent power supply and poor waste management practices present operational inefficiencies. Addressing these challenges requires comprehensive policy reforms, capacity-building initiatives, and strategic investments to enhance the competitiveness of biomanufacturing industries in developing economies.

DOI: 10.4018/979-8-3373-2873-7.ch014

INTRODUCTION

Biomanufacturing—the production of commercially valuable goods through biological systems—has become a powerful driver of global industrial transformation. Encompassing diverse sectors such as pharmaceuticals, agriculture, biofuels, and environmental biotechnology, it offers sustainable alternatives to traditional manufacturing approaches (Shokoohi & Attar, 2024). With its potential to reduce carbon emissions, minimize waste, and foster cleaner production, biomanufacturing is increasingly regarded as a cornerstone of the bioeconomy. For developing economies aiming to diversify industries and achieve sustainable growth, it presents a significant strategic opportunity (Isoko et al., 2024).

Yet, despite its promise, the adoption and scaling of biomanufacturing in these regions face substantial hurdles. Limited access to advanced bioprocessing technologies—often costly and reliant on imports—remains a major constraint. Many countries lack modern equipment, specialized laboratories, and the technical expertise essential for innovation, which hampers research output, slows product development, and delays commercialization (Asghar et al., 2022).

Infrastructure weaknesses compound the problem. Numerous facilities operate with outdated systems, unreliable electricity, and inadequate quality control. The absence of dependable cold chains, waste treatment infrastructure, and secure production environments undermines both scalability and product consistency. Such deficiencies discourage foreign investment and inflate production costs, reducing the global competitiveness of local bio-based products (Ali et al., 2024).

Financial constraints present another critical barrier. Biomanufacturing R&D demands long-term investment, yet public funding in many developing economies is insufficient, and private investment is often deterred by high risks and lengthy development timelines. The elevated cost of importing reagents, enzymes, and engineered strains further strains resources for institutions and startups (Asin-Garcia et al., 2024).

Regulatory and policy challenges also slow progress. Many countries lack coherent biotechnology policies, streamlined approval processes, and effective intellectual property protections (Gregory and Trump, 2023). Uncertainty in regulations can delay market entry, discourage innovation, and hinder compliance with international standards. Bureaucratic inefficiencies and inconsistent enforcement of biosafety protocols further erode confidence in regulatory systems (Gillum et al., 2024).

Human resource gaps remain a pressing issue. Building a skilled biomanufacturing workforce requires specialized academic programs and hands-on training, yet educational systems in many developing economies fall short of industry needs. This shortage of expertise not only affects operational efficiency but also limits participation in advanced research and global collaborations (Evans and Silbey, 2022).

Despite these challenges, encouraging developments are emerging. Several developing economies are beginning to prioritize biomanufacturing through investments in education, research infrastructure, and policy reforms. International partnerships, targeted capacity-building efforts, and public-private collaborations are starting to address technological, financial, and regulatory gaps (Gregory and Trump, 2023). This review examines these complex challenges and explores strategic pathways to enable sustainable growth and technological progress in biomanufacturing.

TECHNOLOGICAL CHALLENGES

Technological limitations represent one of the most critical barriers to the development and sustainability of biomanufacturing in developing economies. The complexity and capital-intensive nature of biomanufacturing processes demand access to advanced tools, well-equipped laboratories, and skilled human resources. Unfortunately, many low- and middle-income countries lack the technological foundation needed to support high-quality, consistent, and scalable bio-based production. The absence of these foundational systems slows innovation, reduces efficiency, and restricts participation in the global bioeconomy.

Limited Access to Advanced Bioprocessing Technologies

Bioprocessing technologies, including upstream and downstream processing systems, are central to producing biopharmaceuticals, enzymes, vaccines, and biofuels. In developing economies, access to such technologies is often restricted due to high acquisition and maintenance costs, lack of domestic manufacturing, and limited knowledge transfer from developed countries. This limitation makes it difficult for researchers and industries to carry out precise fermentation control, real-time monitoring, and purification processes required for large-scale production. Consequently, many potential products remain at the laboratory scale, never reaching commercialization (Matanguihan and Wu, 2022).

Moreover, rapid advances in synthetic biology, CRISPR-based editing tools, and automation systems in developed countries continue to widen the technological gap. Developing nations struggle to keep pace due to poor technology transfer mechanisms and insufficient funding for local adaptation. The inability to adopt and customize these new technologies limits innovation and severely hinders the competitiveness of developing economies in the biomanufacturing sector (Kiran et al., 2024).

Another major technological challenge is the heavy dependence on imported raw materials and equipment. Developing economies often lack local suppliers of critical components such as microbial strains, fermentation media, bioreactor parts, diagnostic kits, and single-use systems. Importation not only increases production costs but also exposes industries to risks related to currency fluctuations, trade barriers, and supply chain disruptions (Hassan et al., 2025).

This dependence reduces resilience and flexibility in responding to local demands and emergencies, such as during pandemics when global supply chains become stressed. Additionally, imported materials are not always suited to the environmental and climatic conditions of developing regions, leading to inefficiencies and lower product yields. The lack of indigenous production capacity also discourages innovation and technology localization, thereby perpetuating reliance on foreign systems (Malik, 2024).

Inadequate Research and Development (R&D) Infrastructure

The absence of well-equipped R&D infrastructure significantly hampers technological advancement in biomanufacturing across many developing economies. Effective R&D requires access to state-of-the-art laboratories, biosafety-level facilities, cold storage systems, analytical tools, and high-throughput screening capabilities. However, many universities and research institutes operate with obsolete equipment and limited access to digital tools for bioinformatics and modeling (Al-Worafi, 2024).

This inadequacy restricts the ability to conduct applied and translational research, which is crucial for converting lab-scale innovations into commercially viable processes. Furthermore, limited R&D facilities discourage international collaboration and make it difficult for local scientists to engage in globally competitive research. The result is a weak innovation pipeline and an inability to meet local and regional bioproduct demands (Khopade and Shah, 2026).

The combined effect of these technological limitations is a sluggish pace of innovation and a bottleneck in commercializing biotechnological discoveries. Startups and academic researchers face delays in testing new ideas, scaling up prototypes, and complying with product quality standards. This disconnects between discovery and application undermines the economic potential of biomanufacturing and contributes to a cycle of underdevelopment in biotechnology sectors (Raza, 2024).

Moreover, technology constraints limit the ability of developing economies to respond quickly to health crises, food insecurity, and environmental degradation—areas where biomanufacturing could offer solutions. Without proactive investment in technology infrastructure, these countries risk being excluded from global value chains and the benefits of the bioeconomy (Shokoohi and Attar, 2024).

Potential Solutions and Pathways Forward

Addressing technological challenges in biomanufacturing requires a multi-pronged approach. Governments and institutions must prioritize investments in modernizing infrastructure and fostering technology transfer agreements. Public-private partnerships can be instrumental in financing the procurement and localization of advanced bioprocessing systems. Incentivizing domestic manufacturing of inputs and supporting local innovation ecosystems can reduce dependence on imports (Asin-Garcia et al., 2025).

Additionally, capacity-building initiatives should focus on training technical personnel, promoting international exchange programs, and establishing regional centers of excellence in biotechnology. By fostering an environment that enables technological growth and innovation, developing economies can gradually overcome their current limitations and realize the full potential of biomanufacturing as shown in Table 1.

Table 1. Technological challenges in biomanufacturing in developing economies

Challenge area	Description	Impact	Possible remedies	References
Limited Access to Bioprocessing Technologies	High cost, poor availability of advanced bioreactors, monitoring tools, and automation systems	Low productivity, poor scale-up potential, outdated practices	Invest in technology transfer, subsidize acquisition, and promote open-access platforms	Kim et al. (2024)
Dependence on Imported Raw Materials & Equipment	Limited local production of biomanufacturing inputs; overreliance on foreign suppliers	High production costs, vulnerability to supply chain disruptions	Develop local supply chains, encourage indigenous production	Whitford et al. (2022)
Inadequate R&D Infrastructure	Obsolete laboratories, limited access to molecular tools, poor data analytics infrastructure	Weak innovation pipeline, low research output, limited commercialization	Upgrade R&D facilities, invest in digital tools, create biotech innovation hubs	Wilson et al. (2022)
Lack of Skilled Technical Workforce	Inadequate training in advanced techniques and systems	Poor process management, inefficient operations	Support academic-industry partnerships, training, and mentoring programs	Mandato and Kulhanek (2022)
Poor Technology Transfer Mechanisms	Weak linkages between research institutions and industry	Slow adoption of new technologies, fragmented innovation ecosystem	Foster industry-academia collaborations, IP frameworks, and incubation centers	Stana et al. (2024)

ECONOMIC AND FINANCIAL CONSTRAINTS

Biomanufacturing in developing economies is severely impeded by economic and financial barriers that affect every stage of the production pipeline—from research to market entry. Unlike traditional manufacturing, biomanufacturing is highly capital-intensive, requiring large investments in research, process development, quality control, and regulatory compliance. The inability to secure sufficient funding or attract investment partners has made it difficult for many developing countries to harness the full economic potential of biomanufacturing technologies.

High Production Costs and Limited Funding Opportunities

One of the primary economic challenges in developing economies is the high cost of production. Biomanufacturing operations often require expensive imported reagents, bioreactor components, enzymes, and genetically engineered microorganisms. Due to limited local manufacturing capabilities, these costs are inflated by import duties, logistics, and currency fluctuations. Additionally, the expense of maintaining good manufacturing practices (GMP) and quality assurance protocols further strains financial resources, especially for small-scale enterprises and research institutions (Shokoohi and Attar, 2024).

Adding to this burden is the limited access to reliable and sustained funding. Government allocations to research and innovation in many developing countries are minimal, and what little exists often gets diverted to traditional sectors such as agriculture or infrastructure. As a result, biomanufacturing projects struggle to survive the long development timelines required to bring products to market. Grant systems, venture capital, and innovation funds that are prevalent in high-income countries are either scarce or non-existent in many developing economies, limiting the pace and scale of biomanufacturing initiatives (Billington, 2016).

Startup companies play a pivotal role in driving innovation and commercialization in the biomanufacturing space. However, in developing economies, these startups often face immense difficulties in securing seed funding or attracting investors willing to support high-risk biotech ventures. Investors typically view biotechnology as a long-term commitment with uncertain returns, especially in environments where regulatory frameworks are weak, infrastructure is inadequate, and exit opportunities (such as public listings or mergers) are limited (Choudhary et al., 2024).

Moreover, many biotechnology startups in developing regions operate within fragmented ecosystems, lacking access to incubators, mentorship, and industry linkages. This isolation results in a limited capacity to pitch competitive business models or demonstrate market readiness. The consequence is a low startup survival rate and missed opportunities for indigenous biotechnological solutions that could address local public health, agricultural, and environmental challenges.

Limited Access to Credit and Financial Instruments

A related issue is the unavailability of tailored financial instruments such as low-interest loans, credit guarantees, or risk-sharing mechanisms for biotech enterprises. Traditional banks and financial institutions are often reluctant to extend credit to biomanufacturing ventures due to their technical complexity and long gestation periods. The lack of risk-tolerant financial ecosystems discourages entrepreneurial activity and hinders the establishment of homegrown biomanufacturing industries.

International funding programs and donor-supported initiatives have made some impact, particularly in health-focused biomanufacturing (e.g., vaccine production), but these efforts are often short-term and project-based rather than systemic and sustainable. To build long-term financial viability, developing economies need to foster inclusive financing models that support early-stage development and facilitate the transition to commercial-scale operations.

Even when biomanufacturing entities in developing economies manage to create viable products, they frequently encounter challenges in accessing markets. Regulatory delays, poor infrastructure for distribution, and lack of consumer awareness all act as barriers to product uptake. Additionally, foreign products often dominate local markets due to their established brand trust, economies of scale, and compliance with international standards, making it difficult for locally produced bioproducts to gain traction.

Another major commercialization hurdle is the absence of efficient value chains and supply networks. Many bio-based products require cold chains, trained personnel, and coordinated logistics for effective delivery—systems that are underdeveloped in many regions. Moreover, local procurement policies often do not prioritize domestically produced biotech goods, instead favoring cheaper imports. This lack of supportive procurement and marketing strategies undercuts local industry growth and limits the return on investment for innovators.

Underdeveloped Innovation-to-Market Ecosystems

The gap between research output and commercial product development is also widened by underdeveloped innovation ecosystems. Few platforms exist in developing economies to bridge the "valley of death"—the critical stage between proof of concept and market readiness. Without mechanisms for technology transfer, licensing, and business development, promising research remains confined to academic journals rather than evolving into accessible, profitable products (Huang et al., 2020).

Additionally, intellectual property (IP) rights enforcement and commercialization support services—such as patent filing, licensing negotiations, and venture development offices—are poorly established. This further discourages private sector engagement and reduces the incentives for innovation. Strengthening these systems is essential for building a resilient and profitable biomanufacturing sector (Mary and Enoch, 2024).

Overcoming the economic and financial constraints facing biomanufacturing in developing economies requires coordinated efforts among governments, investors, academia, and industry. Strategic financial incentives such as tax breaks, innovation grants, and credit support can stimulate entrepreneurship and de-risk investment. Governments should also establish biotech-specific industrial policies that include public procurement mandates, subsidies for local inputs, and infrastructure investment (Fajardo et al., 2025).

Furthermore, regional market integration, harmonized regulatory standards, and the development of biotechnology clusters can enhance economies of scale and improve competitiveness (figure 1). A shift toward demand-driven innovation—where products are designed to meet local market needs—can also accelerate uptake and commercialization. Ultimately, addressing financial and economic barriers is not only crucial for advancing biomanufacturing but also for fostering inclusive economic growth and health security in developing nations.

Figure 1. Four key economic and financial challenges of biomanufacturing in developing economies

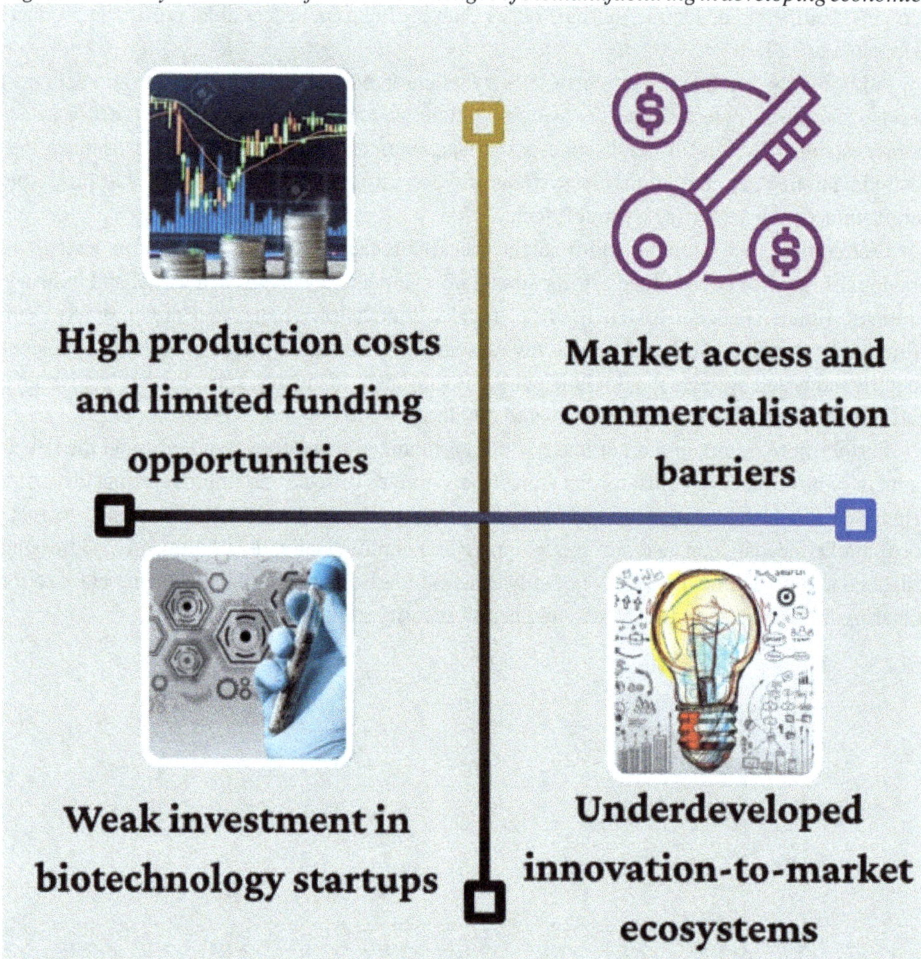

REGULATORY AND POLICY BOTTLENECKS

Biomanufacturing, due to its complex and high-stakes nature, relies heavily on robust regulatory systems and supportive policy frameworks. In many developing economies, these structures remain weak or underdeveloped, creating significant barriers to progress in the biotechnology sector. Regulatory and policy bottlenecks affect not just product approval timelines and manufacturing compliance, but also innovation, intellectual property protection, and global competitiveness.

Weak Policy Frameworks and Regulatory Challenges

In many low- and middle-income countries, biotechnology and biomanufacturing are not yet clearly defined within national policy agendas. The absence of clear, enforceable policies on biosafety, bioethics, and bioproduct commercialization leaves innovators and manufacturers in regulatory limbo. The lack of designated agencies or clear regulatory pathways for approvals delays time-to-market and discourages private sector investment (Sammut, 2021). Furthermore, overlapping jurisdictions and bureaucratic red tape often characterize the regulatory environment in these regions. Multiple agencies may demand compliance for the same process, leading to delays, inefficiencies, and increased costs. The absence of stakeholder engagement in policy formation means that existing regulations often do not reflect the realities or needs of local industry, research institutions, or emerging startups (Khandekar and Ghosh, 2023).

Intellectual Property Rights (IPR) are critical for protecting biotechnological innovations and encouraging investment in research and development. However, in many developing economies, IPR systems are weak or inconsistently enforced. Local inventors often face difficulties in patent registration, protection, and enforcement, which undermines the incentive to innovate (Sinhmar and Purohit, 2025). Furthermore, technology transfer and licensing agreements are often poorly structured or entirely absent. This creates barriers to the commercialization of research outputs and limits the participation of universities and public research institutes in biomanufacturing ventures. Foreign investors and multinational companies also view weak IPR protection as a significant risk, which further reduces the flow of global expertise and partnerships into these economies (Gaitán, 2021).

Barriers to Accessing International Intellectual Property Systems

While some developing countries are signatories to international IP treaties (e.g., the TRIPS agreement under WTO), they frequently lack the institutional capacity or human resources to engage effectively with these frameworks. This creates a disadvantage in negotiating equitable licensing agreements or protecting innovations globally. The high cost of international patent filing also poses a significant financial burden on local innovators (Sundaram, 2025). Additionally, limited awareness about IP among researchers, entrepreneurs, and policymakers means that many valuable biotechnological inventions remain unprotected. This results in the loss of competitive advantage and undermines efforts to build sustainable bioeconomies that rely on home-grown technologies and knowledge systems (Sinhmar and Purohit, 2025).

Compliance with international standards is critical for the global acceptance of bioproducts, yet this remains a persistent challenge in many developing countries. Lack of access to updated protocols and guidelines, inadequate testing facilities, and the absence of accredited quality control laboratories hinder the ability of local manufacturers to meet global regulatory expectations (Hock et al., 2020). Furthermore, developing economies often struggle to comply with the documentation, certification, and traceability standards required by international markets. This not only limits export potential but also affects the credibility of local products in domestic markets. The absence of standardized regulatory processes makes it difficult for local companies to establish mutual recognition agreements or participate in international supply chains (Katsieris, 2024).

Need for Regulatory Capacity Building

To overcome these regulatory gaps, developing economies must invest in building the capacity of national regulatory authorities. This includes training personnel, developing digital regulatory platforms, and creating risk-based, science-driven frameworks that support innovation without compromising safety. International partnerships and donor agencies can play a crucial role by providing technical assistance and harmonizing regulatory standards across regions (Abbott and Snidal, 2021). At the same time, engaging local stakeholders—industry leaders, academic researchers, legal experts, and civil society organizations—in the policymaking process ensures that regulations are both technically sound and contextually appropriate. This inclusive approach enhances regulatory transparency, fosters trust, and encourages compliance among market participants.

Finally, regulatory and policy frameworks must be dynamic and aligned with the needs of the biomanufacturing sector. Policy instruments such as tax incentives, priority review mechanisms, and fast-track approval for critical bioproducts can stimulate innovation and reduce time-to-market. Clear guidelines for biosafety, clinical trials, and environmental impact assessments are also essential for building investor confidence and safeguarding public health (Asin-Garcia et al., 2025).

To drive sustainable growth, developing countries must prioritize biomanufacturing in national development agendas, establish dedicated biotechnology authorities, and promote cross-sectoral collaboration. Strengthening regulatory governance is not just a compliance issue—it is a strategic imperative for unlocking the transformative potential of biomanufacturing in developing economies (table 2).

Table 2. Regulatory and policy bottlenecks in biomanufacturing

Challenge Area	Specific Issues	Impact on Biomanufacturing	Proposed Solutions	References
Weak Policy Frameworks	Lack of national biotech strategies, poor interagency coordination	Delays in approvals, limited investment	Develop clear biotech policies and establish dedicated regulatory bodies	Sammut (2021)
Regulatory Challenges	Bureaucratic delays, redundant processes	High compliance costs, low private sector participation	Streamline regulatory processes; digitize application systems	Khandekar and Ghosh (2023)
Intellectual Property Rights	Poor enforcement, limited IP awareness	Innovation loss, low investor confidence	Strengthen IP systems; conduct awareness campaigns and training	Sinhmar and Purohit (2025)
Licensing and Technology Transfer	Absence of commercialization frameworks	Research outputs remain unused	Create national licensing offices; support academia-industry linkages	Katsieris (2024)
International Standards Compliance	Limited access to certified labs and global protocols	Inability to export or compete globally	Invest in lab accreditation and technical capacity	Hock et al. (2020)
Capacity Gaps in Regulatory Agencies	Lack of trained personnel, outdated procedures	Regulatory bottlenecks	Provide training and international support programs	Abbott and Snidal (2021)

continued on following page

Table 2. Continued

Challenge Area	Specific Issues	Impact on Biomanufacturing	Proposed Solutions	References
Low Stakeholder Involvement	Limited industry and academia engagement in policy	Misaligned regulations and real-world needs	Foster inclusive policy-making processes	
Market Recognition and Trust	Non-compliance with global safety and efficacy standards	Consumer distrust and low uptake	Harmonize with international standards and promote quality assurance	Asin-Garcia et al. (2025)

HUMAN RESOURCE AND CAPACITY GAPS

Human capital forms the foundation of any successful biomanufacturing industry. The availability of a skilled workforce capable of driving innovation, maintaining bioprocessing standards, and ensuring regulatory compliance is essential. Unfortunately, developing economies suffer from pronounced human resource limitations that hinder growth in this high-tech sector. These challenges are interwoven with educational shortfalls, limited training opportunities, and systemic underinvestment in capacity building.

Shortage of Skilled Workforce and Training Deficiencies

A major bottleneck is the lack of adequately trained professionals with expertise in bioprocessing, bioengineering, quality control, regulatory affairs, and industrial microbiology. Most developing countries rely on general science graduates who often lack specialized training tailored to the biomanufacturing industry's specific demands. This creates a mismatch between industry needs and available skillsets, ultimately affecting operational efficiency, innovation, and product quality (Tusé et al., 2020). The problem is compounded by the absence of dedicated technical and vocational programs focusing on biotechnology manufacturing. Institutions that do offer biotechnology courses often emphasize theory over practice, leaving graduates unprepared for real-world applications. Continuous professional development programs, internships, and hands-on industrial training are scarce, widening the skills gap and slowing industrial progress (Delebecque and Philp, 2019).

Even when curricula exist, there is often a lack of qualified trainers, modern laboratories, and pilot-scale production facilities in academic institutions. Without exposure to industry-grade equipment and biomanufacturing processes, students and researchers cannot bridge the gap between academia and industry. This limits innovation and stifles the growth of a dynamic workforce that can respond to evolving sectoral demands (Harrer, 2023). In addition, insufficient funding for research fellowships, laboratory upgrades, and industrial placement programs reduces the ability of institutions to attract and retain competent personnel. These capacity challenges hinder the development of a national talent pool required for scaling up biomanufacturing ventures (Halstead and Sautter, 2023).

Limited Academic-Industry Collaboration

Another critical gap lies in the weak linkage between academia and industry. In many developing economies, universities and research centers operate in isolation, with minimal engagement with the private sector. This disconnection prevents knowledge transfer, inhibits joint problem-solving, and discourages the commercialization of research outputs (Bstieler et al., 2015). Where collaborative efforts exist, they are often informal or fragmented, lacking structured mechanisms such as technology transfer offices, innovation hubs, and public-private research consortia. This undermines the translation of academic innovation into market-ready products and services. Industry players also hesitate to invest in collaborative R&D due to uncertainties about intellectual property rights and lack of trust in institutional capacities (Olaisen and Revang, 2017).

A further challenge is that curricula are rarely aligned with the actual needs of biomanufacturing industries. Outdated course content and inflexible academic structures prevent the co-creation of training modules that reflect industry demands. Without regular input from industry stakeholders, academic programs fail to prepare graduates with job-relevant competencies such as bioprocess validation, GMP (Good Manufacturing Practices), and regulatory compliance (Prestigiacomo et al., 2024). Developing economies need deliberate efforts to create joint training programs, internship schemes, and advisory boards that include industry experts. These strategies can enhance workforce preparedness, encourage innovation, and reduce onboarding costs for employers.

Brain Drain and Retention of Talent

The challenges of workforce development are further compounded by the brain drain phenomenon. Skilled professionals trained in biotechnology often migrate to developed countries in search of better employment prospects, research opportunities, and improved working conditions. This exodus not only depletes the already limited talent pool but also results in financial losses from investments in education and training. Poor remuneration, limited career advancement opportunities, and inadequate research infrastructure are among the factors driving talent migration (Oke, 2025). Young graduates, particularly those with specialized knowledge, perceive local biomanufacturing industries as lacking in innovation, stability, and global competitiveness—further fuelling their desire to leave (Najib et al., 2019).

To reverse brain drain and build local capacity, it is essential to create an enabling environment that motivates professionals to stay and contribute. This includes competitive salaries, mentorship opportunities, continuous learning platforms, and merit-based promotions. Additionally, developing centers of excellence in biomanufacturing research and innovation can serve as magnets for both local and diaspora talent (Latukha et al., 2022). Governments and private institutions should also explore policies to attract returnees through fellowship programs, startup grants, and partnerships with foreign institutions. Such strategic interventions not only boost local capacity but also foster cross-border knowledge exchange and innovation.

INFRASTRUCTURE AND OPERATIONAL CHALLENGES

Biomanufacturing is inherently infrastructure-intensive, relying on stable power supply, sophisticated waste management systems, and efficient logistics to ensure quality and regulatory compliance. However, developing economies frequently face critical infrastructure and operational deficits that significantly hinder the growth and sustainability of biomanufacturing ventures. These challenges not only raise operational costs but also threaten product integrity and environmental safety.

Inconsistent Power Supply and Energy Constraints

A reliable and continuous power supply is a non-negotiable requirement for any biomanufacturing process, which often involves temperature-sensitive fermentation, aseptic environments, and computer-controlled bioreactors. Unfortunately, in many developing countries, power outages and voltage fluctuations are common, forcing facilities to rely heavily on diesel generators. This adds to production costs, increases emissions, and compromises process control (Marqusee and Don II, 2020). Moreover, most regions lack access to renewable or clean energy solutions due to limited investment and policy incentives. The result is a high-carbon production footprint and a reliance on expensive, polluting alternatives that hinder both environmental and economic sustainability. Without guaranteed energy reliability, many small- and medium-scale enterprises find it difficult to scale operations or maintain quality consistency in their bioproducts (Falcone, 2023).

Frequent power disruptions lead to operational downtime, spoilage of sensitive biological products, and equipment damage. The inability to maintain ideal fermentation or storage conditions during outages can result in batch failures, thereby increasing production waste and reducing profitability. In some cases, this leads to the abandonment of large-scale production goals in favor of smaller, risk-averse operations (Elmadhoun et al., 2025). To address these issues, biomanufacturing facilities in developing economies need investment in hybrid power systems, uninterrupted power supply (UPS) units, and energy-efficient technologies. Government subsidies for renewable energy and infrastructure upgrades could also support long-term energy security in the sector (Ali et al., 2024).

Waste Management and Environmental Concerns

Biomanufacturing processes generate a variety of waste streams—ranging from biological waste to chemical byproducts and spent media. In many developing economies, the lack of dedicated biowaste management facilities poses serious public health and environmental risks. Untreated or poorly managed waste can contaminate water bodies, spread diseases, and damage ecosystems (Lynch et al., 2022). Moreover, few facilities operate under strict biosafety level protocols or have access to effluent treatment plants. This can result in regulatory non-compliance and sanctions, further deterring investment. In some cases, waste management is outsourced to third-party vendors with limited oversight, raising concerns about illegal dumping or improper treatment (Kumar et al., 2024).

The absence of national standards or waste disposal guidelines for biomanufacturing adds to the challenge. Most small-scale producers lack the financial or technical capacity to establish in-house treatment plants. Additionally, the lack of recycling and waste valorization technologies means that potentially reusable byproducts are discarded rather than converted into secondary inputs or energy (Hock et al., 2020). Developing economies must invest in green biomanufacturing practices, support waste-to-energy innovations, and develop biosafety regulations that reflect both environmental priorities and industrial realities. Creating incentives for environmental compliance and sustainable operations will encourage responsible production (Ogwu et al., 2025).

Supply Chain and Logistics Issues

A robust supply chain is critical for the timely delivery of raw materials, reagents, and packaging materials—many of which are imported in developing countries. Delays at ports, high transportation costs, and limited cold-chain logistics contribute to frequent production interruptions. These inefficiencies make it difficult for local biomanufacturers to maintain continuous production cycles or respond flexibly to market demands (Rajaeifar et al., 2022). Furthermore, inadequate transport infrastructure—such as poorly maintained roads, limited rail networks, and bottlenecked urban logistics—adds to delivery times and operational unpredictability. For time-sensitive inputs like enzymes or cell cultures, even minor delays can compromise viability and quality (Ojadi and Maiyaki, 2025).

Supply chain unreliability increases operational risks and often forces producers to maintain large inventories, which ties up working capital and reduces agility. Additionally, reliance on imported inputs exposes the sector to exchange rate volatility and global supply disruptions, as seen during the COVID-19 pandemic. This not only raises production costs but also affects the affordability and availability of locally made bioproducts (Tao et al., 2025). To mitigate these challenges, governments and industry stakeholders should invest in local production of bioprocessing inputs, strengthen transportation and storage infrastructure, and create regional hubs for logistics efficiency. Strategic partnerships with international suppliers and digital supply chain management systems can also enhance resilience and transparency.

POTENTIAL STRATEGIES FOR OVERCOMING CHALLENGES

Government Incentives and Policy Reforms

One of the most impactful strategies to address biomanufacturing challenges in developing economies is through robust government incentives and policy reforms. Strategic support, such as tax holidays, subsidized loans, and grants, can significantly lower entry barriers for local firms. Additionally, creating targeted policies that streamline regulatory approvals for biomanufacturing projects can enhance investor confidence and accelerate industrial growth (Rathore and Shereef, 2022). Beyond financial support, governments must institute clear and enforceable biomanufacturing development frameworks that prioritize infrastructure, R&D, and human capacity. National biotechnology policies should integrate biomanufacturing goals into broader industrial, health, and agricultural agendas. Periodic review and adaptation of these policies in line with global trends and local needs are also essential for long-term sustainability (Gregory and Trump, 2023).

Public-private partnerships offer a dynamic platform to combine government backing with private sector efficiency and innovation. Through PPPs, governments can facilitate infrastructure development (e.g., biotech parks, research hubs) while the private sector provides capital, expertise, and commercialization pathways. These partnerships also improve risk-sharing and foster a more collaborative industrial ecosystem (Carbonara and Pellegrino, 2019). In addition, PPPs can enable joint research and demonstration projects, shared access to expensive equipment, and co-development of sustainable bioproducts. Establishing centers of excellence that link universities, industries, and public institutions can ensure continuous innovation and capacity building, particularly in areas such as vaccine production, biofertilizer development, and environmental remediation (Ferasso and Grenier, 2021).

Enhancing Indigenous Innovation and Local Resource Utilization

Developing economies possess vast indigenous biological resources and traditional knowledge systems that remain underutilized. Promoting research that leverages native microbes, plants, and enzymes for biomanufacturing can reduce dependency on imported raw materials and align industrial outputs with local ecological contexts (Ogwu et al., 2025). Governments and academic institutions should fund bio-prospecting initiatives and establish national bioresource banks to conserve and catalogue valuable strains and compounds. By enhancing indigenous innovation, countries can create unique competitive advantages in niche bio-based industries such as herbal pharmaceuticals, microbial enzymes, and region-specific diagnostics (Preetha et al., 2024).

Rather than relying solely on high-end foreign technologies, there should be a focus on local adaptation and frugal innovation. Technologies that are energy-efficient, low-cost, and easily operable under local conditions are more sustainable and scalable in developing economies. Open-source platforms and south-south technology transfer initiatives can support the spread of such adaptable tools (Winkler et al., 2020). Moreover, setting up technology incubation centers and fabrication labs (FabLabs) can allow local startups and research teams to prototype, test, and scale their biomanufacturing innovations. These platforms can also support reverse engineering and improve technical self-reliance (Oppedisano, 2024).

Investment in Biotechnology Education and Research

A foundational strategy is the strengthening of biotechnology education and research systems. Without a knowledgeable and skilled workforce, even the most well-funded industries cannot function effectively. Updating academic curricula, incorporating industry-oriented training, and supporting postgraduate and technical education are crucial. Governments should also allocate more funds to university research and provide competitive grants for applied bioscience innovation. Establishing national research priorities and incentivizing interdisciplinary studies will further improve innovation output. Fellowships, research mobility programs, and industry internships can enhance student exposure and employability (Suzette et al., 2024).

For any reform or investment strategy to work, the regulatory agencies must be equally empowered. This includes training personnel in emerging biomanufacturing trends, upgrading testing laboratories, and developing guidelines in line with international best practices. Strong regulatory institutions ensure public safety, enhance trust in bioproducts, and facilitate export readiness. Furthermore, capacity-building workshops and international collaboration with regulatory bodies such as WHO, FDA, and ISO can provide frameworks for compliance and monitoring. Technical assistance programs can be tailored to specific national priorities, including vaccine production, food biotechnology, or biosafety assessment (Woteki & Buckley, 2020).

Establishing innovation hubs and incubators is another potent strategy for overcoming development bottlenecks. These centers provide early-stage biotech startups with the tools, mentorship, and market access needed to grow (Pustovrh et al., 2020). They also encourage cross-sector innovation, where healthcare, agriculture, and environmental sustainability converge. A successful innovation ecosystem includes venture capital access, intellectual property support, business development services, and linkages to global markets. Governments can catalyze this by providing seed funding and attracting private investors through regulatory ease and co-investment schemes (Rossi et al., 2021).

Regional Collaboration and Knowledge Exchange

Developing economies can benefit immensely from regional collaboration and knowledge sharing. Collaborative platforms between neighboring countries or regional economic blocs can promote standardization, pooling of research infrastructure, and collective policy lobbying at international forums (Stephen, 2021). Platforms such as the African Union Development Agency (AUDA-NEPAD) or ASEAN's Biotechnology Consortium can facilitate joint clinical trials, transboundary regulation harmonization, and shared databases for research. These collaborations reduce redundancy, accelerate innovation, and ensure equitable access to biotechnological advancements (Feng et al., 2024).

Finally, innovative financing models such as impact investing, green bonds, and blended finance can attract both public and private capital into biomanufacturing. These models ensure that investment is not only profit-driven but also aligned with environmental, health, and social goals (Srivastav and Das, 2025). By integrating biomanufacturing into climate adaptation, food security, and health preparedness strategies, governments can tap into multilateral funding from institutions like the World Bank, GAVI, and the Global Environment Facility. Crowdfunding platforms and diaspora engagement can also supplement financing for community-level biotech initiatives.

FUTURE PROSPECTS AND RECOMMENDATIONS

Emerging Trends in Biomanufacturing

Biomanufacturing is evolving rapidly with emerging trends shaping its future trajectory. Notable advancements include the adoption of synthetic biology, automation, artificial intelligence (AI)-assisted bioprocessing, and continuous manufacturing systems. These technologies enable enhanced efficiency, real-time process monitoring, and improved scalability. Additionally, sustainable practices such as green bioprocessing and waste valorization are gaining traction as industries aim to align production with environmental conservation (Mehta et al., 2024). For developing economies, adopting these innovations could revolutionize traditional manufacturing sectors like pharmaceuticals, agriculture, and energy. However, a strategic framework is needed to support the transition from conventional to advanced biomanufacturing practices. This requires building technological literacy, fostering innovation ecosystems, and developing region-specific roadmaps (George and George, 2024).

Another key future prospect is the alignment of biomanufacturing with the circular bioeconomy, where biological waste and renewable biomass are converted into high-value products. This paradigm promotes sustainability, resource efficiency, and minimal environmental impact. Through this model, developing countries can reduce dependency on fossil-based industries and create resilient local economies driven by bio-based innovation (Swaminaathan et al., 2024). To achieve this, policy frameworks must incentivize bio-based product development, recycling technologies, and closed-loop supply chains. Furthermore, integrating sustainability metrics into biomanufacturing performance evaluations will guide industries toward environmentally sound practices (Tsakalova et al., 2024).

Role of International Collaboration and Funding

International partnerships are crucial for the long-term growth of biomanufacturing in developing economies. Multilateral organizations, development banks, and bilateral cooperation frameworks offer vital technical and financial support. For instance, collaboration with institutions like the World Bank, WHO, GAVI, FAO, and global universities can support knowledge transfer, workforce training, and the establishment of state-of-the-art facilities (Asin-Garcia et al., 2025). Joint research programs, access to global intellectual property pools, and participation in international clinical trials will elevate the competitiveness of local industries. Moreover, foreign direct investment (FDI) in biotechnology parks and export-oriented biomanufacturing clusters can accelerate integration into global value chains (Ahmad et al., 2023).

Besides institutional partnerships, diaspora engagement offers untapped potential. Skilled professionals and entrepreneurs abroad can be mobilized to transfer expertise, mentor startups, and co-invest in local ventures. Additionally, private philanthropic organizations, such as the Gates Foundation and Wellcome Trust, can provide catalytic funding for high-impact projects like vaccine production or biofortified crops (Union, 2020). Governments should establish formal diaspora innovation schemes and co-create platforms that facilitate remote collaboration, fundraising, and project incubation. This inclusive approach strengthens domestic innovation while maintaining global relevance.

Roadmap for Sustainable Biomanufacturing Growth

Developing a strategic roadmap (China as a good examples) is essential for guiding biomanufacturing efforts in developing countries. This roadmap must span short-, medium-, and long-term goals, clearly outlining the stages of infrastructure development, human resource enhancement, regulatory reform, and commercialization. It should be tailored to local contexts while remaining aligned with global standards and sustainability objectives (Zhang et al., 2022).

The roadmap must also emphasize intersectoral collaboration—engaging academia, industry, government, and civil society in co-designing policy and implementation strategies. Key performance indicators (KPIs), impact assessments, and regular stakeholder consultations should be embedded to track progress and guide iterative improvements (Table 3).

Table 3. Roadmap for sustainable biomanufacturing growth in developing economies

Timeframe	Strategic Actions	Key Stakeholders	Expected Outcomes
Short-term (1–3 yrs)	Establish national biomanufacturing policy. Launch biotech education and skill programs. Provide seed funding and incentives for startups	Government, Universities, Incubators	Policy foundation, talent pipeline, early-stage innovation
Mid-term (4–7 yrs)	Develop biotechnology parks and labs. Foster public-private partnerships. Streamline regulatory frameworks	Industries, Investors, Regulators	Scaled R&D infrastructure, industry growth, regulatory clarity
Long-term (8–15 yrs)	Integrate into global biotech value chains. Commercialize indigenous innovations. Align with green and circular bioeconomy	Export agencies, Multilateral institutions	Export-driven growth, sustainable production, global recognition

(Zhang et al., 2022)

For the roadmap to be effective, monitoring and evaluation (M&E) mechanisms must be institutionalized. Regular audits, benchmarking with international peers, and impact assessments can inform adaptive policymaking. Open data platforms and transparent reporting systems will further build public and investor confidence in the sector (Kuchenmüller et al., 2022). Developing countries should also consider establishing national biomanufacturing councils or inter-ministerial task forces to coordinate strategy execution, align priorities, and resolve bottlenecks. Such institutional arrangements promote accountability and ensure that growth is inclusive, equitable, and sustainable (Liu, 2025).

CONCLUSION

The future of biomanufacturing in developing economies lies at the intersection of innovation, collaboration, and strategic foresight. By leveraging emerging technologies, fostering global partnerships, and committing to sustainable development, these nations can transform biomanufacturing into a cornerstone of their economic and health resilience. A clear and inclusive roadmap, grounded in local realities and global best practices, will be pivotal in achieving this vision. Addressing human resource and capacity gaps requires a multipronged approach. This involves reforming educational programs, building robust academia-industry linkages, and implementing targeted talent retention strategies. By investing in people—through skill development, mentorship, and professional incentives—developing economies can lay the foundation for a vibrant, innovative, and globally competitive biomanufacturing sector.

REFERENCES

Abbott, K. W., & Snidal, D. (2021). Strengthening international regulation through transnational new governance: Overcoming the orchestration deficit. In *The spectrum of international institutions* (pp. 95–139). Routledge.

Ahmad, H., Shabbir, I., Iqbal, I., & Akhtar, M. M. (2023). The Crossroad between Intellectual Property and Clinical Trials: Balancing Incentives for Innovation with Access to Healthcare. *Trends in Intellectual Property Research, 1*(2). Advance online publication. DOI: 10.69971/tipr.1.2.2023.16

Al-Worafi, Y. M. (2024). Research and Development in Developing Countries: Achievements and Challenges. *Handbook of Medical and Health Sciences in Developing Countries: Education, Practice, and Research*, 1-23. https://doi.org/DOI: 10.1007/978-3-030-74786-2_385-1

Ali, A., Usman, M., Jayamani, E., Soon, K., & bin Ab Wahab, M. K. (2024). Sustainable Biomanufacturing. In *Biomedical Implants* (pp. 195-217). CRC Press.

Ali, A., Usman, M., Jayamani, E., Soon, K., & bin Ab Wahab, M. K. (2024). Sustainable Biomanufacturing. In *Biomedical Implants* (pp. 195-217). CRC Press.

Asghar, A., Sairash, S., Hussain, N., Baqar, Z., Sumrin, A., & Bilal, M. (2022). Current challenges of biomass refinery and prospects of emerging technologies for sustainable bioproducts and bioeconomy. *Biofuels, Bioproducts & Biorefining, 16*(6), 1478–1494. DOI: 10.1002/bbb.2403

Asin-Garcia, E., Fawcett, J. D., Batianis, C., & Dos Santos, V. A. M. (2024). A snapshot of biomanufacturing and the need for enabling research infrastructure. *Trends in Biotechnology*. Advance online publication. DOI: 10.1016/j.tibtech.2024.10.014 PMID: 39592270

Asin-Garcia, E., Fawcett, J. D., Batianis, C., & Dos Santos, V. A. M. (2025). A snapshot of biomanufacturing and the need for enabling research infrastructure. *Trends in Biotechnology, 43*(5), 1000–1014. DOI: 10.1016/j.tibtech.2024.10.014 PMID: 39592270

Billington, J. K. (2016). A new product development partnership model for antibiotic resistance. *American Journal of Law & Medicine, 42*(2-3), 487–523. DOI: 10.1177/0098858816658277 PMID: 29086636

Bstieler, L., Hemmert, M., & Barczak, G. (2015). Trust formation in university–industry collaborations in the US biotechnology industry: IP policies, shared governance, and champions. *Journal of Product Innovation Management, 32*(1), 111–121. DOI: 10.1111/jpim.12242

Carbonara, N., & Pellegrino, R. (2019). The role of public private partnerships in fostering innovation. *Construction Management and Economics, 38*(2), 140–156. DOI: 10.1080/01446193.2019.1610184

Choudhary, V., Patel, K., Niaz, M., Panwala, M., Mehta, A., & Choudhary, K. (2024). Risk Management Strategies for Biotech Startups: A Comprehensive Framework for Early-Stage Projects. In *Recent Trends In Engineering and Science for Resource Optimization and Sustainable Development* (pp. 448-456). CRC Press.

Delebecque, C. J., & Philp, J. (2019). Education and training for industrial biotechnology and engineering biology. *Engineering Biology*, *3*(1), 6–11. DOI: 10.1049/enb.2018.0001

Elmadhoun, B., Alsaidalani, R., & Burczynski, F. (2025). Quality Risk Management in the Final Operational Stage of Sterile Pharmaceutical Manufacturing: A Case Study Highlighting the Management of Sustainable Related Risks in Product Sterilization, Inspection, Labeling, Packaging, and Storage Processes. *Sustainability*, *17*(4), 1670. DOI: 10.3390/su17041670

Evans, J., & Silbey, S. S. (2022). Co-opting regulation: Professional control through discretionary mobilization of legal prescriptions and expert knowledge. *Organization Science*, *33*(5), 2041–2064. DOI: 10.1287/orsc.2021.1525

Fajardo, O., Dorado, F., & Lora, A. (2025). The Potential for Bioeconomy and Biotechnology Transfer and Collaboration Between Colombia and China. *Sustainability*, *17*(11), 5083. DOI: 10.3390/su17115083

Falcone, P. M. (2023). Sustainable energy policies in developing countries: A review of challenges and opportunities. *Energies*, *16*(18), 6682. DOI: 10.3390/en16186682

Feng, K., Miranda, A. V., Obnial, J. C., Ebhodaghe, I. D., & Lucero-Prisno, D. E.III. (2024). Drug regulatory harmonization in the Association of Southeast Asian Nations: Is it time for an ASEAN medicines agency? A policy review. *Clinical Epidemiology and Global Health*, *28*, 101649. DOI: 10.1016/j.cegh.2024.101649

Ferasso, M., & Grenier, C. (2021). Fostering SME's co-development of innovative projects in biotech clusters: Extending the sets of enablers for the knowledge creation process. *Technology in Society*, *67*, 101729. DOI: 10.1016/j.techsoc.2021.101729

Gaitán, M. G. (2021). Licensing as a Central Structure of Technology Transfer Agreements–Joint Venture and Franchising Agreements. *GRUR International*, *70*(5), 427–439. DOI: 10.1093/grurint/ikab032

George, A. S., & George, A. H. (2024). Riding the wave: An exploration of emerging technologies reshaping modern industry. *Partners Universal International Innovation Journal*, *2*(1), 15–38. DOI: 10.5281/zenodo.10613734

Gillum, D. R., Moritz, R., & Koblentz, G. D. (2024). Establishing a national biosafety and biosecurity agency for the United States. *Frontiers in Bioengineering and Biotechnology*, *12*, 1474120. DOI: 10.3389/fbioe.2024.1474120 PMID: 39483610

Gregory, F. D., & Trump, B. D. (2023). The Evolving Landscape of Biotechnology Research: Challenges and Opportunities in Acquisitions, Funding, Education, and Workforce Development for a Productive Bioeconomy. *Advanced Study Institute on NATO ASI on Quantum Nano-Photonics*, 25-50. https://doi.org/DOI: 10.1007/978-94-024-2296-2_2

Gregory, F. D., & Trump, B. D. (2023). The Evolving Landscape of Biotechnology Research: Challenges and Opportunities in Acquisitions, Funding, Education, and Workforce Development for a Productive Bioeconomy. *Advanced Study Institute on NATO ASI on Quantum Nano-Photonics*, 25-50. https://doi.org/DOI: 10.1007/978-94-024-2296-2_2

Halstead, D. C., & Sautter, R. L. (2023). A literature review on how we can address medical laboratory scientist staffing shortages. *Laboratory Medicine*, *54*(1), e31–e36. DOI: 10.1093/labmed/lmac090 PMID: 36149058

Harrer, S. (2023). Attention is not all you need: The complicated case of ethically using large language models in healthcare and medicine. *EBioMedicine*, *90*. Advance online publication. DOI: 10.1016/j.ebiom.2023.104512 PMID: 36924620

Hassan, Y. M., Mohamed, A. S., Hassan, Y. M., & El-Sayed, W. M. (2025). Recent developments and future directions in point-of-care next-generation CRISPR-based rapid diagnosis. *Clinical and Experimental Medicine*, *25*(1), 1–15. DOI: 10.1007/s10238-024-01540-8 PMID: 39789283

Hock, S. C., Kian, S. M., & Wah, C. L. (2020). Global challenges in the manufacture, regulation and international harmonization of GMP and quality standards for biopharmaceuticals. *Generics and Biosimilars Initiative Journal*, *9*(2), 52+. https://link.gale.com/apps/doc/A677574365/AONE?u=anon~82686abc&sid=googleScholar&xid=8b9cb9ef

Huang, X., Ma, L., Li, R., & Liu, Z. (2020). Determinants of innovation ecosystem in underdeveloped areas—Take nanning high-tech zone in western china as an example. *Journal of Open Innovation*, *6*(4), 135. DOI: 10.3390/joitmc6040135

Isoko, K., Cordiner, J. L., Kis, Z., & Moghadam, P. Z. (2024). Bioprocessing 4.0: A pragmatic review and future perspectives. *Digital Discovery*, *3*(9), 1662–1681. DOI: 10.1039/D4DD00127C

Katsieris, D. (2024). Accreditation, Certification, and Inspection: Impact on Global Trade. In *Handbook of Quality System, Accreditation and Conformity Assessment* (pp. 421-437). Singapore: Springer Nature Singapore. https://doi.org/DOI: 10.1007/978-981-97-5750-3_25

Khandekar, P., & Ghosh, P. K. (2023). Bioeconomy: Different Countries, Different Strategies, Multiple Benefits. *Asian Biotechnology and Development Review*, *25*(3).

Khopade, A. J., & Shah, M. (2026). Challenges for Commercial Translation of Nanomedicines: From Lab Scale to Production Scale. In *Commercial Scale Production of Nanomedicines* (pp. 1-40). CRC Press.

Kim, K. J., Lee, S. J., & Kim, D. M. (2024). Cell-free systems for a multi-pronged approach to next-generation therapeutics and diagnostics. *Biotechnology and Bioprocess Engineering; BBE*, *29*(2), 233–239. DOI: 10.1007/s12257-024-00058-w

Kiran, B. R., Prasad, M. N. V., & Mohan, S. V. (2024). Synthetic biology: an emerging field for developing economies. In *Bioremediation and Bioeconomy* (pp. 767–787). Elsevier., DOI: 10.1016/B978-0-443-16120-9.00013-3

Kuchenmüller, T., Chapman, E., Takahashi, R., Lester, L., Reinap, M., Ellen, M., & Haby, M. M. (2022). A comprehensive monitoring and evaluation framework for evidence to policy networks. *Evaluation and Program Planning*, *91*, 102053. DOI: 10.1016/j.evalprogplan.2022.102053 PMID: 35217289

Kumar, S., Tarei, P. K., & Swarnakar, V. (2024). Analyzing barriers to sustainable healthcare waste disposal: A hybrid decision-making framework. *Benchmarking*. Advance online publication. DOI: 10.1108/BIJ-10-2023-0744

Latukha, M., Shagalkina, M., Mitskevich, E., & Strogetskaya, E. (2022). From brain drain to brain gain: The agenda for talent management in overcoming talent migration from emerging markets. *International Journal of Human Resource Management*, *33*(11), 2226–2255. DOI: 10.1080/09585192.2021.1949374

Liu, A. (2025). Toward the effective implementation of the Biosafety Protocol: A Chinese regulatory capacity-building perspective. *Journal of Law and the Biosciences*, *12*(1), lsaf011. Advance online publication. DOI: 10.1093/jlb/lsaf011 PMID: 40463477

Lynch, C., Jordan, L., & O'Connell, J. D. (2022). Redesigning Spent Media from Cell Culture Bioprocess to Feed New Bacterial Fermentations. In *Cell Culture Engineering and Technology: In appreciation to Professor Mohamed Al-Rubeai* (pp. 129-146). Cham: Springer International Publishing. https://doi.org/DOI: 10.1007/978-3-030-79871-0_5

Malik, S. (2024). Emerging Trends in Agricultural Biotechnology: Opportunities and Challenges. *Frontiers in Agriculture*, *1*(2), 356–389.

Mandato, K., & Kulhanek, B. (2022). The impact of inadequate training. In *Healthcare Technology Training: An Evidence-based Guide for Improved Quality* (pp. 11–17). Springer International Publishing., DOI: 10.1007/978-3-031-10322-3_2

Marqusee, J., & Don, D. J.II. (2020). Reliability of emergency and standby diesel generators: Impact on energy resiliency solutions. *Applied Energy*, *268*, 114918. DOI: 10.1016/j.apenergy.2020.114918

Mary, T., & Enoch, O. (2024). Legal Considerations in the Development and Commercialization of Corporate Intellectual Property. *International Journal of Rural Development. Environmental Health Report*, *8*(3), 593109. DOI: 10.22161/ijreh.8.3.1

Matanguihan, C., & Wu, P. (2022). Upstream continuous processing: Recent advances in production of biopharmaceuticals and challenges in manufacturing. *Current Opinion in Biotechnology*, *78*, 102828. DOI: 10.1016/j.copbio.2022.102828 PMID: 36332340

Mehta, A., Niaz, M., Adetoro, A., & Nwagwu, U. (2024). Advancements in manufacturing technology for the biotechnology industry: The role of artificial intelligence and emerging trends. *International Journal of Chemistry. Mathematics and Physics*, *8*(2), 12–18. DOI: 10.22161/ijcmp.8.2.3

Najib, M., Abdullah, S., Narresh, S., & Juni, M. H. (2019). Brain-drain phenomenon among healthcare workers. *International Journal of Public Health and Clinical Sciences*, *6*(3), 90–103.

Ogwu, M. C., Kosoe, E. A., & Osawaru, M. E. (2025). Raw Materials for Sustainable Bioeconomy Development in the Global South. In *Sustainable Bioeconomy Development in the Global South: Volume I Status and Perspectives* (pp. 37-63). Singapore: Springer Nature Singapore. https://doi.org/DOI: 10.1007/978-981-96-0640-5_2

Ogwu, M. C., Kosoe, E. A., & Osawaru, M. E. (2025). Raw Materials for Sustainable Bioeconomy Development in the Global South. In *Sustainable Bioeconomy Development in the Global South: Volume I Status and Perspectives* (pp. 37-63). Singapore: Springer Nature Singapore. https://doi.org/DOI: 10.1007/978-981-96-0640-5_2

Ojadi, F. I., & Maiyaki, S. F. (2025). Logistics Bottlenecks: Port congestion, Shipping Delays, and the Inflationary Effects of Transportation Challenges. In *Supply Chain Disruptions and Impact on Global Inflation* (pp. 115-136). IGI Global Scientific Publishing. https://doi.org/DOI: 10.4018/979-8-3373-1982-7.ch005

Oke, G. (2025). Interdisciplinary cross-sectoral strategies to mitigate health workforce migration in Africa. *Journal of Medicine, Surgery, and Public Health, 100179.* Advance online publication. DOI: 10.1016/j.glmedi.2025.100179

Olaisen, J., & Revang, O. (2017). The dynamics of intellectual property rights for trust, knowledge sharing and innovation in project teams. *International Journal of Information Management*, *37*(6), 583–589. DOI: 10.1016/j.ijinfomgt.2017.05.012

Oppedisano, R. (2024). Innovative FabLabs. In *Collaborative Spaces and FabLabs: A Global Organisational and Collaborative Network* (pp. 31–40). Springer Nature Switzerland., DOI: 10.1007/978-3-031-62829-0_4

Preetha, N., Balakrishnan, V., & Thomas, G. (2024). Bioprospecting from Medicinal Plants and Benefit Sharing. In *Biodiversity and Business: Bio Prospecting and Benefit Sharing* (pp. 247-267). Cham: Springer Nature Switzerland. https://doi.org/DOI: 10.1007/978-3-031-71674-4_15

Prestigiacomo, R., Chan, C. C., & Kark, L. (2024). A biomedical engineering curriculum development: A qualitative study engaging four stakeholders. *European Journal of Education*, *59*(2), e12632. DOI: 10.1111/ejed.12632

Pustovrh, A., Rangus, K., & Drnovšek, M. (2020). The role of open innovation in developing an entrepreneurial support ecosystem. *Technological Forecasting and Social Change*, *152*, 119892. DOI: 10.1016/j.techfore.2019.119892

Rajaeifar, M. A., Ghadimi, P., Raugei, M., Wu, Y., & Heidrich, O. (2022). Challenges and recent developments in supply and value chains of electric vehicle batteries: A sustainability perspective. *Resources, Conservation and Recycling*, *180*, 106144. DOI: 10.1016/j.resconrec.2021.106144

Rathore, A., & Shereef, F. (2022). Innovating manufacturing technology in emerging economies. *Nature Biotechnology*, *40*(12), 1714–1716. DOI: 10.1038/s41587-022-01499-5 PMID: 36171278

Raza, A. (2024). Advances in Biotechnological Innovations: Bridging the Gap Between Laboratory Discoveries and Industrial Applications. *Agricultural and Biotechnological Reflections*, *1*(02), 84–97.

Rossi, M., Martini, E., & Kolte, A. (2021). The role of venture capitalists in an organised innovation ecosystem: Evidence from the USA. *International Journal of Business Environment*, *12*(3), 265–286.

Sammut, S. M. (2021). The role of the biotechnology industry in addressing health inequities in Africa: Strengthening the entire health care value chain. *Journal of Commercial Biotechnology*, *26*(4).

Shokoohi, M., & Attar, T. (2024). Biomanufacturing for a sustainable future: Unleashing the potential of biotechnology in pharmaceutical raw material production. [IJHES]. *International Journal of New Findings in Health and Educational Sciences*, *2*(2), 142–153. DOI: 10.63053/ijhes.81

Shokoohi, M., & Attar, T. (2024). Biomanufacturing for a sustainable future: Unleashing the potential of biotechnology in pharmaceutical raw material production. [IJHES]. *International Journal of New Findings in Health and Educational Sciences*, *2*(2), 142–153. DOI: 10.63053/ijhes.81

Shokoohi, M., & Attar, T. (2024). Biomanufacturing for a sustainable future: Unleashing the potential of biotechnology in pharmaceutical raw material production. [IJHES]. *International Journal of New Findings in Health and Educational Sciences*, *2*(2), 142–153.

Sinhmar, D., & Purohit, R. (2025). Patenting Life: Global Perspectives on Intellectual Property in Genetic and Biotechnological Innovation Amidst Ethical and Legal Challenges. *Journal on Development of Intellectual Property and Research*, *1*(1), 29–40. https://journal.cdipr.ac.in/index.php/jdipr/article/view/5

Srivastav, A. K., & Das, P. (2025). Green Finance and Investment in IoT–Biotechnology Synergies. In *Biotechnology and IoT in Agriculture and Food Production: Green Innovation* (pp. 153-160). Berkeley, CA: Apress. https://doi.org/DOI: 10.1007/979-8-8688-1469-3_17

Stana, A., Rista, A., Mukli, L., & Xhaferra, E. (2024). The Role of the Academic Incubator as an Acceleration Tool to Foster Entrepreneurship and Academic-Industry Connections. *Interdisciplinary Journal of Research and Development*, *11*(3), 104–104.

Stephen, M. D. (2021). China's new multilateral institutions: A framework and research agenda. *International Studies Review*, *23*(3), 807–834. DOI: 10.1093/isr/viaa076

Sundaram, J. (2025). Analysis of TRIPS Agreement and the justification of international IP rights protection in the WTO's multilateral trading system, with particular reference to pharmaceutical patents. *Information & Communications Technology Law*, *24*(2), 121–163. DOI: 10.1080/13600834.2015.1004244

Suzette, T., Gaylan, E. G., Taneo, J. K. B., Bercero, G. I. M. R., Piloton-Narca, M., & Marchee, T. (2024). Challenges in teaching biotechnology in the Philippine STE program. *International Journal of Learning. Teaching and Educational Research*, *23*(3), 367–389.

Swaminaathan, P., Saravanan, A., & Thamarai, P. (2024). Utilization of bioresources for high-value bioproducts production: Sustainability and perspectives in circular bioeconomy. *Sustainable Energy Technologies and Assessments*, *63*, 103672. DOI: 10.1016/j.seta.2024.103672

Tao, J., Aamir, M., Shoaib, M., Yasir, N., & Babar, M. (2025). Bridging the Gap Between Supply Chain Risk and Organizational Performance Conditioning to Demand Uncertainty. *Sustainability*, *17*(6), 2462. DOI: 10.3390/su17062462

Tsakalova, M., Onorato, C., Karathanasis, A. Z., & Deligkiozi, I. (2024). A circular economy framework for the assessment of bio-based value chains. *Sustainable Chemistry for the Environment, 6*, 100099. DOI: 10.1016/j.scenv.2024.100099

Tusé, D., Nandi, S., McDonald, K. A., & Buyel, J. F. (2020). The emergency response capacity of plant-based biopharmaceutical manufacturing-what it is and what it could be. *Frontiers in Plant Science, 11*, 594019. DOI: 10.3389/fpls.2020.594019 PMID: 33193552

Union, A. (2020). The digital transformation strategy for Africa (2020-30). http://www.au.int/

Whitford, B., Jones, D., & Kinnane, S. (2022). Biomanufacturing design: Reducing the environmental burden. *Current Opinion in Biotechnology, 76*, 102717. PMID: 35439701

Wilson, S., Steele, S., & Adeli, K. (2022). Innovative technological advancements in laboratory medicine: Predicting the lab of the future. *Biotechnology & Biotechnological Equipment, 36*(sup1), S9–S21. https://doi.org/DOI: 10.1080/13102818.2021.2011413

Winkler, T., Ulz, A., Knöbl, W., & Lercher, H. (2020). Frugal innovation in developed markets–Adaption of a criteria-based evaluation model. *Journal of Innovation & Knowledge, 5*(4), 251–259. DOI: 10.1016/j.jik.2019.11.004

Woteki, C. E., Buckley, G. J., & National Academies of Sciences, Engineering, and Medicine. (2020). Global Efforts to Strengthen Regulatory Systems. In *Stronger Food and Drug Regulatory Systems Abroad*. National Academies Press (US).

Zhang, X., Zhao, C., Shao, M. W., Chen, Y. L., Liu, P., & Chen, G. Q. (2022). The roadmap of bioeconomy in China. *Engineering Biology, 6*(4), 71–81. DOI: 10.1049/enb2.12026 PMID: 36968339

Chapter 15

Future Trends and Innovations in Bioprocessing and Biomanufacturing: Advancing Towards Sustainable and Smart Bioproduction

Nibedita Bardhan
https://orcid.org/0009-0001-6982-6519
Calcutta University, India

ABSTRACT

Sustainable processing is more important than ever, given the urgent need to meet net-zero objectives and reduce carbon emissions, thereby mitigating the effects of climate change. With the use of inexpensive, renewable materials, nature-inspired, highly selective biocatalysts that function optimally in mild conditions, and a lower energy and carbon footprint, bioprocessing offers all the necessary qualities to address the sustainable processing challenge. There has been a lot of interest lately in creating intensified bioprocesses because the productivity of bioprocessing is still far from ideal for meeting the massive demand for food, medications, biofuels, and bio-based chemicals. Considerable progress has been made in customising and utilising the technologies in the toolbox that are typically used in chemical process intensification. With an emphasis on upstream, bioreactor, and downstream separation phases, this chapter illustrates the diverse array of ongoing bioprocess intensification initiatives.

INTRODUCTION

The phrase "Bioprocessing 4.0," which is gaining popularity quickly, is frequently used to describe the biomanufacturing industry's adoption of Industry 4.0 (I4.0) technology (Pandey et al., 2024). The name is derived from Industrie 4.0, a project that started in Germany about 2010

DOI: 10.4018/979-8-3373-2873-7.ch015

and employed the Industrial Internet of Things (IIoT) to strategically connect business models, supply chains, and processes in order to advance production (Isoko et al., 2024). The initiative's ultimate goal was to create intelligent adaptive factories that could operate independently and provide a more customised and varied range of products (Shokoohi & Attar, 2024). At the time of writing, biomanufacturing is still going through its third industrial revolution, nevertheless, because this manufacturing endeavour did not incorporate bio-manufacturing (Oliver-Cuenca et al., 2024). In recent decades, technologies such as plug-and-play, single-use, and cell-line development breakthroughs have enabled revolutionary productivity increases. For instance, an expression level of 5 g L−1 may be attained using single-use bioreactors and contemporary cell lines, making a 2000 L bioreactor as productive as a (thin space (1/6-em)) 20000 L bioreactor from 20 years ago (Jain et al., 2025) (Patel & Singh, 2021). Modern single-use bioreactors are more appealing since downstream processing is made easier by the decreased working volumes upstream.

Figure 1. A systematic approach for identifying and evaluating key sustainable manufacturing techniques

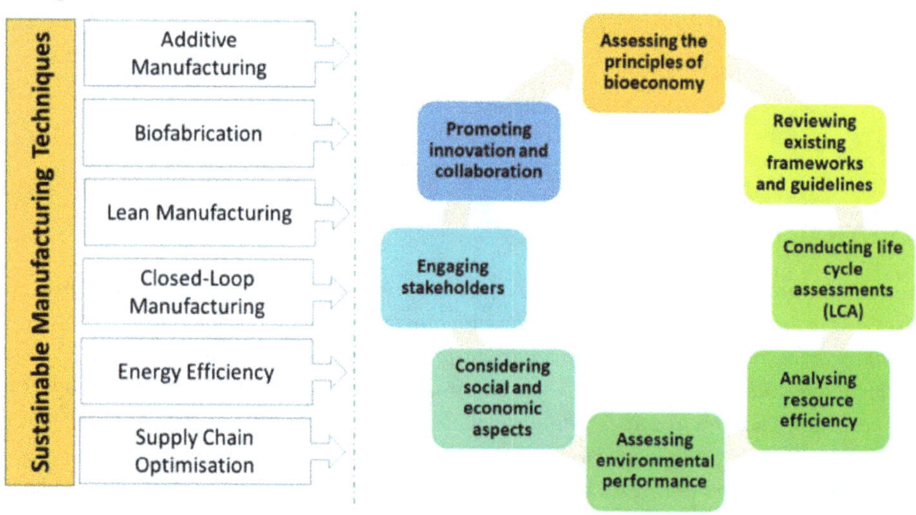

(Tišma et al., 2023)

Furthermore, this trend is being further advanced by the development of end-to-end integrated continuous biomanufacturing (ICB) platforms that include single pass tangential flow filtration, simulated moving beds, multicolumn chromatography, perfusion in production, N-1 bioreactors, and actual moving beds (Gargalo et al., 2020). In 2019, Biosana-Pharma used a fully integrated continuous biomanufacturing process to generate the first monoclonal antibody (mAb), marking the pinnacle of continuous bioprocessing innovation (Gargalo et al., 2020) (Barua, 2025). In comparison to conventional batch manufacturing, Biosana-Pharma asserted that this continuous approach greatly decreased production time, enhanced yield, and decreased costs (Banerjee et al., 2025) (Jain et al., 2024). Even with poor efficiency batch production, many high value-added products—like those in the pharmaceutical industry—made using industrial biotechnology procedures can continue to be lucrative (Rathore et al., 2021).

Table 1. Upcoming advances and trends in bioprocessing and biomanufacturing

Trend / Innovation	Description	Potential Impact	Example Applications
Continuous Bioprocessing	Shift from batch to continuous processes for upstream and downstream operations	Improved efficiency, product quality, and scalability	Monoclonal antibody production
Single-Use Technologies (SUTs)	Disposable bioreactors, mixers, and filters	Reduced contamination risk, lower capital costs	Vaccine and personalized medicine manufacturing
Automation & Process Analytical Technology (PAT)	Integration of sensors and control systems for real-time monitoring	Enhanced process control, reduced human error	Real-time quality assurance in cell culture
Digital Twins and AI in Biomanufacturing	Virtual modeling of bioprocesses using real-time data and machine learning	Predictive analytics, reduced downtime, process optimization	Bioreactor performance prediction
Synthetic Biology & CRISPR Technologies	Genetic modification for enhanced cell lines or new biological pathways	Customized product design, increased yield	Engineered probiotics, synthetic vaccines
Modular Biomanufacturing	Plug-and-play manufacturing units	Faster deployment, scalable production	Mobile vaccine units, disaster response biologics
Advanced Cell Line Engineering	Enhanced productivity and robustness of cell lines	Increased yield and tolerance to stress	High-expression CHO cell lines
3D Bioprinting & Tissue Engineering	Printing living cells and tissues layer by layer	Personalized implants, regenerative medicine	Organ-on-a-chip, printed skin grafts
Sustainable Bioprocessing	Use of green technologies, renewable feedstocks, and waste reduction strategies	Lower environmental impact, circular bioeconomy	Algae-based bioplastics, carbon capture via microbes
Integration with IoT & Cloud Platforms	Connectivity between equipment, cloud storage, and remote access	Data-driven manufacturing, remote process management	Cloud-controlled fermentation systems
Omics and Big Data in Process Optimization	Genomics, proteomics, metabolomics data integration for process understanding	Deep insights into cell behavior, tailored process development	Adaptive bioprocess development
Decentralized/On-Demand Manufacturing	Localized, small-footprint manufacturing units	Faster response to local healthcare needs, reduced logistics	Field hospitals, rural vaccine production

As some bioproducts gain market share, the potential for greater efficiency through truly continuous biomanufacturing is gradually becoming apparent (Palladino et al., 2024). However, this is frequently thwarted by the absence of continuous product recovery and purification processes, especially for complex labile molecules like glycoproteins (Ali et al., 2024) (Barua et al., 2024). An excellent example of BPI is the ongoing isolation of peptide-derived antibiotics, including beta lactams, utilising the Podbielniak centrifugal extractor, which has been in use since the 1940s, in contrast to high molecular weight glycoproteins (Wang et al., 2024). Thus, it is essential to develop a new, comprehensive method for teaching engineers how to design intensified bioprocesses (both upstream and downstream), new equipment for more effective bioprocessing of living cells, and ongoing procedures for isolating increasingly complex molecules like proteins, enzymes, vaccines, and peptides (Jain et al., 2024) (Ahmed & Gupta, 2023). Table 1 presents the upcoming developments and trends in bioprocessing and biomanufacturing.

Figure 2. An outline of CO2 conversion techniques and the use of C1/C2 compounds produced from CO2 for the biomanufacturing of common items. On the left is a summary of energy conversion and the sources that were used. Numerous useful compounds may be biomanufactured using both natural and artificial microbes once CO2 has been transformed from inorganic to organic carbon substrates

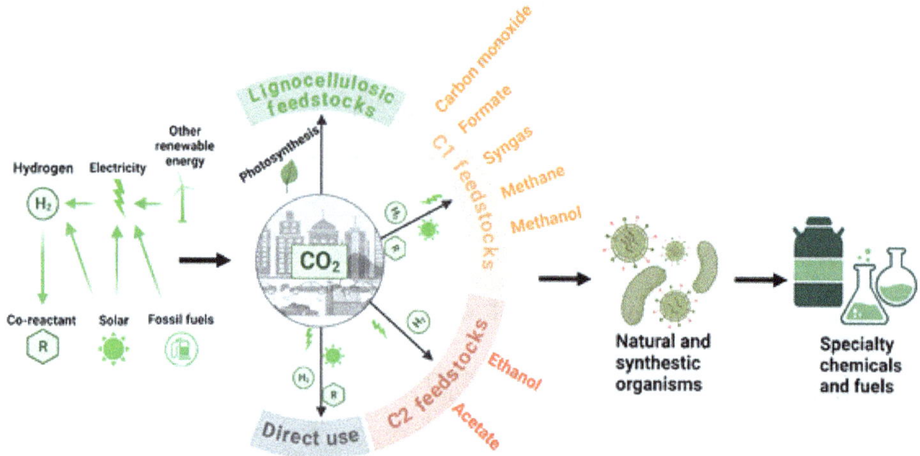

(Kurt et al., 2023)

Our planet, the environment, and our prospects for maintaining our standard of living have all changed in the past ten years. The demand for extremely stable biocatalysts has never been stronger because of factors including population increase, climate change, food supply issues, access to clean water, public health risks, poor sanitation, and declining air and water quality (Khoiruddin et al., 2025) (Jain et al., 2024). To process very large quantities of air, water, and contaminants, as well as to collect and recycle greenhouse gases, recycle resources, and capture solar energy with little energy and water consumption, future biocatalysts must be as stable and effective as chemical catalysts (Borgosz & Dikicioglu, 2024) (Barua., 2024) (Chowdhury et al.,2024). A new requirement emerged unexpectedly during the previous year: to quickly create, test in clinical trials, and scale up the production of hundreds of millions of doses of vaccines and distribute them for worldwide immunisation in order to prevent a novel coronavirus pandemic. Current market economics does not drive any of these global concerns. Using biological catalysts' selectivity to meet the aforementioned worldwide objectives will need a completely new engineering strategy. For usage in large-scale bioprocessing, new composite devices or sophisticated materials created for other sectors would need to be modified. Existing bioprocesses that produce food components (amino acids, organic acids, flavours, fragrances, and fine chemicals), alcohols, solvents, lipid modifications, new antibiotics, pharmaceutical or chemical intermediates, enzymes (food grade, industrial, or therapeutic), high-value human biological medicines (antibodies), or live cells for regenerative medicine will not be able to process the volume of material needed to meet future global challenges. These extremely important worldwide demands can only be met by expanding the use of highly stable biological catalysts and creating continuous bioprocesses using innovative techniques.

Figure 3. An overview of the one-step CO2 fixation and conversion process using microbial electro-synthesis

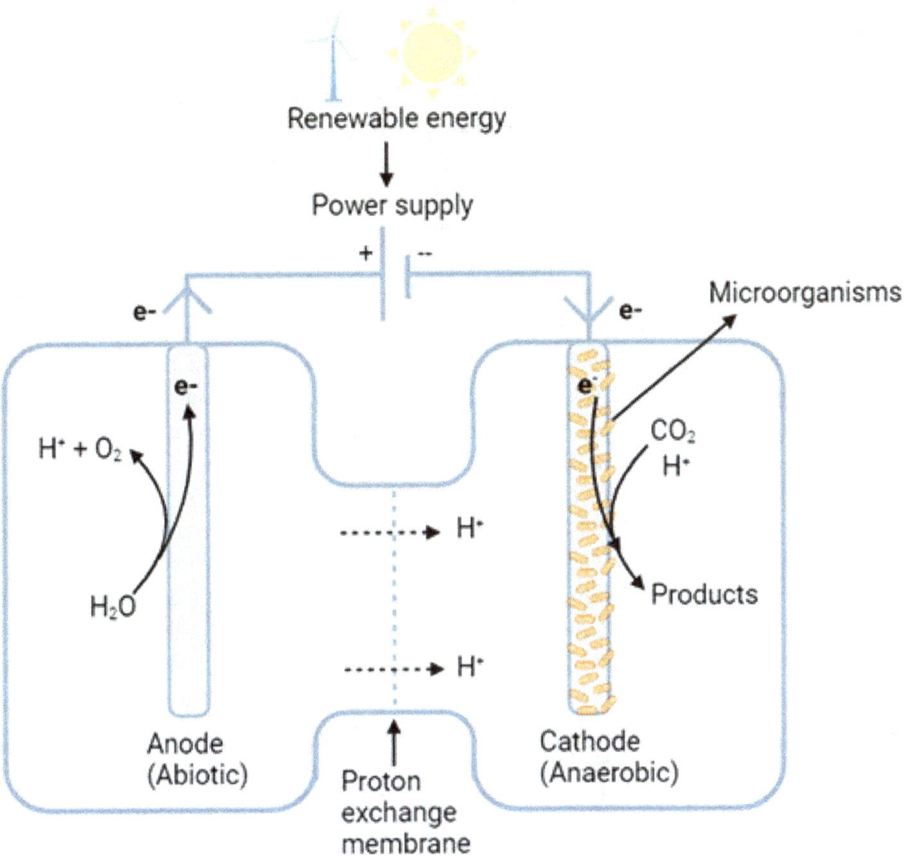

(Liu et al.,2023)

BIOPROCESSING 4.0 AND BIOMANUFACTURING

With the growing demand for bioproducts worldwide, the biomanufacturing sector is always changing (Pandey et al., 2024). Newer technologies must be adopted in order to produce bioproducts more efficiently and at a lower cost. The bioprocessing sector has been keenly aware of the growing trend of incorporating large-scale applications of big data, automation, and computational intelligence and analytics (Gonzalez & Martinez, 2023) (Banerjee & Barua, 2024). This tendency further conceptualises the new paradigm of Bio-processing 4.0. Connected end-to-end continuous bioprocessing is the result of revolutionary developments brought about by the tremendous strain of mass manufacturing of biobased goods, as well as their growing significance, timeliness, and achieving market competency for offering affordable sustainable solutions. There are significant obstacles to the feasibility, commercialisation, and acceptability of advanced biomanufacturing, despite the growing interest and investment in this field. The promise of many of these technologies in the context of industry is heavily hyped due to the rapid and abrupt development of engineering biology paradigms and the use of potentially deceptive parallels and simplifications when marketing the science. The need for new products (like artificial food, renewable energy, and regenerative medicines) and new research tools (like induced pluripotent stem cells (iPSC), metabolic engineering, synthetic biology, systems biology, cascade biocatalysis, etc.) at the start of this century will lead to a new biomanufacturing revolution. This revolution will either produce new products (like new functional tissues or drugs) or produce existing products in a far more efficient way than current platforms in terms of product yield, volumetric productivity, product titer, feasibility of scale-up, etc. In order to restore normal functioning, regenerative medicines replace, engineer, or create damaged human cells, tissues, or organs (35). In order to restore previously irreparable tissues or organisms, research first concentrated on engineering injured tissues and organisms by promoting the body's natural repair processes. The majority of subsequent research is on safely implanting cells, tissues, and organs in patients once they have been grown in vitro. Transplantation using regenerated cells, tissues, or organs from the patient themself may be able to address the concerns of transplant rejection and the scarcity of donor organisms.

When promoting the industrial sector's adoption of several biomanufacturing techniques, there is now a distinction between what is technically and financially realistic and what is theoretically possible. Bioproducts that need to be rigorously controlled are produced and purified through upstream and downstream processes (Kumar., 2023) (Barua., 2024). To design, optimise, and regulate, quality by design (QbD), process analytical technology (PAT), and continuous process verification (CPV) are used (Lee & Park, 2023). The enormous volume of data produced by these intricate processes need sophisticated technical and computational techniques for analysis and interpretation (Barua., 2024) (Patel & Kumar, 2023). The combination of the four "Cs"—control, connect, collaborate, and collect—allows for equipment interoperability, equipment interconnection, information transparency, technical support, and decentralised decision-making, all of which contribute to the notable increase in bioproduct productivity (Nikita et al., 2024) (Abdi et al., 2025). As a result, Bioprocessing 4.0 is a cutting-edge strategy that transforms biomanufacturing capabilities by creating a digital ecosystem.

The most obvious method to gauge the success of any fermentation is to measure the amount of biomass and measure the amount of microbial growth. The generating centre of every fermentation process is the microbial biomass, which is often the product itself. However, off-line analysis is largely the only method available for biomass measurement and quantification. The very early and late stages of fermentation, when extremely low and very high biomass concentrations are present, respectively, hinder the efficacy of online growth monitoring methods, even if they are used. Information on cell concentration and morphological dynamics, including cell size distribution and the distribution of single cells, budding cells, and cell clusters, may be obtained through recent technical advancements like the oCelloScope equipment. For instance, the latter could be associated with insulin synthesis, which is very important for yeast-based insulin manufacturing methods. Additionally, investigating how pertinent process events that commonly complicate process operation—like aeration or stirring failure—affect cell morphology may be very beneficial for integrated troubleshooting. These discoveries might result in new image-based production-scale monitoring techniques. Both business and academics are interested in developing smart technologies because of the potential for increased efficiency that smart biomanufacturing offers. However, considerable further work will be needed to really deploy these technologies in an industrial context. To guarantee that sufficiently big data sets can be obtained, significant technological obstacles still need to be addressed, as the first two case studies demonstrate. The variety and range of applications that may be created has expanded due to recent developments in energy regeneration processes and the manufacture of cell-free extract. As a result, the cell-free platform has developed from a simple exploratory research tool to a viable substitute for the live systems that are often employed in biological research and biomanufacturing. Together with the development of synthetic biology, cell-free systems have emerged as a promising technology for just-in-time production of high-value small molecules and therapeutically significant biologics. They have also been used for metabolic engineering, biosensing, and genetic part prototyping. A new method for research and point-of-care production of a variety of macromolecular and small molecule products is cell-free biology. The lack of cellular development and maintenance is a characteristic of cell-free systems that enables the direct allocation of energy and carbon resources towards a desired outcome. Furthermore, it is possible to quickly adjust the response conditions in cell-free systems since they are easier to observe and control than live systems. From their usage as an investigative tool in the early 1950s, cell-free systems have developed into a sophisticated platform that may be used to a wide range of synthetic biology, bioengineering, and biomanufacturing applications. Cell-free systems are becoming a competitive alternative to conventional live cells in a number of application fields due to recent developments in extract preparation, enhancements in energy regeneration processes, and the capacity to carry out high-throughput continuous reactions in microfluidic chips. For instance, because of their tunability and unrestricted access to metabolism without the cell wall's obstruction, they have emerged as useful investigative tools for metabolic engineering research. Cell-free application optimisation is still a significant hurdle, though. Computational and mathematical modelling is a vital tool that might advance the platform in the face of this difficulty. In addition to promoting the development of metabolic engineering strategies—such as helping to make the proper genetic alteration for a particular function, which is not always intuitive—models also make it easier to comprehend the significance of systems-level factors and interactions. Several experimental and computational options that may be explored in future study were brought to light by the extensive evaluation of the literature that was given here. Growing needs for biopharmaceuticals have fuelled the development of synthetic biology and metabolic engineering techniques for the biomanufacturing of bioactive natural materials. By building and expressing known and newly discovered biosynthetic genes, mostly from model and non-model plants, a range of natural products, such as terpenes, flavonoids, alkaloids, and cannabinoids, have been produced using metabolically modified microbes as the bioproduction hosts. A crucial debottlenecking strategy for enhancing and simplifying the biomanufacturing of natural products is the use of omics technology and machine learning (ML) platforms as high throughput analytical tools. These tools have been used more and more to support data-guided optimisation of specific biosynthetic pathways and the expansion of microbial production capacity. In general, biomanufacturing is the industrial manufacture of biomolecules and materials for use in treatments using scalable, proven procedures that incorporate microorganisms and biological systems such as animal, plant, or stem cells. Therefore, while the goal of biomanufacturing firms is to enhance human well-being by creating new goods based on organic germs, such as stem cell treatments, genome sequencing, and pharmaceuticals, artificial intelligence also plays a significant role. The use of single or multiple omics in natural product research has significantly increased the number of metabolites, biosynthetic genes, and regulatory elements from both model and non-model plants that have been discovered using omics. The production of several natural products from previously unfinished and gapped pathways, including the opiate alkaloid noscapine and cannabinoids, in microbial hosts through the use of transcriptome-guided gene mining and microbial engineering techniques has created new and exciting opportunities in the biomanufacturing of natural products using bioengineered microbes as the preferred biological manufacturing system.

Figure 4. Advantages of automation in the process of biomanufacturing

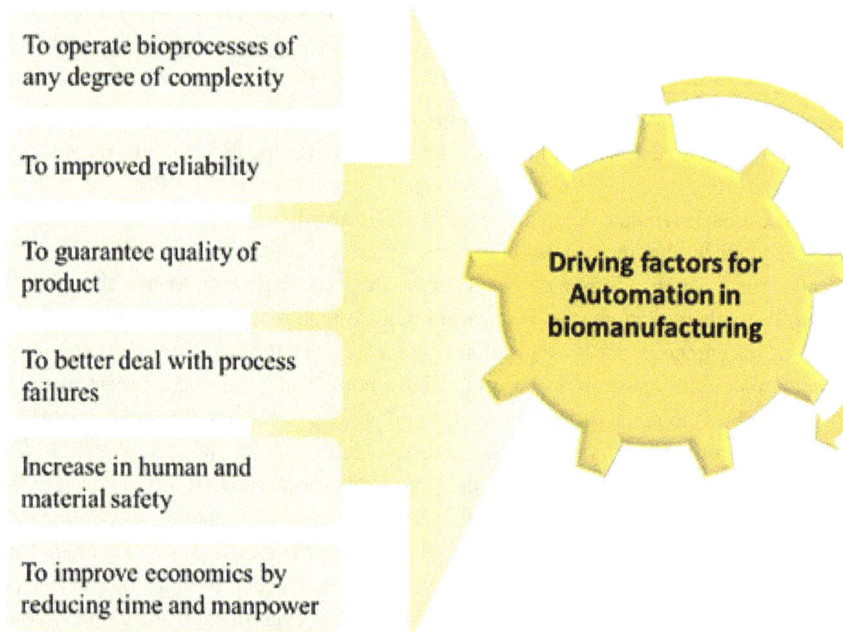

(Rathore et al., 2021)

Step change increases in the resultant process parameters and, hence, intensification may be achieved in bioprocesses by improving the biocatalyst. The unique and unique significance of biocatalyst modification using various recombinant approaches to improve bioprocesses has been highlighted in a number of reviews (Ali et al., 2024). These changes are especially effective and have the potential to lead to further process improvements. The abundance of tools available is aptly demonstrated by a recent overview of prospective microbial alteration strategies (Barua et al., 2025). Biocomposite materials (flexible or nonflexible) enable innovative bioreactor and photobioreactor designs that require less water and less electricity for mass transfer of O_2, CO_2, and nutrients, increased micro mixing. Coating architecture can promote consistent lighting of photosynthetic microorganisms, as well as increase product separation and purification. The conversion of suspended chemical catalytic unit operations to surface catalysis flow ways is comparable to this method of BPI. The use of thin biocoating immobilisation methods is restricted to bioprocesses that create secreted products, break down liquid wastes, or absorb or generate gases. Microalgae bioprocesses may benefit greatly from the usage of biocomposites (Berliner et al., 2022). Immobilised cell survival depends on the creation of a biocoating nanoporosity architecture and maintaining porosity and adhesion after rehydration. New coating microstructure techniques have recently improved light penetration and produced permanent coating nanoporosity (Ahmed & Gupta, 2023). It is also difficult to understand the biology of coating-entrapped cells that are restricted by nutrition, process conditions, or synthetic biology to not divide after immobilisation. The biology of non-growing nutrient-limited cells and how to maintain their activity and survival remain largely understood, despite the fact that "resting cells" have been used as suspended biocatalysts by the chemical and pharmaceutical intermediate industries for decades (Patel & Kumar, 2023).

Figure 5. Bioeconomy-integrated bionic production using an integrated approach to sustainable manufacturing

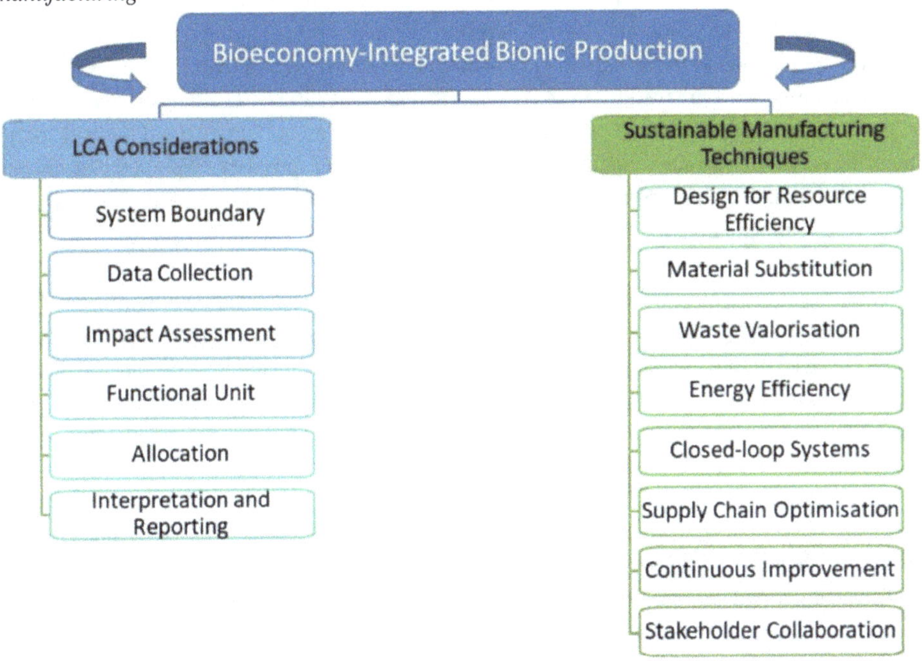

(Tišma et al., 2023)

THE DIGITAL REVOLUTION IN BIOPROCESSING 4.0

In biomanufacturing, digital transformation is the process of switching from paper-based or semi-automated manufacturing to digital, autonomous manufacturing (Pandey et al., 2024). This method centres on implementing an IIoT infrastructure that enables real-time access to all business events for the appropriate individuals. However, neither the engineering execution nor the business evaluation of digital transformation should be viewed as a project. Therefore, achieving technical breakthroughs with a short time to value is essential for a successful digital transformation strategy (Ahmed & Gupta, 2023). This ensures a quick return on investment (ROI) to demonstrate the initiative's commercial worth early on. Agile work practices and the use of early and regular stakeholder feedback to direct technology development can help achieve this (Patel & Kumar, 2023). When creating a centralised perspective for their clinical trials, Novartis, Nerve Live107, and Pfizer used this iterative and incremental strategy in an effort to increase manufacturing productivity while consuming less resources. This makes it possible for management to understand the importance of every stage of the digital transformation strategy since it shows measurable business outcomes as it develops (Pandey et al., 2024). With its emphasis on continuous improvement and brief, iterative innovation cycles, this methodology is in line with lean manufacturing and IT project management philosophies. This is a significant departure from the waterfall approach currently used in many engineering projects in biomanufacturing (Ahmed & Gupta, 2023). Businesses and systems integrators are working together more and more to create bespoke digital solutions. Tulip is a prime example of this strategy, having adopted the Industry 4.0 paradigm by emphasising operator-centric solutions and working with the ISPE to match their products with the Pharma 4.0 vision (Pandey et al., 2024). The Industry 4.0 paradigm states that a world that is vendor-centric and isolated is inefficient. Because end users of manufacturing software systems frequently have to create expensive, proprietary point solutions, this is accurate. This strategy restricts the capacity to take use of the greatest knowledge since it prevents communication, cooperation, and the transfer of previously produced solutions across various businesses. The integrator supplies the infrastructure required for this solution, enabling customised adaptation according to the particular requirements of managers and operators (Ahmed & Gupta, 2023). Digital Twin (DT) integration in bioprocessing has emerged as a key industrial priority. The bioprocessing industry is interested in using this technology despite the difficulties in putting it into practice. This is because it has the power to improve overall profitability and process efficiency. The potential for online monitoring, control, and optimisation, which would enable products with exact and desirable qualities, is what motivates the use of DTs. Researchers suggest a fresh approach to DT implementation in bioprocessing in order to achieve this goal. This entails creating a hybrid model that blends machine learning (ML) methods with first principal models. This strategy successfully overcomes the drawbacks of earlier techniques and creates a closed control loop system that continually monitors the system and modifies input variables to provide the best results. With the specific goal of boosting productivity and profitability across a range of sectors, traditional technologies have been converted into innovative digital technologies in Industry 4.0. Additionally, it offers industries a great chance to strengthen their competitive edge and adjust to the changing needs of the global economy. For example, sensors in biomanufacturing monitor the conditions of the bioreactor in real time and measure important process parameters like temperature, pH, and nutrient levels. The efficiency of DTs depends on the collection, transmission, and analysis of the data produced by these sensors. This is where the Internet of Things and advancements in data collecting systems come into play, allowing for the seamless integration of data from various sources to guarantee that DTs always have access to the most up-to-date and correct information. Furthermore, the application of ML algorithms and hybrid modelling approaches is improving DTs' capacity to more accurately mimic intricate processes and forecast results. A strong tool for tracking, managing, and improving bioprocesses is DT. It could serve as a link between the third and fourth industrial revolutions for bioprocesses. Industries are encouraged to create smart technologies because digital technology in bioprocessing processes carry the potential of greater productivity and efficiency. A DT enables improved decision-making and performance optimisation by simulating and monitoring the real-world equivalent in real-time. Fundamentally, DT depends on three elements: modelling, data collecting, and sensors. These elements form the foundation of the DT framework, promoting its efficacy and utility in a variety of fields. System integration problems may arise when DTs are implemented in the bioprocess sector. This speaks to the difficulty of switching from antiquated to contemporary technologies. It includes harmonising different parts of present systems and incorporating new systems into the ones that already exist. The integration issue increases with the age of these systems. Furthermore, security is another area of worry with regard to DT deployment, especially in light of recent high-profile data breaches. It is difficult to provide this real-time connection, particularly when handling large amounts of data in real-time. Additionally, internal decisions made by a corporation are crucial to the growth of DT. Data security, integration, and quality are all jeopardised by poor data management, which results in scattered, isolated, and infrequently updated data. Therefore, businesses need to set up a strong data management system for a successful digital transformation using DTs. Developments in simulation software have made it easier to create intricate models that faithfully replicate real-world items. Techniques like reduced-order models (ROMs) are used to improve simulation performance. These technical developments improve model accuracy while reducing the time and money required for DT creation. Additionally, difficulties with data quality are being addressed by advancements in communication and software technology. It is essential to guarantee the quality, availability, and correctness of the data for DTs. A thorough foundation must be established in order to facilitate effective data transmission between the physical entity and its DT and reduce any possible effects on DT performance brought on by these difficulties. Data validity and quality are guaranteed when dependable communication protocols are used in conjunction with cloud and edge computing. Data quality is further improved by centralised databases, particularly when obtaining from many sources. Adopting Industry 4.0 standards gives businesses a strong foundation for developing DT. Additionally, by encouraging the development of new DT techniques, tools, and standards, workforce training improves the environment. Technologies that facilitate knowledge and sophisticated design methodologies are used to address organisational difficulties. Businesses may keep up to speed with the latest technological developments by retraining employees and implementing Industry 4.0 standards. This guarantees a sufficient flow of DT knowledge, enabling well-informed choices. Making educated judgements on data management and relevant technologies before DT development begins is also facilitated by clearly outlining DT needs. Performance-wise, detailed digital representations of physical assets employing advanced simulation and machine learning models are made possible by the increasing availability of reliable hardware, falling prices, and increasing processing power. This ensures seamless real-time communication between digital and physical twins. Tools called digital twins (DTs) are used to forecast how a system would behave based on past data. The mathematical models that the DT use must accurately represent the system in order for these predictions to be correct. The difficulty is in developing models for certain uses and situations. For bioprocess operations, a number of mathematical models have been developed; these models might be data-centric, knowledge-centric, or grounded on fundamental ideas. Körber Pharma are also delivering varied Industry 4.0 solutions to interface with current fragmented systems.

Some businesses decide to develop their digital solutions in-house. Notable examples are data42, a data lake program that uses clinical trial data to improve knowledge of illnesses and patient insights, and Novartis, as previously discussed with Nerve Live. In a similar vein, GSK's technology stack development shows a tendency towards internal development for more customised and business-specific digital solutions. However, most biomanufacturing enterprises cannot use these solutions since they frequently demand a profound grasp of digital technologies. Open systems that use interoperability and data sharing standards, including open platform communications (OPC) and other relevant standards that have not yet been created, will free data in the new industrial world. After then, data may be contextualised and linked for usage in a wide range of applications. Facilitating improved decision-making, spotting areas for improvement, and eventually optimising operations are the objectives. Connected data in bioprocessing may increase efficiency in the following areas. Numerous industrial revolutions have occurred since the beginning of manufacturing, all made possible by notable increases in productivity. Every revolution signalled a significant change in the economy and altered how businesses operate to satisfy consumer needs. The advent of computers on production lines was the final significant revolution. The emergence of automation, which boosts productivity and speed, replaced this. It also reduces human-induced process variability. The pharmaceutical business continues to research methods to employ automation to improve quality and speed to market, while adopting technology more slowly than other industries. The industry's approach to medication manufacture is currently undergoing another revolution that will open the door for even more adjustments.

Figure 6. A blueprint for producing bionics with the bioeconomy integrated

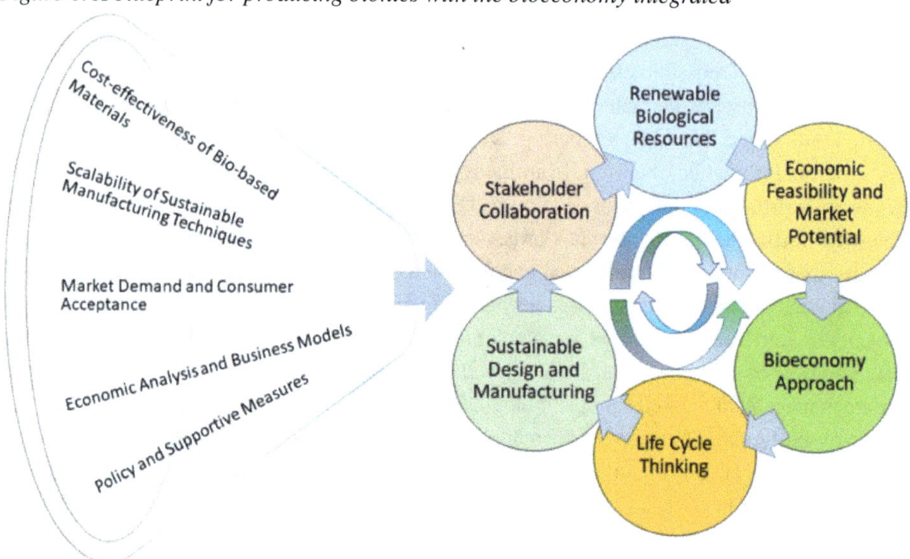

(Tišma et al., 2023)

FUTURE PERSPECTIVES

A big but doable change is the move from an Integrated Continuous Biomanufacturing (ICB) platform to a smart factory. Although switching from batch to continuous processes presented many difficulties, other sectors have already overcome the main technological obstacles to integrating smart factories (Pandey et al., 2024). A solid basis has been formed by solutions like OPC UA for connection and interoperability, cloud computing for data storage in data lakes offered by cloud service providers, and well-known AI algorithms for big data analysis. Numerous frameworks and roadmaps as well as a broad spectrum of commercial relationships also assist its progress (Gonzalez & Martinez, 2023). It is difficult to defend an expectation of the orders of magnitude in productivity improvements promised by any industrial revolution, though, as Industry 4.0 has become somewhat of a catchphrase since its beginnings. This could be explained by the strategies' inadequate implementation (Ahmed & Gupta, 2023). Despite the interdependence of industrial processes, the absence of a single hub and enterprise-wide FAIR data standards may hinder businesses from realising efficiency advantages. It's possible that strategy and technology are not aligned (Gonzalez & Martinez, 2023). Instead of concentrating just on large production quantities, the future factory seeks to increase efficiency in sectors like biomanufacturing where flexibility, product personalisation, and variety are the desired business goals (Patel & Kumar, 2023). This may also be explained by the fact that a smart factory makes operations considerably more nimble over time. Additionally, even if medication approval rates are currently slowing down, the impacts of increased access to high-quality historical data are still being seen (Pandey et al., 2024). Ultimately, since Industry 4.0 was introduced less than 15 years ago, it is still too early to draw any firm conclusions regarding its effects. In an effort to make sustainable processing a reality, business and academic researchers are interested in bioprocess intensification, a technique that is founded on the tried-and-true ideas of chemical process intensification. Up until now, a lot of focus has been on applications pertaining to the pharmaceutical processing of medications, vaccines, etc., as well as the large-scale production of biofuels, biobased chemicals, biopolymers, food components, etc., all of which produce a product that is valuable to society and driven by the market. Significant and as-yet-unrealized potential exists in bioprocessing to address contemporary environmental issues like CO_2 collection, but this depends on large-scale bioprocesses being significantly more efficient. It can be difficult to navigate the intricacies of bioprocesses while simulating their general features and unpredictability, especially given the scarcity of trustworthy online sensors. The majority of process variables are evaluated either online or offline, which raises expenses and results in ineffective information delivery. Data collection is further complicated by the human operations of online sensors and the robustness of online sensors under challenging conditions. To save experimental effort, modelling tools should be used to evaluate new technologies based on the bioprocess intensification philosophy. When assessing the realistic results of simulated commercial-scale processes that are based on laboratory-scale testing, this is particularly crucial (Pandey et al., 2024). In addition to the intricate biological processes, this will necessitate sophisticated models for every stage of the whole process chain. Frameworks that facilitate the deployment of trustworthy predictive models are desperately needed, particularly for emerging technologies. The productivity and yield model results will allow the BPI technologies to be compared to the costs and performance of traditional methods. The digital manufacturing tools of Bioprocessing 4.0 will become indispensable as continuous processing becomes more widely used in today's and tomorrow's bioprocessing industries (Gonzalez & Martinez, 2023). This will necessitate further development and integration of automated hardware as well as innovative, online and in-line process analytics technologies (PAT) (Ahmed & Gupta, 2023). Effective cooperation between several disciplines, including synthetic biology, biotechnology, material science, chemical and process engineering, process systems engineering, and control engineering, is necessary to further develop the subject of bioprocess intensification. In biomanufacturing, digital transformation is the process of switching from paper-based or semi-automated manufacturing to digital, autonomous manufacturing. This method centres on implementing an IIoT infrastructure that enables real-time access to all business events for the appropriate individuals. However, neither the engineering execution nor the business evaluation of digital transformation should be viewed as a project. The creation of new technologies should, above all, be the responsibility of university research as well as industrial collaboration to facilitate the testing of novel theories and concepts. In this case, it is critical that academics have a thorough understanding of the technical requirements and constraints of the industry and that additional measures be taken to facilitate long-term, sustainable partnerships in order to create promising solutions for implementation at higher TRL levels. Digital tools for process development optimisation have been addressed thus far. But in the upcoming years, the growing tendency of employing these tools to enhance bioprocesses in operation may cause a disruption in the biomanufacturing sector. This is due to the fact that digital technologies can provide autonomous UPS operation, which may result in more lucrative, environmentally friendly, and effective services.

CONCLUSION

Sustainable processing is more important than ever in light of the urgent need to meet net zero objectives in order to reduce carbon emissions and the effects of climate change. With the use of inexpensive, renewable materials, nature-inspired, highly selective biocatalysts that function best in mild settings, and a lower energy and carbon footprint, bioprocessing offers all the necessary qualities to meet the sustainable processing problem. It is difficult to defend an expectation of the orders of magnitude in productivity improvements promised by any industrial revolution, though, as Industry 4.0 has become somewhat of a catchphrase since its beginnings. This could be explained by the strategies' inadequate implementation. Despite the interdependence of industrial processes, the absence of a single hub and enterprise-wide FAIR data standards may hinder businesses from realising efficiency advantages. It's possible that strategy and technology are not aligned. There has been a lot of interest lately in creating intensified bioprocesses because the productivity of bioprocessing is still far from ideal for meeting the massive demand for food, medications, biofuels, and bio-based chemicals. Considerable progress has been made in customising and utilising the technologies in the toolbox that are typically used in chemical process intensification. Instead of concentrating just on large production quantities, the future factory seeks to increase efficiency in sectors like biomanufacturing where flexibility, product personalisation, and variety are the desired business goals. This may also be explained by the fact that a smart factory makes operations considerably more nimble over time. Additionally, even if medication approval rates are currently slowing down, the impacts of increased access to high-quality historical data are still being seen. Industrial biotechnology has a bright future if it prioritises sustainability, fosters multidisciplinary cooperation, and makes use of developing technologies. The next generation of bioseparation technologies will be greatly influenced by the combination of biotechnology, sophisticated materials science, bioinformatics, and process engineering. We anticipate that the articles in this Special Issue will stimulate greater bioseparation and bioprocessing research and development, opening the door to a biotechnological environment that is more effective, sustainable, and profitable. Businesses will create distinctive digital twins that contain all process knowledge and are updated when new information becomes available. Only information-rich tests recommended by the model will be carried out by experimental teams, and the digital twin will be employed for autonomous operation within verified ranges. With the aid of AR and VR technologies combined with data from MES and centralised data hubs, engineers will concentrate on troubleshooting and advanced analysis.

REFERENCES

Abdi, H., Jahanian, A., & Nozari, H. (2025). Digital Twin-Enabled Bioreactors: Transforming Industrial Biotechnology in Smart Economies. In *Dynamic and Safe Economy in the Age of Smart Technologies* (pp. 105-120). IGI Global Scientific Publishing.

Ahmed, T., & Gupta, R. (2023). Challenges in scaling biobased nanocomposite production for medical applications. *Journal of Advanced Materials*, *10*(2), 112–120.

. Ali, A., Usman, M., Jayamani, E., Soon, K., & bin Ab Wahab, M. K. (2024). Sustainable Biomanufacturing. In *Biomedical Implants* (pp. 195-217). CRC Press.

Ali, M., Shabbir, K., Ali, S., Mohsin, M., Kumar, A., Aziz, M., & Sultan, H. M. (2024). A New Era of Discovery: How Artificial Intelligence has Revolutionized the Biotechnology. *Nepal Journal of Biotechnology*, *12*(1), 1–11.

. Banerjee, A., & Barua, R. (2024). A Comprehensive Overview of Carbon-Based Nanofluids and Related Progress for Heat Transfer Uses. *Environmental Applications of Carbon-Based Materials*, 196-217.

Banerjee, D., Barua, R., Datta, S., & Pathote, D. (2025). The Use of Artificial Neural Networks in Biomedical Engineering. In *Expert Artificial Neural Network Applications for Science and Engineering* (pp. 33–50). IGI Global Scientific Publishing.

Barua, R. (2024). Advanced Biomimetic Compound Continuum Robot for Minimally Invasive Surgical Applications. In *Modeling, Simulation, and Control of AI Robotics and Autonomous Systems* (pp. 213-231). IGI Global.

Barua, R. (2024). An Investigation of AI Techniques for Detecting Kidney Stones in CT Scan Images Through Advanced Image Processing. In *Enhancing Medical Imaging with Emerging Technologies* (pp. 133–150). IGI Global.

Barua, R. (2024). Exploring Artificial Intelligence in Evolving Healthcare Environments: A Comprehensive Analysis. In *Advances in Computational Intelligence for the Healthcare Industry 4.0* (pp. 123-138). IGI Global.

Barua, R. (2024). The Emerging Role of Artificial Intelligence in Organ-on-a-Chip (OOAC) Biomedical Devices. In *Reshaping Healthcare with Cutting-Edge Biomedical Advancements* (pp. 369-381). IGI Global.

Barua, R. (2025). Unleashing Human Potential: Exploring the Advantage of Biomechanics in Sport Performance. In *Global Innovations in Physical Education and Health* (pp. 409-436). IGI Global.

Barua, R., & Datta, S. (2025). Revolutionizing Nerve Repair: The Transformative Role of Nanoparticles in Peripheral Nerve Regeneration. In *Nanomaterials and the Nervous System* (pp. 275-300). IGI Global.

Barua, R., Datta, S., & Jain, N. (2024). Novel Power Generation Technology Based on Renewable Energy. In *Optimization Techniques for Hybrid Power Systems: Renewable Energy, Electric Vehicles, and Smart Grid* (pp. 407-425). IGI Global.

Berliner, A. J., Lipsky, I., Vengerova, G., & Arkin, A. P. (2022). Towards the Future of Space Bioprocess Engineering.

Borgosz, L., & Dikicioglu, D. (2024). Industrial internet of things: What does it mean for the bioprocess industries? *Biochemical Engineering Journal*, *201*, 109122.

Chowdhury, S., Jain, N., Waidi, Y. O., Barua, R., Das, S., Prasad, A., & Datta, S. (2024). Biological Smart Biomaterials: Materials for Biomedical Applications. In *Applications of Biotribology in Biomedical Systems* (pp. 313–325). Springer Nature Switzerland.

Garcia, L., & Martinez, R. (2023). Enhancing mechanical properties of biobased polymers through nanocomposite formation. *Journal of Sustainable Materials*, *15*(3), 245–260.

Gargalo, C. L., Udugama, I., Pontius, K., Lopez, P. C., Nielsen, R. F., Hasanzadeh, A., & Gernaey, K. V. (2020). Towards smart biomanufacturing: A perspective on recent developments in industrial measurement and monitoring technologies for bio-based production processes. *Journal of Industrial Microbiology & Biotechnology: Official Journal of the Society for Industrial Microbiology and Biotechnology*, *47*(11), 947–964. PMID: 32895764

Gonzalez, R., & Martinez, H. (2023). The role of biobased polymers in achieving sustainable development goals. *Journal of Green Chemistry*, *12*(5), 345–362.

Isoko, K., Cordiner, J. L., Kis, Z., & Moghadam, P. Z. (2024). Bioprocessing 4.0: A pragmatic review and future perspectives. *Digital Discovery*, *3*(9), 1662–1681.

Jain, N., Barua, R., & Datta, S. (2025). Functional Nanomaterials and their Applications in Biomedicine. In *Bioabsorbable Polymers for Drug Carriers and Fixation Devices* (pp. 61–79). Apple Academic Press.

Jain, N., Waidi, Y. O., Barua, R., Das, S., Vannaladsaysy, V., Prasad, A., & Datta, S. (2024). Bioinspired Nanocomposites: Multifunctional Materials towards Sustainable Alternatives. In *Nanomanufacturing Techniques in Sustainable Healthcare Applications* (pp. 78-93). CRC Press.

Jain, N., Waidi, Y. O., Barua, R., Vannaladsaysy, V., Prasad, A., & Datta, S. (2024). Plastic recycling for energy production. *Biodegradable Waste Processing for Sustainable Developments*, 113.

Jain, N., Waidi, Y. O., Chowdhury, S., Barua, R., Das, S., Prasad, A., & Datta, S. (2024). Medical Devices Tribology. In *Applications of Biotribology in Biomedical Systems* (pp. 235–250). Springer Nature Switzerland.

Khoiruddin, K., Boopathy, R., Kawi, S., & Wenten, I. G. (2025). Towards next-generation membrane bioreactors: Innovations, challenges, and future directions. *Current Pollution Reports*, *11*(1), 15.

Kumar, P. (2023). Role of Industry 4.0 in Biotechnology to Produce Environmentally Sustainable Biotechnology Products. *Asian Biotechnology and Development Review*, *25*(3).

Kurt, E., Qin, J., Williams, A., Zhao, Y., & Xie, D. (2023). Perspectives for Using CO_2 as a Feedstock for Biomanufacturing of Fuels and Chemicals. *Bioengineering (Basel, Switzerland)*, *10*(12), 1357. PMID: 38135948

Lee, J., & Park, H. (2023). Advances in nanoclay-polymer drug delivery systems. *Journal of Nanomedicine*, *17*(3), 102–118.

Liu, Z., Xue, X., Cai, W., Cui, K., Patil, S. A., & Guo, K. (2023). Recent progress on microbial electrosynthesis reactor designs and strategies to enhance the reactor performance. *Biochemical Engineering Journal*, *190*, 108745.

Nikita, S., Banerjee, S., Jesubalan, N. G., Kulkarni, A., Gupta, K., & Rathore, A. S. (2024). Holistic process control framework for smart biomanufacturing: A deep learning driven approach. *Computers & Chemical Engineering*, *187*, 108742.

Oliver-Cuenca, V., Salaris, V., Muñoz-Gimena, P. F., Agüero, Á., Peltzer, M. A., Montero, V. A., Arrieta, M. P., Sempere-Torregrosa, J., Pavon, C., Samper, M. D., Crespo, G. R., Kenny, J. M., López, D., & Peponi, L. (2024). Bio-Based and Biodegradable Polymeric Materials for a Circular Economy. *Polymers*, *16*(21), 3015. PMID: 39518225

Palladino, F., Marcelino, P. R. F., Schlogl, A. E., José, Á. H. M., Rodrigues, R. D. C. L. B., Fabrino, D. L., & Rosa, C. A. (2024). Bioreactors: Applications and Innovations for a sustainable and healthy future—a critical review. *Applied Sciences (Basel, Switzerland)*, *14*(20), 9346.

Pandey, K., Pandey, M., Kumar, V., Aggarwal, U., & Singhal, B. (2024). Bioprocessing 4.0 in biomanufacturing: Paving the way for sustainable bioeconomy. *Systems Microbiology and Biomanufacturing*, *4*(2), 407–424.

Patel, M., & Singh, A. (2021). Reducing medical waste through biodegradable polymers: Current trends and future prospects. *Journal of Green Chemistry*, *27*(5), 403–420.

Patel, S., & Kumar, A. (2023). Biobased polymers: A review of sources, properties, and applications. *International Journal of Polymer Science*, *15*(6), 291–312.

Rathore, A. S., Mishra, S., Nikita, S., & Priyanka, P. (2021). Bioprocess control: Current progress and future perspectives. *Life (Chicago, Ill.)*, *11*(6), 557. PMID: 34199245

Shokoohi, M., & Attar, T. (2024). Biomanufacturing for a sustainable future: Unleashing the potential of biotechnology in pharmaceutical raw material production. (IJHES). *International Journal of New Findings in Health and Educational Sciences*, *2*(2), 142–153.

Tišma, S., & Škrtić, M. M. (2023). Integrating Bioeconomy Principles in Bionic Production: Enhancing Sustainability and Environmental Performance. *Journal of Risk and Financial Management*, *16*(10), 437.

Wang, G., Mohsin, A., Chu, J., Zhuang, Y., & Zhang, S. (2024). Advances and prospects for advanced biomanufacturing. *Scale-up and Chemical Process for Microbial Production of Plant-Derived Bioactive Compounds*, 1-16.

Compilation of References

Abbasi, B. A., Iqbal, J., Kiran, F., Ahmad, R., Kanwal, S., Munir, A., & Mahmood, T. (2020). Green formulation and chemical characterizations of Rhamnella gilgitica aqueous leaves extract conjugated NiONPs and their multiple therapeutic properties. *Journal of Molecular Structure*, *1218*, 128490.

Abbasi, B. A., Iqbal, J., Mahmood, T., Qyyum, A., & Kanwal, S. (2019). Biofabrication of iron oxide nanoparticles by leaf extract of Rhamnus virgata: Characterization and evaluation of cytotoxic, antimicrobial and antioxidant potentials. *Applied Organometallic Chemistry*, *33*(7), e4947.

Abbott, K. W., & Snidal, D. (2021). Strengthening international regulation through transnational new governance: Overcoming the orchestration deficit. In *The spectrum of international institutions* (pp. 95–139). Routledge.

Abdallah, Y. K., & Estévez, A. T. (2023). 3D-printed bioreceptive tiles of reaction–diffusion (Gierer–Meinhardt model) for multi-scale algal strains' passive immobilization. *Buildings (Basel, Switzerland)*, *13*(8), 1972. DOI: 10.3390/buildings13081972

Abdi, H., Jahanian, A., & Nozari, H. (2025). Digital Twin-Enabled Bioreactors: Transforming Industrial Biotechnology in Smart Economies. In *Dynamic and Safe Economy in the Age of Smart Technologies* (pp. 105-120). IGI Global Scientific Publishing.

Abdul Manan, M. (2025). Progress in Probiotic Science: Prospects of Functional Probiotic-Based Foods and Beverages. *International Journal of Food Sciences*, *2025*(1), 5567567.

Abdul-Fattah, A. M., & Truong, V. L. (2010). Drying process methods for biopharmaceutical products: an overview. *Formulation and process development strategies for manufacturing biopharmaceuticals*, 705-738.

Abdullah, B., Muhammad, S. A. F. A. S., Shokravi, Z., Ismail, S., Kassim, K. A., Mahmood, A. N., & Aziz, M. M. A. (2019). Fourth generation biofuel: A review on risks and mitigation strategies. *Renewable & Sustainable Energy Reviews*, *107*, 37–50. DOI: 10.1016/j.rser.2019.02.018

Abo-Zaid, G. A., Soliman, N. A., Abdullah, A. S., El-Sharouny, E. E., Matar, S. M., & Sabry, S. A. (2020). Maximization of siderophores production from biocontrol agents, *Pseudomonas aeruginosa* F2 and *Pseudomonas fluorescens* JY3 using batch and exponential fed-batch fermentation. *Processes (Basel, Switzerland)*, *8*(4), 455. Advance online publication. DOI: 10.3390/pr8040455

Abreu, T., Sousa, P., Gonçalves, J., Hontman, N., Teixeira, J., Câmara, J. S., & Perestrelo, R. (2024). Grape pomace as a renewable natural biosource of value-added compounds with potential food industrial applications. *Beverages, 10*(2), 45.

Abufalgha, A. A., Clarke, K. G., & Pott, R. W. (2020). Characterisation of bubble diameter and gas hold-up in simulated hydrocarbon-based bioprocesses in a bubble column reactor. *Biochemical Engineering Journal, 158*, 107577.

Abu, R., Gundersen, M. T., & Woodley, J. M. (2015). Thermodynamic calculations for systems biocatalysis. In *Computer aided chemical engineering* (Vol. 37, pp. 233–238). Elsevier., DOI: 10.1016/B978-0-444-63576-1.50037-6

Achar, S. S., Mohanty, S. K., Indu, B. K., Suhasa, G., & Shilpa, P. (2025). Bioreactors. In *In Vitro Production of Plant Secondary Metabolites: Theory and Practice* (pp. 205–226). Springer Nature Singapore.

Acharya, P., Fasim, A., More, V. S., Shivaram, A. K., & More, S. S. (2023). Enzyme technology in value addition of dairy and milk production. In *Value-addition in beverages through enzyme technology* (pp. 77–96). Elsevier.

Achmad, G. N., Yudaruddin, R., Nugroho, B. A., Fitrian, Z., Suharsono, S., Adi, A. S., Hafsari, P., & Fitriansyah, F. (2023). Government support, eco-regulation and eco-innovation adoption in SMEs: The mediating role of eco-environmental. *Journal of Open Innovation, 9*(4), 100158.

Adebami, G. E., Kuila, A., Ajunwa, O. M., Fasiku, S. A., & Asemoloye, M. D. (2022). Genetics and metabolic engineering of yeast strains for efficient ethanol production. *Journal of Food Process Engineering, 45*(7), e13798.

Adeniyi, A. G., Ighalo, J. O., & Onifade, D. V. (2018). Biofuels from microalgae biomass: A review of conversion processes and procedures. *Arabian Journal of Chemistry, 15*(6), 103791. DOI: 10.1016/j.arabjc.2022.103791

Adhikari, M. (2017). Recent advances in bacterial fermentation for the production of therapeutic proteins. *Biotechnology Advances, 35*(3), 391–403.

Afeyan, N. B., & Cooney, C. L. (2006). Professor Daniel I.C. Wang: A legacy of education, innovation, publication, and leadership. *Biotechnology and Bioengineering, 95*(2), 206–217. DOI: 10.1002/bit.21078

Agapakis, C. M., Boyle, P. M., & Silver, P. A. (2012). Natural strategies for the spatial optimization of metabolism in synthetic biology. *Nature Chemical Biology, 8*(6), 527–535. PMID: 22596204

Agarwal, A., Jaiswal, N., Tripathi, A. D., & Paul, V. (2020). Downstream processing; applications and recent updates. In *Bioprocessing for Biofuel Production: Strategies to Improve Process Parameters* (pp. 29-55). Springer.

Agarwal, A. K., Gupta, J. G., & Dhar, A. (2017). Potential and challenges for large-scale application of biodiesel in automotive sector. *Progress in Energy and Combustion Science, 61*, 113–149. DOI: 10.1016/j.pecs.2017.03.002

Agarwal, A., Liu, Y., Dooley, L., McDowell, C., & Thaysen, M. (2022). Large-scale industrial fermenter foaming control: Automated machine learning for antifoam prediction and defoaming process implementation. *Industrial & Engineering Chemistry Research*, *61*(15), 5227–5238.

Aggarwal, N., Pham, H. L., Ranjan, B., Saini, M., Liang, Y., Hossain, G. S., Ling, H., Foo, J. L., & Chang, M. W. (2024). Microbial engineering strategies to utilize waste feedstock for sustainable bioproduction. *Nature Reviews Bioengineering*, *2*(2), 155–174.

Aglave, G., Yerram, S., Patnam, J. D., Ajmal, C., Nizam, V. M., Joga, R., Raghuvanshi, R. S., & Srivastava, S. (2024). Proactive Approaches to cGMP Compliance: Insights and Key Takeaways from USFDA Warning Letters to Pharmaceutical Industries Between 2019 and 2024. *Journal of Pharmaceutical Innovation*, *19*(4), 49.

Agrawal, R. (2024). Downstream Processing. In *Textbook of Industrial Microbiology* (pp. 279–295). Springer.

Aguilar-Gallardo, C., & Bonora-Centelles, A. (2023). Blockchain technology for advanced therapy medicinal products: Applications in tracking, data sharing, and supply chain automation. *Journal of Pharmaceutical and Biopharmaceutical Research*, *5*(2), 430–443.

Ahmad, H., Shabbir, I., Iqbal, I., & Akhtar, M. M. (2023). The Crossroad between Intellectual Property and Clinical Trials: Balancing Incentives for Innovation with Access to Healthcare. *Trends in Intellectual Property Research*, *1*(2). Advance online publication. DOI: 10.69971/tipr.1.2.2023.16

Ahmad, J., Marsidi, N., Sheikh Abdullah, S. R., Hasan, H. A., Othman, A. R., Ismail, N., & Kurniawan, S. B. (2024). Integrating phytoremediation and mycoremediation with biosurfactant-producing fungi for hydrocarbon removal and the potential production of secondary resources. *Chemosphere*, *349*, 140881. DOI: 10.1016/j.chemosphere.2023.140881 PMID: 38048826

Ahmad, M., Ali, A., Ullah, Z., Sher, H., Dai, D. Q., Ali, M., & Ali, I. (2022). Biosynthesized silver nanoparticles using Polygonatum geminiflorum efficiently control fusarium wilt disease of tomato. *Frontiers in Bioengineering and Biotechnology*, *10*, 988607. PMID: 36159677

Ahmad, M., Rajapaksha, A. U., Lim, J. E., Zhang, M., Bolan, N., Mohan, D., Vithanage, M., Lee, S. S., & Ok, Y. S. (2014). Biochar as a sorbent for contaminant management in soil and water: A review. *Chemosphere*, *99*, 19–33. DOI: 10.1016/j.chemosphere.2013.10.071 PMID: 24289982

Ahmed, I., Zia, M. A., Afzal, H., Ahmed, S., Ahmad, M., Akram, Z., Sher, F., & Iqbal, H. M. (2021). Socio-economic and environmental impacts of biomass valorisation: A strategic drive for sustainable bioeconomy. *Sustainability*, *13*(8), 4200.

Ahmed, T., & Gupta, R. (2023). Challenges in scaling biobased nanocomposite production for medical applications. *Journal of Advanced Materials*, *10*(2), 112–120.

Ajayeoba, T. A., & Ijabadeniyi, O. A. (2025). Transforming Food for the Future: Precision Fermentation as a Key to Sustainability, Nutrition, and Health. *Nutrition and Health (Berkhamsted, Hertfordshire)*.

Ajayi, R. (2025). Integrating IoT and cloud computing for continuous process optimization in real-time systems. *Int J Res Publ Rev*, *6*(1), 2540–2558.

Alam, A. M. (2024). Analyzing FDA form 483 data of 2023: Identifying trends and areas of concern in regulatory compliance. *Journal of Pharmaceutical and Biological Sciences, 12*(1), 3-7.

Alexandre-Franco, M. F., Kouider, R., Kassir Al-Karany, R., Cuerda-Correa, E. M., & Al-Kassir, A. (2024). Recent Advances in Polymer Science and Fabrication Processes for Enhanced Microfluidic Applications: An Overview. *Micromachines, 15*(9), 1137. PMID: 39337797

Ali, A., Usman, M., Jayamani, E., Soon, K., & bin Ab Wahab, M. K. (2024). Sustainable Biomanufacturing. In *Biomedical Implants* (pp. 195-217). CRC Press.

Ali, A., Usman, M., Jayamani, E., Soon, K., & bin Ab Wahab, M. K. (2024). Sustainable Biomanufacturing. In Biomedical Implants (pp. 195-217). CRC Press. https://doi.org/DOI: 10.1201/9781003375098-12

Ali, F., & Nollet, L. M. L. (2024). *Global Regulations of Medicinal, Pharmaceutical, and Food Products*. Springer.

Ali, H., Khan, E., & Ilahi, I. (2019). Environmental chemistry and ecotoxicology of hazardous heavy metals: Environmental persistence, toxicity, and bioaccumulation. *Journal of Chemistry, 6730305*. Advance online publication. DOI: 10.1155/2019/6730305

Ali, I., Ding, W., & Zhang, Z. (2023). Microalgae-based bioplastics: A comprehensive review. *Renewable & Sustainable Energy Reviews, 178*, 113247. DOI: 10.1016/j.rser.2023.113247

Ali, M., Shabbir, K., Ali, S., Mohsin, M., Kumar, A., Aziz, M., & Sultan, H. M. (2024). A New Era of Discovery: How Artificial Intelligence has Revolutionized the Biotechnology. *Nepal Journal of Biotechnology, 12*(1), 1–11.

Ali, M., Shabbir, K., Ali, S., Mohsin, M., Kumar, A., Aziz, M., Zubair, M., & Sultan, H. M. (2024). A new era of discovery: How artificial intelligence has revolutionized biotechnology. *Nepal Journal of Biotechnology, 12*(1), 1–1. DOI: 10.3126/njb.v12i1.67165

Ali, S. S., Elsamahy, T., Abdelkarim, E. A., Al-Tohamy, R., Kornaros, M., Ruiz, H. A., Zhao, T., Li, F., & Sun, J. (2022). Biowastes for biodegradable bioplastics production and end-of-life scenarios in circular bioeconomy and biorefinery concept. *Bioresource Technology, 363*, 127869. PMID: 36064080

Al-Maqtari, Q. A., Waleed, A., & Mahdi, A. A. (2019). Microbial enzymes produced by fermentation and their applications in the food industry-A review. *International Journal of Agriculture Innovation and Research, 8*(1), 2319–1473.

Alonso-Gutierrez, J., Chan, R., Batth, T. S., Adams, P. D., Keasling, J. D., Petzold, C. J., & Lee, T. S. (2-13). Metabolic engineering of *Escherichia coli* for limonene and perillyl alcohol production. *Metabolic Engineering, 19*, 33–41.

Alper, H. S., & Stephanopoulos, G. (2009). Engineering yeasts for biofuels production: From strains to systems. *Bioresource Technology, 100*(4), 2335–2341.

Alsharari, N. M., & Aljohani, M. S. (2024). The benchmarking implementation and management control process as influenced by interplay of environmental and cultural factors: Institutional and contingency perspectives. *Benchmarking, 31*(9), 3327–3348.

Altamirano, C., Paredes, C., Cairó, J. J., & Gòdia, F. (2006). Improvement of CHO cell culture medium formulation: Simultaneous substitution of glucose and glutamine. *Biotechnology Progress*, *22*(3), 609–617. PMID: 16739940

Altman, A. (2003). From plant tissue culture to biotechnology: Scientific revolutions, abiotic stress tolerance, and forestry. *In Vitro Cellular & Developmental Biology. Plant*, *39*, 75–84. DOI: 10.1079/IVP2002379

Alves, S. S., & Vasconcelos, J. M. T. (1996). Optimisation of agitation and aeration in fermenters. *Bioprocess Engineering*, *14*(3), 119–123.

Al-Worafi, Y. M. (2024). Research and Development in Developing Countries: Achievements and Challenges. *Handbook of Medical and Health Sciences in Developing Countries: Education, Practice, and Research*, 1-23. https://doi.org/DOI: 10.1007/978-3-030-74786-2_385-1

Al-Yasiri, A. J. (2021). Global Energy Demand For Different Energy Sources: Current Status and Future Prospects. *Akkad Journal Of Contemporary Economic Studies*, *1*(4), 186–196. DOI: 10.55202/ajces.v1i4.96

Amgen. (2021). *Amgen's Next-Generation Biomanufacturing*. https://www.amgen.com/stories/2021/06/next-generation-biomanufacturing

Aminizadeh, S., Heidari, A., Dehghan, M., Toumaj, S., Rezaei, M., Navimipour, N. J., & Unal, M. (2024). Opportunities and challenges of artificial intelligence and distributed systems to improve the quality of healthcare service. *Artificial Intelligence in Medicine*, *149*, 102779. PMID: 38462281

Anas, M.. (2025). Mitigating heavy metal pollution in agriculture: A multi-omics and nanotechnology approach to safeguard global wheat production. *Journal of Hazardous Materials Advances*, *17*, 100584. https://doi.org/https://doi.org/10.1016/j.hazadv.2024.100584

Anastasopoulou, A.. (2020). Environmental impact assessment of monoclonal antibody manufacturing using Life Cycle Assessment. *Biotechnology Progress*, *36*(2), e2924.

Andersen, R. L., Jensen, K. M., & Mikkelsen, M. J. (2015). Continuous Ethanol Fermentation of Pretreated Lignocellulosic Biomasses, Waste Biomasses, Molasses and Syrup Using the Anaerobic, Thermophilic Bacterium Thermoanaerobacter italicus Pentocrobe 411. *PLoS One*, *10*(8), e0136060. DOI: 10.1371/journal.pone.0136060

Andres, Y., Dumont, E., Le Cloirec, P., & Ramirez-Lopez, E. (2006). Wood bark as packing material in a biofilter used for air treatment. *Environmental Technology*, *27*(12), 1297–1301. DOI: 10.1080/09593332708618747 PMID: 17285934

Andrews, G. F., & Przezdziecki, J. (1986). Design of fluidized-bed fermentors. *Biotechnology and Bioengineering*, *28*(6), 802–810. PMID: 18555396

Anfossi, L., Di Nardo, F., Cavalera, S., Giovannoli, C., & Baggiani, C. (2018). Multiplex lateral flow immunoassay: An overview of strategies towards high-throughput point-of-need testing. *Biosensors (Basel)*, *9*(1), 2. PMID: 30587769

Anilionyte, O., Liang, H., Ma, X., Yang, L., & Zhou, K. (2018). Short, auto-inducible promoters for well-controlled protein expression in Escherichia coli. *Applied Microbiology and Biotechnology*, *102*(16), 7007–7015. DOI: 10.1007/s00253-018-9141-z

Anjum, N. A., Ahmad, I., & Duarte, A. C. (Eds.). (2012). *The plant family Brassicaceae: Contribution towards phytoremediation*. Springer., https://www.researchgate.net/publication/230729665_The_Plant_Family_Brassicaceae_Contribution_Towards_Phytoremediation

Anyshchenko, A., & Yarnold, J. (2021). From 'mad cow' crisis to synthetic biology: Challenges to EU regulation of GMOs beyond the European context. *International Environmental Agreement: Politics, Law and Economics, 21*(3), 391–404.

Aon, M. A., & Cortassa, S. (2015). Systems biology of the fluxome. *Processes (Basel, Switzerland), 3*(3), 607–618. DOI: 10.3390/pr3030607

Appels, L., Lauwers, J., Degrève, J., Helsen, L., Lievens, B., Willems, K., & Dewil, R. (2011). Anaerobic digestion in global bio-energy production: Potential and research challenges. *Renewable & Sustainable Energy Reviews, 15*(9), 4295–4301. DOI: 10.1016/j.rser.2011.07.121

Arendt, E. K., Moroni, A., & Zannini, E. (2011). Medical nutrition therapy: use of sourdough lactic acid bacteria as a cell factory for delivering functional biomolecules and food ingredients in gluten free bread. *Microbial Cell Factories, 10 Suppl 1*(Suppl 1), S15. https://doi.org/DOI: 10.1186/1475-2859-10-S1-S15

Aretz, I., & Meierhofer, D. (2016). Advantages and pitfalls of mass spectrometry based metabolome profiling in systems biology. *International Journal of Molecular Sciences, 17*(5), 632. PMID: 27128910

Armstrong, R. N. (1987). Enzyme-catalyzed detoxication reactions: Mechanisms and stereochemistr. *Critical Reviews in Biochemistry, 22*(1), 39–88. PMID: 3115676

Arratia-Quijada, J., Nuño, K., Ruíz-Santoyo, V., & Andrade-Espinoza, B. A. (2024). Nanoencapsulation of probiotics: Need and critical considerations to design new non-dairy probiotic products. *Journal of Functional Foods, 116*, 106192. DOI: 10.1016/j.jff.2024.106192

Arulrajah, P., Lievonen, A. E., Subaşı, D., Pagal, S., Weuster-Botz, D., & Heins, A. L. (2025). Scale-down bioreactors—Comparative analysis of configurations. *Bioprocess and Biosystems Engineering*. Advance online publication. DOI: 10.1007/s00449-025-03158-4

Arvelli, S., Jia, L., Zhang, M., & Zhao, J. (2025). Review of Advanced Technologies and Circular Pathways for Food Waste Valorization. *Journal of Agricultural and Food Chemistry, 73*(26), 16085–16108. DOI: 10.1021/acs.jafc.5c03394 PMID: 40549968

Asar, R., Erenler, S., Devecioglu, D., Ispirli, H., Karbancioglu-Guler, F., Ozturk, H. I., & Dertli, E. (2025). Understanding the Functionality of Probiotics on the Edge of Artificial Intelligence (AI) Era. *Fermentation (Basel, Switzerland), 11*(5), 259.

Asghar, A., Sairash, S., Hussain, N., Baqar, Z., Sumrin, A., & Bilal, M. (2022). Current challenges of biomass refinery and prospects of emerging technologies for sustainable bioproducts and bioeconomy. *Biofuels, Bioproducts & Biorefining, 16*(6), 1478–1494. DOI: 10.1002/bbb.2403

Ashok, A., Doriya, K., Rao, D. R. M., & Kumar, D. S. (2017). Design of solid state bioreactor for industrial applications: An overview to conventional bioreactors. *Biocatalysis and Agricultural Biotechnology, 9*, 11–18. DOI: 10.1016/j.bcab.2016.10.014

Asin-Garcia, E., Fawcett, J. D., Batianis, C., & Dos Santos, V. A. M. (2024). A snapshot of biomanufacturing and the need for enabling research infrastructure. *Trends in Biotechnology*. Advance online publication. DOI: 10.1016/j.tibtech.2024.10.014 PMID: 39592270

Atsumi, S., Cann, A. F., Connor, M. R., Shen, C. R., Smith, K. M., Brynildsen, M. P., Chou, K. J. Y., Hanai, T., & Liao, J. C. (2007). Metabolic engineering of *Escherichia coli* for 1-butanol production. *Metabolic Engineering*, *10*(6), 305–311. DOI: 10.1016/j.ymben.2007.08.003 PMID: 17942358

Attal-Juncqua, A., Getz, J., Morhard, R., & Gronvall, G. K. (2024). Integrating safety, security, sustainability, and social responsibility principles into the U.S. bioeconomy. *MSphere*, *9*(5), e0008424. DOI: 10.1128/msphere.00084-24 PMID: 38687115

Austin, H. P., Allen, M. D., Donohoe, B. S., Rorrer, N. A., Kearns, F. L., Silveira, R. L., Pollard, B. C., Dominick, G., Duman, R., El Omari, K., Mykhaylyk, V., Wagner, A., Michener, W. E., Amore, A., Skaf, M. S., Crowley, M. F., Thorne, A. W., Johnson, C. W., Woodcock, H. L., & Beckham, G. T. (2018). Characterization and engineering of a plastic-degrading aromatic polyesterase. *Proceedings of the National Academy of Sciences of the United States of America*, *115*(19), E4350–E4357. DOI: 10.1073/pnas.1718804115 PMID: 29666242

Averesch, N. J., Berliner, A. J., Nangle, S. N., Zezulka, S., Vengerova, G. L., Ho, D., & Arkin, A. P. (2023). Microbial biomanufacturing for space-exploration—What to take and when to make. *Nature Communications*, *14*(1), 2311. DOI: 10.1038/s41467-023-37910-1 PMID: 37085475

Ayala, J. C., Pimienta, E., Rodríguez, C., Anné, J., Vallín, C., Milanés, M. T., King-Batsios, E., Huygen, K., & Van Mellaert, L. (2013). Use of Strep-tag II for rapid detection and purification of Mycobacterium tuberculosis recombinant antigens secreted by Streptomyces lividans. *Journal of Microbiological Methods*, *94*(3), 192–198. DOI: 10.1016/j.mimet.2013.06.004

Ayoglu, B., Häggmark, A., Neiman, M., Igel, U., Uhlén, M., Schwenk, J. M., & Nilsson, P. (2011). Systematic antibody and antigen-based proteomic profiling with microarrays. *Expert Review of Molecular Diagnostics*, *11*(2), 219–234. DOI: 10.1586/erm.10.110 PMID: 21405972

Azad, A. K., Rasul, M. G., Khan, M. M. K., Sharma, S. C., & Hazrat, M. A. (2015). Prospect of biofuels as an alternative transport fuel in Australia. *Renewable & Sustainable Energy Reviews*, *43*, 331–351. DOI: 10.1016/j.rser.2014.11.047

Azubuike, C. C., Chikere, C. B., & Okpokwasili, G. C. (2016). Bioremediation techniques—Classification based on site of application: Principles, advantages, limitations and prospects. *World Journal of Microbiology & Biotechnology*, *32*(11), 180. Advance online publication. DOI: 10.1007/s11274-016-2137-x

Bäcker, M., Delle, L., Poghossian, A., Biselli, M., Zang, W., Wagner, P., & Schöning, M. J. (2011). Electrochemical sensor array for bioprocess monitoring. *Electrochimica Acta*, *56*(26), 9673–9678.

Bailey, J. E., & Ollis, D. F. (2018). *Biochemical engineering fundamentals* (2nd ed.). McGraw-Hill.

Bailey, R. C., Kwong, G. A., Radu, C. G., Witte, O. N., & Heath, J. R. (2007). DNA-encoded antibody libraries: A unified platform for multiplexed cell sorting and detection of genes and proteins. *Journal of the American Chemical Society*, *129*(7), 1959–1967. DOI: 10.1021/ja065930i PMID: 17260987

Bajić, B., Vučurović, D., Vasić, Đ., Jevtić-Mučibabić, R., & Dodić, S. (2022). Biotechnological production of sustainable microbial proteins from agro-industrial residues and by-products. *Foods*, *12*(1), 107. DOI: 10.3390/foods12010107 PMID: 36613323

Bakeev, K. A. (Ed.). (2010). *Process Analytical Technology: Spectroscopic Tools and Implementation Strategies for the Chemical and Pharmaceutical Industries*. Wiley.

Balaji, S. G., Penubaka, K. K. R., Kumar, M., Goel, P., Jadhav, A. B., & Mohakud, S. (2025). Circular economy strategies for resource efficiency and sustainable development in manufacturing industries. *Journal of Neonatal Surgery*, *14*(13s). https://www.researchgate.net/publication/390598115

Balan, V., Mihai, C. T., Cojocaru, F. D., Uritu, C. M., Dodi, G., Botezat, D., & Gardikiotis, I. (2019). Vibrational spectroscopy fingerprinting in medicine: From molecular to clinical practice. *Materials (Basel)*, *12*(18), 2884. PMID: 31489927

Bala, S., Garg, D., Thirumalesh, B. V., Sharma, M., Sridhar, K., Inbaraj, B. S., & Tripathi, M. (2022). Recent Strategies for Bioremediation of Emerging Pollutants: A Review for a Green and Sustainable Environment. *Toxics*, *10*(8), 484. DOI: 10.3390/toxics10080484 PMID: 36006163

Balat, M. (2008). Potential importance of hydrogen as a future solution to environmental and transportation problems. *International Journal of Hydrogen Energy*, *33*(15), 4013–4029. DOI: 10.1016/j.ijhydene.2008.05.047

Baldanta, S., Guevara, G., & Navarro-Llorens, J. M. (2022). SEVA-Cpf1, a CRISPR-Cas12a vector for genome editing in cyanobacteria. *Microbial Cell Factories*, *21*(1), 103. DOI: 10.1186/s12934-022-01830-4

Banerjee, D., Barua, R., Datta, S., & Pathote, D. (2025). The Use of Artificial Neural Networks in Biomedical Engineering. In *Expert Artificial Neural Network Applications for Science and Engineering* (pp. 33–50). IGI Global Scientific Publishing.

Bankar, S. B., Survase, S. A., Singhal, R. S., & Granström, T. (2012). Continuous two stage acetone–butanol–ethanol fermentation with integrated solvent removal using Clostridium acetobutylicum B 5313. *Bioresource Technology*, *106*, 110–116. DOI: 10.1016/j.biortech.2011.12.005

Bano, S., Singh, K., Chaudhary, A., & Chandra, R. (2025). Innovative methods for the valorisation of solid wastes from sugar mill and refineries for sustainable development: A review. *Cleaner Waste Systems*, *10*, 100230. DOI: 10.1016/j.clwas.2025.100230

Bao, J., Ye, Q., & Zhong, J. J. (Eds.). (2016). *Bioreactor engineering research and industrial applications II*. Springer., DOI: 10.1007/978-3-662-48347-3

Baratta, M., Jian, W., Hengel, S., Kaur, S., Cunliffe, J., Boer, J., Hughes, N., Kar, S., Kellie, J., & Kim, Y. J. (2024). 2023 White Paper on Recent Issues in Bioanalysis: Deuterated Drugs; LNP; Tumor/FFPE Biopsy; Targeted Proteomics; Small Molecule Covalent Inhibitors; Chiral Bioanalysis; Remote Regulatory Assessments; Sample Reconciliation/Chain of Custody (PART 1A–Recommendations on Mass Spectrometry, Chromatography, Sample Preparation Latest Developments, Challenges, and Solutions and BMV/Regulated Bioanalysis PART 1B-Regulatory Agencies' Inputs on Regulated Bioanalysis/BMV, Biomarkers/IVD/CDx/BAV, Immunogenicity, Gene & Cell Therapy and Vaccine). *Bioanalysis*, *16*(9), 307–364. PMID: 38913185

Barcelos, M. C., Ramos, C. L., Kuddus, M., Rodriguez-Couto, S., Srivastava, N., Ramteke, P. W., Mishra, P. K., & Molina, G. (2020). Enzymatic potential for the valorization of agro-industrial by-products. *Biotechnology Letters*, *42*(10), 1799–1827.

Bari, M. L., & Zaman, S. (2021). Microbial biotechnology in food and health: present and future food safety regulation. In *Microbial Biotechnology in Food and Health* (pp. 1–20). Elsevier.

Barone, A. S., Maragoni-Santos, C., de Farias, P. M., Cortat, C. M. G., Maniglia, B. C., Ongaratto, R. S., Ferreira, S., & Fai, A. E. C. (2025). Rethinking single-use plastics: Innovations, polices, consumer awareness and market shaping biodegradable solutions in the food packaging industry. *Trends in Food Science & Technology*, •••, 104906.

Barone, P. W., Avgerinos, S., Ballard, R., Brussel, A., Clark, P., Dowd, C., Gerentes, L., Hart, I., Keumurian, F. J., Kindermann, J., & Leung, J. C. (2019). Biopharmaceutical industry approaches to facility segregation for viral safety: An effort from the consortium on adventitious agent contamination in biomanufacturing. *PDA Journal of Pharmaceutical Science and Technology*, *73*(2), 191–203. DOI: 10.5731/pdajpst.2018.009118

Barrangou, R., & Doudna, J. A. (2016). Applications of CRISPR technologies in research and beyond. *Nature Biotechnology*, *34*(9), 933–941. DOI: 10.1038/nbt.3659

Barua, R. (2024). Advanced Biomimetic Compound Continuum Robot for Minimally Invasive Surgical Applications. In *Modeling, Simulation, and Control of AI Robotics and Autonomous Systems* (pp. 213-231). IGI Global.

Barua, R. (2024). Exploring Artificial Intelligence in Evolving Healthcare Environments: A Comprehensive Analysis. In *Advances in Computational Intelligence for the Healthcare Industry 4.0* (pp. 123-138). IGI Global.

Barua, R. (2024). The Emerging Role of Artificial Intelligence in Organ-on-a-Chip (OOAC) Biomedical Devices. In *Reshaping Healthcare with Cutting-Edge Biomedical Advancements* (pp. 369-381). IGI Global.

Barua, R. (2025). Unleashing Human Potential: Exploring the Advantage of Biomechanics in Sport Performance. In *Global Innovations in Physical Education and Health* (pp. 409-436). IGI Global.

Barua, R., & Datta, S. (2025). Revolutionizing Nerve Repair: The Transformative Role of Nanoparticles in Peripheral Nerve Regeneration. In *Nanomaterials and the Nervous System* (pp. 275-300). IGI Global.

Barua, R., Datta, S., & Jain, N. (2024). Novel Power Generation Technology Based on Renewable Energy. In *Optimization Techniques for Hybrid Power Systems: Renewable Energy, Electric Vehicles, and Smart Grid* (pp. 407-425). IGI Global.

Barua, R. (2024). An Investigation of AI Techniques for Detecting Kidney Stones in CT Scan Images Through Advanced Image Processing. In *Enhancing Medical Imaging with Emerging Technologies* (pp. 133–150). IGI Global.

Basaran, P. (2024). Plant Molecular Farming for the Bulk Production of Industrial Enzymes. In *Applications of Plant Molecular Farming* (pp. 69–110). Springer.

Bashiardes, S., Godneva, A., Elinav, E., & Segal, E. (2018). Towards utilization of the human genome and microbiome for personalized nutrition. *Current Opinion in Biotechnology*, *51*, 57–63.

Bastian, F., Bernard, C., Lyon, U., Cohen, A., Piccoli, P., Luna, M. V., Bastián, F., Luna, V., Baraldi, R., & Bottini, R. (1998). Production of indole-3-acetic acid and gibberellins A_1 and A_3 by Acetobacter diazotrophicus and Herbaspirillum seropedicae in chemically-defined culture media Production of indole-3-acetic acid and gibberellins A 1 and A 3 by Acetobacter diazotrophicus and Herbaspirillum seropedicae in chemically-defined culture media. In *Plant Growth Regulation* (Vol. 24, Issue 7). https://www.researchgate.net/publication/263453138

Baumann, P., & Hubbuch, J. (2017). Downstream process development strategies for effective bioprocesses: Trends, progress, and combinatorial approaches. *Engineering in Life Sciences*, *17*(11), 1142–1158. PMID: 32624742

Beeckman, D. S. A., & Rüdelsheim, P. (2020). Biosafety and biosecurity in containment: A regulatory overview. *Frontiers in Bioengineering and Biotechnology*, *8*, 650. DOI: 10.3389/fbioe.2020.00650 PMID: 32719780

Beleno, M. T., & Ramos, R. T. (2024). Agro-industrial waste valorization: An environmental improvement strategy. In Agro-industrial environmental improvement models [Chapter]. Autonomous University of Baja California. https://doi.org/DOI: 10.13140/RG.2.2.27769.28005

Bell, E. L., Hutton, A. E., Burke, A. J., O'Connell, A., Barry, A., O'Reilly, E., & Green, A. P. (2024). Strategies for designing biocatalysts with new functions. *Chemical Society Reviews*, *53*(6), 2851–2862. DOI: 10.1039/d3cs00972f PMID: 38353665

Beltrán-Velasco, A. I., & Clemente-Suárez, V. J. (2025). Harnessing gut microbiota for biomimetic innovations in health and biotechnology. *Biomimetics*, *10*(2), 73.

Ben Yahia, B., Piednoir, A., Dahomais, T., Eggermont, S., & Paul, W. (2023). "Organized stress" for robust scale-up of intensified production process with fed-batch seed bioreactor. *Biotechnology and Bioengineering*, *120*(9), 2509–2522. DOI: 10.1002/bit.28487

Benavides, P. T., Balchandani, S., & Gracida-Alvarez, U. R. (2024). Environmental analysis of biotechnologies for biofuels, bioplastics, and bioproducts: A greenhouse gas (GHG) emissions review. *Biotechnology for the Environment*, *1*(1), 10. DOI: 10.1186/s44314-024-00010-5

Benn, N., & Zitomer, D. (2018). Pretreatment and anaerobic co-digestion of selected PHB and PLA bioplastics. *Frontiers in Environmental Science*, *5*, 93. DOI: 10.3389/fenvs.2017.00093

Benz, G. T. (2022). *Agitator Design Technology for Biofuels and Renewable Chemicals*. John Wiley & Sons.

Berliner, A. J., Lipsky, I., Vengerova, G., & Arkin, A. P. (2022). Towards the Future of Space Bioprocess Engineering.

Bermúdez-Humarán, L. G., Kharrat, P., Chatel, J.-M., & Langella, P. (2011). Lactococci and lactobacilli as mucosal delivery vectors for therapeutic proteins and DNA vaccines. *Microbial Cell Factories*, *10*(S1), S4. DOI: 10.1186/1475-2859-10-S1-S4

Bezbradica, D., Crovic, M. J., Tanaskovic, S., Lukovic, N., Carevic, M., Milivojevic, A., & Knezevic-Jugovic, Z. (2017). Enzymatic syntheses of esters-Green chemistry for valuable food, fuel and fine chemicals. *Current Organic Chemistry*, *21*(2), 104–138.

Bhardwaj, D., Ansari, M. W., Sahoo, R. K., & Tuteja, N. (2014). Biofertilizers function as key player in sustainable agriculture by improving soil fertility, plant tolerance and crop productivity. *Microbial Cell Factories*, *13*, 66. Advance online publication. DOI: 10.1186/1475-2859-13-66

Bhat, R. (2021). Valorization of agri-food wastes and by-products: recent trends, innovations and sustainability challenges.

Bhatia, S. K., Bhatia, S., Inda-Webb, M. E., Kourmentza, K., Moon, T. S., Singh, V., & Zhao, J. (2024). Biotechnology for sustainable materials: Innovating today for a greener tomorrow. *Biotechnology for Sustainable Materials*, *1*(1), 3. DOI: 10.3390/su16198515

Bhatia, S. K., Kim, J. H., Song, H. S., Jeon, J. M., Kim, Y. G., & Yang, Y. H. (2022). Waste to bioenergy: A sustainable approach for production of biohydrogen using organic waste. *Bioresource Technology*, *344*, 126203.

Bhatia, S. K., Otari, S. V., Jeon, J. M., & Yang, Y. H. (2019). Biowaste-to-bioplastic (polyhydroxyalkanoates): Conversion technologies, strategies, and challenges. *Bioresource Technology*, *298*, 122393. DOI: 10.1016/j.biortech.2019.122393 PMID: 33494006

Bhattacharyya, P., Roychoudhury, N., & Banerjee, S. (2021). Bioremediation of heavy metals using microbial consortia: Recent trends and applications. *Environmental Technology & Innovation*, *24*, 101893. DOI: 10.1007/978-981-16-0602-1_12

Bianchetti, G., De Maio, F., Abeltino, A., Serantoni, C., Riente, A., Santarelli, G., Sanguinetti, M., Delogu, G., Martinoli, R., & Barbaresi, S. (2023). Unraveling the gut microbiome–diet connection: Exploring the impact of digital precision and personalized nutrition on microbiota composition and host physiology. *Nutrients*, *15*(18), 3931.

Bibra, M., Krishnaraj, R. N., & Sani, R. K. (2021). Fermentation strategies in the food and beverage industry. *Biomolecular Engineering Solutions for Renewable Specialty Chemicals: Microorganisms, Products, and Processes*, 141-164.

Bikram, P. U., Linda, C. D., & Lew, P. C. (2014). Metabolic engineering as a tool for enhanced lactic acid production. *Trends in Biotechnology*, *32*(12), 637–644. DOI: 10.1016/j.tibtech.2014.10.005

Bilal, M., & Iqbal, H. M. (2020). State-of-the-art strategies and applied perspectives of enzyme biocatalysis in food sector—Current status and future trends. *Critical Reviews in Food Science and Nutrition*, *60*(12), 2052–2066.

Billington, J. K. (2016). A new product development partnership model for antibiotic resistance. *American Journal of Law & Medicine*, *42*(2-3), 487–523. DOI: 10.1177/0098858816658277 PMID: 29086636

BioFabUSA. (2021). *Enabling Next-Generation Biomanufacturing. Advanced Regenerative Manufacturing Institute*. ARMI.

Biogen. (2020). *Innovation in Biomanufacturing*. https://www.biogen.com/en_us/responsibility/manufacturing.html

Biological Weapons Convention (BWC). (1972). *Convention on the Prohibition of the Development, Production and Stockpiling of Biological and Toxin Weapons.* https://www.un.org/disarmament/biological-weapons/

Blasi, A., Verardi, A., Lopresto, C. G., Siciliano, S., & Sangiorgio, P. (2023). Lignocellulosic agricultural waste valorization to obtain valuable products: An overview. *Recycling*, *8*(4), 61.

Błaszak, B., Dorawa, P., Sudoł, P., Fabiszak, K., Świadek, M., Witucka, K., Zimnicka, J., Brudnicki, M., Maciejewski, B., & Bovkun, D. (2024). Kombucha fermentation in coffee: Application of constant air flow reactor. *Processes (Basel, Switzerland)*, *12*(10), 2159.

Blazej, R. G., Kumaresan, P., & Mathies, R. A. (2006). Microfabricated bioprocessor for integrated nanoliter-scale Sanger DNA sequencing. *Proceedings of the National Academy of Sciences of the United States of America*, *103*(19), 7240–7245. DOI: 10.1073/pnas.0602476103 PMID: 16648246

Bokelmann, C., Bromley, J., & Takors, R. (2025). Pros and cons of airlift and bubble column bioreactors: How internals improve performance. *Biochemical Engineering Journal*, *213*, 109539. DOI: 10.1016/j.bej.2024.109539

Bommer, G. T., Van Schaftingen, E., & Veiga-da-Cunha, M. (2020). Metabolite repair enzymes control metabolic damage in glycolysis. *Trends in Biochemical Sciences*, *45*(3), 228–243.

Borgosz, L., & Dikicioglu, D. (2024). Industrial internet of things: What does it mean for the bioprocess industries? *Biochemical Engineering Journal*, *201*, 109122.

Bornscheuer, U. T., Huisman, G. W., Kazlauskas, R. J., Lutz, S., Moore, J. C., & Robins, K. (2012). Engineering the third wave of biocatalysis. *Nature*, *485*(7397), 185–194. DOI: 10.1038/nature11117

Borys, M. C., Linzer, D. I. H., & Papoutsakis, E. T. (2019). Culture of CHO cells for recombinant protein production. In Smith, E. (Ed.), *Biopharmaceutical Production Technology* (Vol. 1, pp. 41–82). Wiley-VCH.

Botta, C., Tsoureki, D., Gautam, A., Patz, S., Pissaridi, K., Ferrocino, I., Franciosa, I., Cocolin, L., Huson, D. H., & Rantsiou, K. (2024). The pros and cons of tracking the microbial contamination in infant food processing chain through amplicon sequencing and metagenomics. In *Food System Microbiomes* (pp. 1–161). Abstracts Book.

Bowler, A. L., Bakalis, S., & Watson, N. J. (2020). A review of in-line and on-line measurement techniques to monitor industrial mixing processes. *Chemical Engineering Research & Design*, *153*, 463–495.

Bowyer, J., Bratkovich, S., Frank, M., Fernholz, K., & Howe, J. (2018). *Biofuels: A review of the life cycle literature*. Dovetail Partners Inc.

Bremenkamp, I., & Sousa Gallagher, M. J. (2025). Edible coatings for ready-to-eat products: Critical review of recent studies, sustainable packaging perspectives, challenges and emerging trends. *Polymers*, *17*(3), 376.

Brett, C. M. (2022). Electrochemical impedance spectroscopy in the characterisation and application of modified electrodes for electrochemical sensors and biosensors. *Molecules (Basel, Switzerland)*, *27*(5), 1497. PMID: 35268599

Brignoli, Y., Freeland, B., Cunningham, D., & Dabros, M. (2020). Control of specific growth rate in fed-batch bioprocesses: Novel controller design for improved noise management. *Processes (Basel, Switzerland), 8*(6), 679. Advance online publication. DOI: 10.3390/pr8060679

Brindhadevi, K., Shanmuganathan, R., Pugazhendhi, A., Gunasekar, P., & Manigandan, S. (2021). Biohydrogen production using horizontal and vertical continuous stirred tank reactor-a numerical optimization. *International Journal of Hydrogen Energy, 46*(20), 11305–11312. DOI: 10.1016/j.ijhydene.2020.06.155

Broad, G. M. (2023). Improving the agri-food biotechnology conversation: Bridging science communication with science and technology studies. *Agriculture and Human Values, 40*(3), 929–938.

Brorson, K. A., & Xu, Y. (2010). Virus filtration of biotechnology products. *Biotechnology and Bioengineering, 106*(2), 203–212. PMID: 20178120

Bstieler, L., Hemmert, M., & Barczak, G. (2015). Trust formation in university–industry collaborations in the US biotechnology industry: IP policies, shared governance, and champions. *Journal of Product Innovation Management, 32*(1), 111–121. DOI: 10.1111/jpim.12242

Buchner, E. (1897). Alkoholische Gärung ohne Hefezellen. *Berichte der Deutschen Chemischen Gesellschaft, 30*(1), 117–124. DOI: 10.1002/cber.18970300121

Buchner, E., & Rapp, R. (1899). Alkoholische gährung ohne hefezellen. *Berichte der Deutschen Chemischen Gesellschaft, 32*(1), 127–137. DOI: 10.1002/cber.18990320120

Bud, R. (1994). *The uses of life: A history of biotechnology*. Cambridge University Press.

Budzianowski, W. M., & Postawa, K. (2017). Total chain integration of sustainable biogas production. *Renewable Energy, 106*, 41–56. DOI: 10.1016/j.renene.2016.12.073

Buecherl, L., & Myers, C. J. (2022). Engineering genetic circuits: Advancements in genetic design automation tools and standards for synthetic biology. *Current Opinion in Microbiology, 68*, 102155. DOI: 10.1016/j.mib.2022.102155 PMID: 35588683

Bulcha, J. T., Wang, Y., Ma, H., Tai, P. W., & Gao, G. (2021). Viral vector platforms within the gene therapy landscape. *Signal Transduction and Targeted Therapy, 6*(1), 53. PMID: 33558455

Buller, A. R., Brinkmann-Chen, S., Garcia-Borràs, M., Houk, K. N., & Arnold, F. H. (2023). Enzyme engineering and biocatalysis for green chemistry. *Nature Reviews. Chemistry, 7*(1), 45–60. DOI: 10.1038/s41570-022-00440-8 PMID: 38123688

Buller, R., Lutz, S., Kazlauskas, R., Snajdrova, R., Moore, J., & Bornscheuer, U. (2023). From nature to industry: Harnessing enzymes for biocatalysis. *Science, 382*(6673), eadh8615. PMID: 37995253

Bunnak, P., Allmendinger, R., Ramasamy, S. V., Lettieri, P., & Titchener-Hooker, N. J. (2016). Life-cycle and cost of goods assessment of fed-batch and perfusion-based manufacturing processes for mAbs. *Biotechnology Progress, 32*(5), 1324–1335. DOI: 10.1002/btpr.2323

Burns, N. K., Theakstone, A. G., Zhu, H., O'Dell, L. A., Pearson, J. R., Ashton, T. D., & Conlan, X. A. (2020). The identification of synthetic cannabinoids surface coated on herbal substrates using solid-state nuclear magnetic resonance spectroscopy. *Analytica Chimica Acta, 1104*, 105–109. PMID: 32106940

Busse, C., Biechele, P., de Vries, I., Reardon, K. F., Solle, D., & Scheper, T. (2017). Sensors for disposable bioreactors. *Engineering in Life Sciences, 17*(8), 940–952. DOI: 10.1002/elsc.201700049 PMID: 32624843

Butler, M. (2005). Animal cell cultures: Recent achievements and perspectives in the production of biopharmaceuticals. *Applied Microbiology and Biotechnology, 68*(3), 283–291. DOI: 10.1007/s00253-005-1980-8

Byrne, K. (2014). High density CHO cell cultures: Improved productivity and product quality. A thesis submitted to Dublin City University, Dublin, Ireland.

Călinoiu, L.-F., Ştefănescu, B. E., Pop, I. D., Muntean, L., & Vodnar, D. C. (2019). Chitosan coating applications in probiotic microencapsulation. *Coatings, 9*(3), 194.

Callegari, A., & Capodaglio, A. G. (2018). Properties and beneficial uses of (bio)chars, with special attention to products from sewage sludge pyrolysis. *Resources, 7*(1), 20. DOI: 10.3390/resources7010020

Callihan, D. R., Downing, M., Meyer, E., Ochoa, L. A., Petuch, B., Tranchell, P., & White, D. (2021). Considerations for laboratory biosafety and biosecurity during the coronavirus disease 2019 pandemic: applying the ISO 35001: 2019 standard and high-reliability organizations principles. *Applied Biosafety : Journal of the American Biological Safety Association, 26*(3), 113–122. PMID: 36035545

Camacho, E. F., & Bordons, C. (2007). *Model Predictive Control*. Springer.

Candia-Sanchez, L. F., Álvarez-Cervantes, J., Díaz, R., & Díaz-Godínez, G. (2017). Uso potencial de biorreactores para la producción de lacasas de hongos basidiomicetos. *Mexican Journal of Biotechnology, 2*(1), 15–36. DOI: 10.29267/mxjb.2017.2.1.15

Cankar, K., van Houwelingen, A., Bosch, D., Sonke, T., Bouwmeester, H., & Beekwilder, J. (2015). A chicory cytochrome P450 mono-oxygenase CYP71AV8 for the oxidation of (+)-valencene. *FEBS Letters, 589*(1), 9–16. DOI: 10.1016/j.febslet.2014.11.020 PMID: 21115006

Cappia, J. M. (2004). Principles of steam-in-place. *Pharmaceutical Technology, 24*(Suppl.), S40.

Carbonara, N., & Pellegrino, R. (2019). The role of public private partnerships in fostering innovation. *Construction Management and Economics, 38*(2), 140–156. DOI: 10.1080/01446193.2019.1610184

Carbonell, P., Jervis, A. J., Robinson, C. J., Yan, C., Dunstan, M., & Swainston, N. (2018). An automated Design–Build–Test–Learn pipeline for enhanced microbial production of fine chemicals. *Communications Biology, 1*(1), 66. DOI: 10.1038/s42003-018-0076-9 PMID: 30271948

Carlsen, L., & Bruggemann, R. (2022). The 17 United Nations' sustainable development goals: A status by 2020. *International Journal of Sustainable Development and World Ecology, 29*(3), 219–229. https://ui.adsabs.harvard.edu/link_gateway/2022IJSDW.29.219C/doi:10.1080/13504509.2021.1948456

Carpenter, C. B. (2018). Safety considerations for working with animal models involving human health hazards. *Animal Models and Experimental Medicine*, *1*(2), 91–99. PMID: 30891553

Carter, H. E., Clark, R. K., Dickman, S. R., Loo, Y. H., Skell, I. S., & Strong, W. A. (1945). *ISOLATION AND PURIFICATION OF STREPTOMYCIN**.

Casini, A., Storch, M., Baldwin, G. S., & Ellis, T. (2015). Bricks and blueprints: Methods and standards for DNA assembly. *Nature Reviews. Molecular Cell Biology*, *16*(9), 568–576. DOI: 10.1038/nrm4014 PMID: 26081612

Castro-Criado, D., Rivera-Flores, O., Abdullah, J. A. A., Castro-Osorto, E., Alonso-González, M., Ramos-Casco, L., Perez-Puyana, V. M., Sánchez-Barahona, M., Sánchez-Cid, P., Jiménez-Rosado, M., & Romero, A. (2023). Valorization of Honduran Agro-Food Waste to Produce Bioplastics. *Polymers*, *15*(12), 2625. DOI: 10.3390/polym15122625 PMID: 37376271

Cauchon, N. S., Oghamian, S., & Hassanpour, S.. (2019). Innovation in Chemistry, Manufacturing, and Controls—A Regulatory Perspective from Industry. *Journal of Pharmaceutical Sciences*, *108*(1), 1–12. https://www.sciencedirect.com/science/article/pii/S0022354919300929 PMID: 30794794

CDC. (2009). *Biosafety in Microbiological and Biomedical Laboratories* (5th ed.). https://www.cdc.gov/labs/BMBL.html

Cecconet, D., Molognoni, D., Callegari, A., & Capodaglio, A. G. (2018). Agro-food industry wastewater treatment with microbial fuel cells: Energetic recovery issues. *International Journal of Hydrogen Energy*, *43*(1), 500–511. DOI: 10.1016/j.ijhydene.2017.07.231

Cecilia, J. A., García-Sancho, C., Maireles-Torres, P., & Luque, R. (2019). Industrial food waste valorization: A general overview. In Bastidas-Oyanedel, J.-R., & Schmidt, J. E. (Eds.), *Biorefinery* (pp. 253–272). Springer., DOI: 10.1007/978-3-030-10961-5_11

Ceroni, F., Algar, R., Stan, G.-B., & Ellis, T. (2015). Quantifying cellular capacity identifies gene expression designs with reduced burden. *Nature Methods*, *12*(5), 415–418. DOI: 10.1038/nmeth.3339

Cerrone, F., & O'Connor, K. E. (2025). Cultivation of filamentous fungi in airlift bioreactors: Advantages and disadvantages. *Applied Microbiology and Biotechnology*, *109*(1), 41. DOI: 10.1007/s00253-025-13422-4 PMID: 39928147

Chaachouay, N., & Zidane, L. (2024). Plant-derived natural products: A source for drug discovery and development. *Drugs and Drug Candidates*, *3*(1), 184–207. DOI: 10.3390/ddc3010011

Chabanon, M., Duval, H., Grenier, J., Beauchesne, C., Goyeau, B., & David, B. (2019). Histological method to study the effect of shear stress on cell proliferation and tissue morphology in a bioreactor. *Tissue Engineering and Regenerative Medicine*, *16*, 225–235. DOI: 10.1007/s13770-019-00181-3 PMID: 31205852

Chai, W. Y., Teo, K. T. K., Tan, M. K., & Tham, H. J. (2022). Fermentation process control and optimization. *Chemical Engineering & Technology*, *45*(10), 1731–1747.

Challener, C. A. (2023). *The future is continuous: Accelerating the shift in biomanufacturing*. Pharma's Almanac.

Chandrababu, K. B., Kannan, A., Savage, J. R., Stadmiller, S., Ryle, A. E., Cheung, C., Kelley, R. F., Maa, Y. F., Saggu, M., & Bitterfield, D. L. (2024). Stability comparison between microglassification and lyophilization using a monoclonal antibody. *Journal of Pharmaceutical Sciences, 113*(4), 1054–1060. DOI: 10.1016/j.xphs.2023.11.022

Chandrasekaran, M., Basheer, S. M., Chellappan, S., Krishna, J. G., & Beena, P. (2015). Enzymes in food and beverage production: An overview. *Enzym Food Beverage Process CRC Press, 25*, 133–154.

Chandrashekhar, H., & Rao, J. V. (2010). An overview of fermenter and the design considerations to enhance its productivity. *Pharmacologyonline, 1*, 261–301.

Chang, C. C., Ryu, D. D. Y., Park, C. S., Kim, J. Y., & Ogrydziak, D. M. (1998). Recombinant bioprocess optimization for heterologous protein production using two-stage, cyclic fed-batch culture. *Applied Microbiology and Biotechnology, 49*(5), 531–537. PMID: 9650251

Chan-Yam, K., Meyer, T., Scott, J. A., & Basiliko, N. (2022). Methane production potential of pulp mill sludges: Microbial community and substrate constraints. *FEMS Microbiology Letters, 368*(21-24), fnab161. Advance online publication. DOI: 10.1093/femsle/fnab161 PMID: 34994385

Chaudhary, A. K., & Lee, E. Y. (2015). Tightly regulated and high level expression vector construction for Escherichia coli BL21 (DE3). *Journal of Industrial and Engineering Chemistry, 31*, 367–373. DOI: 10.1016/j.jiec.2015.07.011

Cheang, B., & Zydney, A. L. (2004). A two-stage ultrafiltration process for fractionation of whey protein isolate. *Journal of Membrane Science, 231*(1-2), 159–167.

Chen, W., & Hang, F. (2019). Lactic acid bacteria starter. In *Lactic Acid Bacteria: Bioengineering and Industrial Applications* (pp. 93-143). Springer.

Chen, C. K., & Blaschek, H. P. (1999). Acetate enhances solvent production and prevents degeneration in *Clostridium beijerinckii* BA101. *Applied Microbiology and Biotechnology, 52*(2), 170–173. DOI: 10.1007/s002530051504 PMID: 10499256

Chen, C. W., Lin, H. F., Kuo, C. L., Tsai, H. L., & Tsai, J. F. Y. (1988). Cloning and expression of a DNA sequence conferring cephamycin C production. *Bio/technology, 6*(10), 1222–1224.

Chen, G. Q., & Jiang, X. R. (2018). Engineering microorganisms for improving polyhydroxyalkanoate biosynthesis. *Current Opinion in Biotechnology, 53*, 20–25. DOI: 10.1016/j.copbio.2017.11.003 PMID: 29169056

Cheng, L., Yang, X., Li, S., Fu, Q., Fu, S., Wang, J., Li, F., Lei, L., & Shen, Z. (2017). Impact of gene modification of phosphotransferase system on expression of glutamate dehydrogenase protein of *Streptococcus suis* in *Escherichia coli. Biotechnology, Biotechnological Equipment, 31*(3), 612–618. DOI: 10.1080/13102818.2017.1304179

Chen, N. Y. (1990). The design of airlift fermenters for use in biotechnology. *Biotechnology & Genetic Engineering Reviews, 8*(1), 379–396.

Chenthamarakshan, A., Parambayil, N., Miziriya, N., Soumya, P. S., Lakshmi, M. K., Ramgopal, A., & Nambisan, P. (2017). Optimization of laccase production from Marasmiellus palmivorus LA1 by Taguchi method of design of experiments. *BMC Biotechnology, 17*(1), 12. PMID: 28193272

Chen, X., Dong, Y., Huang, Y., Fan, J., Yang, M., & Zhang, J. (2021). Whole-genome resequencing using next-generation and Nanopore sequencing for molecular characterization of T-DNA integration in transgenic poplar 741. *BMC Genomics*, *22*, 329. DOI: 10.1186/s12864-021-07625-y PMID: 33957867

Chen, X., Hu, R., Hu, L., Huang, Y., Shi, W., Wei, Q., & Li, Z. (2020). Portable analytical techniques for monitoring volatile organic chemicals in biomanufacturing processes: Recent advances and limitations. *Frontiers in Chemistry*, *8*, 837. PMID: 33024746

Chen, X., Zhou, L., Tian, K., Kumar, A., Singh, S., Prior, B. A., & Wang, Z. (2013). Metabolic engineering of *Escherichia coli*: A sustainable industrial platform for bio-based chemical production. *Biotechnology Advances*, *31*(8), 1200–1223. DOI: 10.1016/j.biotechadv.2013.08.009

Chen, Y., Yang, O., Sampat, C., Bhalode, P., Ramachandran, R., & Ierapetritou, M. (2020). Digital twins in pharmaceutical and biopharmaceutical manufacturing: A literature review. *Processes (Basel, Switzerland)*, *8*(9), 1088. Advance online publication. DOI: 10.3390/pr8091088

Chettri, D., Verma, A. K., Chirania, M., & Verma, A. K. (2024). Optimization Strategies for Enhanced Production of Microbial Products. In *Industrial Microbiology and Biotechnology: A New Horizon of the Microbial World* (pp. 465–487). Springer Nature Singapore., DOI: 10.1007/978-981-97-6270-5_15

Chien, F., Ngo, Q. T., Hsu, C. C., Chau, K. Y., & Iram, R. (2021). Assessing the mechanism of barriers towards green finance and public spending in small and medium enterprises from developed countries. *Environmental Science and Pollution Research International*, *28*(43), 60495–60510. DOI: 10.1007/s11356-021-14907-1

Chisti, Y., & Moo-Young, M. (2006). Bioreactor design. *Basic biotechnology, 3*, 181-200. ISBN 978-0-521-54958-5

Chitnis, A. V., Nair, L. L., Gupta, D., & Dhoble, A. S. (2024). Non-sterile cultivation of oleaginous organisms. *Trends in Biotechnology*, *42*(12), 1583–1587. DOI: 10.1016/j.tibtech.2024.06.004

Cho, A., Yun, H., Park, J. H., Lee, S. Y., & Park, S. (2010). Prediction of novel synthetic pathways for the production of desired chemicals. *BMC Systamatic Biology*, *4*(1), 35.

Choi, K. R., Jang, W. D., Yang, D., Cho, J. S., Park, D., & Lee, S. Y. (2020). Systems metabolic engineering strategies: Integrating systems and synthetic biology with metabolic engineering. *Trends in Biotechnology*, *38*(7), 760–772. DOI: 10.1016/j.tibtech.2019.12.015 PMID: 30737009

Choi, S. Y., Song, C. W., Shin, J. H., & Lee, S. Y. (2019). Biorefineries for the production of top building block chemicals and their derivatives. *Metabolic Engineering*, *28*, 223–239. PMID: 25576747

Choi, Y. J., & Lee, S. Y. (2013). Insect cell culture and its application in biopharmaceutical production. *Biotechnology Advances*, *31*(6), 996–1008.

Choi, Y. J., Shin, S.-H., & Shin, H. S. (2022). Immunomodulatory Effects of Bifidobacterium spp. and Use of Bifidobacterium breve and Bifidobacterium longum on Acute Diarrhea in Children. *Journal of Microbiology and Biotechnology*, *32*(9), 1186.

Chomać-Pierzecka, E. (2025). Innovation as an Attribute of the Sustainable Development of Pharmaceutical Companies. *Sustainability, 17*(6), 2417. DOI: 10.3390/su17062417

Chong, J. W. R., Tan, X., Khoo, K. S., Ng, H. S., Jonglertjunya, W., Yew, G. Y., & Show, P. L. (2022). Microalgae-based bioplastics: Future solution towards mitigation of plastic wastes. *Environmental Research, 206*, 112620. DOI: 10.1016/j.envres.2021.112620 PMID: 34968431

Choudhary, V., Patel, K., Niaz, M., Panwala, M., Mehta, A., & Choudhary, K. (2024). Risk Management Strategies for Biotech Startups: A Comprehensive Framework for Early-Stage Projects. In *Recent Trends In Engineering and Science for Resource Optimization and Sustainable Development* (pp. 448-456). CRC Press.

Chowdhury, S., Jain, N., Waidi, Y. O., Barua, R., Das, S., Prasad, A., & Datta, S. (2024). Biological Smart Biomaterials: Materials for Biomedical Applications. In *Applications of Biotribology in Biomedical Systems* (pp. 313–325). Springer Nature Switzerland.

Christiansen, G. D. (2020). Quality control and quality assurance issues in biopharmaceutical processing. In *Biotechnology* (pp. 33–71). CRC Press.

Christiansen, G. D. (2020). *Quality Control and Quality Assurance Issues in Biopharmaceutical Processing*. Taylor and Francis., DOI: 10.1201/9781003055297-3

Christopher, L. P., Kapatral, V., Vaisvil, B., Emel, G., & DeVeaux, L. C. (2014). Draft Genome Sequence of a New Homofermentative, Lactic Acid-Producing *Enterococcus faecalis* Isolate, CBRD01. *Genome Announcements*, *2*(2), e00147–e14. DOI: 10.1128/genomea.00147-14

Chukwunweike, J., Anang, A. N., Adeniran, A. A., & Dike, J. (2024). Enhancing manufacturing efficiency and quality through automation and deep learning: addressing redundancy, defects, vibration analysis, and material strength optimization Vol. 23. *World Journal of Advanced Research and Reviews. GSC Online Press.*

Chu, S. S., Nguyen, H. A., Zhang, J., Tabassum, S., & Cao, H. (2022). Towards multiplexed and multimodal biosensor platforms in real-time monitoring of metabolic disorders. *Sensors (Basel)*, *22*(14), 5200. PMID: 35890880

Clementschitsch, F., & Bayer, K. (2006). Improvement of bioprocess monitoring: Development of novel concepts. *Microbial Cell Factories*, *5*, 19. Advance online publication. DOI: 10.1186/1475-2859-5-19

Clomburg, J. M., Crumbley, A. M., & Gonzalez, R. (2017a). Industrial biomanufacturing: The future of chemical production. *Science*, *355*(6320), aag0804. PMID: 28059717

Colwill, J. A., Wright, E. I., Rahimifard, S., & Clegg, A. J. (2012). Bio-based plastics in the automotive industry. *Journal of Biobased Materials and Bioenergy*, *6*(3), 274–281. DOI: 10.1166/jbmb.2012.1213

Connelly, S., Shin, S. G., Dillon, R. J., Ijaz, U. Z., Quince, C., Sloan, W. T., & Collins, G. (2017). Bioreactor scalability: Laboratory-scale bioreactor design influences performance, ecology, and community physiology in expanded granular sludge bed bioreactors. *Frontiers in Microbiology*, *8*, 664. DOI: 10.3389/fmicb.2017.00664 PMID: 28507535

Connor, M. R., & Liao, J. C. (2008). Engineering of an *Escherichia coli* strain for the production of 3-methyl-1-butanol. *Applied and Environmental Microbiology, 74*(18), 5769–5775. DOI: 10.1128/AEM.00468-08 PMID: 18676713

Constantinides, A., Spencer, J. L., & Gaden, E. L.Jr. (1970). Optimization of batch fermentation processes. I. Development of mathematical models for batch penicillin fermentations. *Biotechnology and Bioengineering, 12*(5), 803–830. PMID: 5489784

Cordiner, J. L., Kis, Z., Moghadam, P. Z., & Isoko, K. (2024). Bioprocessing 4.0: A Pragmatic Review and Future Perspectives. *Digital Discovery, 3*, 1662–1681. DOI: 10.1039/d4dd00127c

Cosenza, M. E. (2021). *Global Regulatory Expectations and Interactions.* In *Translational Medicine* (pp. 103–122). CRC Press.

Cosme, F., Nunes, F. M., & Filipe-Ribeiro, L. (2024). *Winemaking: Advanced Technology and Flavor Research* (Vol. 13). MDPI.

Costa, R., Conceição, M. M., da Silva, A. R., & Conceição, J. T. P. (2021). Marketing verde–A importância do consumo sustentável para as empresas. Research. *Social Development, 10*(7), e26310716812–e26310716812. DOI: 10.33448/rsd-v10i7.16812

Covarrubias, C. E., Rivera, T. A., Soto, C. A., Deeks, T., & Kalergis, A. M. (2022). Current GMP standards for the production of vaccines and antibodies: An overview. *Frontiers in Public Health, 10*, 1021905. PMID: 36743162

Cristofoli, N. L., Lima, A. R., Tchonkouang, R. D., Quintino, A. C., & Vieira, M. C. (2023). Advances in the food packaging production from agri-food waste and by-products: Market trends for a sustainable development. *Sustainability, 15*(7), 6153. Advance online publication. DOI: 10.3390/su15076153

Cui, S., Hu, M., Sun, Y., Mao, B., Zhang, Q., Zhao, J., Tang, X., & Zhang, H. (2022). Effect of trehalose and lactose treatments on the freeze-drying resistance of lactic acid bacteria in high-density culture. *Microorganisms, 11*(1), 48.

Cui, Z., Zhong, Y., Sun, Z., Jiang, Z., Deng, J., Wang, Q., Nielsen, J., Hou, J., & Qi, Q. (2023). Reconfiguration of the reductive TCA cycle enables high-level succinic acid production by Yarrowia lipolytica. *Nature Communications, 14*(1), 8480. DOI: 10.1038/s41467-023-44245-4

D'Almeida, A. P., & de Albuquerque, T. L. (2024). Innovations in Food Packaging: From Bio-Based Materials to Smart Packaging Systems. *Processes (Basel, Switzerland), 12*(10), 2085. DOI: 10.3390/pr12102085

da Silva Fernandes, F., de Souza, É. S., Carneiro, L. M., Alves Silva, J. P., de Souza, J. V. B., & da Silva Batista, J. (2022). Current ethanol production requirements for the yeast Saccharomyces cerevisiae. *International Journal of Microbiology, 2022*(1), 7878830.

da Silva, F. V. S., Murtagh, J., & Mu'azzam, K. (2024). *A roadmap for model-based bioprocess development. Biotechnology Advances.* https://www.sciencedirect.com/science/article/pii/S0734975024000727

Dahiya, A., Singh, K., & Ashish, A., Nipun, Bhadyaria, A., Thakur, S., Kumar, M., Das Gupta, G., Das Kurmi, B., & Pal, R. R. (2025). Global harmonization in advanced therapeutics: Balancing innovation, safety, and access. *Personalized Medicine*, ●●●, 1–11. PMID: 40277251

Dahlgren, G., & Hausner, D. B. (2023). *ICH Q13 and what is next for continuous manufacturing*. Pharmaceutical Engineering.

Daisley, B. A., & Allen-Vercoe, E. (2024). Microbes as medicine. *Annals of the New York Academy of Sciences*, *1541*(1), 63–82.

Dai, Y., Chen, Y., Lin, X., & Zhang, S. (2024). Recent Applications and Prospects of Enzymes in Quality and Safety Control of Fermented Foods. *Foods*, *13*(23), 3804. PMID: 39682876

Dalton, B., Bhagabati, P., De Micco, J., Padamati, R. B., & O'Connor, K. (2022). A review on biological processes for pharmaceuticals and personal care products removal. *Chemosphere*, *286*, 131716. DOI: 10.1016/j.chemosphere.2021.131716

Dang, B. T., Bui, X. T., Tran, D. P., Ngo, H. H., & Nghiem, L. D. (2022). Current application of algae derivatives for bioplastic production: A review. *Bioresource Technology*, *347*, 126698. DOI: 10.1016/j.biortech.2022.126698 PMID: 35026424

Daniel, C., Roussel, Y., Kleerebezem, M., & Pot, B. (2011). Recombinant lactic acid bacteria as mucosal biotherapeutic agents. *Trends in Biotechnology*, *29*(10), 499–508. DOI: 10.1016/j.tibtech.2011.05.002

Darvishi, F., & Abolhasan Moghaddami, N. (2019). Optimization of an industrial medium from molasses for bioethanol production using the Taguchi statistical experimental-design method. *Fermentation (Basel, Switzerland)*, *5*(1), 14.

Das, D., Panesar, P. S., Panesar, G., & Timilsena, Y. (2022). Sources, composition, and characterization of agro-industrial byproducts. In *Valorization of Agro-Industrial Byproducts* (pp. 11–30). CRC Press.

Das, P. K., Sahoo, A., & Veeranki, V. D. (2025). Modeling and Optimization of Recombinant Tocilizumab Production From Pichia pastoris Using Response Surface Methodology and Artificial Neural Network. *Biotechnology and Bioengineering*. PMID: 40371610

Das, S. P., Das, D., & Goyal, A. (2014). Statistical optimization of fermentation process parameters by Taguchi orthogonal array design for improved bioethanol production. *Journal of Fuels*, *2014*(1), 419674.

Das, S., & Dash, H. R. (2014). Microbial bioremediation: A potential tool for restoration of contaminated areas. *Environmental Science and Pollution Research International*, *21*(17), 10255–10272. DOI: 10.1007/978-981-16-0602-1_17

Dassau, E., Zadok, I., & Lewin, D. R. (2006). Combining six-sigma with integrated design and control for yield enhancement in bioprocessing. *Industrial & Engineering Chemistry Research*, *45*(25), 8299–8309.

David, F., Steinwand, M., Hust, M., Bohle, K., Ross, A., Dübel, S., & Franco-Lara, E. (2011). Antibody production in *Bacillus megaterium*: Strategies and physiological implications of scaling from microtiter plates to industrial bioreactors. *Biotechnology Journal*, *6*(12), 1516–1531. DOI: 10.1002/biot.201000417

De Felice, F., Petrillo, A., Cioffi, R., & Calabrese, M. (2022). Digital transformation and regulatory compliance in biopharmaceutical manufacturing: A framework proposal. *Technovation*, *117*, 102526.

de Matas, M., De Beer, T., Folestad, S., Ketolainen, J., Lindén, H., Lopes, J. A., Oostra, W., Weimer, M., Öhrngren, P., & Rantanen, J. (2016). Strategic framework for education and training in Quality by Design (QbD) and process analytical technology (PAT). *European Journal of Pharmaceutical Sciences*, *90*, 2–7. PMID: 27112991

de Mello, A. F., de Souza Vandenberghe, L. P., Herrmann, L. W., Letti, L. A., Burgos, W. J., Scapini, T., Manzoki, M. C., de Oliveira, P. Z., & Soccol, C. R. (2024). Strategies and engineering aspects on the scale-up of bioreactors for different bioprocesses. *Systems Microbiology and Biomanufacturing*, *4*(2), 365–385. DOI: 10.1007/s43393-023-00230-9

De Melo, A. C., de Castro, H. F., & de Moraes, F. F. (2014). Enzymatic synthesis of biodiesel via alcoholysis of palm oil. *Applied Biochemistry and Biotechnology*, *173*(6), 1365–1375. DOI: 10.1007/s12010-014-0934-y

de Mélo, A. H., Nunes, A. L., Carvalho, P. H., da Silva, M. F., Teixeira, G. S., & Goldbeck, R. (2023). Evaluation of Saccharomyces cerevisiae modified via CRISPR/Cas9 as a cellulosic platform microorganism in simultaneously saccharification and fermentation processes. *Bioprocess and Biosystems Engineering*, *46*(8), 1111–1119.

de Souza, N. R. D., Groenestege, M., Spekreijse, J., Ribeiro, C., Matos, C. T., Pizzol, M., & Cherubini, F. (2024). Challenges and opportunities toward a sustainable bio-based chemical sector in Europe. *Wiley Interdisciplinary Reviews. Energy and Environment*, *13*(5), e534. DOI: 10.1002/wene.534

de Vos, W. M. (2011). Systems solutions by lactic acid bacteria: From paradigms to practice. *Microbial Cell Factories*, *10*(Suppl 1), S2. DOI: 10.1186/1475-2859-10-S1-S2

Deb, P., Talukdar, S. A., Mohsina, K., Sarker, P. K., & Sayem, S. A. (2013). Production and partial characterization of extracellular amylase enzyme from *Bacillus amyloliquefaciens* P-001. *SpringerPlus*, *2*(1), 154. DOI: 10.1186/2193-1801-2-154

Deckers, M., Deforce, D., Fraiture, M.-A., & Roosens, N. H. (2020). Genetically modified microorganisms for industrial food enzyme production: An overview. *Foods*, *9*(3), 326.

Dederer, H.-G. (2016). The challenge of regulating genetically modified organisms in the European Union: trends and issues. In *Contemporary Issues in Environmental Law: The EU and Japan* (pp. 139-168). Springer.

Deeba, F., Pruthi, V., & Negi, Y. S. (2016). Converting paper mill sludge into neutral lipids by oleaginous yeast *Cryptococcus vishniaccii* for biodiesel production. *Bioresource Technology*, *213*, 96–102. DOI: 10.1016/j.biortech.2016.02.105 PMID: 26965670

Del Hierro, A. G., Moreno-Cid, J. A., & Casey, E. (2024). Continuous biomanufacturing for sustainable bioeconomy applications. *EFB Bioeconomy Journal, 4*, 100071. DOI: 10.1016/j.bioeco.2024.100071

Delebecque, C. J., & Philp, J. (2019). Education and training for industrial biotechnology and engineering biology. *Engineering Biology, 3*(1), 6–11. DOI: 10.1049/enb.2018.0001

DeLisa, M., Kargi, F., & Shuler, M. (2017). *Bioprocess engineering: Basic concepts* (3rd ed.). Pearson.

Delvigne, F., & Goffin, P. (2014). Microbial heterogeneity affects bioprocess robustness: Dynamic single-cell analysis contributes to understanding of microbial populations. *Biotechnology Journal, 9*(1), 61–72. DOI: 10.1002/biot.201300119 PMID: 24408611

Delvigne, F., Takors, R., Mudde, R., van Gulik, W., & Noorman, H. (2017). Bioprocess scale-up/down as integrative enabling technology: From fluid mechanics to systems biology and beyond. *Microbial Biotechnology, 10*(5), 1267–1274. DOI: 10.1111/1751-7915.12782

Demain, A. L. (2007). REVIEWS: The business of biotechnology. *Industrial Biotechnology (New Rochelle, N.Y.), 3*(3), 269–283. DOI: 10.1089/ind.2007.3.269

Demain, A. L., & Elander, R. P. (1999). The β-lactam antibiotics: Past, present, and future. *Antonie van Leeuwenhoek, 75*(1), 5–19. DOI: 10.1023/A:1001790109552

Demain, A. L., & Vaishnav, P. (2009). Production of recombinant proteins by microbes and higher organisms. *Biotechnology Advances, 27*(3), 297–306. DOI: 10.1016/j.biotechadv.2009.01.008

Demirbas, A. (2011). Competitive liquid biofuels from biomass. *Applied Energy, 88*(1), 17–28. DOI: 10.1016/j.apenergy.2010.07.016

Desai, P. D., & Zimmerman, W. B. (2023). Microbubble Intensification of Bioprocessing: The role of direct microorganism and bubble interactions. *Johnson Matthey Technology Review, 67*(4), 371–401.

Dhakal, D., Dhakal, Y., & Sohng, J. K. (2017). Book review: antibody-drug conjugates: fun- damentals, drug development, and clinical outcomes to target cancer. *Frontiers in Pharmacology, 8*, 771.

Dhiman, P., Aggarwal, S., & Sethi, M. (2025). Technological innovations in food waste valorisation. *Discover Sustainability, 6*, 45. DOI: 10.1007/s43621-025-01073-4

Dhiman, S., Kaur, S., Thakur, B., Singh, P., & Tripathi, M. (2025). Nutritional Enhancement of Plant-Based Fermented Foods: Microbial Innovations for a Sustainable Future. *Fermentation (Basel, Switzerland), 11*(6), 346.

Di Bartolo, A., Infurna, G., & Dintcheva, N. T. (2021). A review of bioplastics and their adoption in the circular economy. *Polymers, 13*(8), 1229. DOI: 10.3390/polym13081229 PMID: 33920269

Diederich, S. (2025). *Biosafety Level 4 (BSL4)–Virus research at the highest level of biosafety and biosecurity* (Vol. 122). Academic Press.

Diehl, M., Bock, H. G., Schlöder, J. P., Findeisen, R., Nagy, Z., & Allgöwer, F. (2002). Real-time optimization and nonlinear model predictive control of processes governed by differential-algebraic equations. *Journal of Process Control, 12*(4), 577–585.

DiGiandomenico, K., Dunn, E., Sadowski, C., Godwin, S., Keeler, M., Preston, F., Niven, P., Ramsey, P., & Hay, H. (2020). Environmental health and biosafety risk assessment guidance for commercial-scale cell and gene therapy manufacturing. *Applied Biosafety : Journal of the American Biological Safety Association, 25*(4), 201–213. PMID: 36032393

Dilkes-Hoffman, L. S., Pratt, S., Lant, P. A., & Laycock, B. (2019). The role of biodegradable plastic in solving plastic solid waste accumulation. In *Plastics to energy* (pp. 469–505). William Andrew Publishing., DOI: 10.1016/b978-0-12-813140-4.00019-4

Ding, S., Cargill, A. A., Medintz, I. L., & Claussen, J. C. (2015). Increasing the activity of immobilized enzymes with nanoparticle conjugation. *Current Opinion in Biotechnology, 34*, 242–250. DOI: 10.1016/j.copbio.2015.04.005

Dkhar, D. S., Kumari, R., Malode, S. J., Shetti, N. P., & Chandra, P. (2023). Integrated lab-on-a-chip devices: Fabrication methodologies, transduction system for sensing purposes. *Journal of Pharmaceutical and Biomedical Analysis, 223*, 115120. PMID: 36343538

Donato, K., Medori, M., Stuppia, L., Beccari, T., Dundar, M., Marks, R., Michelini, S., Borghetti, E., Zuccato, C., & Seppilli, L. (2023). Unleashing the potential of biotechnology for sustainable development. *European Review for Medical and Pharmacological Sciences, 27*(6, Suppl), 100–113.

Dong, L., Liu, Z., & Bian, Y. (2021). Match circular economy and urban sustainability: Re-investigating circular economy under sustainable development goals (SDGs). *Circular Economy and Sustainability, 1*, 243–256. DOI: 10.1007/s43615-021-00021-2

Doran, P. M. (1995). *Bioprocess engineering principles*. Elsevier.

Dragone, G., Fernandes, B., Vicente, A. A., & Teixeira, J. A. (2010). Third generation biofuels from microalgae. In Méndez-Vilas, A. (Ed.), *Current research, technology and education topics in applied microbiology and microbial biotechnology* (pp. 1355–1366). FORMATEX., https://www.researchgate.net/publication/236006059_Third_generation_biofuels_from_microalgae

Dragosits, M., & Mattanovich, D. (2013). Adaptive laboratory evolution—Principles and applications for biotechnology. *Microbial Cell Factories, 12*, 64. Advance online publication. DOI: 10.1186/1475-2859-12-64

Drandev, S., Penev, K. I., & Karamanev, D. (2016). Study of the hydrodynamics and mass transfer in a rectangular air-lift bioreactor. *Chemical Engineering Science, 146*, 180–188. DOI: 10.1016/j.ces.2016.02.041

Drexler, D. M., Reily, M. D., & Shipkova, P. A. (2011). Advances in mass spectrometry applied to pharmaceutical metabolomics. *Analytical and Bioanalytical Chemistry, 399*(8), 2645–2653. DOI: 10.1007/s00216-010-4370-8 PMID: 21107980

Duarte, J. G., Duarte, M. G., Piedade, A. P., & Mascarenhas-Melo, F. (2025). Rethinking Pharmaceutical Industry with Quality by Design: Application in Research, Development, Manufacturing, and Quality Assurance. *The AAPS Journal, 27*(4), 96. PMID: 40389714

Du, C., Zhang, Y., Gao, X., Liu, Q., & Wang, X. (2022). Model-based optimization in large-scale fermentation: Recent advances and future prospects. *Bioengineering (Basel, Switzerland)*, *9*(9), 473. PMID: 36135019

Dudley, Q. M., Karim, A. S., & Jewett, M. C. (2015). Cell-free metabolic engineering: Biomanufacturing beyond the cell. *Biotechnology Journal*, *10*(1), 69–82.

Dutta, D., Kumar, P., Singh, A., & Khade, S. (2024). Bioprocess strategies for enhanced performance in single-use bioreactors for biomolecule synthesis: A biokinetic approach. *Food Bioengineering*, *3*(3), 337–351.

Dutta, K., Daverey, A., & Lin, J. G. (2014). Evolution retrospective for alternative fuels: First to fourth generation. *Renewable Energy*, *69*, 114–122. DOI: 10.1016/j.renene.2014.02.044

Du, Y. H., Wang, M. Y., Yang, L. H., Tong, L. L., Guo, D. S., & Ji, X. J. (2022). Optimization and scale-up of fermentation processes driven by models. *Bioengineering (Basel, Switzerland)*, *9*(9), 473. Advance online publication. DOI: 10.3390/bioengineering9090473

Dwivedi, C. M. (2006). Validation of Cell Culture-Based Processes. In *Cell Culture Technology for Pharmaceutical and Cell-Based Therapies*. Taylor and Francis.

Ecker, D. M., Jones, S. D., & Levine, H. L. (2015). The therapeutic monoclonal antibody market. *mAbs*, *7*(1), 9–14. DOI: 10.4161/19420862.2014.989042

Eckerstorfer, M. F., Engelhard, M., Heissenberger, A., Simon, S., & Teichmann, H. (2019). Plants developed by new genetic modification techniques—Comparison of existing regulatory frameworks in the EU and non-EU countries. *Frontiers in Bioengineering and Biotechnology*, *7*, 26.

Eggeling, L., & Bott, M. (Eds.). (2005). *Handbook of Corynebacterium glutamicum*. CRC Press., DOI: 10.1201/9781420039696

Eibl, R., Eibl, D., Pörtner, R., Catapano, G., Czermak, P., Catapano, G., & Pörtner, R. (2009). Bioreactor design and scale-up. *Cell and Tissue Reaction Engineering: With a Contribution by Martin Fussenegger and Wilfried Weber*, 173-259. https://doi.org/DOI: 10.1007/978-3-540-68182-3_5

Eibl, R., & Eibl, D. (Eds.). (2019). *Single-use technology in biopharmaceutical manufacture* (2nd ed.). John Wiley & Sons.

Eibl, R., Kaiser, S., Lombriser, R., & Eibl, D. (2010). Disposable bioreactors: The current state-of-the-art and recommended applications in biotechnology. *Applied Microbiology and Biotechnology*, *86*(1), 41–49. DOI: 10.1007/s00253-009-2420-4 PMID: 20094714

Elahi, A., Bukhari, D. A., Shamim, S., & Rehman, A. (2021). Plastics degradation by microbes: A sustainable approach. *Journal of King Saud University. Science*, *33*(6), 101538. DOI: 10.1016/j.jksus.2021.101538

Ellis, J. T., Hengge, N. N., Sims, R. C., & Miller, C. D. (2012). Acetone, butanol, and ethanol production from wastewater algae. *Bioresource Technology*, *111*, 491–495. DOI: 10.1016/j.biortech.2012.02.002 PMID: 22366611

Ellis, T., Adie, T., & Baldwin, G. S. (2011). DNA assembly for synthetic biology: From parts to pathways and beyond. *Integrative Biology, 3*(2), 109–118. DOI: 10.1039/C0IB00070A PMID: 21246151

Elmadhoun, B., Alsaidalani, R., & Burczynski, F. (2025). Quality Risk Management in the Final Operational Stage of Sterile Pharmaceutical Manufacturing: A Case Study Highlighting the Management of Sustainable Related Risks in Product Sterilization, Inspection, Labeling, Packaging, and Storage Processes. *Sustainability, 17*(4), 1670. DOI: 10.3390/su17041670

El-Malek, F. A., Khairy, H., Farag, A., & Omar, S. (2020). The sustainability of microbial bioplastics, production and applications. *International Journal of Biological Macromolecules, 157*, 319–328. DOI: 10.1016/j.ijbiomac.2020.04.076 PMID: 32315677

Elsayed, A., Jaber, N., Al-Remawi, M., & Abu-Salah, K. (2023). From cell factories to patients: Stability challenges in biopharmaceuticals manufacturing and administration with mitigation strategies. *International Journal of Pharmaceutics, 645*, 123360. Advance online publication. DOI: 10.1016/j.ijpharm.2023.123360

EMA. (2018). *Guideline on the requirements for quality documentation concerning biological investigational medicinal products in clinical trials*. European Medicines Agency. https://www.ema.europa.eu

EMA. (2019). Guideline on the Use of Process Analytical Technology (PAT) in the Manufacture of Medicinal Products.

EMA. (2020). Guideline on process validation for the manufacture of biotechnology-derived active substances and data to be provided in the regulatory submission.

EMA. (2022). *Marketing Authorisation Procedures in the EU*. European Medicines Agency. https://www.ema.europa.eu

Emadian, S. M., Onay, T. T., & Demirel, B. (2017). Biodegradation of bioplastics in natural environments. Waste management, 59, 526-536. https://doi.org/DOI: 10.1016/j.wasman.2016.10.006

Embden, G., Meyerhof, O., & Parnas, J. (1934). Glycolysis and the Embden-Meyerhof pathway. *Biochemische Zeitschrift, 273*, 416–429.

Escandell, J. M., Pais, D. A., Carvalho, S. B., & Vincent, K. (2022). *Leveraging rAAV bioprocess understanding and next generation bioanalytics development. Trends in Biotechnology*. https://www.sciencedirect.com/science/article/pii/S0958166921002421

Eslami, T., & Jungbauer, A. (2024). Control strategy for biopharmaceutical production by model predictive control. *Biotechnology Progress, 40*(2), 3426. PMID: 38199980

Esmaeilnejad-Ahranjani, P., & Hajimoradi, M. (2022). Optimization of industrial-scale centrifugal separation of biological products: Comparing the performance of tubular and disc stack centrifuges. *Biochemical Engineering Journal, 178*, 108281.

Estevez, A. T., & Navarro, D. (2017). Biomanufacturing the future: Biodigital architecture & genetics. *Procedia Manufacturing, 12*, 7–16. DOI: 10.1016/j.promfg.2017.08.002

Esvelt, K. M., & Wang, H. H. (2013). Genome-scale engineering for systems and synthetic biology. *Molecular Systems Biology, 9*(1), 641. DOI: 10.1038/msb.2012.66 PMID: 23340847

European Commission. (2015). EudraLex - Volume 4 - Good Manufacturing Practice (GMP) guidelines. https://ec.europa.eu/health/documents/eudralex_en

Evans, H. M. (2019). A New Age of Evolution: Protecting the Consumer's Moral and Legal Right to Know through the Clear and Transparent Labeling of All Genetically Modified Foods. *Journal of Law and Health, 33*, vi.

Evans, J., & Silbey, S. S. (2022). Co-opting regulation: Professional control through discretionary mobilization of legal prescriptions and expert knowledge. *Organization Science, 33*(5), 2041–2064. DOI: 10.1287/orsc.2021.1525

Ezemba, C., Ekwegbalu, E. A., & Ezemba, A. S. (2022). Fermentation, types of fermenters, design & uses of fermenters and optimization of the fermentation process. *Department of Microbiology, Chukwuemeka Odumegwu Ojukwu UniversityPress.* https://www.researchgate.net/publication/358265321_FERMENTATION_TYPES OF_FERMENTERS_DESIGN_USES_OF_FERMENTERS_AND_OPTIMZATI ON_OF_FERMENTATION_PROCESS. ISBN: 978-620-2-05649-6

Fabricio, M. F., Vargas, B. K., Tischer, B., Wagner, R., Ribeiro, S. R., Cordeiro, N., Flôres, S. H., & Ayub, M. A. Z. (2023). Revamping kombucha production: Achieving consistency and probiotic potential through a tailor-made microbial consortium. *International Journal of Gastronomy and Food Science, 34*, 100844.

Fadlallah, H., Jarrahi, M., Herbert, E., Ferrari, R., Mejean, A., & Peerhossaini, H. (2016). Effects of shear stress on the growth rate of micro-organisms in agitated reactors. In *Fluids Engineering Division Summer Meeting* (Vol. 50282, p. V01AT13A006). American Society of Mechanical Engineers. https://doi.org/DOI: 10.1115/FEDSM2016-7590

Fagerberg, L., Strömberg, S., El-Obeid, A., Gry, M., Nilsson, K., Uhlén, M., Pontén, F., & Asplund, A. (2011). Large-scale protein profiling in human cell lines using antibody-based proteomics. *Journal of Proteome Research, 10*(9), 4066–4075. DOI: 10.1021/pr200263f PMID: 21726073

Fajardo, O., Dorado, F., & Lora, A. (2025). The Potential for Bioeconomy and Biotechnology Transfer and Collaboration Between Colombia and China. *Sustainability, 17*(11), 5083. DOI: 10.3390/su17115083

Falcone, P. M. (2023). Sustainable energy policies in developing countries: A review of challenges and opportunities. *Energies, 16*(18), 6682. DOI: 10.3390/en16186682

Fallahi, P., Habte-Tsion, H.-M., & Rossi, W. (2018). Depolymerizating enzymes in human food: bakery, dairy products, and drinks. In *Enzymes in human and animal nutrition* (pp. 211–237). Elsevier.

Fallde, M., & Eklund, M. (2015). Towards a sustainable socio-technical system of biogas for transport: The case of the city of Linköping in Sweden. *Journal of Cleaner Production, 98*, 17–28. DOI: 10.1016/j.jclepro.2014.08.015

Falzarano, M., Polettini, A., Pomi, R., Rossi, A., & Zonfa, T. (2023). Anaerobic Biodegradability of Commercial Bioplastic Products: Systematic Bibliographic Analysis and Critical Assessment of the Latest Advances. *Materials (Basel, Switzerland), 16*(6), 2216. DOI: 10.3390/ma16062216 PMID: 36984096

Famili, P., & Cleary, S. (2022). Laboratory Information Management System (LIMS) and Electronic Data. *Analytical Testing for the Pharmaceutical GMP Laboratory*, 345-373.

Farid, S. S. (2007). Process economics of industrial monoclonal antibody manufacture. *Journal of Chromatography. B, Analytical Technologies in the Biomedical and Life Sciences, 848*(1), 8–18. PMID: 16899415

FDA. (2004). *Guidance for Industry: PAT — A Framework for Innovative Pharmaceutical Development, Manufacturing, and Quality Assurance*. U.S. Food and Drug Administration. https://www.fda.gov

FDA. (2006). Guidance for Industry: Q8(R2) Pharmaceutical Development. U.S. Food and Drug Administration. https://www.fda.gov

FDA. (2017). *Advancement of Emerging Technology Applications for Pharmaceutical Innovation and Modernization*. U.S. Food and Drug Administration.

FDA. (2018). *Cybersecurity for Networked Medical Devices Containing Off-the-Shelf (OTS) Software*. U.S. Food and Drug Administration.

FDA. (2020). *Guidance for Industry: CGMP for Phase 1 Investigational Drugs*. U.S. Food and Drug Administration. https://www.fda.gov

FDA. (2021). *Guidance for Industry: Quality Metrics Reporting Program*. https://www.fda.gov/media/90320/download

FDA. (2023). *FDA Guidance for Industry: Expedited Programs for Serious Conditions – Drugs and Biologics*. https://www.fda.gov/media/86377/download

Feidl, F., Garbellini, S., Luna, M. F., Vogg, S., Souquet, J., Broly, H., Morbidelli, M., & Butté, A. (2019). Combining mechanistic modeling and Raman spectroscopy for monitoring antibody chromatographic purification. *Processes (Basel, Switzerland), 7*(10), 683. Advance online publication. DOI: 10.3390/pr7100683

Feldgarden, M., Brover, V., Haft, D. H., Prasad, A. B., Slotta, D. J., Tolstoy, I., Tyson, G. H., Zhao, S., Hsu, C.-H., & McDermott, P. F. (2019). Validating the AMRFinder tool and resistance gene database by using antimicrobial resistance genotype-phenotype correlations in a collection of isolates. *Antimicrobial Agents and Chemotherapy, 63*(11), 00483–00419. DOI: 10.1128/aac

Feng, K., Miranda, A. V., Obnial, J. C., Ebhodaghe, I. D., & Lucero-Prisno, D. E.III. (2024). Drug regulatory harmonization in the Association of Southeast Asian Nations: Is it time for an ASEAN medicines agency? A policy review. *Clinical Epidemiology and Global Health, 28*, 101649. DOI: 10.1016/j.cegh.2024.101649

Ferasso, M., & Grenier, C. (2021). Fostering SME's co-development of innovative projects in biotech clusters: Extending the sets of enablers for the knowledge creation process. *Technology in Society, 67*, 101729. DOI: 10.1016/j.techsoc.2021.101729

Ferremi Leali, N., Binati, R. L., Martelli, F., Gatto, V., Luzzini, G., Salini, A., Slaghenaufi, D., Fusco, S., Ugliano, M., & Torriani, S. (2022). Reconstruction of simplified microbial consortia to modulate sensory quality of kombucha tea. *Foods, 11*(19), 3045.

Ferrer-Miralles, N., & Villaverde, A. (2013). Bacterial cell factories for recombinant protein production; expanding the catalogue. *Microbial Cell Factories, 12*(1), 113. DOI: 10.1186/1475-2859-12-113

Filippi, M., Mekkattu, M., & Katzschmann, R. K. (2025). Sustainable biofabrication: From bioprinting to AI-driven predictive methods. *Trends in Biotechnology, 43*(2), 290–303. DOI: 10.1016/j.tibtech.2024.07.008

Fink, B. A. (2023). Codex Alimentarius at home and abroad: the regulatory costs of developing and implementing international and national food-safety standards. In *Research Handbook on International Food Law* (pp. 347–367). Edward Elgar Publishing.

Fischer, E. (1894). Einfluss der Configuration auf die Wirkung der Enzyme. *Berichte der Deutschen Chemischen Gesellschaft, 27*(3), 2985–2993. DOI: 10.1002/cber.18940270364

Fisher, A. C., Franco, R. D., & Ho, C. (2021). Biomanufacturing in the age of COVID-19: Advances and challenges in vaccine production. *Trends in Biotechnology, 39*(11), 1164–1176.

Fisher, A. C., Kamga, M. H., Agarabi, C., & Brorson, K. (2019). Integrated Continuous Biomanufacturing. *Trends in Biotechnology, 37*(8), 802–815. DOI: 10.1016/j.tibtech.2019.01.013

Fisher, A. C., Kamga, M. H., Agarabi, C., Brorson, K., Lee, S. L., & Yoon, S. (2019). The current scientific and regulatory landscape in advancing integrated continuous biopharmaceutical manufacturing. *Trends in Biotechnology, 37*(3), 253–267. PMID: 30241924

Fleet, G. H. (2008). Wine yeasts for the future. *FEMS Yeast Research, 8*(7), 979–995. DOI: 10.1111/j.1567-1364.2008.00427.x

Food and Drug Administration. (2004). *PAT—A framework for innovative pharmaceutical development, manufacturing, and quality assurance.* U.S. Food and Drug Administration. https://www.fda.gov/regulatory-information/search-fda-guidance-documents/pat-framework-innovative-pharmaceutical-development-manufacturing-and-quality-assurance

Formenti, L. R., Nørregaard, A., Bolic, A., Hernandez, D. Q., Hagemann, T., Heins, A. L., Larsson, H., Mears, L., Mauricio-Iglesias, M., & Krühne, U. (2014). Challenges in industrial fermentation technology research. *Biotechnology Journal, 9*(6), 727–738.

Forti, V., Balde, C. P., Kuehr, R., & Bel, G. (2020). The Global E-waste Monitor 2020: Quantities, flows and the circular economy potential. https://ewastemonitor.info/wp-content/uploads/2020/11/GEM_2020_def_july1_low.pdf

Frangopol, D. M., & Liu, M. (2019). Maintenance and management of civil infrastructure based on condition, safety, optimization, and life-cycle cost. *Structures and infrastructure systems*, 96-108.

Fredi, G., & Dorigato, A. (2021). Recycling of bioplastic waste: A review. *Advanced Industrial and Engineering Polymer Research, 4*(3), 159–177. DOI: 10.1016/j.aiepr.2021.06.006

Freitag, R. (2013). Chromatographic techniques in the downstream processing of proteins in biotechnology. In *Animal Cell Biotechnology* (pp. 419–458). Methods and Protocols.

Frestedt, J. L. (2018). Foods, food additives, and generally regarded as safe (GRAS) food assessments. *Food control and biosecurity*, 543-565.

Frick, S., Kramell, R., & Kutchan, T. M. (2007). Metabolic engineering with a morphine biosynthetic P450 in opium poppy surpasses breeding. *Metabolic Engineering*, *9*(2), 169–176. DOI: 10.1016/j.ymben.2006.10.004 PMID: 17189709

Fuentes, L. G., Lara, A. R., Martínez, L. M., Ramírez, O. T., Martínez, A., Bolívar, F., & Gosset, G. (2013). Modification of glucose import capacity in Escherichia coli: Physiologic consequences and utility for improving DNA vaccine production. *Microbial Cell Factories*, *12*(1), 42. DOI: 10.1186/1475-2859-12-42

Fuentes-Ramírez, L. E., Bustillos-Cristales, R., Tapia-Hernández, A., Jiménez-Salgado, T., Wang, E. T., Martínez-Romero, E., & Caballero-Mellado, J. (2001). Novel nitrogen-fixing acetic acid bacteria, Gluconacetobacter johannae sp. nov. and Gluconacetobacter azotocaptans sp. nov., associated with coffee plants. *International Journal of Systematic and Evolutionary Microbiology*, *51*(4), 1305–1314. DOI: 10.1099/00207713-51-4-1305

Fuller, A., Fan, Z., Day, C., & Barlow, C. (2020). Digital twin: Enabling technologies, challenges and open research. *IEEE Access : Practical Innovations, Open Solutions*, *8*, 108952–108971.

Fu, R., Kang, L., Zhang, C., & Fei, Q. (2023). Application and progress of techno-economic analysis and life cycle assessment in biomanufacturing of fuels and chemicals. *Green Chemical Engineering*, *4*(2), 189–198. DOI: 10.1016/j.gce.2022.06.002

Gadde, B., Bonnet, S., Menke, C., & Garivait, S. (2009). Air pollutant emissions from rice straw open field burning in India, Thailand and the Philippines. *Environmental Pollution*, *157*(5), 1554–1558. DOI: 10.1016/j.envpol.2009.01.004 PMID: 19201513

Gadd, G. M. (2010). Metals, minerals and microbes: Geomicrobiology and bioremediation. *Microbiology (Reading, England)*, *156*(Pt 3), 609–643. DOI: 10.1099/mic.0.037143-0 PMID: 20019082

Gaitán, M. G. (2021). Licensing as a Central Structure of Technology Transfer Agreements–Joint Venture and Franchising Agreements. *GRUR International*, *70*(5), 427–439. DOI: 10.1093/grurint/ikab032

Galan, E. A., Zhao, H., Wang, X., Dai, Q., Huck, W. T., & Ma, S. (2020). Intelligent microfluidics: The convergence of machine learning and microfluidics in materials science and biomedicine. *Matter*, *3*(6), 1893–1922.

Galbraith, S. C., Bhatia, H., Liu, H., & Yoon, S. (2018). Media formulation optimization: Current and future opportunities. *Current Opinion in Chemical Engineering*, *22*, 42–47.

Galindo Casas, M., Stargardt, P., Mairhofer, J., & Wiltschi, B. (2020). Decoupling Protein Production from Cell Growth Enhances the Site-Specific Incorporation of Noncanonical Amino Acids in *E. coli*. *ACS Synthetic Biology*, *9*(11), 3052–3066. DOI: 10.1021/acssynbio.0c00298

Ganesh, S., Su, Q., Nagy, Z., & Reklaitis, G. (2020). Advancing smart manufacturing in the pharmaceutical industry. In *Smart manufacturing* (pp. 21–57). Elsevier.

Ganigué, R., Puig, S., Batlle-Vilanova, P., Balaguer, M. D., & Colprim, J. (2015). Microbial electrosynthesis of butyrate from carbon dioxide. *Chemical Communications*, *51*(15), 3235–3238. DOI: 10.1039/C4CC10121A PMID: 25608945

Gao, J. Q., Li, D., & Qiao, G. H. (2024). Circular economy strategies in supply chains: Enhancing resource efficiency and sustainable development goals. *Environmental Science and Pollution Research International*, *31*(7), 8751–8767. DOI: 10.1007/s11356-023-31551-z PMID: 38180660

Garbeva, P., Hol, W. H. G., & de Boer, W. (2018). The role of volatile compounds in microbial interactions. *Trends in Microbiology*, *26*(11), 942–953. DOI: 10.1016/j.tim.2018.06.002

García Martínez, J. B., Pearce, J. M., Throup, J., Cates, J., Lackner, M., & Denkenberger, D. C. (2022). Methane single cell protein: Potential to secure a global protein supply against catastrophic food shocks. *Frontiers in Bioengineering and Biotechnology*, *10*, 906704.

García-Fruitós, E. (2012). Lactic acid bacteria: A promising alternative for recombinant protein production. *Microbial Cell Factories*, *11*(1), 157. DOI: 10.1186/1475-2859-11-157

Garcia, L., & Martinez, R. (2023). Enhancing mechanical properties of biobased polymers through nanocomposite formation. *Journal of Sustainable Materials*, *15*(3), 245–260.

Garcia-Ochoa, F., & Gomez, E. (2009). Bioreactor scale-up and oxygen transfer rate in microbial processes: An overview. *Biotechnology Advances*, *27*(2), 153–176. DOI: 10.1016/j.biotechadv.2008.10.006

Garcia-Ochoa, F., Gomez, E., Santos, V. E., & Merchuk, J. C. (2010). Oxygen uptake rate in microbial processes: An overview. *Biochemical Engineering Journal*, *49*(3), 289–307. DOI: 10.1016/j.bej.2010.01.011

Garcıa-Ochoa, F., Santos, V. E., Casas, J. A., & Gómez, E. (2000). Xanthan gum: Production, recovery, and properties. *Biotechnology Advances*, *18*(7), 549–579. DOI: 10.1016/S0734-9750(00)00050-1 PMID: 14538095

Gargalo, C. L., Udugama, I., Pontius, K., Lopez, P. C., Nielsen, R. F., Hasanzadeh, A., & Gernaey, K. V. (2020). Towards smart biomanufacturing: A perspective on recent developments in industrial measurement and monitoring technologies for bio-based production processes. *Journal of Industrial Microbiology & Biotechnology: Official Journal of the Society for Industrial Microbiology and Biotechnology*, *47*(11), 947–964. PMID: 32895764

Garg, V., Velumani, D., Lin, Y.-C., & Haye, A. (2024). A comprehensive review of probiotic claim regulations: Updates from the Asia-Pacific regions, the United States, and Europe. *PharmaNutrition*, •••, 100423.

Garlapati, V. K., Shankar, U., & Budhiraja, A. (2016). Bioconversion technologies of crude glycerol to value added industrial products. *Biotechnology Reports (Amsterdam, Netherlands)*, *9*, 9–14. PMID: 28352587

Gawel, E., Pannicke, N., & Hagemann, N. (2019). A path transition towards a bioeconomy—The crucial role of sustainability. *Sustainability*, *11*(11), 3005.

Gawin, A., Ertesvåg, H., Hansen, S. A. H., Malmo, J., & Brautaset, T. (2020). Translational regulation of periplasmic folding assistants and proteases as a valuable strategy to improve production of translocated recombinant proteins in Escherichia coli. *BMC Biotechnology*, *20*(1), 24. DOI: 10.1186/s12896-020-00615-0

Geada, P., Vicente, A. A., & Teixeira, J. A. (2024) Bioreactor: General Configuration, Classification, and Bioreactor Types. In *Bioreactor Technology in Food Processing* (pp. 36-58). CRC Press. https://doi.org/DOI: 10.1201/9780429424236

Gee, A. P. (2021). Development and Maintenance of a Quality Program. In *Cell Therapy: cGMP Facilities and Manufacturing* (pp. 195–208). Springer.

Geigert, J. (2023). *Regulatory Pathways Impacting Biopharmaceuticals*. In *The Challenge of CMC Regulatory Compliance* (pp. 35–56). Springer. Link

Gellissen, G., Kunze, G., Gaillardin, C., Cregg, J. M., Berardi, E., Veenhuis, M., & van der Klei, I. (2005). New yeast expression platforms based on methylotrophic *Hansenula polymorpha* and *Pichia pastoris* and on dimorphic *Arxula adeninivorans* and *Yarrowia lipolytica*—A comparison. *FEMS Yeast Research*, *5*(11), 1079–1096. DOI: 10.1016/j.femsyr.2005.06.004 PMID: 16144775

George, A. S., & George, A. H. (2024). Riding the wave: An exploration of emerging technologies reshaping modern industry. *Partners Universal International Innovation Journal*, *2*(1), 15–38. DOI: 10.5281/zenodo.10613734

Gérard, A., Woolfe, A., Mottet, G., Reichen, M., Castrillon, C., Menrath, V., & Brenan, C. (2020). High-throughput single-cell activity-based screening and sequencing of antibodies using droplet microfluidics. *Nature Biotechnology*, *38*(6), 715–721. PMID: 32231335

Germain, E., & Stephenson, T. (2005). Biomass characteristics, aeration and oxygen transfer in membrane bioreactors: Their interrelations explained by a review of aerobic biological processes. *Reviews in Environmental Science and Biotechnology*, *4*, 223–233. DOI: 10.1007/s11157-005-2097-3

Gervais, J., & Wang, C. (2025). Flocculation and Filtration. *BioProcess International*, *23*, 3.

Ghaderi, H., Arasteh, J., & Hesampour, A. (2018). Using response surface methodology in combination with Plackett–Burman design for optimization of culture media and extracellular expression of Trichoderma reesei synthetic endoglucanase II in Escherichia coli. *Molecular Biology Reports*, *45*(5), 1197–1208. PMID: 30032381

Ghanemi, A. (2015). Cell cultures in drug development: Applications, challenges and limitations. *Saudi Pharmaceutical Journal : SPJ : the Official Publication of the Saudi Pharmaceutical Society*, *23*(4), 453–454. DOI: 10.1016/j.jsps.2014.04.002

Ghasemi, M., Kanani, M., & Rahimnejad, M. (2021). Recent advances in biopharmaceuticals production with flexible and smart manufacturing systems. *Biotechnology Letters*, *43*(3), 519–532.

Ghasemi, R., & Behzadnia, N. (2018). Real-time monitoring and control strategies in biopharmaceutical manufacturing. *Journal of Industrial Microbiology & Biotechnology*, *45*(7), 593–606.

Ghobashy, M. M., Elhady, M. A., & El-Sawy, N. M. (2021). Radiation crosslinking of modifying biodegradable plastics for sustainable future: A review. *Journal of Polymer Research*, *28*(10), 389. DOI: 10.1007/s10965-021-02751-3

Ghosh, R.. (2020). Artificial intelligence and machine learning in biomanufacturing: A review. *Biotechnology Journal*, *15*(9), 1900566.

Ghosh, R.. (2020). Artificial intelligence and machine learning inbiomanufacturing: A review. *Biotechnology Journal*, *15*(9), 1900566.

Giacomucci, L., Raddadi, N., Soccio, M., Lotti, N., & Fava, F. (2020). Biodegradation of polyvinyl chloride plastic films by enriched anaerobic marine consortia. *Marine Environmental Research*, *158*, 104949. DOI: 10.1016/j.marenvres.2020.104949 PMID: 32217303

Gibbons, L., Maslanka, F., Le, N., Magill, A., Singh, P., Mclaughlin, J., Madden, F., Hayes, R., McCarthy, B., Rode, C., & O'Mahony, J. (2023). An assessment of the impact of Raman-based glucose feedback control on CHO cell bioreactor process development. *Biotechnology Progress*, *39*(5), e3371. Advance online publication. DOI: 10.1002/btpr.3371

Gillespie, P. F., Wang, Y., Yin, K., Groegler, E., Cunningham, N., Stiving, A. Q., Raffaele, J., Marusa, N., Tubbs, C. M., Loughney, J. W., & Winters, M. A. (2024). Automated, quantitative capillary Western blots to analyze host cell proteins in COVID-19 vaccine produced in Vero cell line. *Vaccines*, *12*(12), 1373. Advance online publication. DOI: 10.3390/vaccines12121373

Gillum, D. R., Moritz, R., & Koblentz, G. D. (2024). Establishing a national biosafety and biosecurity agency for the United States. *Frontiers in Bioengineering and Biotechnology*, *12*, 1474120. DOI: 10.3389/fbioe.2024.1474120 PMID: 39483610

Giri, N. A., Sakhale, B. K., & Nirmal, N. P. (2023). Functional beverages: an emerging trend in beverage world. *Recent Frontiers of Phytochemicals*, 123-142.

Glick, B. R. (1995). Metabolic load and heterologous gene expression. *Biotechnology Advances*, *13*(2), 247–261. DOI: 10.1016/0734-9750(95)00004-A PMID: 14537822

Glick, B. R. (2010). Using soil bacteria to facilitate phytoremediation. *Biotechnology Advances*, *28*(3), 367–374. DOI: 10.1016/j.biotechadv.2010.02.001 PMID: 20149857

Godbolea, A., Awate, S., Varadana, O. N., & Suresha, S. (2018). Biomass to Biofuel: A Review of Technologies of Production and Future Prospects. *International Journal of Engineering Research & Technology (Ahmedabad)*, *7*, 24–32. DOI: 10.17577/IJERTV7IS040017

Goeddel, D. V., Kleid, D. G., Bolivar, F., Heyneker, H. L., Yansura, D. G., Crea, R., Hirose, T., Kraszewski, A., Itakura, K., & Riggs, A. D. (1979). Expression in *Escherichia coli* of chemically synthesized genes for human insulin. *Proceedings of the National Academy of Sciences of the United States of America*, *76*(1), 106–110. DOI: 10.1073/pnas.76.1.106

Goker, M., Kurbanoglu, S., Huri, P. Y., Sezgintürk, M. K., & Ozkan, S. A. (2020). Bioprocess monitoring by biosensor-based technologies. In *Commercial Biosensors and Their Applications* (pp. 259–285). Elsevier.

Goldrick, S., Duran-Villalobos, C. A., Jankauskas, K., Lovett, D., Farid, S. S., & Lennox, B. (2019). Modern day monitoring and control challenges outlined on an industrial-scale benchmark fermentation process. *Computers & Chemical Engineering*, *130*, 106471.

Gomaa, A. (2018). Application of enzymes in brewing. *J. Nutr. Food Sci. Forecast*, *1*(5).

Gomes, D. G., Coelho, E., Silva, R., Domingues, L., & Teixeira, J. A. (2023). Bioreactors and engineering of filamentous fungi cultivation. In *Current developments in biotechnology and bioengineering* (pp. 219–250). Elsevier., DOI: 10.1016/B978-0-323-91872-5.00018-1

Gomes, T. A., Zanette, C. M., & Spier, M. R. (2020). An overview of cell disruption methods for intracellular biomolecules recovery. *Preparative Biochemistry & Biotechnology*, *50*(7), 635–654. PMID: 32074000

Gonçalves, G. C. V., Weis, C. M. S. C., Wolff, É. R., Alves, V., Sanches, F. L., Tormen, L., Treichel, H., & Bertan, L. C. (2025). Vegan fermented drinks as an alternative to milk: Trend or challenge? *Food Science and Engineering*, 1-26.

González-Gloria, K. D., Rodríguez-Jasso, R. M., Saxena, R., Sindhu, R., Ali, S. S., Singhania, R. R., & Ruiz, H. A. (2022). Bubble column bioreactor design and evaluation for bioethanol production using simultaneous saccharification and fermentation strategy from hydrothermally pretreated lignocellulosic biomass. *Biochemical Engineering Journal*, *187*, 108645.

Gonzalez, R., & Martinez, H. (2023). The role of biobased polymers in achieving sustainable development goals. *Journal of Green Chemistry*, *12*(5), 345–362.

Goodman, A.-L. (2019). A Natural Stand Off between the Food and Drug Administration and the Courts: The Rise in Food-Labeling Litigation & the Need for Regulatory Reform. *BCL Rev.*, *60*, 271.

Goshtasbi, H., Okolodkov, Y. B., Movafeghi, A., Awale, S., Safary, A., Barar, J., & Omidi, Y. (2023). Harnessing microalgae as sustainable cellular factories for biopharmaceutical production. *Algal Research*, *74*, 103237.

Gottschalk, U. (2017). *Process scale purification of antibodies*. CRC Press.

Gottschalk, U., Brorson, K., & Shukla, A. A. (2012). The need for innovation in biomanufacturing. *Nature Biotechnology*, *30*(6), 489–492. DOI: 10.1038/nbt.2263

Gouda, M. K., Swellam, A. E., & Omar, S. H. (2024). Production of biodiesel by enzymatic transesterification [Review]. *Energy Sources. Part A, Recovery, Utilization, and Environmental Effects*, *46*(1), 1–21. DOI: 10.1080/15567036.2023.2283993

Goulet, D. R., & Atkins, W. M. (2020). Considerations for the design of antibody-based therapeutics. *Journal of Pharmaceutical Sciences*, *109*(1), 74–103. DOI: 10.1016/j.xphs.2019.05.031 PMID: 31173761

Gramer, M. J. (2014). Product quality considerations for mammalian cell culture process development and manufacturing. *Advances in Biochemical Engineering/Biotechnology*, *139*, 123–166. PMID: 23748351

Graumann, K., & Premstaller, A. (2006). Manufacturing of recombinant therapeutic proteins in microbial systems. *Biotechnology Journal, 1*(2), 164–186. DOI: 10.1002/biot.200500051

Gregory, F. D., & Trump, B. D. (2023). The Evolving Landscape of Biotechnology Research: Challenges and Opportunities in Acquisitions, Funding, Education, and Workforce Development for a Productive Bioeconomy. *Advanced Study Institute on NATO ASI on Quantum Nano-Photonics*, 25-50. https://doi.org/DOI: 10.1007/978-94-024-2296-2_2

Gronemeyer, P., Ditz, R., & Strube, J. (2014). Trends in upstream and downstream process development for antibody manufacturing. *Bioengineering (Basel, Switzerland), 1*(4), 188–212. PMID: 28955024

Gronemeyer, P., Ditz, R., & Strube, J. (2014). Trends in Upstream and Downstream Process Development for Antibody Manufacturing. *Bioengineering (Basel, Switzerland), 1*(4), 188–212. PMID: 28955024

GSK. (2021). *Artificial Intelligence and Machine Learning in Biomanufacturing*. Retrieved from https://www.gsk.com/en-gb/media/press-releases/gsk-uses-ai-in-manufacturing

GSK. (2022). *Digital Transformation in Vaccine Manufacturing*. GSK Innovation Reports.

Guieysse, B., Quijano Govantes, G., & Muñoz Torre, R. (2011). Airlift bioreactors—Bioreactors design. In *Comprehensive biotechnology* (2nd ed., pp. 159–170). Elsevier., DOI: 10.1016/B978-0-08-088504-9.00107-7

Guo, W., Sheng, J., & Feng, X. (2015). 13C-metabolic flux analysis: An accurate approach to demystify microbial metabolism for biochemical production. *Bioengineering (Basel, Switzerland), 3*(1), 3. PMID: 28952565

Guo, X.-Q., Wei, Y.-M., & Yu, B. (2012). Recombinant Mycobacterium smegmatis expressing Hsp65–hIL–2 fusion protein and its influence on lymphocyte function in mice. *Asian Pacific Journal of Tropical Medicine, 5*(5), 347–351. DOI: 10.1016/S1995-7645(12)60056-X

Guo, Z., Zhou, Y., Li, J., Liu, D., Huang, Y., Zhang, Y., Yu, R., & Zhu, J. (2025). Dihydroartemisinic acid dehydrogenase-mediated alternative route for artemisinin biosynthesis. *Nature Communications, 16*(1), 3888. DOI: 10.1038/s41467-025-59312-1 PMID: 40274872

Gupta, A., & Zahir, F. (2020). Biosafety Issues for Scientists and Laboratory Workers. In *Introduction to Occupational Health Hazards* (pp. 114–157). Bentham Science Publishers.

Gupta, K., Karihaloo, J. L., & Khetarpal, R. K. (2014). *Biosafety regulations for GM crops in Asia-Pacific*. Asia-Pacific Association of Agricultural Research Institutions.

Gupta, N., Wijenayake, W. P. T., Roy, D., Kumar, R., Rangot, M., Chugh, P., Santoyo, G., Chattaraj, S., Bhaskar, S. S., Andjelković, S., & Guerra-Sierra, B. E. (2025). Smart Recycling and Sustainable Lignocellulosic Waste Management. In *Value Addition and Utilization of Lignocellulosic Biomass: Through Novel Technological Interventions* (pp. 221–250). Springer Nature Singapore.

Gurawalia, H., Shinde, P. B., & Sharma, K. K. (2024). Embracing Industry 4.0 Ingredients in Synthetic Biology for the Development of Carbon–Neutral Economy. In *Biorefinery and Industry 4.0: Empowering Sustainability* (pp. 215–252). Springer Nature Switzerland.

Gurunathan, M. K., Navasingh, R. J. H., Selvam, J. D. R., & Čep, R. (2025). Development and characterization of starch bioplastics as a sustainable alternative for packaging. *Scientific Reports, 15*(1), 15264. DOI: 10.1038/s41598-025-00221-0 PMID: 40312412

Gyorgypal, A., Yang, O., & Chopda, V. (2022). *Recent advances in integrated process analytical techniques and control strategies for monoclonal antibody biomanufacturing. Journal of Chemical Technology and Biotechnology*. https://www.researchgate.net/publication/351056378

Haider, S. I., & Asif, S. E. (2016). *Quality Control Training Manual: Comprehensive Training Guide for API, Finished Pharmaceutical and Biotechnologies Laboratories*. CRC Press.

Halim-Lim, S. A., Jamaludin, A. A., Islam, A. T., Weerabahu, S., & Priyono, A. (2025). Unlocking potential for a circular bioeconomy transition through digital innovation, lean manufacturing and green practices: A review. *Management of Environmental Quality, 36*(1), 130–154.

Halstead, D. C., & Sautter, R. L. (2023). A literature review on how we can address medical laboratory scientist staffing shortages. *Laboratory Medicine, 54*(1), e31–e36. DOI: 10.1093/labmed/lmac090 PMID: 36149058

Hamid, K. A., Elsayed, E. A., El Enshasy, H. A., Esawy, M., & Malek, R. A. (2018). Bioprocess optimization for levan production by Bacillus subtilis B58. *Journal of Scientific and Industrial Research, 77*, 386–393.

Hang, Y., Boryczka, J., & Wu, N. (2022). Visible-light and near-infrared fluorescence and surface-enhanced Raman scattering point-of-care sensing and bio-imaging: A review. *Chemical Society Reviews, 51*(1), 329–375. PMID: 34897302

Hansen, E. H., Møller, B. L., Kock, G. R., Bünner, C. M., Kristensen, C., Jensen, O. R., Okkels, F. T., Olsen, C. E., Motawia, M. S., & Hansen, J. (2009). De novo biosynthesis of vanillin in fission yeast (*Schizosaccharomyces pombe*) and baker's yeast (*Saccharomyces cerevisiae*). *Applied and Environmental Microbiology, 75*(9), 2765–2774. DOI: 10.1128/AEM.02681-08 PMID: 19286778

Harding, K. G., Dennis, J. S., von Blottnitz, H., & Harrison, S. T. L. (2017). A life-cycle comparison between inorganic and biological catalysis for the production of biodiesel. *Journal of Cleaner Production, 142*, 3157–3169. DOI: 10.1016/j.jclepro.2016.10.134

Haris, M., Fatima, N., Iqbal, J., Chalgham, W., Mumtaz, A. S., El-Sheikh, M. A., & Tavafoghi, M. (2023). Oscillatoria limnetica mediated green synthesis of iron oxide (Fe2O3) nanoparticles and their diverse in vitro bioactivities. *Molecules (Basel, Switzerland), 28*(5), 2091. PMID: 36903337

Harrer, S. (2023). Attention is not all you need: The complicated case of ethically using large language models in healthcare and medicine. *EBioMedicine, 90*. Advance online publication. DOI: 10.1016/j.ebiom.2023.104512 PMID: 36924620

Harvey, A. L., Edrada-Ebel, R., & Quinn, R. J. (2015). The re-emergence of natural products for drug discovery in the genomics era. *Nature Reviews. Drug Discovery, 14*(2), 111.

Hasegawa, S., Suda, M., Uematsu, K., Natsuma, Y., Hiraga, K., Jojima, T., Inui, M., & Yukawa, H. (2013). Engineering of Corynebacterium glutamicum for High-Yield <scp>l</scp> -Valine Production under Oxygen Deprivation Conditions. *Applied and Environmental Microbiology, 79*(4), 1250–1257. DOI: 10.1128/AEM.02806-12

Hassane, A. M., Obiedallah, M., Karimi, J., Khattab, S. M., Hussein, H. R., Abo-Dahab, Y., Eltoukhy, A., Abo-Dahab, N. F., & Abouelela, M. E. (2025). Unravelling fungal genome editing revolution: Pathological and biotechnological application aspects. *Archives of Microbiology, 207*(7), 150.

Hassan, Y. M., Mohamed, A. S., Hassan, Y. M., & El-Sayed, W. M. (2025). Recent developments and future directions in point-of-care next-generation CRISPR-based rapid diagnosis. *Clinical and Experimental Medicine, 25*(1), 1–15. DOI: 10.1007/s10238-024-01540-8 PMID: 39789283

HD, A., & Vijayan P. U, H. (2025). Bio-green Evolution: The Journey of Microalgae Products from Lab to Market—An Overview of Microalgae-Based Processes and Products—Part I. *Microalgae Horizons: Fundamentals, Innovations, and Industrial Applications*, 185-275.

Hekmat, D. (2015). Large-scale crystallization of proteins for purification and formulation. *Bioprocess and Biosystems Engineering, 38*(7), 1209–1231. PMID: 25700885

Hemmerich, J., Noack, S., Wiechert, W., & Oldiges, M. (2018). Microbioreactor systems for accelerated bioprocess development. *Biotechnology Journal, 13*(4), 1700141. DOI: 10.1002/biot.201700141 PMID: 29283217

Herdlevær, K. M., & Barth, T. (2024). Optimizing formic acid-assisted Co-HTL of digested sewage sludge and lignocellulosic waste for enhanced bio-crude yield and energy recovery. *Energies, 17*(1), 258. DOI: 10.3390/en17010258

Hernández-Longoria, R., Hernández-Ruiz, Y., Gutiérrez-Jasso, F., & Zarazúa, A. (2021). Validation of an analytical method for the quantification of human fibrinogen in pharmaceutical products by size-exclusion liquid chromatography (SEC-HPLC). *International Journal of Hematology, 113*(4), 480–492. DOI: 10.1007/s12185-020-03045-5

He, Y., Degraeve, P., & Oulahal, N. (2024). Bioprotective yeasts: Potential to limit postharvest spoilage and to extend shelf life or improve microbial safety of processed foods. *Heliyon, 10*(3).

HHS. (2022). *Healthcare Cybersecurity and Risk Mitigation Guide*. Department of Health and Human Services.

Hickey, J. M., Santiago, M. G., & Carlson, E. D. (2020). Flexible biomanufacturing: Industry perspectives on single-use technologies and facility design. *Biotechnology Advances, 44*, 107608.

Hidalgo-Fuentes, B., de Jesús-José, E., Cabrera-Hidalgo, A. J., Sandoval-Castilla, O., Espinosa-Solares, T., González-Reza, R. M., Zambrano-Zaragoza, M. L., Liceaga, A. M., & Aguilar-Toalá, J. E. (2024). Plant-based fermented beverages: Nutritional composition, sensory properties, and health benefits. *Foods, 13*(6), 844.

Hirani, A. H., Javed, N., Asif, M., Basu, S. K., & Kumar, A. (2018). A review on first-and second-generation biofuel productions. Biofuels: greenhouse gas mitigation and global warming: next generation biofuels and role of biotechnology, 141-154. http://dx.doi.org/DOI: 10.1007/978-81-322-3763-1_8

Hirasawa, T., & Maeda, T. (2022). Adaptive laboratory evolution of microorganisms: Methodology and application for bioproduction. *Microorganisms, 11*(1), 92.

Hirst, M. B., & Richter, C. L. (2016). Review of aroma formation through metabolic pathways of *Saccharomyces cerevisiae* in beverage fermentations. *American Journal of Enology and Viticulture, 67*(4), 361–370. DOI: 10.5344/ajev.2016.15098

Hoang, A. T., Nižetić, S., Ng, K. H., Papadopoulos, A. M., Le, A. T., Kumar, S., Hadiyanto, H., & Pham, V. V. (2022). Microbial fuel cells for bioelectricity production from waste as sustainable prospect of future energy sector. *Chemosphere, 287*(Pt 3), 132285. DOI: 10.1016/j.chemosphere.2021.132285 PMID: 34563769

Hoang, P. H., Hoang, H. H., & Chung, W. (2022). Extraction and characterization of polyhydroxyalkanoates from microbial biomass. *Journal of Environmental Chemical Engineering, 10*(3), 107419. DOI: 10.1016/j.jece.2022.107419

Hock, S. C., Kian, S. M., & Wah, C. L. (2020). Global challenges in the manufacture, regulation and international harmonization of GMP and quality standards for biopharmaceuticals. *Generics and Biosimilars Initiative Journal, 9*(2), 52+. https://link.gale.com/apps/doc/A677574365/AONE?u=anon~82686abc&sid=googleScholar&xid=8b9cb9ef

Hodgman, C. E., & Jewett, M. C. (2012). Cell-free synthetic biology: Thinking outside the cell. *Metabolic Engineering, 14*(3), 261–269. DOI: 10.1016/j.ymben.2011.09.002 PMID: 21946161

Hoff, B., Plassmeier, J., Blankschien, M., Letzel, A. C., Kourtz, L., Schröder, H., Koch, W., & Zelder, O. (2021). Unlocking nature's biosynthetic power—Metabolic engineering for the fermentative production of chemicals. *Angewandte Chemie International Edition, 60*(5), 2258–2278.

Holland, I., & Davies, J. A. (2020). Automation in the life science research laboratory. *Frontiers in Bioengineering and Biotechnology, 8*, 571777. PMID: 33282848

Holzer, R., Bloch, W., & Brinkmann, C. (2020). Minimally invasive electrochemical patch-based sensor system for monitoring glucose and lactate in the human body—A survey-based analysis of the end-user's perspective. *Sensors (Basel), 20*(20), 5761. PMID: 33050656

Hong, M., Chen, E. Y. X., & Chen, X. (2021). Towards truly sustainable polymers: A metal-free recyclable polyester from biorenewable non-strained γ-butyrolactone. *Nature Chemistry, 13*(11), 1043–1049. DOI: 10.1038/s41557-021-00748-5

Hopewell, J., Dvorak, R., & Kosior, E. (2009). Plastics recycling: Challenges and opportunities. *Philosophical Transactions of the Royal Society of London. Series B, Biological Sciences, 364*(1526), 2115–2126. DOI: 10.1098/rstb.2008.0311 PMID: 19528059

Ho, S. H., Huang, S. W., Chen, C. Y., Hasunuma, T., Kondo, A., & Chang, J. S. (2013). Bioethanol production using carbohydrate-rich microalgae biomass as feedstock. *Bioresource Technology, 135*, 191–198. DOI: 10.1016/j.biortech.2012.10.015 PMID: 23116819

Hosinski, G. **(2022).** *IoT at Amgen – Evaluating and piloting Industry 4.0 technology in biomanufacturing* (Master's thesis, Massachusetts Institute of Technology).

Hosoya, Y., Okamoto, S., Muramatsu, H., & Ochi, K. (1998). Acquisition of Certain Streptomycin-Resistant (*str*) Mutations Enhances Antibiotic Production in Bacteria. *Antimicrobial Agents and Chemotherapy, 42*(8), 2041–2047. DOI: 10.1128/AAC.42.8.2041

Hossain, M. M., Kabir, M. H., & Kim, J. H. (2023). Application of AI in biomanufacturing: Challenges and future prospects. *Computers in Biology and Medicine*, *155*, 106554.

Howell, J. (2023). Regulatory considerations of encapsulation used in the food industry. In *Microencapsulation in the Food Industry* (pp. 419–425). Elsevier.

Hsu, P. D., Scott, D. A., & Weinstein, J. A. (2013). DNA targeting specificity of RNA-guided Cas9 nucleases. *Nature Biotechnology*, *31*(9), 827–832. DOI: 10.1038/nbt.2647

Huang, M. nan, Lu, X. yao, Zong, H., Zhuge, B., & Shen, W. (2018). Bioproduction of trans-10,cis-12-Conjugated Linoleic Acid by a Highly Soluble and Conveniently Extracted Linoleic Acid Isomerase and an Extracellularly Expressed Lipase from Recombinant Escherichia coli Strains. *Journal of Microbiology and Biotechnology*, *28*(5), 739–747. DOI: 10.4014/jmb.1802.02007

Huang, X., Ma, L., Li, R., & Liu, Z. (2020). Determinants of innovation ecosystem in underdeveloped areas—Take nanning high-tech zone in western china as an example. *Journal of Open Innovation*, *6*(4), 135. DOI: 10.3390/joitmc6040135

Huang, Y. M., Hu, W., Rustandi, E., Chang, K., Yusuf-Makagiansar, H., & Ryll, T. (2010). Maximizing productivity of CHO cell culture using chemically defined media in fed-batch culture. *Biotechnology Progress*, *26*(5), 1400–1410. PMID: 20945494

Huang, Y. M., Hu, W., Rustandi, E., Chang, K., Yusuf-Makagiansar, H., & Ryll, T. (2010). Maximizing productivity of CHO cell-based fed-batch culture using chemically defined media in stirred-tank bioreactors. *Biotechnology and Bioengineering*, *106*(4), 804–814. PMID: 21404255

Hundleby, P. A. C., & Sack, M. (2018). Biosafety, Risk Assessment and Regulation of Molecular Farming. In *Plant Biotechnology and Emerging Areas*. Wiley., DOI: 10.1002/9781118801512.ch13

Hunt, M. M., Meng, G., Rancourt, D. E., Gates, I. D., & Kallos, M. S. (2014). Factorial experimental design for the culture of human embryonic stem cells as aggregates in stirred suspension bioreactors reveals the potential for interaction effects between bioprocess parameters. *Tissue Engineering. Part C, Methods*, *20*(1), 76–89. PMID: 23668683

Hu, Q., Qi, H., Bai, Z., Dou, M., Zeng, J., Zhang, F., & Zhang, H. (2007). Biosorption of cadmium by a Cd 2+-hyperresistant Bacillus cereus strain HQ-1 newly isolated from a lead and zinc mine. *World Journal of Microbiology & Biotechnology*, *23*, 971–976. DOI: 10.1007/s11274-006-9322-2

Hu, Q., Sommerfeld, M., Jarvis, E., Ghirardi, M., Posewitz, M., Seibert, M., & Darzins, A. (2008). Microalgal triacylglycerols as feedstocks for biofuel production: Perspectives and advances. *The Plant Journal*, *54*(4), 621–639. DOI: 10.1111/j.1365-313X.2008.03492.x PMID: 18476868

Hu, S., Kong, J., Sun, Z., Han, L., Kong, W., & Yang, P. (2011). Heterologous protein display on the cell surface of lactic acid bacteria mediated by the s-layer protein. *Microbial Cell Factories*, *10*(1), 86. DOI: 10.1186/1475-2859-10-86

Hussain, Z., Mishra, J., & Vanacore, E. (2020). Waste to energy and circular economy: The case of anaerobic digestion. *Journal of Enterprise Information Management*, *33*(4), 817–838.

Ibrahim, H. M., Yusoff, W. M. W., Hamid, A. A., Illias, R. M., Hassan, O., & Omar, O. (2005). Optimization of medium for the production of β-cyclodextrin glucanotransferase using Central Composite Design (CCD). *Process Biochemistry*, *40*(2), 753–758.

ICH Q9. (2023). *Quality Risk Management.* International Council for Harmonisation. https://www.ich.org/page/quality-guidelines

ICH. (2021). *ICH Q12: Technical and Regulatory Considerations for Pharmaceutical Product Lifecycle Management.* International Council for Harmonisation. https://www.ich.org

Imamoglu, E. (2024). Artificial Intelligence and/or Machine Learning Algorithms in Microalgae Bioprocesses. *Bioengineering (Basel, Switzerland), 11*(11), 1143. PMID: 39593803

Ingrao, C., Gigli, M., & Siracusa, V. (2017). An attributional Life Cycle Assessment application experience to highlight environmental hotspots in the production of foamy polylactic acid trays for fresh-food packaging usage. *Journal of Cleaner Production, 150*, 93–103. DOI: 10.1016/j.jclepro.2017.03.007

Iowa State University. (2001). *Plant Sciences Institute update. Iowa State University Plant Sciences Institute Newsletter, 2*(1).

Ishwarya, S. P., Anandharamakrishnan, C., & Stapley, A. G. (2015). Spray-freeze-drying: A novel process for the drying of foods and bioproducts. *Trends in Food Science & Technology, 41*(2), 161–181.

Isoko, K., Cordiner, J. L., Kis, Z., & Moghadam, P. Z. (2024). Bioprocessing 4.0: A pragmatic review and future perspectives. *Digital Discovery, 3*(9), 1662–1681. DOI: 10.1039/D4DD00085B

ISPE. (2020). *Pharmaceutical Workforce of the Future: Education and Training for Advanced Manufacturing*. International Society for Pharmaceutical Engineering.

Issaoui, M., Jellali, S., Zorpas, A. A., & Dutournie, P. (2022). Membrane technology for sustainable water resources management: Challenges and future projections. *Sustainable Chemistry and Pharmacy, 25*, 100590.

Jacquemart, R., Lin, Y. H., & Kamen, A. A. (2016). Biomanufacturing of viral vectors: Industrial challenges and opportunities. *Biotechnology Journal, 11*(4), 473–484. PMID: 26632496

Jacquemart, R., Lin, Y. H., Stern, B., Azouz, A., & Kamen, A. (2016). Manufacturing of adenovirus vectors: Part I. Upstream processes. *Pharmaceutical Bioprocessing, 4*(3), 183–197.

Jadhav, R. R., & Khare, D. (2024). Green biotherapeutics: Overcoming challenges in plant-based expression platforms. *Plant Biotechnology Reports, 18*(4), 465–486.

Jagschies, G., Lindskog, E., Łącki, K., & Galliher, P. (2018). *Biopharmaceutical processing: Development, design, and implementation of manufacturing processes*. Elsevier.

Jahangirian, H., Lemraski, E. G., Webster, T. J., Rafiee-Moghaddam, R., & Abdollahi, Y. (2020). A review of environmentally friendly synthesis of pharmaceuticals using biocatalysis and green chemistry principles. *Biotechnology Advances, 38*, 107322.

Jain, N., Waidi, Y. O., Barua, R., Das, S., Vannaladsaysy, V., Prasad, A., & Datta, S. (2024). Bioinspired Nanocomposites: Multifunctional Materials towards Sustainable Alternatives. In *Nanomanufacturing Techniques in Sustainable Healthcare Applications* (pp. 78-93). CRC Press.

Jain, N., Waidi, Y. O., Barua, R., Vannaladsaysy, V., Prasad, A., & Datta, S. (2024). Plastic recycling for energy production. *Biodegradable Waste Processing for Sustainable Developments*, 113.

Jain, N., Barua, R., & Datta, S. (2025). Functional Nanomaterials and their Applications in Biomedicine. In *Bioabsorbable Polymers for Drug Carriers and Fixation Devices* (pp. 61–79). Apple Academic Press.

Jain, S. (2016). Regulatory Requirements for New Drug Approval in Different Countries: An Overview. [Link to PDF]. *World Journal of Pharmaceutical Research*, *5*(6), 786–816.

Jairoun, A. A., Al-Hemyari, S. S., Shahwan, M., Alkhoujah, S., El-Dahiyat, F., Jaber, A. A. S., & Zyoud, S. H. (2025). Towards eco-friendly pharmaceuticals: Regulatory and policy approaches for sustainable medicines use. *Exploratory Research in Clinical and Social Pharmacy*, *17*, 100576. DOI: 10.1016/j.rcsop.2025.100576 PMID: 40026320

Jaiswal, S., Sharma, B., & Shukla, P. (2020). Integrated approaches in microbial degradation of plastics. *Environmental Technology & Innovation*, *17*, 100567. DOI: 10.1016/j.eti.2019.100567

Jana, S. C., Madhusree, C., & Utpal, R. (2019). Optimization of media and culture conditions for improved production of bacteriocin by using conventional one-factor-at-a-time (OFAT) method. *EC Microbiology*, *15*, 251–258.

Janković, T., Straathof, A. J., & Kiss, A. A. (2024). Eco-efficient downstream processing of 1, 3-propanediol applicable to various fermentation processes. *Process Biochemistry*, *143*, 210–224.

Jannah, S. R., Rahayu, E. S., Yanti, R., Suroto, D. A., & Wikandari, R. (2022). Study of Viability, Storage Stability, and Shelf Life of Probiotic Instant Coffee Lactiplantibacillus plantarum Subsp. plantarum Dad-13 in Vacuum and Nonvacuum Packaging at Different Storage Temperatures. *International Journal of Food Sciences*, *2022*(1), 1663772.

Jansen, M. L. A., Bracher, J. M., Papapetridis, I., Verhoeven, M. D., de Bruijn, H., de Waal, P. P., van Maris, A. J. A., Klaassen, P., & Pronk, J. T. (2017). Saccharomyces cerevisiae strains for second-generation ethanol production: From academic exploration to industrial implementation. *FEMS Yeast Research*, *17*(5). Advance online publication. DOI: 10.1093/femsyr/fox044

Jariyasakoolroj, T., Tashiro, K., & Wang, H. (2020). Advanced supramolecular design for direct ink writing of soft materials. *Advanced Materials*, *32*(39), 2003760. DOI: 10.1002/adma.202003760

Jayakody, L. N., Ferdouse, J., & Hayashi, K. (2022). Alginate-based composites for packaging applications: A review. *Journal of Polymers and the Environment*, *30*(5), 1747–1767. DOI: 10.1007/s10924-021-02315-w

Jayakrishnan, A., Wan Rosli, W. R., Tahir, A. R. M., Razak, F. S. A., Kee, P. E., Ng, H. S., Chew, Y.-L., Lee, S.-K., Ramasamy, M., & Tan, C. S. (2024). Evolving paradigms of recombinant protein production in pharmaceutical industry: A rigorous review. *Sci*, *6*(1), 9.

Jenkins, T. E. (2013). *Aeration control system design: a practical guide to energy and process optimization*. John Wiley & Sons.

Jenzsch, M., Bell, C., Buziol, S., Kepert, F., Wegele, H., & Hakemeyer, C. (2018). Trends in process analytical technology: Present state in bioprocessing. In *New bioprocessing strategies: Development and manufacturing of recombinant antibodies and proteins* (pp. 211–252). Springer., DOI: 10.1007/10_2017_48

Jeong, H., Barbe, V., Lee, C. H., Vallenet, D., Yu, D. S., Choi, S.-H., Couloux, A., Lee, S.-W., Yoon, S. H., Cattolico, L., Hur, C.-G., Park, H.-S., Ségurens, B., Kim, S. C., Oh, T. K., Lenski, R. E., Studier, F. W., Daegelen, P., & Kim, J. F. (2009). Genome Sequences of Escherichia coli B strains REL606 and BL21(DE3). *Journal of Molecular Biology*, *394*(4), 644–652. DOI: 10.1016/j.jmb.2009.09.052

Jeyachandran, S., Vibhute, P., Kumar, D., & Ragavendran, C. (2024). Random mutagenesis as a tool for industrial strain improvement for enhanced production of antibiotics: A review. *Molecular Biology Reports*, *51*(1), 19.

Jia, H., Harikumar, P., Atkinson, E., Rigsby, P., & Wadhwa, M. (2021). The first WHO international standard for harmonizing the biological activity of bevacizumab. *Biomolecules*, *11*(11), 1610. Advance online publication. DOI: 10.3390/biom11111610

Jiang, J., Ma, Y., Zhou, L., Han, W., Liang, Y., Dong, J., Ding, Y., Li, W., Lei, Q., & Li, J. (2025). Synergistic Genetic and Chemical Engineering of Probiotics for Enhanced Intestinal Microbiota Regulation and Ulcerative Colitis Treatment. *Advanced Materials*, ●●●, 2417050.

Jiang, W., Bikard, D., Cox, D., Zhang, F., & Marraffini, L. A. (2013). RNA-guided editing of bacterial genomes using CRISPR-Cas systems. *Nature Biotechnology*, *31*(3), 233–239. DOI: 10.1038/nbt.2508 PMID: 23360965

Jiménez-González, C., & Woodley, J. M. (2010). Bioprocesses: Modeling needs for process evaluation and sustainability assessment. *Computers & Chemical Engineering*, *34*(7), 1009–1017. DOI: 10.1016/j.compchemeng.2010.03.004

Jing, J., Chen, Y., Sheng, L., & Wu, M. (2018). Optimized production of insulin variant, a recombinant platelet aggregation inhibitor, by high cell-density fermentation of recombinant Escherichia coli. *Protein Expression and Purification*, *152*, 7–12. PMID: 30033357

Jin, H., Cantin, G. T., Maki, S., Chew, L. C., Resnick, S. M., Ngai, J., & Retallack, D. M. (2011). Soluble periplasmic production of human granulocyte colony-stimulating factor (G-CSF) in Pseudomonas fluorescens. *Protein Expression and Purification*, *78*(1), 69–77. DOI: 10.1016/j.pep.2011.03.002

Jin, M., Slininger, P. J., Dien, B. S., Waghmode, S., Moser, B. R., Orjuela, A., & Balan, V. (2018). Microbial lipid-based lignocellulosic biorefinery: Feasibility and challenges. *Trends in Biotechnology*, *36*(3), 281–297. DOI: 10.1016/j.tibtech.2017.10.020 PMID: 30278987

Joga, R., Srivastava, S., & Nagpal, K. (2024). Regulatory Landscape and Challenges in CAR-T Cell Therapy Development in the US, EU, Japan, and India. *European Journal of Pharmaceutical Sciences*, *2024*. Advance online publication. DOI: 10.1016/j.ejps.2024.106557

Johnson, T. J., Katuwal, S., Anderson, G. A., Gu, L., Zhou, R., & Gibbons, W. R. (2018). Photobioreactor cultivation strategies for microalgae and cyanobacteria. *Biotechnology Progress*, *34*(4), 811–827.

Johnston, C. W., Wyatt, M. A., Li, X., Ibrahim, A., Shuster, J., Southam, G., & Magarvey, N. A. (2013). Gold biomineralization by a metallophore from a gold-associated microbe. *Nature Chemical Biology*, *9*(4), 241–243. DOI: 10.1038/nchembio.1179 PMID: 23377039

Jones, D. T., & Woods, D. R. (1986). Acetone-butanol fermentation revisited. *Microbiological Reviews*, *50*(4), 484–524. DOI: 10.1128/mr.50.4.484-524.1986

Jones, J. A., Toparlak, Ö. D., & Koffas, M. A. (2015). Metabolic pathway balancing and its role in the production of biofuels and chemicals. *Current Opinion in Biotechnology*, *33*, 52–59. DOI: 10.1016/j.copbio.2014.11.013 PMID: 25445548

Jönsson, A. S., & Trägårdh, G. (1990). Ultrafiltration applications. *Desalination*, *77*, 135–179.

Joshi, S., & Mishra, S. (2022). Recent advances in biofuel production through metabolic engineering. *Bioresource Technology*, *352*, 127037. DOI: 10.1016/j.biortech.2022.127037 PMID: 35318143

Jossen, V., Eibl, R., & Eibl, D. (2019). Single-use bioreactors–an overview. *Single-use technology in biopharmaceutical manufacture*, 37-52. https://doi.org/DOI: 10.1002/9781119477891.ch4

Jothyswarupha, K., Venkataraman, S., Rajendran, D. S., Shri, S. S., Sivaprakasam, S., Yamini, T., Karthik, P., & Kumar, V. V. (2025). Immobilized enzymes: Exploring its potential in food industry applications. *Food Science and Biotechnology*, *34*(7), 1533–1555. PMID: 40129709

Julien, C., & Whitford, W. (2007). Bioreactor monitoring, modeling, and simulation. *BioProcess International*, *5*(01), S10–S17.

Jungbauer, A. (2013). Product purification: Protein A chromatography. In Harnisch, J. P. (Ed.), *Biopharmaceutical Manufacturing* (pp. 151–176). Wiley.

Jung, H. N., Lee, S.-Y., Lee, S., Youn, H., & Im, H.-J. (2022). Lipid nanoparticles for delivery of RNA therapeutics: Current status and the role of *in vivo* imaging. *Theranostics*, *12*(17), 7509–7531. DOI: 10.7150/thno.77259

Jung, I. S., Oh, M. K., Cho, Y. C., & Kong, I. S. (2011). The viability to a wall shear stress and propagation of Bifidobacterium longum in the intensive membrane bioreactor. *Applied Microbiology and Biotechnology*, *92*, 939–949. DOI: 10.1007/s00253-011-3387-z PMID: 21681403

Junker, B. H. (2021). Scale-up methodologies for *Escherichia coli* and yeast fermentation processes. *Journal of Bioscience and Bioengineering*, *131*(3), 245–256. DOI: 10.1016/j.jbiosc.2020.11.011 PMID: 16233642

Junne, S., & Neubauer, P. (2018). How scalable and suitable are single-use bioreactors? *Current Opinion in Biotechnology*, *53*, 240–247. DOI: 10.1016/j.copbio.2018.04.003 PMID: 29753977

Kabeyi, M. J. B., & Olanrewaju, O. A. (2022). Technologies for biogas to electricity conversion. *Energy Reports*, *8*, 774–786. DOI: 10.1016/j.egyr.2022.11.007

Kai, Y., Hasegawa, M., & Ohta, T. (2016). Production of fatty acids in *Saccharomyces cerevisiae*. *Journal of Biotechnology*, *222*, 69–77. DOI: 10.1016/j.jbiotec.2016.02.017

Kakadellis, S., & Harris, Z. M. (2020). Don't scrap the waste: The need for broader system boundaries in bioplastic food packaging life-cycle assessment. *The Science of the Total Environment*, *727*, 138831. DOI: 10.1016/j.scitotenv.2020.138831

Kakko, N., Ivanona, N., & Rantasalo, A. (2016). Cell disruption methods. *CHEM-E3140. Bioprocess Technology*, *II*, 11–13.

Kalil, S. J., Maugeri, F., & Rodrigues, M. I. (2000). Response surface analysis and simulation as a tool for bioprocess design and optimization. *Process Biochemistry*, *35*(6), 539–550.

Kanagesan, K., Abdulla, R., & Derman, E. (2022). Ulvan, a bioactive marine polysaccharide as a green ingredient for functional food and pharmaceutical applications. *Molecules (Basel, Switzerland)*, *27*(20), 7035. DOI: 10.3390/molecules27207035 PMID: 36296626

Kang, H. J., Yu, H. H., Cho, C. W., Rhee, Y. K., Kim, T. W., & Chin, Y. W. (2024). Optimization of medium composition and fluidized bed drying conditions for efficient production of dry yeast. *Microorganisms*, *13*(1), 22. PMID: 39858790

Kang, M., Choe, D., Kim, K., Cho, B.-K., & Cho, S. (2020). Synthetic biology approaches in the development of engineered therapeutic microbes. *International Journal of Molecular Sciences*, *21*(22), 8744.

Känsäkoski, M., Kurkinen, M., von Weymarn, N., Niemelä, P., Neubauer, P., Juuso, E., & Suhonen, P. (2006). Process analytical technology (PAT) needs and applications in the bioprocess industry. *VTT Technical Research Centre of Finland*, *60*, 99.

Karim, A. S., & Jewett, M. C. (2016). A cell-free framework for rapid biosynthetic pathway prototyping and enzyme discovery. *Metabolic Engineering*, *36*, 116–126. DOI: 10.1016/j.ymben.2016.03.002 PMID: 26996382

Karkaria, V., Tsai, Y. K., Chen, Y. P., & Chen, W. (2025). An optimization-centric review on integrating artificial intelligence and digital twin technologies in manufacturing. *Engineering Optimization*, *57*(1), 161–207.

Karlsen, F., & Skov, P. V. (2022). Review–Potentials and limitations of utilising brewer's spent grain as a protein source in aquaculture feeds. *Journal of Cleaner Production*, *357*, 131986.

Karmakar, R., Behera, N. R., Mandal, A., Sharma, P. K., Toomey, J. B., Kundu, K., & Kumar, R. (2025). State-of-the-Art in algal biofuel research: Waste-algae as a sustainable energy solution. *Journal of Solid Waste Technology Management*, *51*(3), 385–404.

Kartik, A., Akhil, D., Lakshmi, D., Gopinath, K. P., Arun, J., Sivaramakrishnan, R., & Pugazhendhi, A. (2021). A critical review on production of biopolymers from algae biomass and their applications. *Bioresource Technology*, *329*, 124868. DOI: 10.1016/j.biortech.2021.124868 PMID: 33707076

Kasari, M., Kasari, V., Kärmas, M., & Jõers, A. (2022). Decoupling Growth and Production by Removing the Origin of Replication from a Bacterial Chromosome. *ACS Synthetic Biology*, *11*(8), 2610–2622. DOI: 10.1021/acssynbio.1c00618

Katakhade, R., Sahoo, S., Anerao, K., & Poshadri, A. (2023). Bacteriocin as a bio-preservative and its applications in food products. *Pharma Innov. J*, *12*, 2226–2231.

Katsieris, D. (2024). Accreditation, Certification, and Inspection: Impact on Global Trade. In *Handbook of Quality System, Accreditation and Conformity Assessment* (pp. 421-437). Singapore: Springer Nature Singapore. https://doi.org/DOI: 10.1007/978-981-97-5750-3_25

Kaur, I., & Sharma, A. D. (2021). Bioreactor: Design, functions and fermentation innovations. *Res. Rev. Biotechnol. Biosci*, *8*, 34–43.

Kaur, P., & Chugh, A. (2021). Challenges in governance of Synthetic Biology: Biorisk assessment. *Asian Biotechnology and Development Review, 23*(3).

Kay, J. E., & Jewett, M. C. (2015). Lysate of engineered Escherichia coli supports high-level conversion of glucose to 2,3-butanediol. *Metabolic Engineering, 30*, 190–200. DOI: 10.1016/j.ymben.2015.06.004 PMID: 26428449

Keasling, J. D. (2010). Advanced biofuel production in microbes. *Biotechnology Journal, 5*(2), 147–162. DOI: 10.1002/biot.200900233 PMID: 20084640

Keasling, J. D. (2010). Manufacturing molecules through metabolic engineering. *Science, 330*(6009), 1355–1358. DOI: 10.1126/science.1193990 PMID: 21127247

Keasling, J. D. (2017). Synthetic biology and the development of tools for metabolic engineering. *Metabolic Engineering, 44*, 177–185. DOI: 10.1016/j.ymben.2017.10.004 PMID: 22314049

Kelley, B. (2009). Industrialization of mAb production technology: The bioprocessing industry at a crossroads. *mAbs, 1*(5), 443–452. PMID: 20065641

Kendall, E. C. (2022). *Bioreactors: Design, background, and applications* (No. LA-UR-22-29370). Los Alamos National Laboratory (LANL), Los Alamos, NM (United States). https://doi.org/DOI: 10.2172/1887112

Khafaga, D. S. R., Muteeb, G., Elgarawany, A., Aatif, M., Farhan, M., Allam, S., Almatar, B. A., & Radwan, M. G. (2024). Green nanobiocatalysts: Enhancing enzyme immobilization for industrial and biomedical applications. *PeerJ, 12*, e17589. DOI: 10.7717/peerj.17589

Khalid, M., De la ROsa, D., & Fikre, B. (2020). *Enhancing environmental sustainability in slow fashion apparel industry: Risk identification and supply chain mapping of bio-based polymer fibers.*

Khalid, M. Y., Arif, Z. U., Ahmed, W., & Arshad, H. (2022). Recent trends in recycling and reusing techniques of different plastic polymers and their composite materials. *Sustainable Materials and Technologies, 31*, e00382. DOI: 10.1016/j.susmat.2021.e00382

Khalil, A. S., & Collins, J. J. (2010). Synthetic biology: Applications come of age. *Nature Reviews. Genetics, 11*(5), 367–379. DOI: 10.1038/nrg2775 PMID: 20395970

Khanal, O., & Lenhoff, A. M. (2021). Developments and opportunities in continuous biopharmaceutical manufacturing. *mAbs, 13*(1). Advance online publication. DOI: 10.1080/19420862.2021.1903664

Khanal, S. K., Tarafdar, A., & You, S. (2023). Artificial intelligence and machine learning for smart bioprocesses. *Bioresource Technology, 375*, 128826. PMID: 36871700

Khandekar, P., & Ghosh, P. K. (2023). Bioeconomy: Different Countries, Different Strategies, Multiple Benefits. *Asian Biotechnology and Development Review, 25*(3).

Khang, A., & Akhai, S. (2024). Green intelligent and sustainable manufacturing: Key advancements, benefits, challenges, and applications for transforming industry. In *Machine vision and industrial robotics in manufacturing* (pp. 405–417). CRC Press., DOI: 10.1201/9781032788487-20

Khan, M. I., Shin, J. H., & Kim, J. D. (2018). The promising future of microalgae: Current status, challenges, and optimization of a sustainable and renewable industry for biofuels, feed, and other products. *Microbial Cell Factories*, *17*(1), 36. DOI: 10.1186/s12934-018-0879-x PMID: 29506528

Khanna, S., Goyal, A., & Moholkar, V. S. (2011). Production of n-butanol from biodiesel derived crude glycerol using *Clostridium pasteurianum* immobilized on amberlite. *Fuel*, *102*(1), 211–219. DOI: 10.1016/j.fuel.2012.07.011

Khan, S., Ullah, M. W., Siddique, R., Nabi, G., Manan, S., Yousaf, M., & Hou, H. (2016). Role of recombinant DNA technology to improve life. *International Journal of Genomics*, *2016*(1), 2405954.

Khan, S., Ullah, M. W., Siddique, R., Nabi, G., Manan, S., Yousaf, M., & Hou, H. (2016). Role of Recombinant DNA Technology to Improve Life. *International Journal of Genomics*, *2016*, 1–14. DOI: 10.1155/2016/2405954

Khoiruddin, K., Boopathy, R., Kawi, S., & Wenten, I. G. (2025). Towards next-generation membrane bioreactors: Innovations, challenges, and future directions. *Current Pollution Reports*, *11*(1), 15.

Khopade, A. J., & Shah, M. (2026). Challenges for Commercial Translation of Nanomedicines: From Lab Scale to Production Scale. In *Commercial Scale Production of Nanomedicines* (pp. 1-40). CRC Press.

Khorana, H. G., Buchi, H., Ghosh, H., Gupta, N., Jacob, T. M., Kossel, H., Morgan, R., Narang, S. A., Ohtsuka, E., & Wells, R. D. (1980). Total synthesis of a gene for an alanine transfer RNA from yeast. *Nature*, *283*(5743), 273–278. DOI: 10.1038/283273a0

Kilduff, J. E., Mattaraj, S., Wigton, A., Kitis, M., & Karanfil, T. (2004). Effects of reverse osmosis isolation on reactivity of naturally occurring dissolved organic matter in physicochemical processes. *Water Research*, *38*(4), 1026–1036. PMID: 14769423

Kim, E. J., Kim, J. H., Kim, M. S., Jeong, S. H., & Choi, D. H. (2021). Process analytical technology tools for monitoring pharmaceutical unit operations: A control strategy for continuous process verification. *Pharmaceutics*, *13*(6), 919. PMID: 34205797

Kim, H. W., Hong, S. H., & Choi, H. (2020). Effect of nitrate and perchlorate on selenate reduction in a sequencing batch reactor. *Processes (Basel, Switzerland)*, *8*(3), 344. Advance online publication. DOI: 10.3390/pr8030344

Kim, J. K., Kim, D. Y., & Lee, N. K. (2020). A review on the properties and applications of carrageenan. *Polymer Korea*, *44*(6), 707–719. DOI: 10.7317/pk.2020.44.6.707

Kim, J. Y., Kim, Y. G., & Lee, G. M. (2012). CHO cells in biotechnology for production of recombinant proteins: Current state and further potential. *Applied Microbiology and Biotechnology*, *93*(3), 917–930. PMID: 22159888

Kim, K. J., Lee, S. J., & Kim, D. M. (2024). Cell-free systems for a multi-pronged approach to next-generation therapeutics and diagnostics. *Biotechnology and Bioprocess Engineering; BBE*, *29*(2), 233–239. DOI: 10.1007/s12257-024-00058-w

Kim, S. K., Lee, D.-H., Kim, O. C., Kim, J. F., & Yoon, S. H. (2017). Tunable Control of an *Escherichia coli* Expression System for the Overproduction of Membrane Proteins by Titrated Expression of a Mutant *lac* Repressor. *ACS Synthetic Biology*, *6*(9), 1766–1773. DOI: 10.1021/acssynbio.7b00102

Kim, S., Jang, Y.-S., Ha, S.-C., Ahn, J.-W., Kim, E.-J., Hong Lim, J., Cho, C., Shin Ryu, Y., Kuk Lee, S., Lee, S. Y., & Kim, K.-J. (2015). Redox-switch regulatory mechanism of thiolase from Clostridium acetobutylicum. *Nature Communications*, *6*(1), 8410. DOI: 10.1038/ncomms9410

Kim, T., Chung, H. S., Lee, H.-S., Uthaman, S., Park, I.-K., & Park, K. (2023). Effects of retinoid-loaded hyaluronic acid nanomicelles on vaginal epithelium in a murine menopause model. *Investigative and Clinical Urology*, *64*(2), 182. DOI: 10.4111/icu.20220366

Kiran, B. R., Prasad, M. N. V., & Mohan, S. V. (2024). Synthetic biology: an emerging field for developing economies. In *Bioremediation and Bioeconomy* (pp. 767–787). Elsevier., DOI: 10.1016/B978-0-443-16120-9.00013-3

Kirar, S., Mohne, D., Singh, M., Sagar, V., Bhise, A., Goswami, S., & Bhaumik, J. (2024). Eco-friendly lignin nanocomposite films as advanced UV protective and antimicrobial sustainable packaging materials. *Sustainable Materials and Technologies*, *40*, e00864. DOI: 10.1016/j.susmat.2024.e00864

Kirk, T. V., & Szita, N. (2013). Oxygen transfer characteristics of miniaturized bioreactor systems. *Biotechnology and Bioengineering*, *110*(4), 1005–1019. DOI: 10.1002/bit.24824 PMID: 23280578

Kittler, S., Müller, F., Elshazly, M., Wandrey, G. B., Klein, T., Daub, A., Spadiut, O., & Kopp, J. (2025). Transferability of bioprocessing modes for recombinant protease production: From fed-batch to continuous cultivation with *Bacillus licheniformis*. *BMC Biotechnology*, *25*(1), 13. Advance online publication. DOI: 10.1186/s12896-025-00897-8

Kjeldsen, T., Andersen, A. S., Hubálek, F., Johansson, E., Kreiner, F. F., Schluckebier, G., & Kurtzhals, P. (2023). Molecular engineering of insulin for recombinant expression in yeast. *Trends in Biotechnology*, *42*(4), 464–478. DOI: 10.1016/j.tibtech.2023.09.012 PMID: 37880066

Ko, C. L., & Wang, F. S. (2006). Run-to-run fed-batch optimization for protein production using recombinant Escherichia coli. *Biochemical Engineering Journal*, *30*(3), 279–285.

Koczoń, P., Hołaj-Krzak, J. T., Palani, B. K., Bolewski, T., Dąbrowski, J., Bartyzel, B. J., & Gruczyńska-Sękowska, E. (2023). The analytical possibilities of FT-IR spectroscopy powered by vibrating molecules. *International Journal of Molecular Sciences*, *24*(2), 1013. PMID: 36674526

Ko, H., Kang, M., Kim, M.-J., Yi, J., Kang, J., Bae, J.-H., Sohn, J.-H., & Sung, B. H. (2021). A novel protein fusion partner, carbohydrate-binding module family 66, to enhance heterologous protein expression in Escherichia coli. *Microbial Cell Factories*, *20*(1), 232. DOI: 10.1186/s12934-021-01725-w

Köhler, G., & Milstein, C. (1975). Continuous cultures of fused cells secreting antibody of pre-defined specificity. *Nature*, *256*(5517), 495–497. PMID: 1172191

Kohlstedt, M., & Wittmann, C. (2019). GC-MS-based 13C metabolic flux analysis resolves the parallel and cyclic glucose metabolism of *Pseudomonas putida* KT2440 and *Pseudomonas aeruginosa* PAO1. *Metabolic Engineering, 54*, 35–53. DOI: 10.1016/j.ymben.2019.01.008 PMID: 30831266

Kolber, N. S., Fattal, R., Bratulic, S., Carver, G. D., & Badran, A. H. (2021). Orthogonal translation enables heterologous ribosome engineering in E. coli. *Nature Communications, 12*(1), 599. DOI: 10.1038/s41467-020-20759-z

Konstantinov, K. B., & Cooney, C. L. (2015). White paper on continuous bioprocessing. *May 20, 2015*. American Institute of Chemical Engineers (AIChE). https://www.aiche.org

Konstantinov, K. B., & Cooney, C. L. (2015). White paper on continuous bioprocessing. *Journal of Pharmaceutical Sciences, 104*(3), 813–820. DOI: 10.1002/jps.24252

Koul, B., Yakoob, M., & Shah, M. P. (2022). Agricultural waste management strategies for environmental sustainability. *Environmental Research, 206*, 112285. PMID: 34710442

Kourmentza, K., Kachrimanidou, V., Psaki, O., Pateraki, C., Ladakis, D., & Koutinas, A. (2020). Competitive advantage and market introduction of PHA polymers and potential use of PHA monomers. In *The Handbook of Polyhydroxyalkanoates* (pp. 167–202). CRC Press.

Kozitsina, A. N., Svalova, T. S., Malysheva, N. N., Okhokhonin, A. V., Vidrevich, M. B., & Brainina, K. Z. (2018). Sensors based on bio and biomimetic receptors in medical diagnostic, environment, and food analysis. *Biosensors (Basel), 8*(2), 35. PMID: 29614784

Kraemer, M., Reed, J., & Tobin, S. (2011). Global regulatory challenges in biopharmaceutical manufacturing. *Pharmaceutical Technology Europe, 23*(4), 42–47.

Krämer, I., & Federici, M. (2020). Implementation and microbiological stability of dose-banded ganciclovir infusion bags prepared in series by a robotic system. *European Journal of Hospital Pharmacy. Science and Practice, 27*(4), 209–215. DOI: 10.1136/ejhpharm-2019-001925

Krause, D., Birle, S., Hussein, M. A., & Becker, T. (2011). Bioprocess monitoring and control via adaptive sensor calibration. *Engineering in Life Sciences, 11*(4), 402–416. DOI: 10.1002/elsc.201000141

Krebs, H. A., & Johnson, W. A. (1937). The role of citric acid in intermediate metabolism in animal tissues. *Enzymologia, 4*, 148–156.

Kroll, P.. (2017). Model Predictive Control of Bioprocesses: A Review. *Journal of Process Control, 56*, 1–14.

Krömer, J. O., Ferreira, R. G., Petrides, D., & Kohlheb, N. (2020). Economic process evaluation and environmental life-cycle assessment of bio-aromatics production. *Frontiers in Bioengineering and Biotechnology, 8*, 403. Advance online publication. DOI: 10.3389/fbioe.2020.00403

Krunic, T., & Osmokrovic, A. (2025). Effect of pretreatment, lyophilization parameters and different cryoprotectants on the efficiency of probiotic freeze-drying immobilization. *Hemijska Industrija*.

Krywko-Cendrowska, A., Szweda, D., & Szweda, R. (2020). Well-defined conjugated macromolecules based on oligo(arylene ethynylene)s in sensing. *Processes (Basel, Switzerland), 8*(5), 539. Advance online publication. DOI: 10.3390/pr8050539

Kuchenmüller, T., Chapman, E., Takahashi, R., Lester, L., Reinap, M., Ellen, M., & Haby, M. M. (2022). A comprehensive monitoring and evaluation framework for evidence to policy networks. *Evaluation and Program Planning, 91*, 102053. DOI: 10.1016/j.evalprogplan.2022.102053 PMID: 35217289

Kumar, T. P., Rahul, M., & Chandrajit, B. (2011). Biofiltration of volatile organic compounds (VOCs): an overview. Res J Chem Sci, 2231, 606X. https://isca.me/rjcs/Archives/vol1/I8/ISCA-RJCS-2011-174-15.pdf

Kumar, J., Chauhan, A. S., Shah, R. L., Gupta, J. A., & Rathore, A. S. (2020). Amino acid supplementation for enhancing recombinant protein production in *E. coli. Biotechnology and Bioengineering, 117*(8), 2420–2433. DOI: 10.1002/bit.27371

Kumar, M. U., Jeyasundar, P. G. S. A., Das, M. A., Azeem, M., Mani, V. M., & Ayswaria, R. (2025). *Recombinant DNA Technology in the Improvement of Microbial Enzyme Production.* Microbial Enzymes.

Kumar, P. (2023). Role of Industry 4.0 in Biotechnology to Produce Environmentally Sustainable Biotechnology Products. *Asian Biotechnology and Development Review, 25*(3).

Kumar, R., Gupta, G., Hussain, A., Rani, A., Thapliyal, A., Gunsola, D., & Mitra, D. (2025a). Pioneering zero-waste technologies utilization and its framework on sustainable management: International, national and state level. *Discover Applied Sciences, 7*(3), 224.

Kumar, R., Kamboj, N., & Mitra, D. (2024). Microbial innovations in agriculture: Interdisciplinary approaches to leveraging microbes for food sustainability and security. *Indian Journal of Microbiology Research, 11*(3), 129–139.

Kumar, R., Kamboj, N., Mitra, D., & Ray, A. (2025b). Strengthening Local Communities Through Advanced Recycling Technology for Sustainable Growth. In Mitra, D., Choudhury, T., Madan, A., Chattaraj, S., & Pellegrini, M. (Eds.), *AI Technologies for Enhancing Recycling Processes* (pp. 393–420). IGI Global Scientific Publishing.

Kumar, R., Lakhera, A., Gulati, M., Rani, A., Thapliyal, A., Gunsola, D., & Mitra, D. (2025d). Genome Mining of Biocontrol Agents for Bioprospecting Action Modes. In Mitra, D., de los Santos Villalobos, S., Rani, A., Elena Guerra Sierra, B., & Andjelković, S. (Eds.), *Bio-control Agents for Sustainable Agriculture*. Springer.

Kumar, R., Sangwan, K. S., Herrmann, C., & Thakur, S. (2023). A cyber physical production system framework for online monitoring, visualization and control by using cloud, fog, and edge computing technologies. *International Journal of Computer Integrated Manufacturing, 36*(10), 1507–1525.

Kumar, S., Tarei, P. K., & Swarnakar, V. (2024). Analyzing barriers to sustainable healthcare waste disposal: A hybrid decision-making framework. *Benchmarking*. Advance online publication. DOI: 10.1108/BIJ-10-2023-0744

Kumar, V., Bhalla, A., & Rathore, A. S. (2014). Design of experiments applications in bioprocessing: Concepts and approach. *Biotechnology Progress, 30*(1), 86–99. PMID: 24123959

Kumar, V., Kothari, R., Pathak, V. V., & Tyagi, S. (2018). Optimization of substrate concentration for sustainable biohydrogen production and kinetics from sugarcane molasses: Experimental and economical assessment. *Waste and Biomass Valorization, 9*(2), 273–281.

Kumar, V., Nanda, M., Joshi, H. C., Singh, A., Sharma, S., & Verma, M. (2018). Production of biodiesel and bioethanol using algal biomass harvested from fresh water river. *Renewable Energy, 116*, 606–612. DOI: 10.1016/j.renene.2017.10.016

Kumar, V., & Verma, P. (2024). Microbial valorization of kraft black liquor for production of platform chemicals, biofuels, and value-added products: A critical review. *Journal of Environmental Management, 366*, 121631. PMID: 38986370

Kumar, V., Verma, P., de Freitas, F. A., Srivastava, P. K., Vashishth, A., & Américo-Pinheiro, J. H. P. (2025). A critical review on biofuels generation from pulp-paper mill sludge with emphasis on pretreatment methods: Renewable energy for environmental sustainability. *BMC Environmental Science, 2*(1), 2. DOI: 10.1186/s44329-024-00016-0

Kuo, C. C., Lin, Y. T., & Liu, C. H. (2018). Glycosylation of therapeutic proteins in mammalian cells. *Current Opinion in Chemical Engineering, 22*, 1–7.

Kurosawa, K., Plassmeier, J., Kalinowski, J., Rückert, C., & Sinskey, A. J. (2015). Engineering l-arabinose metabolism in triacylglycerol-producing Rhodococcus opacus for lignocellulosic fuel production. *Metabolic Engineering, 30*, 89–95. DOI: 10.1016/j.ymben.2015.04.006

Kurt, E., Qin, J., Williams, A., Zhao, Y., & Xie, D. (2023). Perspectives for Using CO2 as a Feedstock for Biomanufacturing of Fuels and Chemicals. *Bioengineering (Basel, Switzerland), 10*(12), 1357. PMID: 38135948

Kusuktham, B., & Srinophakun, P. (2014). Improvement of butanol production from palm empty fruit bunch by *Clostridium beijerinckii. Energy Procedia, 52*, 627–632. DOI: 10.1016/j.egypro.2014.07.118

Kwon, T., Leroux, A. C., Zang, H., Pollard, D., Zehe, C., & Akbari, S. (2024). Cell-based shear stress sensor for bioprocessing. *Journal of Biotechnology, 390*, 71–79. DOI: 10.1016/j.jbiotec.2024.05.007

Ladu, L., & Quitzow, R. (2017). Bio-based economy: Policy framework and foresight thinking. *Food Waste Reduction and Valorisation: Sustainability Assessment and Policy Analysis*, 167–195.

Lakshmi, D. S., Trivedi, N., & Reddy, C. R. K. (2020). Synthesis and characterization of seaweed cellulose derived carboxymethylcellulose. *Carbohydrate Polymers, 250*, 116904. DOI: 10.1016/j.carbpol.2020.116904

Lalor, F., Fitzpatrick, J., Sage, C., & Byrne, E. (2019). Sustainability in the biopharmaceutical industry: Seeking a holistic perspective. *Biotechnology Advances, 37*(5), 698–707. DOI: 10.1016/j.biotechadv.2019.03.015 PMID: 30922993

Lan, E. I., & Liao, J. C. (2013). Microbial synthesis of n-butanol, isobutanol, and other higher alcohols from diverse resources. *Bioresource Technology*, *135*, 339–349. DOI: 10.1016/j.biortech.2012.09.104

Lang, D. A., Meyer, T., & Smith, C. D. (2020). Robotics in Biopharmaceutical Fill-Finish Operations: Benefits and Considerations. *Pharmaceutical Engineering*, *40*(3), 58–65.

Langdon, S. P., Wyld, D., & Reeves, J. R. (2009). Contamination in cell culture: Risks and preventive measures. *Methods in Molecular Biology (Clifton, N.J.)*, *946*, 15–28.

Lange, I., Kourentzi, K., & Willson, R. C. (2022). Supply chain resilience in the biopharmaceutical industry. *Biotechnology Journal*, *17*(7), 2100425.

Länge, K. (2019). Bulk and surface acoustic wave sensor arrays for multi-analyte detection: A review. *Sensors (Basel)*, *19*(24), 5382. PMID: 31817599

Langer, E. S. (2015). Biopharmaceutical Manufacturing Trends. *BioProcess International*, *13*(4), 24–30.

Langer, E. S., & Rader, R. A. (2014). Single-use bioprocessing: A technology that is revolutionizing the biomanufacturing industry. *BioProcess International*, *12*(6), 24–30.

Latukha, M., Shagalkina, M., Mitskevich, E., & Strogetskaya, E. (2022). From brain drain to brain gain: The agenda for talent management in overcoming talent migration from emerging markets. *International Journal of Human Resource Management*, *33*(11), 2226–2255. DOI: 10.1080/09585192.2021.1949374

Lazim, N. A. M., & Nazir, N. M. (2025). Biotechnology and Genetic Engineering: Unlocking New Possibilities. In *Evolving Landscapes of Research and Development: Trends, Challenges, and Opportunities* (pp. 109-122). IGI Global Scientific Publishing. https://doi.org/DOI: 10.4018/979-8-3693-7101-5.ch005

Le Borgne, S., & Baquerizo, G. (2019). Microbial Ecology of Biofiltration Units Used for the Desulfurization of Biogas. *ChemEngineering*, *3*(3), 72. DOI: 10.3390/chemengineering3030072

Lee, J. S., Kallehauge, T. B., Pedersen, L. E., & Kildegaard, H. F. (2018). Site-specific genome engineering for high-level protein production in CHO cells. *Biotechnology Journal*, *13*(3), 1700645.

Lee, J. W., Yi, J., Kim, T. Y., Choi, S., Ahn, J. H., Song, H., Lee, M.-H., & Lee, S. Y. (2016). Homo-succinic acid production by metabolically engineered Mannheimia succiniciproducens. *Metabolic Engineering*, *38*, 409–417. DOI: 10.1016/j.ymben.2016.10.004

Lee, J.. (2018). Industrial big data analytics and cyber-physical systems for future manufacturing systems. *Annual Reviews in Control*, *45*, 1–10.

Lee, J., Bagheri, B., & Kao, H. A. (2015). A cyber-physical systems architecture for Industry 4.0-based manufacturing systems. *Manufacturing Letters*, *3*, 18–23.

Lee, J., Kim, H., Lim, H. R., Kim, Y. S., Hoang, T. T. T., Choi, J., & Yeo, W. H. (2024). Large-scale smart bioreactor with fully integrated wireless multivariate sensors and electronics for long-term in situ monitoring of stem cell culture. *Science Advances*, *10*(7), eadk6714. Advance online publication. DOI: 10.1126/sciadv.adk6714 PMID: 38354246

Lee, J., Lapira, E., Bagheri, B., & Kao, H. A. (2020). *Industrial AI: Applications with Sustainable Performance*. Springer.

Lee, J., & Park, H. (2023). Advances in nanoclay-polymer drug delivery systems. *Journal of Nanomedicine, 17*(3), 102–118.

Lee, K. Y., Buldum, G., Mantalaris, A., & Bismarck, A. (2014). More than meets the eye in bacterial cellulose: Biosynthesis, bioprocessing, and applications in advanced fiber composites. *Macromolecular Bioscience, 14*(1), 10–32. DOI: 10.1002/mabi.201300298 PMID: 23897676

Lee, P. C., Lee, S. Y., Hong, S. H., Chang, H. N., & Park, S. C. (2003). Biological conversion of wood hydrolysate to succinic acid by Anaerobiospirillum succiniciproducens. *Biotechnology Letters, 25*(2), 111–114. DOI: 10.1023/A:1021907116361

Lee, S. L.. (2015). Modernizing pharmaceutical manufacturing: From batch to continuous production. *Journal of Pharmaceutical Innovation, 10*(3), 191–199.

Lee, S. Y. (1996). High cell-density culture of *Escherichia coli. Trends in Biotechnology, 14*(3), 98–105. DOI: 10.1016/0167-7799(96)80930-9

Lee, S. Y., Kim, H. U., Chae, T. U., Cho, J. S., Kim, J. W., & Shin, J. H. (2019). A comprehensive metabolic map for production of bio-based chemicals. *Nature Catalysis, 2*(1), 18–33. DOI: 10.1038/s41929-018-0212-4

Lee, S. Y., Lee, D. Y., & Kim, T. Y. (2005). Systems biotechnology for strain improvement. *Trends in Biotechnology, 23*(7), 349–358. PMID: 15923052

Lee, S. Y., Park, J. H., Jang, S. H., Nielsen, L. K., Kim, J., & Jung, K. S. (2008). Fermentative butanol production by clostridia. *Biotechnology and Bioengineering, 101*(2), 209–228. DOI: 10.1002/bit.22003

Lengare, R. R., Arjun, Y. N., & Bais, S. K. (2024). A Review on Quality Control and Quality Assurance in Pharmaceuticals. [PDF Link]. *International Journal of Pharmacy and Herbal Technology, 2*(4), 2507–2520.

Leong, H. Y., Chang, C.-K., Khoo, K. S., Chew, K. W., Chia, S. R., Lim, J. W., Chang, J.-S., & Show, P. L. (2021). Waste biorefinery towards a sustainable circular bioeconomy: A solution to global issues. *Biotechnology for Biofuels, 14*, 1–15. PMID: 33827663

Levine, H. L.. (2019). Continuous Biomanufacturing: Modern Approaches and Technologies. *BioProcess International, 17*(4), 42–49.

Liang, B., Zhao, Y., & Yang, J. (2020). Recent Advances in Developing Artificial Autotrophic Microorganism for Reinforcing CO2 Fixation. *Frontiers in Microbiology, 11*, 592631. DOI: 10.3389/fmicb.2020.592631 PMID: 33240247

Liang, L., Tan, H., & Liu, R. (2025). Emerging gene editing in industrial microbiology beyond CRISPR-Cas9. *Trends in Biotechnology, 43*(4), 742–744. DOI: 10.1016/j.tibtech.2024.09.012

Lian, J., Chao, R., & Zhao, H. (2014). Metabolic engineering of a Saccharomyces cere- visiae strain capable of simultaneously utilizing glucose and galactose to pro- duce enantiopure (2r, 3r)-butanediol. *Metabolic Engineering, 23*, 92–99.

Liao, B. Q., Lin, H. J., Langevin, S. P., Gao, W. J., & Leppard, G. G. (2011). Effects of temperature and dissolved oxygen on sludge properties and their role in bioflocculation and settling. *Water Research, 45*(2), 509–520. PMID: 20875910

Liao, J. C., Mi, L., Pontrelli, S., & Luo, S. (2016). Fuelling the future: Microbial engineering for the production of sustainable biofuels. *Nature Reviews. Microbiology, 14*(5), 288–304. DOI: 10.1038/nrmicro.2016.32 PMID: 27026253

Lidén, G. (2002). Understanding the bioreactor. *Bioprocess and Biosystems Engineering, 24*, 273–279. DOI: 10.1007/s004490100263

Liese, A., & Hilterhaus, L. (2013). Evaluation of immobilized enzymes for industrial applications. *Chemical Society Reviews, 42*(15), 6236. DOI: 10.1039/c3cs35511j

Liew, F. E., Nogle, R., Abdalla, T., Rasor, B. J., Canter, C., Jensen, R. O., Wang, L., Strutz, J., Chirania, P., De Tissera, S., Mueller-Cajar, O., & Köpke, M. (2022). Carbon-negative production of acetone and isopropanol by gas fermentation at industrial pilot scale. *Nature Biotechnology, 40*(3), 335–344. DOI: 10.1038/s41587-021-01195-w PMID: 35190685

Li, F., Vijayasankaran, N., Shen, A., Kiss, R., & Amanullah, A. (2010). Cell culture processes for monoclonal antibody production. *mAbs, 2*(5), 466–479. PMID: 20622510

Li, G., Chen, K., Wei, Y., Zeng, J., Yang, Y., He, F., & Ouyang, P. (2022). Mass transfer, gas holdup, and kinetic models of batch and continuous fermentation in a novel rectangular dynamic membrane airlift bioreactor. *Engineering, 13*, 153–163. DOI: 10.1016/j.eng.2021.07.025

Li, J., & Neubauer, P. (2020). *Escherichia coli* as a cell factory for heterologous production of nonribosomal peptides and polyketides. *New Biotechnology, 59*, 1–11. DOI: 10.1016/j.nbt.2020.06.003 PMID: 24704144

Lim, E. J., & Abd Rahim, M. H. (2025). Fermentation for Enhanced Biosynthesis and Bioavailability of Micronutrients, Prebiotics, Bioactive Peptides and Functional Fatty Acids in Food Products. *International Journal of Advanced Research in Food Science and Agriculture Technology, 4*(1), 9–27.

Lindberg, P., Park, S., & Melis, A. (2010). Engineering a platform for photosynthetic iso- prene production in cyanobacteria, using Synechocystis as the model organism. *Metabolic Engineering, 12*(1), 70–79.

Lin, P. P., Rabe, K. S., Takasumi, J. L., Kadisch, M., Arnold, F. H., & Liao, J. C. (2015). Isobutanol production at elevated temperatures in thermophilic *Geobacillus thermoglucosidasius. Metabolic Engineering, 24*, 1–8. DOI: 10.1016/j.ymben.2014.03.006 PMID: 24721011

Lin, Y. H., & Gu, Y. J. (2021). Biodegradation kinetic studies of phenol and P-cresol in a batch and continuous stirred-tank bioreactor with Pseudomonas putida ATCC 17484 cells. *Processes (Basel, Switzerland), 9*(1), 133. DOI: 10.3390/pr9010133

Li, Q., Zhang, W., Liao, S., Xing, D., Xiao, Y., Zhou, D., & Yang, Q. (2023). Mechanism of lead adsorption by a Bacillus cereus strain with indole-3-acetic acid secretion and inorganic phosphorus dissolution functions. *BMC Microbiology, 23*(1), 57. DOI: 10.1186/s12866-023-02795-z PMID: 36869296

Lisci, S. (2023). Development of monitoring and control systems for biotechnological processes.

Lisci, S., Grosso, M., & Tronci, S. (2020). A geometric observer-assisted approach to tailor state estimation in a bioreactor for ethanol production. *Processes (Basel, Switzerland)*, *8*(4), 480. Advance online publication. DOI: 10.3390/pr8040480

Liu, A. (2025). Toward the effective implementation of the Biosafety Protocol: A Chinese regulatory capacity-building perspective. *Journal of Law and the Biosciences*, *12*(1), lsaf011. Advance online publication. DOI: 10.1093/jlb/lsaf011 PMID: 40463477

Liu, H. (2015). Impact of glycosylation on the efficacy and safety of monoclonal antibodies. *mAbs*, *7*(2), 256–263.

Liu, K., Atiyeh, H. K., Stevenson, B. S., Tanner, R. S., Wilkins, M. R., & Huhnke, R. L. (2014). Continuous syngas fermentation for the production of ethanol, n-propanol and n-butanol. *Bioresource Technology*, *151*, 69–77. DOI: 10.1016/j.biortech.2013.10.059

Liu, L., Bilal, M., Duan, X., & Iqbal, H. M. N. (2019). Mitigation of environmental pollution by genetically engineered bacteria - Current challenges and future perspectives. *The Science of the Total Environment*, *667*, 444–454. DOI: 10.1016/j.scitotenv.2019.02.390 PMID: 30833243

Liu, L., Li, Y., Li, S., Du, G., & Chen, J. (2018). Renewable bio-resources: A review on microbial production of platform chemicals. *Biotechnology Advances*, *36*(6), 1423–1440.

Liu, P., Xu, H., & Zhang, X. (2022). Metabolic engineering of microorganisms for L-alanine production. *Journal of Industrial Microbiology & Biotechnology*, *49*(2). Advance online publication. DOI: 10.1093/jimb/kuab057

Liu, Q., Liu, Y., & Qi, Q. (2016). Microbial production of natural and non-natural flavors: Pathways, engineering, and challenges. *Current Opinion in Biotechnology*, *70*, 1–9. DOI: 10.1016/j.copbio.2020.10.010

Liu, Q., Shen, Q., Bian, X., Chen, H., Fu, J., Wang, H., Lei, P., Guo, Z., Chen, W., Li, D., & Zhang, Y. (2016). Simple and rapid direct cloning and heterologous expression of natural product biosynthetic gene cluster in *Bacillus subtilis* via Red/ET recombineering. *Scientific Reports*, *6*, 34623. DOI: 10.1038/srep34623 PMID: 27687863

Liu, S., Yu, J.-M., Gan, Y.-C., Qiu, X.-Z., Gao, Z.-C., Wang, H., Chen, S.-X., Xiong, Y., Liu, G.-H., Lin, S.-E., McCarthy, A., John, J. V., Wei, D.-X., & Hou, H.-H. (2023). Biomimetic natural biomaterials for tissue engineering and regenerative medicine: New biosynthesis methods, recent advances, and emerging applications. *Military Medical Research*, *10*(1), 16. DOI: 10.1186/s40779-023-00448-w

Liu, Y., Tang, Y., Gao, H., Zhang, W., Jiang, Y., Xin, F., & Jiang, M. (2021). Challenges and Future Perspectives of Promising Biotechnologies for Lignocellulosic Biorefinery. *Molecules (Basel, Switzerland)*, *26*(17), 5411. DOI: 10.3390/molecules26175411 PMID: 34500844

Liu, Z., Xue, X., Cai, W., Cui, K., Patil, S. A., & Guo, K. (2023). Recent progress on microbial electrosynthesis reactor designs and strategies to enhance the reactor performance. *Biochemical Engineering Journal*, *190*, 108745.

Li, W., Huang, C., & Chen, J. (2022). The application of CRISPR/Cas mediated gene editing in synthetic biology: Challenges and optimizations. *Frontiers in Bioengineering and Biotechnology, 10*, 890155. PMID: 36091445

Li, Y., Wang, Y., Wang, R., Yan, X., Wang, J., Wang, X., Chen, S., Bai, F., He, Q., & Yang, S. (2022). Metabolic engineering of *Zymomonas mobilis* for continuous co-production of bioethanol and poly-3-hydroxybutyrate (PHB). *Green Chemistry, 24*(6), 2588–2601. DOI: 10.1039/D1GC04522A

Li, Z., & Rinas, U. (2020). Recombinant protein production associated growth inhibition results mainly from transcription and not from translation. *Microbial Cell Factories, 19*(1), 83. DOI: 10.1186/s12934-020-01343-y

Li, Z., Zhang, W., & Wang, Y. (2022). Valorization of lignocellulosic biomass into value-added products via microbial fermentation. *Bioresource Technology, 363*, 127975. DOI: 10.1016/j.biortech.2022.127975

Löffelholz, C., Kaiser, S. C., Kraume, M., Eibl, R., & Eibl, D. (2014). Dynamic single-use bioreactors used in modern liter-and m 3-scale biotechnological processes: engineering characteristics and scaling up. *Disposable bioreactors II*, 1-44. https://doi.org/DOI: 10.1007/10_2013_187

Löffelholz, C., Husemann, U., Greller, G., Meusel, W., Kauling, J., Ay, P., & Eibl, D. (2013). Bioengineering parameters for single-use bioreactors: Overview and evaluation of suitable methods. *Chemieingenieurtechnik (Weinheim), 85*(1-2), 40–56. DOI: 10.1002/cite.201200125

Lokko, Y., Heijde, M., Schebesta, K., Scholtès, P., Van Montagu, M., & Giacca, M. (2018). Biotechnology and the bioeconomy—Towards inclusive and sustainable industrial development. *New Biotechnology, 40*, 5–10.

Love, J. (2022). Microbial pathways for advanced biofuel production. *Biochemical Society Transactions, 50*(2), 987–1001. DOI: 10.1042/BST20210764 PMID: 35411379

Love, J. C., Reynolds, E. B., Goldston, D., & Frye, H. E. (2025). Biomanufacturing in the US: A MIT. *Policy Brief.*

Lovley, D. R. (2006). Bug juice: Harvesting electricity with microorganisms. *Nature Reviews. Microbiology, 4*(7), 497–508. DOI: 10.1038/nrmicro1442 PMID: 16778836

Lozano, F. J., Lozano, R., Freire, P., Jiménez-Gonzalez, C., Sakao, T., Ortiz, M. G., Trianni, A., Carpenter, A., & Viveros, T. (2018). New perspectives for green and sustainable chemistry and engineering: Approaches from sustainable resource and energy use, management, and transformation. *Journal of Cleaner Production, 172*, 227–232.

Lu, C., Liu, Y., Li, J., Liu, L., & Du, G. (2019). Engineering of biosynthesis pathway and NADPH supply for improved L-5-methyltetrahydrofolate production by Lactococcus lactis. *Journal of Microbiology and Biotechnology, 31*(1), 154.

Lucio, M., & Fermentec, L. (2008). Continuous and batch fermentation processes: Advantages and disadvantages of these processes in the Brazilian ethanol production. In *Article in International Sugar Journal.* https://www.researchgate.net/publication/289874380

Lu, J., Sheahan, C., & Fu, P. (2021). Metabolic engineering of algae for fourth generation biofuels production. *Energy & Environmental Science*, *4*(7), 2451–2466. DOI: 10.1039/C0EE00593B

Luka, G., Ahmadi, A., Najjaran, H., Alocilja, E., DeRosa, M., Wolthers, K., & Hoorfar, M. (2015). Microfluidics integrated biosensors: A leading technology towards lab-on-a-chip and sensing applications. *Sensors (Basel)*, *15*(12), 30011–30031. PMID: 26633409

Luo, H., Liu, Z., Xie, F., Bilal, M., Liu, L., Yang, R., & Wang, Z. (2021). Microbial production of gamma-aminobutyric acid: Applications, state-of-the-art achievements, and future perspectives. *Critical Reviews in Biotechnology*, *41*(4), 491–512.

Luo, X., Reiter, M. A., d'Espaux, L., Wong, J., Denby, C. M., Lechner, A., Zhang, Y., Grzybowski, A. T., Harth, S., Lin, W., Lee, H., Yu, C., Shin, J., Deng, K., Benites, V. T., Wang, G., Baidoo, E. E. K., Chen, Y., Dev, I., & Keasling, J. D. (2019). Complete biosynthesis of cannabinoids and their unnatural analogues in yeast. *Nature*, *567*(7746), 123–126. DOI: 10.1038/s41586-019-0978-9

Luu, X. C., Shida, Y., Suzuki, Y., Kuwahara, D., Fujimoto, T., Takahashi, Y., Sato, N., Nakamura, A., & Ogasawara, W. (2023). Ultrahigh-throughput screening of *Trichoderma reesei* strains capable of carbon catabolite repression release and cellulase hyperproduction using a microfluidic droplet platform. *Bioscience, Biotechnology, and Biochemistry*, *87*(11), 1393–1406. DOI: 10.1093/bbb/zbad108 PMID: 37550222

Lv, Y., Li, W., Liao, W., Jiang, H., Liu, Y., Cao, J., Lu, W., & Feng, Y. (2024). Nano-Drug Delivery Systems Based on Natural Products. *International Journal of Nanomedicine*, *19*, 541–569. DOI: 10.2147/IJN.S443692

Lynch, C., Jordan, L., & O'Connell, J. D. (2022). Redesigning Spent Media from Cell Culture Bioprocess to Feed New Bacterial Fermentations. In *Cell Culture Engineering and Technology: In appreciation to Professor Mohamed Al-Rubeai* (pp. 129-146). Cham: Springer International Publishing. https://doi.org/DOI: 10.1007/978-3-030-79871-0_5

Machireddy, J. R., Rachakatla, S. K., & Ravichandran, P. (2021). Leveraging AI and machine learning for data-driven business strategy: A comprehensive framework for analytics integration. *African Journal of Artificial Intelligence and Sustainable Development*, *1*(2), 12–150.

Macwan, A., Desai, D., Vandra, N., Mishra, K. K., & Jha, Y. (2025). Biotechnology for Global Sustainability: Innovations, Applications, and Challenges. *Int. Res. J. Adv. Eng. Manag*, 59-65.

Madigan, M. T., Bender, K. S., Buckley, D. H., Sattley, W. M., & Stahl, D. A. (2018). Microbial growth and its control. In *Brock biology of microorganisms* (15th ed., pp. 173–208). Pearson.

Madondo, N. I., Rathilal, S., Bakare, B. F., & Tetteh, E. K. (2023). Application of bioelectrochemical systems and anaerobic additives in wastewater treatment: A conceptual review. *International Journal of Molecular Sciences*, *24*(5), 4753. PMID: 36902185

Mahakur, B., Bedaprabha, A., Barik, D. P., Gupta, S., Kumar, R., Mitra, D., & Verma, D. (2025). Hairy Root Culture: An Effective Method for Production of Plant Bioactive Compounds. Genetic Improvement and Conservation Practices of Medicinal Plants. First Edition (2025) | CRC Press, Pages: 9 | eBook ISBN: 9781003482659

Maharaj, K., Bradfield, M. F. A., & Nicol, W. (2014). Succinic acid-producing biofilms of Actinobacillus succinogenes: Reproducibility, stability and productivity. *Applied Microbiology and Biotechnology, 98*(17), 7379–7386. DOI: 10.1007/s00253-014-5779-3

Mahmoodi, M., & Nassireslami, E. (2022). Control algorithms and strategies of feeding for fed-batch fermentation of Escherichia coli: A review of 40 years of experience. *Preparative Biochemistry & Biotechnology, 52*(7), 823–834.

Mahmood, T., Hussain, N., Shahbaz, A., Mulla, S. I., Iqbal, H. M., & Bilal, M. (2023). Sustainable production of biofuels from the algae-derived biomass. *Bioprocess and Biosystems Engineering, 46*(8), 1077–1097. PMID: 36331626

Majhi, B. K. (2025). Cyanobacteria: Photosynthetic cell factories for biofuel production. *Journal of Bioresources and Bioproducts, 10*(2), 128–144. DOI: 10.1016/j.jobab.2024.10.001

Malakar, S., Paul, S. K., & Pou, K. J. (2020). Biotechnological interventions in beverage production. In *Biotechnological progress and beverage consumption* (pp. 1–37). Elsevier.

Malcata, F. X. (1989). CSTR's in Biochemical Reactions: An Optimization Problem. *Chemical Engineering Education, 23*(2), 112–128.

Malik, S. (2024). Emerging Trends in Agricultural Biotechnology: Opportunities and Challenges. *Frontiers in Agriculture, 1*(2), 356–389.

Malvido, M. C., González, E. A., Bazán Tantaleán, D. L., Bendaña Jácome, R. J., & Guerra, N. P. (2019). Batch and fed-batch production of probiotic biomass and nisin in nutrient-supplemented whey media. *Brazilian Journal of Microbiology : Publication of the Brazilian Society for Microbiology, 50*(4), 915–925.

Ma, N., Mollet, M., & Chalmers, J. J. (2005). Aeration, mixing and hydrodynamics in bioreactors. In *Cell culture technology for pharmaceutical and cell-based therapies* (pp. 243–266). CRC Press., DOI: 10.1201/9780849351068

Manara, P., & Zabaniotou, A. (2016). Co-valorization of crude glycerol waste streams with conventional and/or renewable fuels for power generation and industrial symbiosis perspectives. *Waste and Biomass Valorization, 7*, 135–150.

Mandato, K., & Kulhanek, B. (2022). The impact of inadequate training. In *Healthcare Technology Training: An Evidence-based Guide for Improved Quality* (pp. 11–17). Springer International Publishing., DOI: 10.1007/978-3-031-10322-3_2

Mandenius, C. F., & Brundin, A. (2008). Bioprocess optimization using design-of-experiments methodology. *Biotechnology Progress, 24*(6), 1191–1203. PMID: 19194932

Mandenius, C. F., & Brundin, A. (2008). Bioprocess optimization using design-of-experiments methodology. *Biotechnology Progress, 24*(6), 1191–1203. PMID: 19194932

Mantle, J. L., Rammohan, J., & Romantseva, E. F.. (2019). Cyberbiosecurity for Biopharmaceutical Products. *Frontiers in Bioengineering and Biotechnology, 7*, 116. DOI: 10.3389/fbioe.2019.00116 PMID: 31214582

Mao, B., Gu, J., Li, D., Cui, S., Zhao, J., Zhang, H., & Chen, W. (2018). Effects of different doses of fructooligosaccharides (FOS) on the composition of mice fecal microbiota, especially the Bifidobacterium composition. *Nutrients, 10*(8), 1105.

Marcello, K. M. (2024). *Unraveling the genomic and adaptive strategies of Antarctic cyanobacteria: A bioinformatic analysis of survival mechanisms in extreme cold environments* [Doctoral dissertation, University of California, Davis]. ProQuest Dissertations Publishing.

Marimon, F., & Casadesús, M. (2017). Reasons to adopt ISO 50001 energy management system. *Sustainability, 9*(10), 1740.

Mariyes, T. C., Ju, E.-J., & Lee, J.-H. (2024). Enhancing microbial resilience: The role of adaptive laboratory evolution in industrial biotechnology. *Journal of Life Science, 34*(10), 730–743.

Maroof, L., Khan, I., Yoo, H. S., Kim, S., Park, H. T., Ahmad, B., & Azam, S. (2021). Identification and characterization of low density polyethylene-degrading bacteria isolated from soils of waste disposal sites. *Environmental Engineering Research, 26*(3). Advance online publication. DOI: 10.4491/eer.2020.167

Marques, M. P. C., Fernandes, P., & Cabral, J. M. S. (2010). Bioreactor design for microbial and cell cultures: A review on the major scale-up issues. *Journal of Chemical Technology and Biotechnology, 85*(10), 1184–1194.

Marqusee, J., & Don, D. J.II. (2020). Reliability of emergency and standby diesel generators: Impact on energy resiliency solutions. *Applied Energy, 268*, 114918. DOI: 10.1016/j.apenergy.2020.114918

Martin, G. J., & Chan, S. (2024). Future production of yeast biomass for sustainable proteins: A critical review. *Sustainable Food Technology.*

Mary, T., & Enoch, O. (2024). Legal Considerations in the Development and Commercialization of Corporate Intellectual Property. *International Journal of Rural Development. Environmental Health Report, 8*(3), 593109. DOI: 10.22161/ijreh.8.3.1

Masoumi, S. J., Mehrabani, D., Saberifiroozi, M., Fattahi, M. R., Moradi, F., & Najafi, M. (2021). The effect of yogurt fortified with Lactobacillus acidophilus and Bifidobacterium sp. probiotic in patients with lactose intolerance. *Food Science & Nutrition, 9*(3), 1704–1711.

Massoud, M. A., Fayad, R., Kamleh, R., & El-Fadel, M. (2010). *Environmental management system (ISO 14001) certification in developing countries: Challenges and implementation strategies.*

Masud, M. A. A., Shin, W. S., Sarker, A., Septian, A., Das, K., Deepo, D. M., Iqbal, M. A., Islam, A. R. M. T., & Malafaia, G. (2023). A critical review of sustainable application of biochar for green remediation: Research uncertainty and future directions. *The Science of the Total Environment, 904*, 166813. DOI: 10.1016/j.scitotenv.2023.166813 PMID: 37683867

Matanguihan, C., & Wu, P. (2022). Upstream continuous processing: Recent advances in production of biopharmaceuticals and challenges in manufacturing. *Current Opinion in Biotechnology, 78*, 102828. DOI: 10.1016/j.copbio.2022.102828 PMID: 36332340

Matsuda, F., Toya, Y., & Shimizu, H. (2017). Learning from quantitative data to understand central carbon metabolism. *Biotechnology Advances, 35*(8), 971–980. DOI: 10.1016/j.biotechadv.2017.09.006 PMID: 28928003

Matsumoto, T., Tanaka, T., & Kondo, A. (2017). Engineering metabolic pathways in *Escherichia coli* for constructing a "microbial chassis" for biochemical production. *Bioresource Technology, 245*(Pt B), 1362–1368. https://doi.org/DOI: 10.1016/j.biortech.2017.05.171

Ma, X., Liang, H., Panda, S., Fung, V. K. Y., Zhou, J. F. J., & Zhou, K. (2022). C2 feedstock-based biomanufacturing of value-added chemicals. *Current Opinion in Biotechnology, 73*, 240–245. DOI: 10.1016/j.copbio.2021.08.017 PMID: 34536659

Mazzola, P. G., Lopes, A. M., Hasmann, F. A., Jozala, A. F., Penna, T. C., Magalhaes, P. O., & Pessoa, A.Jr. (2008). Liquid–liquid extraction of biomolecules: an overview and update of the main techniques. *Journal of Chemical Technology & Biotechnology: International Research in Process. Environmental & Clean Technology, 83*(2), 143–157.

McDonnell, G. E. (2020). *Antisepsis, disinfection, and sterilization: Types, action, and resistance* (2nd ed.). John Wiley & Sons.

McElwain, L., Phair, K., Kealey, C., & Brady, D. (2022). Current trends in biopharmaceuticals production in Escherichia coli. *Biotechnology Letters, 44*(8), 917–931. DOI: 10.1007/s10529-022-03276-5

McGovern, P. E., Zhang, J., Tang, J., Zhang, Z., Hall, G. R., Moreau, R. A., Nuñez, A., Butrym, E. D., Richards, M. P., Wang, C., Cheng, G., Zhao, Z., & Wang, C. (2004). Fermented beverages of pre- and proto-historic China. *Proceedings of the National Academy of Sciences of the United States of America, 101*(51), 17593–17598. DOI: 10.1073/pnas.0407921102

McShan, D. C., Rao, S., & Shah, I. (2003). Pathminer: Predicting metabolic pathways by heuristic search. *Bioinformatics (Oxford, England), 19*(13), 1692–1698.

Medina, C. (2016). A cGMP Risk Assessment and Management Strategy: Guidelines for the Pre-Approval Inspection. In *Preparing for FDA Pre-Approval Inspections* (pp. 107–147). CRC Press.

Meena, K. K., Taneja, N. K., Ojha, A., & Meena, S. (2023). Application of spray-drying and freeze-drying for microencapsulation of lactic acid bacteria: A review. *Annals of Phytomedicine, 12*(1), 706–716.

Meereboer, K. W., Misra, M., & Mohanty, A. K. (2020). Review of recent advances in the biodegradability of polyhydroxyalkanoate (PHA) bioplastics and their composites. *Green Chemistry, 22*(17), 5519–5558.

Megharaj, M., Ramakrishnan, B., Venkateswarlu, K., Sethunathan, N., & Naidu, R. (2011). Bioremediation approaches for organic pollutants: A critical perspective. *Environment International, 37*(8), 1362–1375. DOI: 10.1016/j.envint.2011.06.003 PMID: 21722961

Meghwanshi, G. K., Kaur, N., Verma, S., Dabi, N. K., Vashishtha, A., Charan, P., Purohit, P., Bhandari, H., Bhojak, N., & Kumar, R. (2020). Enzymes for pharmaceutical and therapeutic applications. *Biotechnology and Applied Biochemistry, 67*(4), 586–601. PMID: 32248597

Meghwanshi, G. K., Kaur, N., Verma, S., Gupta, N., Kumar, R., & Prakash, V. (2020). Enzymes for pharmaceutical and therapeutic applications. *Biotechnology Reports (Amsterdam, Netherlands), 25*, e00427. DOI: 10.1016/j.btre.2020.e00427 PMID: 32248597

Mehendale, N., Jenne, F., Joshi, C., Sharma, S., Masakapalli, S. K., & MacKinnon, N. (2020). A nuclear magnetic resonance (NMR) platform for real-time metabolic monitoring of bioprocesses. *Molecules (Basel, Switzerland), 25*(20), 4675. PMID: 33066296

Mehta, A., Niaz, M., Adetoro, A., & Nwagwu, U. (2024). Advancements in manufacturing technology for the biotechnology industry: The role of artificial intelligence and emerging trends. *International Journal of Chemistry. Mathematics and Physics, 8*(2), 12–18. DOI: 10.22161/ijcmp.8.2.3

Menacho-Melgar, R., Moreb, E. A., Efromson, J. P., Yang, T., Hennigan, J. N., Wang, R., & Lynch, M. D. (2020). Improved two-stage protein expression and purification via autoinduction of both autolysis and auto DNA/RNA hydrolysis conferred by phage lysozyme and DNA/RNA endonuclease. *Biotechnology and Bioengineering, 117*(9), 2852–2860. DOI: 10.1002/bit.27444

Menzel, K., Zeng, A.-P., & Deckwer, W.-D. (1997). High concentration and productivity of 1,3-propanediol from continuous fermentation of glycerol by Klebsiella pneumoniae. *Enzyme and Microbial Technology, 20*(2), 82–86. DOI: 10.1016/S0141-0229(96)00087-7

Meramo, S., Fantke, P., & Sukumara, S. (2022). Advances and opportunities in integrating economic and environmental performance of renewable products. *Biotechnology for Biofuels, 15*, 144. DOI: 10.1186/s13068-022-02239-2 PMID: 36550529

Merck & Co. (2019). *Digital Transformation in Manufacturing*. Retrieved from https://www.merck.com/news/digital-manufacturing-initiatives

Meyer, H. P., Minas, W., & Schmidhalter, D. (2017). Industrial-scale fermentation. Industrial biotechnology: products and processes, 1-53. http://dx.doi.org/DOI: 10.1002/9783527807833.ch1

Michels, P., & Rosazza, J. (2009). The evolution of microbial transformations for industrial applications. *SIM News*, 36–59.

Minervini, F., Comitini, F., De Boni, A., Fiorino, G. M., Rodrigues, F., Tlais, A. Z. A., Carafa, I., & De Angelis, M. (2022). Sustainable and Health-Protecting Food Ingredients from Bioprocessed Food by-Products and Wastes. *Sustainability, 14*(22), 15283.

Minton, N. P. (1984). Improved plasmid vectors for the isolation of translational lac gene fusions. *Gene, 31*(1–3), 269–273. DOI: 10.1016/0378-1119(84)90220-8

Mirakhori, F., & Niazi, S. K. (2025). Harnessing the AI/ML in Drug and Biological Products Discovery and Development: The Regulatory Perspective. *Pharmaceuticals, 18*(1), 47. PMID: 39861110

Mirsalami, S. M., & Mirsalami, M. (2025). Advances in genetically engineered microorganisms: Transforming food production through precision fermentation and synthetic biology. *Future Foods : a Dedicated Journal for Sustainability in Food Science, 11*, 100601. DOI: 10.1016/j.fufo.2025.100601

Mirzadeh, K., Martínez, V., Toddo, S., Guntur, S., Herrgård, M. J., Elofsson, A., Nørholm, M. H. H., & Daley, D. O. (2015). Enhanced Protein Production in *Escherichia coli* by Optimization of Cloning Scars at the Vector–Coding Sequence Junction. *ACS Synthetic Biology*, *4*(9), 959–965. DOI: 10.1021/acssynbio.5b00033

Mirzadeh, K., Shilling, P. J., Elfageih, R., Cumming, A. J., Cui, H. L., Rennig, M., Nørholm, M. H. H., & Daley, D. O. (2020). Increased production of periplasmic proteins in Escherichia coli by directed evolution of the translation initiation region. *Microbial Cell Factories*, *19*(1), 85. DOI: 10.1186/s12934-020-01339-8

Mishra, B., Mohanta, Y. K., Reddy, C. N., Reddy, S. D. M., Mandal, S. K., Yadavalli, R., & Sarma, H. (2023). Valorization of agro-industrial biowaste to biomaterials: An innovative circular bioeconomy approach. *Circular Economy*, *2*, 100050. DOI: 10.1016/j.cec.2023.100050

Mishra, B., Varjani, S., Kumar, G., Awasthi, M. K., Awasthi, S. K., Sindhu, R., & Zhang, Z. (2021). Microbial approaches for remediation of pollutants: Innovations, future outlook, and challenges. *Energy & Environment*, *32*(6), 1029–1058. DOI: 10.1177/0958305X19896781

Mitchell, A. H., Pannell, M. A., Arbury, S., Thomas, R., & Hodgson, M. J. (2019). Bloodborne pathogens standard enforcement at the occupational safety and health administration: The first twenty-five years. *New Solutions*, *29*(2), 172–185. PMID: 30917759

Mitchell, D. A., Ruiz, H. A., & Krieger, N. (2023). A critical evaluation of recent studies on packed-bed bioreactors for solid-state fermentation. *Processes (Basel, Switzerland)*, *11*(3), 872. DOI: 10.3390/pr11030872

Mitra, S., & Murthy, G. S. (2022). Bioreactor control systems in the biopharmaceutical industry: A critical perspective. *Systems Microbiology and Biomanufacturing*, , 1–22. DOI: 10.1007/s43393-021-00048-6 PMID: 38624976

Mittal, P., Brindle, J., Stephen, J., Plotkin, J. B., & Kudla, G. (2018). Codon usage influences fitness through RNA toxicity. *Proceedings of the National Academy of Sciences of the United States of America*, *115*(34), 8639–8644. DOI: 10.1073/pnas.1810022115

Mohamed, H., Shah, A. M., & Song, Y. (2021). Conversion of agro-industrial wastes into value-added products. In *Conversion of renewable biomass into bioproducts* (pp. 197–217). ACS Publications.

Mohammadian Fazli, M., Soleimani, N., Mehrasbi, M., Darabian, S., Mohammadi, J., & Ramazani, A. (2015). Highly cadmium tolerant fungi: Their tolerance and removal potential. *Journal of Environmental Health Science & Engineering*, *13*, 19. DOI: 10.1186/s40201-015-0176-0 PMID: 25806110

Mohammed, A., Rivers, A., Stuckey, D. C., & Ward, K. (2023). Alginate-based bioplastics: A review. *International Journal of Biological Macromolecules*, *233*, 123550. DOI: 10.1016/j.ijbiomac.2023.123550

Mollah, A. H. (2005). Application of failure mode and effect analysis (FMEA) for process risk assessment. *BioProcess International*, *5*, 12–20.

Monod, J. (2012). The growth of bacterial cultures. In *Selected papers in molecular biology by Jacques Monod* (pp. 606–626). Academic Press. (Original work published 1949), DOI: 10.1016/B978-0-12-460482-7.50047-0

Monod, J., Changeux, J. P., & Jacob, F. (1961). Allosteric proteins and cellular control systems. *Journal of Molecular Biology*, *6*(4), 306–329. DOI: 10.1016/S0022-2836(63)80091-1 PMID: 13936070

Monteiro, M., Fadda, S., & Kontoravdi, C. (2023). Towards advanced bioprocess optimization: A multiscale modelling approach. *Computational and Structural Biotechnology Journal, 21*, 3639–3655. PMID: 37520284

Morales, M., Ma, J., Al-Rub, K. A., & Scheper, T. (2008). Challenges in downstream processing: From clarification to purification. *Biotechnology Journal*, *3*(3), 327–337.

Morello, E., Bermúdez-Humarán, L. G., Llull, D., Solé, V., Miraglio, N., Langella, P., & Poquet, I. (2008). <i>Lactococcus lactis,</i> an Efficient Cell Factory for Recombinant Protein Production and Secretion. *Microbial Physiology, 14*(1–3), 48–58. https://doi.org/DOI: 10.1159/000106082

Moresi, M. (1981). Optimal design of airlift fermenters. *Biotechnology and Bioengineering*, *23*(11), 2537–2560.

Morgado, G., Gerngross, D., Roberts, T. M., & Panke, S. (2018). Synthetic biology for cell-free biosynthesis: Fundamentals of designing novel in vitro multi-enzyme reaction networks. In *Synthetic biology—Metabolic engineering* (pp. 117–146). Springer., DOI: 10.1007/10_2016_46

Moriya, Y., Shigemizu, D., Hattori, M., Tokimatsu, T., Kotera, M., Goto, S., & Kanehisa, M. (2010). Pathpred: An enzyme-catalyzed metabolic pathway prediction server. *Nucleic Acids Research*, *38*(2), W138–W143.

Mortensen, D. N., & Williams, E. R. (2016). Surface-induced protein unfolding in submicron electrospray emitters. *Analytical Chemistry*, *88*(19), 9662–9668. DOI: 10.1021/acs.analchem.6b02512

Moser, A. (1988). The principles of bioprocess technology. In *Bioprocess Technology* (pp. 13–65). Kinetics and Reactors.

Mujahid, M., Wakeel, M., Ali, A. M., Saeed, S., Nawaz, A. S., & Hafeez, K. (2024). Food fermentation: Traditional practices and modern applications in food industry. *International Journal of Food and Fermentation Technology*, *14*(1), 239–273.

Mujtaba, M., Fernandes Fraceto, L., Fazeli, M., Mukherjee, S., Savassa, S. M., Araujo de Medeiros, G., do Espírito Santo Pereira, A., Mancini, S. D., Lipponen, J., & Vilaplana, F. (2023). Lignocellulosic biomass from agricultural waste to the circular economy: A review with focus on biofuels, biocomposites and bioplastics. *Journal of Cleaner Production*, *402*, 136815. Advance online publication. DOI: 10.1016/j.jclepro.2023.136815

Mukherjee, A., Gómez-Sala, B., O'Connor, E. M., Kenny, J. G., & Cotter, P. D. (2022). Global regulatory frameworks for fermented foods: A review. *Frontiers in Nutrition*, *9*, 902642.

Müller, E., Berger, R., Blass, E., Sluyts, D., & Pfennig, A. (2000). *Liquid–liquid extraction*. Ullmann's Encyclopedia of Industrial Chemistry.

Müller, M., Mentel, M., van Hellemond, J. J., Henze, K., Woehle, C., Gould, S. B., & Martin, W. F. (2012). Biochemistry and evolution of anaerobic energy metabolism in eukaryotes. *Microbiology and Molecular Biology Reviews : MMBR*, *76*(2), 444–495. PMID: 22688819

Müller-Späth, T., Morbidelli, M., & Hubbuch, J. (2008). Purification of therapeutic proteins using simulated moving bed chromatography. *Journal of Chromatography. A*, *1171*(1-2), 46–58.

Mulukutla, B. C., Yongky, A., Le, T., Mashek, D. G., & Hu, W. S. (2016). Regulation of glucose metabolism–a perspective from cell bioprocessing. *Trends in Biotechnology*, *34*(8), 638–651. PMID: 27265890

Muncan, J., Tei, K., & Tsenkova, R. (2020). Real-time monitoring of yogurt fermentation process by aquaphotomics near-infrared spectroscopy. *Sensors (Basel)*, *21*(1), 177.

Munro, G. (2017). ICH Q7 good manufacturing practice guide for active pharmaceutical ingredients (APIs). In *ICH quality guidelines: An implementation guide* (pp. 509–534). John Wiley & Sons. https://doi.org/DOI: 10.1002/9781118971147.ch17

Mustapää, T., Nummiluikki, J., & Viitala, R. (2022). Digitalization of calibration data management in pharmaceutical industry using a multitenant platform. *Applied Sciences (Basel, Switzerland)*, *12*(15), 7531.

Myung, S., Zhang, X., & Percival Zhang, Y.-H. (2011). Ultra-stable phosphoglucose isomerase through immobilization of cellulose-binding module-tagged thermophilic enzyme on low-cost high-capacity cellulosic adsorbent. *Biotechnology Progress*, *27*(4), 969–975. DOI: 10.1002/btpr.606

Nadal-Rey, G., McClure, D. D., Kavanagh, J. M., Cassells, B., Cornelissen, S., Fletcher, D. F., & Gernaey, K. V. (2022). Computational fluid dynamics modelling of hydrodynamics, mixing and oxygen transfer in industrial bioreactors with Newtonian broths. *Biochemical Engineering Journal*, *177*, 108265. DOI: 10.1016/j.bej.2021.108265

Nadal-Rey, G., McClure, D. D., Kavanagh, J. M., Cornelissen, S., Fletcher, D. F., & Gernaey, K. V. (2021). Understanding gradients in industrial bioreactors. *Biotechnology Advances*, *46*, 107660. DOI: 10.1016/j.biotechadv.2020.107660 PMID: 33221379

Naik, S. N., Goud, V. V., Rout, P. K., & Dalai, A. K. (2010). Production of first and second generation biofuels: A comprehensive review. *Renewable & Sustainable Energy Reviews*, *14*(2), 578–597. DOI: 10.1016/j.rser.2009.10.003

Najib, M., Abdullah, S., Narresh, S., & Juni, M. H. (2019). Brain-drain phenomenon among healthcare workers. *International Journal of Public Health and Clinical Sciences*, *6*(3), 90–103.

Nakamura, C. E., & Whited, G. M. (2003). Metabolic engineering for the microbial production of 1,3-propanediol. *Current Opinion in Biotechnology*, *14*(5), 454–459. DOI: 10.1016/j.copbio.2003.08.005

Nambiar, A., & Mundra, D. (2022). An overview of data warehouse and data lake in modern enterprise data management. *Big Data and Cognitive Computing*, *6*(4), 132.

Namjoshi, S., Dabbaghi, M., Roberts, M. S., Grice, J. E., & Mohammed, Y. (2020). Quality by design: Development of the quality target product profile (QTPP) for semisolid topical products. *Pharmaceutics*, *12*(3), 287. PMID: 32210126

Nanda, S., Kumar, V., & Vij, R. K. (2023). A review on thermochemical and biochemical conversion of biomass to biofuels. *BioEnergy Research, 16*(1), 1–26. DOI: 10.1007/s12155-022-10526-x

Nanov, M., Despotovska, S., Mitrovska, G., Koceva, V. D., & Acevska, J. (2024). Advantages of trend analysis in stability studies for prediction of potential OOS result within estimated shelf life of medicinal product. *Macedonian Pharmaceutical Bulletin/Makedonsko Farmacevtski Bilten, 70*(1).

Narancic, T., Cerrone, F., Beagan, N., & O'Connor, K. E. (2020). Recent advances in bioplastics: Application and biodegradation. *Polymers, 12*(4), 920. DOI: 10.3390/polym12040920 PMID: 32326661

Narayanan, H.. (2021). Industry 4.0 in pharmaceutical manufacturing: A systematic review. *Journal of Industrial Information Integration, 24*, 100224.

Nargund, S., Mauch, K., & Esswein, S. (2024). *Biopharma 4.0: Digital technologies driving smart manufacturing. Springer*. https://link.springer.com/chapter/10.1007/978-3-031-45669-5_11

Närhi, M., & Nordström, K. (2005). Manufacturing, regulatory and commercial challenges of biopharmaceuticals production: A Finnish perspective. *European Journal of Pharmaceutics and Biopharmaceutics, 59*(3), 397–405. PMID: 15760720

Narisetty, V. R. R., Maitra, S., Tarafdar, A., Alphy, M. P., Kumar, A. N., Madhavan, A., Sirohi, R., Awasthi, M. K., Sindhu, R., Varjani, S., & Binod, P. (2023). Waste-Derived Fuels and Renewable Chemicals for Bioeconomy Promotion: A Sustainable Approach. *BioEnergy Research, 16*(1), 16–32. DOI: 10.1007/s12155-022-10428-y PMID: 35350609

Nascimento, A. P. S., & Barros, A. N. (2025). Sustainable Innovations in Food Microbiology: Fermentation, Biocontrol, and Functional Foods. *Foods, 14*(13), 2320.

Naseem, Z., Mir, S. A., Wani, S. M., Rouf, M. A., Bashir, I., & Zehra, A. (2023). Probiotic-fortified fruit juices: Health benefits, challenges, and future perspective. *Nutrition (Burbank, Los Angeles County, Calif.), 115*, 112154.

Naveen, A. K., & Sontakke, M. (2024). A review on regulatory aspects, challenges and public perception in acceptance of genetically modified foods. *Food Science and Biotechnology, 33*(4), 791–804.

Nehal, N., Mathur, A., Ganguli, M., & Singh, P. (2022). Fermentation Process Versus Nanotechnology. In *Nanomaterials in Clinical Therapeutics* (pp. 115–175). Wiley., DOI: 10.1002/9781119857747.ch4

Neidhardt, F. C., Ingraham, J. L., & Schaechter, M. (1990). *Physiology of the bacterial cell: A molecular approach.* Sinauer Associates.

Nejatishahidein, N., & Zydney, A. L. (2021). Depth filtration in bioprocessing—New opportunities for an old technology. *Current Opinion in Chemical Engineering, 34*, 100746.

Ngongolo, K., & Mmbando, G. S. (2024). Harnessing biotechnology and breeding strategies for climate-resilient agriculture: Pathways to sustainable global food security. *Discover Sustainability, 5*(1), 431.

Nguyen, D. M. N. (2018). Understanding the redox metabolism of pyrococcus furiosus for efficient metabolic engineering.

Nguyen, N. T., Vo, T. S., Tran-Nguyen, P. L., Nguyen, M. N., Pham, V. H., Matsuhashi, R., & Vo, T. T. B. C. (2024). A comprehensive review of aeration and wastewater treatment. *Aquaculture (Amsterdam, Netherlands), 741113.* Advance online publication. DOI: 10.1016/j.aquaculture.2024.741113

Nguyen, P. Q., Courchesne, N. M. D., Duraj-Thatte, A., Praveschotinunt, P., & Joshi, N. S. (2018). Engineered living materials: Prospects and challenges for using biological systems to direct the assembly of smart materials. *Advanced Materials, 30*(19), 1704847.

Nguyen, T.-T., Nguyen, H. A., Arreola, S. L., Mlynek, G., Djinović-Carugo, K., Mathiesen, G., Nguyen, T.-H., & Haltrich, D. (2012). Homodimeric β-Galactosidase from Lactobacillus delbrueckii subsp. *bulgaricus* DSM 20081: Expression in Lactobacillus plantarum and Biochemical Characterization. *Journal of Agricultural and Food Chemistry, 60*(7), 1713–1721. DOI: 10.1021/jf203909e

Nguyen, V. T., Flanagan, B., Gidley, M. J., & Dykes, G. A. (2008). Characterization of Cellulose Production by a Gluconacetobacter xylinus Strain from Kombucha. *Current Microbiology, 57*(5), 449–453. DOI: 10.1007/s00284-008-9228-3

Nielsen, D. R., Leonard, E., Yoon, S. H., Tseng, H. C., Yuan, C., & Prather, K. L. J. (2009). Engineering alternative butanol production platforms in heterologous bacteria. *Metabolic Engineering, 11*(4–5), 262–273. DOI: 10.1016/j.ymben.2009.05.003 PMID: 19464384

Nielsen, J., & Keasling, J. D. (2016). Engineering cellular metabolism. *Cell, 164*(6), 1185–1197. DOI: 10.1016/j.cell.2016.02.004

Nienow, A. W. (2006). Reactor engineering in large scale animal cell culture. *Cytotechnology, 50*(1), 9–33. DOI: 10.1007/s10616-006-9005-0

Nienow, A. W. (2014). Stirring and stirred-tank reactors. *Chemieingenieurtechnik (Weinheim), 86*(12), 2063–2074. DOI: 10.1002/cite.201400087

Nieto-Taype, M. A., Garcia-Ortega, X., Albiol, J., Montesinos-Seguí, J. L., & Valero, F. (2020). Continuous cultivation as a tool toward the rational bioprocess development with Pichia Pastoris cell factory. *Frontiers in Bioengineering and Biotechnology, 8*, 632. PMID: 32671036

Nie, Z., Luo, H., Li, J., Sun, H., Xiao, Y., Jia, R., Liu, T., Chang, Y., Yu, H., & Shen, Z. (2020). High-Throughput Screening of T7 Promoter Mutants for Soluble Expression of Cephalosporin C Acylase in E. coli. *Applied Biochemistry and Biotechnology, 190*(1), 293–304. DOI: 10.1007/s12010-019-03113-y

NIH. (2019). *Guidelines for Research Involving Recombinant or Synthetic Nucleic Acid Molecules.* https://osp.od.nih.gov/biotechnology/nih-guidelines/

Nikita, S., Banerjee, S., Jesubalan, N. G., Kulkarni, A., Gupta, K., & Rathore, A. S. (2024). Holistic process control framework for smart biomanufacturing: A deep learning driven approach. *Computers & Chemical Engineering, 187*, 108742.

Nikolados, E. M., Weiße, A. Y., Ceroni, F., & Oyarzún, D. A. (2019). Growth defects and loss-of-function in synthetic gene circuits. *ACS Synthetic Biology*, *8*(6), 1231–1240. DOI: 10.1021/acssynbio.8b00531 PMID: 31181895

Nikoloudaki, O., Aheto, F., Di Cagno, R., & Gobbetti, M. (2024). Synthetic microbial communities: A gateway to understanding resistance, resilience, and functionality in spontaneously fermented food microbiomes. *Food Research International*, *192*, 114780.

Nishal, S., Kumar, V., Phogat, P., Garg, V., & Dureja, H. (2024). Selection of Design of PAT. In *Introduction to Quality by Design (QbD) From Theory to Practice* (pp. 59–89). Springer Nature Singapore.

Niyigaba, T., Küçükgöz, K., Kołożyn-Krajewska, D., Krolikowski, T., & Trząskowska, M. (2025). Advances in fermentation technology: A focus on health and safety. *Applied Sciences (Basel, Switzerland)*, *15*(6), 3001.

Noda, S., Shirai, T., Mori, Y., Oyama, S., & Kondo, A. (2017). Engineering a synthetic pathway for maleate in *Escherichia coli. Nature Communications*, *8*, 1153. DOI: 10.1038/s41467-017-01253-9 PMID: 29074856

Noens, E. E., Williams, C., Anandhakrishnan, M., Poulsen, C., Ehebauer, M. T., & Wilmanns, M. (2011). Improved mycobacterial protein production using a Mycobacterium smegmatis groEL1ΔCexpression strain. *BMC Biotechnology*, *11*(1), 27. DOI: 10.1186/1472-6750-11-27

Noori, R., Perwez, M., & Sardar, M. (2019). Cross-linked enzyme aggregates: current developments and applications. *Biocatalysis: Enzymatic basics and applications*, 83-112.

O'Donnell, K., & Kartoglu, U. (2024). QRM, Knowledge Management, and the Importance of ICH Q9 (R1).

O'Mara, P., Farrell, A., Bones, J., & Twomey, K. (2018). Staying alive! Sensors used for monitoring cell health in bioreactors. *Talanta*, *176*, 130–139. DOI: 10.1007/978-981-97-8808-8_16 PMID: 28917732

Odetunde, A., Adekunle, B. I., & Ogeawuchi, J. C. (2022). Using Predictive Analytics and Automation Tools for Real-Time Regulatory Reporting and Compliance Monitoring. *Int. J. Multidiscip. Res. Growth Eval*, *3*(2), 650–661.

Ögmundarson, Ó., Sukumara, S., Herrgård, M. J., & Fantke, P. (2020). Combining environmental and economic performance for bioprocess optimization. *Trends in Biotechnology*, *38*(11), 1203–1214. DOI: 10.1016/j.tibtech.2020.04.011

Ogwu, M. C., Kosoe, E. A., & Osawaru, M. E. (2025). Raw Materials for Sustainable Bioeconomy Development in the Global South. In *Sustainable Bioeconomy Development in the Global South: Volume I Status and Perspectives* (pp. 37-63). Singapore: Springer Nature Singapore. https://doi.org/DOI: 10.1007/978-981-96-0640-5_2

Ojadi, F. I., & Maiyaki, S. F. (2025). Logistics Bottlenecks: Port congestion, Shipping Delays, and the Inflationary Effects of Transportation Challenges. In *Supply Chain Disruptions and Impact on Global Inflation* (pp. 115-136). IGI Global Scientific Publishing. https://doi.org/DOI: 10.4018/979-8-3373-1982-7.ch005

Ojeih, C. A., Ogidan, O., Oluwajobi, Y. F., & Adebayo, B. O. (2024). Biotechnology Regulatory Conundrum: Balancing Innovation and Oversight. *Journal of Sustainable Development Law and Policy (The)*, *15*(3), 120–144.

Oke, G. (2025). Interdisciplinary cross-sectoral strategies to mitigate health workforce migration in Africa. *Journal of Medicine, Surgery, and Public Health, 100179*. Advance online publication. DOI: 10.1016/j.glmedi.2025.100179

Okolie, O., Kumar, A., Edwards, C., Lawton, L. A., Oke, A., McDonald, S., Thakur, V. K., & Njuguna, J. (2023). Bio-Based Sustainable Polymers and Materials: From Processing to Biodegradation. *Journal of Composites Science*, *7*(6), 213. DOI: 10.3390/jcs7060213

Okpala, C. O. R., & Korzeniowska, M. (2023). Understanding the relevance of quality management in agro-food product industry: From ethical considerations to assuring food hygiene quality safety standards and its associated processes. *Food Reviews International*, *39*(4), 1879–1952.

Olaisen, J., & Revang, O. (2017). The dynamics of intellectual property rights for trust, knowledge sharing and innovation in project teams. *International Journal of Information Management*, *37*(6), 583–589. DOI: 10.1016/j.ijinfomgt.2017.05.012

Olguin-Maciel, E., Singh, A., Chable-Villacis, R., Tapia-Tussell, R., & Ruiz, H. A. (2020). Consolidated bioprocessing, an innovative strategy towards sustainability for biofuels production from crop residues: An overview. *Agronomy (Basel)*, *10*(11), 1834.

Oliver-Cuenca, V., Salaris, V., Muñoz-Gimena, P. F., Agüero, Á., Peltzer, M. A., Montero, V. A., Arrieta, M. P., Sempere-Torregrosa, J., Pavon, C., Samper, M. D., Crespo, G. R., Kenny, J. M., López, D., & Peponi, L. (2024). Bio-Based and Biodegradable Polymeric Materials for a Circular Economy. *Polymers*, *16*(21), 3015. PMID: 39518225

Olszewska-Widdrat, A., Alexandri, M., López-Gómez, J. P., Schneider, R., & Venus, J. (2020). Batch and Continuous Lactic Acid Fermentation Based on A Multi-Substrate Approach. *Microorganisms*, *8*(7), 1084. DOI: 10.3390/microorganisms8071084

Oosterhuis, N. M., & Junne, S. (2016). Design, Applications, and Development of Single-Use Bioreactors. *Bioreactors: Design, Operation and Novel Applications*, 261-294. https://doi.org/ DOI: 10.1002/9783527683369.ch9

Oppedisano, R. (2024). Innovative FabLabs. In *Collaborative Spaces and FabLabs: A Global Organisational and Collaborative Network* (pp. 31–40). Springer Nature Switzerland., DOI: 10.1007/978-3-031-62829-0_4

Osman, A. I., Chen, Z., Elgarahy, A. M., Farghali, M., Mohamed, I. M., Priya, A., Hawash, H. B., & Yap, P. (2024). Membrane technology for energy saving: Principles, techniques, applications, challenges, and prospects. *Advanced Energy and Sustainability Research*, *5*(5), 2400011.

Osman, Y., Elrazak, A. A., & Khater, W. (2016). Bioprocess optimization of microbial biopolymer production. *Journal of Biobased Materials and Bioenergy*, *10*(2), 119–128.

Ouranidis, A., Davidopoulou, C., Tashi, R. K., & Kachrimanis, K. (2021). Pharma 4.0 continuous mRNA drug products manufacturing. *Pharmaceutics*, *13*(9), 1371. Advance online publication. DOI: 10.3390/pharmaceutics13091371

Ou, Y. J., Ren, Q. Q., Fang, S. T., Wu, J. G., Jiang, Y. X., Chen, Y. R., Zhang, Y., & Song, J. (2020). Complete genome insights into *Lactococcus petauri* CF11 isolated from a healthy human gut using second- and third-generation sequencing. *Frontiers in Genetics*, *11*, 119. DOI: 10.3389/fgene.2020.00119 PMID: 32174973

Ou, Y., & Guo, S. (2023). Safety risks and ethical governance of biomedical applications of synthetic biology. *Frontiers in Bioengineering and Biotechnology*, *11*. Advance online publication. DOI: 10.3389/fbioe.2023.1292029

Overton, H. K., & Yang, F. (2023). Do information disputes work: The effect of perceived risk, news disputes and credibility on consumer attitudes and trust toward biotechnology companies. *Journal of Communication Management (London)*.

Pachaiappan, R., Cornejo-Ponce, L., Rajendran, R., Manavalan, K., Femilaa Rajan, V., & Awad, F. (2022). A review on biofiltration techniques: Recent advancements in the removal of volatile organic compounds and heavy metals in the treatment of polluted water. *Bioengineered*, *13*(4), 8432–8477. DOI: 10.1080/21655979.2022.2050538 PMID: 35260028

Painter, H. J., Altenhofen, L. M., Kafsack, B. F., & Llinás, M. (2013). Whole-genome analysis of *Plasmodium* spp. utilizing a new Agilent Technologies DNA microarray platform. *Methods in Molecular Biology (Clifton, N.J.)*, *923*, 213–219. DOI: 10.1007/978-1-62703-026-7_14 PMID: 22990780

Palladino, F., Marcelino, P. R. F., Schlogl, A. E., José, Á. H. M., Rodrigues, R. C. L. B., Fabrino, D. L., Santos, I. J. B., & Rosa, C. A. (2024). Bioreactors: Applications and innovations for a sustainable and healthy future—a critical review. *Applied Sciences (Basel, Switzerland)*, *14*(20), 9346.

Palladino, F., Marcelino, P. R. F., Schlogl, A. E., José, Á. H. M., Rodrigues, R. D. C. L. B., Fabrino, D. L., & Rosa, C. A. (2024). Bioreactors: Applications and Innovations for a sustainable and healthy future—a critical review. *Applied Sciences (Basel, Switzerland)*, *14*(20), 9346.

Palladino, F., Marcelino, P. R. F., Schlogl, A. E., José, Á. H. M., Rodrigues, R. D. C. L. B., Fabrino, D. L., & Rosa, C. A. (2024). Bioreactors: Applications and Innovations for a sustainable and healthy future-a critical review. *Applied Sciences (Basel, Switzerland)*, *14*(20), 9346. DOI: 10.3390/app14209346

Panahi, H. K. S., Dehhaghi, M., Guillemin, G. J., Gupta, V. K., Lam, S. S., Aghbashlo, M., & Tabatabaei, M. (2022). Bioethanol production from food wastes rich in carbohydrates. *Current Opinion in Food Science*, *43*, 71–81.

Panda, S. K., & Shetty, P. H. (2018). *Innovations in technologies for fermented food and beverage industries*. Springer.

Pandey, A., Srivastava, S., & Rai, P. (2022). Polyhydroxyalkanoates (PHAs): A review on biosynthesis, properties, and applications. *Bioresource Technology Reports*, *19*, 101163. DOI: 10.1016/j.biteb.2022.101163

Pandey, K., Pandey, M., Kumar, V., Aggarwal, U., & Singhal, B. (2024). Bioprocessing 4.0 in biomanufacturing: Paving the way for sustainable bioeconomy. *Systems Microbiology and Biomanufacturing*, *4*(2), 407–424. DOI: 10.1007/s43393-023-00206-y

Pant, D., Joshi, D., Upreti, M. K., & Kotnala, R. K. (2012). Chemical and biological extraction of metals present in E waste: A hybrid technology. *Waste Management (New York, N.Y.), 32*(5), 979–990. DOI: 10.1016/j.wasman.2011.12.002 PMID: 22217552

Papong, S., Malakul, P., Trungkavashirakun, R., Wenunun, P., Chom-in, T., Nithitanakul, M., & Sarobol, E. (2014). Comparative assessment of the environmental profile of PLA and PET drinking water bottles from a life cycle perspective. *Journal of Cleaner Production, 65*, 539–550. DOI: 10.1016/j.jclepro.2013.09.030

Paradis, F. W., Warren, R. A. J., Kilburn, D. G., & Miller, R. C. (1987). The expression of Cellulomonas fimi cellulase genes in Brevibacterium lactofermentum. *Gene, 61*(2), 199–206. DOI: 10.1016/0378-1119(87)90114-4

Paranthaman, S. R., & Karthikeyan, B. (2015). Bioremediation of heavy metal in paper mill effluent using Pseudomonas spp. *International Journal of Microbiology, 1*(1), 1–5. https://microbiozjournals.com/abstract-bioremediation-of-heavy-metal-in-paper-mill-effluent-using-pseudomonas-spp/

Parapouli, M., Vasileiadis, A., Afendra, A. S., & Hatziloukas, E. (2020). *Saccharomyces cerevisiae* and its industrial applications. *AIMS Microbiology, 6*(1), 1–31. DOI: 10.3934/microbiol.2020001

Parekh, S., Vinci, V. A., & Strobel, R. J. (2000). Improvement of microbial strains and fermentation processes. *Applied Microbiology and Biotechnology, 54*(3), 287–301. PMID: 11030563

Parhi, P., Song, K. P., & Choo, W. S. (2022). Growth and survival of Bifidobacterium breve and Bifidobacterium longum in various sugar systems with fructooligosaccharide supplementation. *Journal of Food Science and Technology, 59*(10), 3775–3786.

Park, S. H., Zarrinpar, A., & Lim, W. A. (2003). Rewiring MAP kinase pathways using alternative scaffold assembly mechanisms. *Science, 299*(5609), 1061–1064. DOI: 10.1126/science.1076979 PMID: 12511654

Pasrija, R., & Kumari, D. (2025). Introduction to BSL-2 Facilities. In *Protocols for Studying Pathogenic Fungi* (pp. 1-25). Springer.

Pasteur, L. (1857). Mémoire sur la fermentation appelée lactique. *Annales de Chimie et de Physique, 52*(3), 404–418.

Patarroyo, J. L., Florez-Rojas, J. S., Pradilla, D., Valderrama-Rincón, J. D., Cruz, J. C., & Reyes, L. H. (2020). Formulation and characterization of gelatin-based hydrogels for the encapsulation of Kluyveromyces lactis—Applications in packed-bed reactors and probiotics delivery in humans. *Polymers, 12*(6), 1287.

Patel, A. K., Dong, C. D., Chen, C. W., Pandey, A., & Singhania, R. R. (2023). Production, purification, and application of microbial enzymes. In *Biotechnology of microbial enzymes* (pp. 25–57). Academic Press.

Patel, D., Koç, J. R., & Otegbeye, F. (2025). Creating a GMP cell processing program: A focus on quality and regulation. *Best Practice & Research Clinical Haematology. Article, 101614*. Advance online publication. DOI: 10.1016/j.beha.2025.101614

Patel, M., & Singh, A. (2021). Reducing medical waste through biodegradable polymers: Current trends and future prospects. *Journal of Green Chemistry*, *27*(5), 403–420.

Patel, S. K. S., Choi, S. H., & Kang, Y. C. (2020). Recent developments in process analytical technologies (PATs) for biopharmaceutical production. *Biotechnology Journal*, *15*(5), 1900569.

Patel, S., & Kumar, A. (2023). Biobased polymers: A review of sources, properties, and applications. *International Journal of Polymer Science*, *15*(6), 291–312.

Pathodiya, M. (2025). Quality Risk Management: Degree of formality, Formal and Informal QRM. *Journal of Drug Delivery and Therapeutics*, *15*(2).

Paul, S., Bera, S., Dasgupta, R., Mondal, S., & Roy, S. (2021). Review on the recent structural advances in open and closed systems for carbon capture through algae. *Energy Nexus*, *4*, 100032.

Pauly, M., & Keegstra, K. (2008). Cell-wall carbohydrates and their modification as a resource for biofuels. *The Plant Journal*, *54*(4), 559–568. DOI: 10.1111/j.1365-313X.2008.03463.x PMID: 18476863

Pauwels, E., Breuer, L., & Lander, B. (2021). The pandemic and the global biopharmaceutical supply chain. *Nature Biotechnology*, *39*(7), 749–752.

Pazhayattil, A. B., & Sharma, S. (2025). Post-RCA Impact Assessment, CAPA, and Effectiveness Checks. In *Pharmaceutical Manufacturing Deviation and Failure Investigations: Principles, Practices, and Case Studies* (pp. 77-91). Springer.

Pazhayattil, A. B., Sharma, S., Philip, J. P., Gischewski-Silva, M., & Ingram, M. (2023). Qualification, Continued Process Verification, and Lifecycle Management. In *Technology Transfer: Drug Product Manufacturing Process* (pp. 97-117). Springer.

Peebo, K., & Neubauer, P. (2018). Application of Continuous Culture Methods to Recombinant Protein Production in Microorganisms. *Microorganisms*, *6*(3), 56. DOI: 10.3390/microorganisms6030056

Pejcz, E. (2024). Biotechnological approach of technological advancements for sustainable probiotic bread production. *Sustainability*, *16*(8), 3275.

Peña-Montenegro, T. D., Lozano, L., & Dussán, J. (2015). Genome sequence and description of the mosquitocidal and heavy metal tolerant strain Lysinibacillus sphaericus CBAM5. *Standards in Genomic Sciences*, *10*, 2. DOI: 10.1186/1944-3277-10-2 PMID: 25685257

Peng, Y., Wu, P., Schartup, A. T., & Zhang, Y. (2021). Plastic waste release caused by COVID-19 and its fate in the global ocean. *Proceedings of the National Academy of Sciences of the United States of America*, *118*(47), e2111530118. DOI: 10.1073/pnas.2111530118 PMID: 34751160

PENNELL. R. B. (1960). Fractionation and isolation of purified components by precipitation methods. In *The plasma proteins*, 9-50.

Peralta-Yahya, P. P., Ouellet, M., Chan, R., Mukhopadhyay, A., Keasling, J. D., & Lee, T. S. (2011). Identification and microbial production of a terpene-based advanced biofuel. *Nature Communications*, *2*, 483. DOI: 10.1038/ncomms1494 PMID: 21952217

Perkins, B. A., Sherr, J. L., & Mathieu, C. (2021). Type 1 diabetes glycemic management: Insulin therapy, glucose monitoring, and automation. *Science, 373*(6554), 522–527. PMID: 34326234

Pesch, H. (2023). *Exploring the use of plant factories for the production of biomass for the biorefining industry.*

Peterbauer, C., Maischberger, T., & Haltrich, D. (2011). Food-grade gene expression in lactic acid bacteria. *Biotechnology Journal, 6*(9), 1147–1161. DOI: 10.1002/biot.201100034

Peter, J., Chiara, M. D., Friedrich, A., Yue, J., Pflieger, D., Bergström, A., Sigwalt, A., Barre, B., Freel, K., & Llored, A.. (2018). Genome evolution across 1,011 *Saccharomyces cerevisiae* isolates. *Nature, 556*(7701), 339–344. DOI: 10.1038/s41586-018-0030-5 PMID: 29643504

Petrides, D. (2000). Bioprocess design and economics. In *Bioseparations science and engineering* (pp. 1–83). Oxford University Press.

Pfeifer, B. A., Beitelshees, M., Hill, A., & Jones, C. H. (2023). Harnessing synthetic biology for advancing RNA therapeutics and vaccine design. *npj Systems Biology and Applications, 9*, 60. https://doi.org/DOI: 10.1038/s41540-023-00323-3

Pfizer. (2021). *Pfizer's Manufacturing Response to COVID-19.* https://www.pfizer.com/news/hot-topics/manufacturing-response-covid-19

Philippini, R. R., Martiniano, S. E., Ingle, A. P., Franco Marcelino, P. R., Silva, G. M., Barbosa, F. G., Dos Santos, J. C., & da Silva, S. S. (2020). Agroindustrial byproducts for the generation of biobased products: Alternatives for sustainable biorefineries. *Frontiers in Energy Research, 8*, 152.

Phillips, J. A. (2020). "Novel" sensors for the monitoring of fermentation processes. In *Computer control of fermentation processes* (pp. 15-72). CRC Press.

Pilon-Smits, E. (2005). Phytoremediation. *Annual Review of Plant Biology, 56*, 15–39. DOI: 10.1146/annurev.arplant.56.032604.144214 PMID: 15862088

Pinela, J., Añibarro-Ortega, M., & Barros, L. (2024). Food waste biotransformation into food ingredients: A brief overview of challenges and opportunities. *Foods, 13*(21), 3389.

Pino, M. S., Rodríguez-Jasso, R. M., Michelin, M., Flores-Gallegos, A. C., Morales-Rodriguez, R., Teixeira, J. A., & Ruiz, H. A. (2018). Bioreactor design for enzymatic hydrolysis of biomass under the biorefinery concept. *Chemical Engineering Journal, 347*, 119–136. DOI: 10.1016/j.cej.2018.04.057

Pinto, A. R. O. (2024). *A Framework for Leveraging IT Audit Using Artificial Intelligence.* Universidade NOVA de Lisboa.

Pirt, S. J. (1975). *Principles of microbe and cell cultivation.* Blackwell Scientific.

Pisal, D. S., Kosloski, M. P., & Balu-Iyer, S. V. (2010). Delivery of therapeutic proteins. *Journal of Pharmaceutical Sciences, 99*(6), 2557–2575. PMID: 20049941

Pitzalis, M. F., & Sadler, J. C. (2025). Chemical bio-manufacture from diverse C-rich waste polymeric feedstocks using engineered microorganisms. *RSC Sustainability, 3*(4), 1672–1684. DOI: 10.1039/D5SU00013K

Plavec, T. V., & Berlec, A. (2019). Engineering of lactic acid bacteria for delivery of therapeutic proteins and peptides. *Applied Microbiology and Biotechnology, 103*(5), 2053–2066.

Polakovič, M., Báleš, V., Dluhý, M., & Štefuca, V. (1993). Optimization of a packed bed bioreactor with immobilized cells using experimental design. *Bioprocess Engineering, 9*(5), 225–230.

Pollard, D., & Woodley, J. M. (2007). Biocatalysis for pharmaceutical intermediates: The future is now. *Trends in Biotechnology, 25*(2), 66–73. PMID: 17184862

Pontes, D. S., de Azevedo, M. S. P., Chatel, J.-M., Langella, P., Azevedo, V., & Miyoshi, A. (2011). Lactococcus lactis as a live vector: Heterologous protein production and DNA delivery systems. *Protein Expression and Purification, 79*(2), 165–175. DOI: 10.1016/j.pep.2011.06.005

Pörtner, R., Nagel-Heyer, S., Goepfert, C., Adamietz, P., & Meenen, N. M. (2005). Bioreactor design for tissue engineering. *Journal of Bioscience and Bioengineering, 100*(3), 235–245. DOI: 10.1263/jbb.100.235 PMID: 16243271

Poshadri, A., HW, D., UM, K., & SD, K. (2022). Bacillus coagulans and its spore as potential probiotics in the production of novel shelf-stable foods. *Current Research in Nutrition and Food Science, 10*(3).

Prajapati, N., Patel, J., Singh, S., Yadav, V. K., Joshi, C., Patani, A., Prajapati, D., Sahoo, D. K., & Patel, A. (2023). Postbiotic production: Harnessing the power of microbial metabolites for health applications. *Frontiers in Microbiology, 14*, 1306192.

Pratiwi, R., Rahayu, D., & Barliana, M. I. (2017). Characterization of Bioplastic from Rice Straw Cellulose. *Research Journal of Pharmaceutical, Biological and Chemical Sciences, 8*, 217–221. https://www.rjpbcs.com/pdf/2017_8(1S)/[32].pdf

Praveen, M., & Brogi, S. (2025). Microbial fermentation in food and beverage industries: Innovations, challenges, and opportunities. *Foods, 14*(1), 114.

Preetha, N., Balakrishnan, V., & Thomas, G. (2024). Bioprospecting from Medicinal Plants and Benefit Sharing. In *Biodiversity and Business: Bio Prospecting and Benefit Sharing* (pp. 247-267). Cham: Springer Nature Switzerland. https://doi.org/DOI: 10.1007/978-3-031-71674-4_15

Prestigiacomo, R., Chan, C. C., & Kark, L. (2024). A biomedical engineering curriculum development: A qualitative study engaging four stakeholders. *European Journal of Education, 59*(2), e12632. DOI: 10.1111/ejed.12632

Prithviraj, D., Deboleena, K., Neelu, N., Noor, N., Aminur, R., Balasaheb, K., & Abul, M. (2014). Biosorption of nickel by Lysinibacillus sp. BA2 native to bauxite mine. *Ecotoxicology and Environmental Safety, 107*, 260–268. DOI: 10.1016/j.ecoenv.2014.06.009 PMID: 25011123

Priya, A. K., Jalil, A. A., Vadivel, S., Dutta, K., Rajendran, S., Fujii, M., & Soto-Moscoso, M. (2022). Heavy metal remediation from wastewater using microalgae: Recent advances and future trends. *Chemosphere, 305*, 135375. DOI: 10.1016/j.chemosphere.2022.135375 PMID: 35738200

Puligundla, P., & Mok, C. (2021). Recent advances in biotechnological valorization of brewers' spent grain. *Food Science and Biotechnology, 30*(3), 341–353.

Pustovrh, A., Rangus, K., & Drnovšek, M. (2020). The role of open innovation in developing an entrepreneurial support ecosystem. *Technological Forecasting and Social Change*, *152*, 119892. DOI: 10.1016/j.techfore.2019.119892

Puttarat, N., Ladda, B., Kasorn, A., Tanasupawat, S., & Taweechotipatr, M. (2021). Cholesterol-lowering activity and functional characterization of lactic acid bacteria isolated from traditional Thai foods for their potential used as probiotics. *Songklanakarin Journal of Science and Technology*, *43*(5).

Puumala, L. S., Grist, S. M., Morales, J. M., Bickford, J. R., Chrostowski, L., Shekhar, S., & Cheung, K. C. (2022). Biofunctionalization of multiplexed silicon photonic biosensors. *Biosensors (Basel)*, *13*(1), 53. PMID: 36671887

Qadir, A. (2023). Beyond specialization: The interconnected web of sciences and technological advancements. *SAUS-Journal of IT and Computer Sciences*, *1*(1), 15–19.

Qattan, S. Y. (2025). Harnessing bacterial consortia for effective bioremediation: Targeted removal of heavy metals, hydrocarbons, and persistent pollutants. *Environmental Sciences Europe*, *37*(1), 1–35. DOI: 10.1186/s12302-025-01103-y

Qiao, K., Wasylenko, T. M., Zhou, K., Xu, P., & Stephanopoulos, G. (2017). Lipid production in Yarrowia lipolytica is maximized by engineering cytosolic redox metabolism. *Nature Biotechnology*, *35*(2), 173–177. DOI: 10.1038/nbt.3763

Qin, S. J., & Badgwell, T. A. (2003). A survey of industrial model predictive control technology. *Control Engineering Practice*, *11*(7), 733–764.

Qin, Y., Li, Q., Fan, L., Ning, X., Wei, X., & You, C. (2023). *Biomanufacturing by In Vitro Biotransformation (ivBT)*. Using Purified Cascade Multi-enzymes., DOI: 10.1007/10_2023_231

Qumsani, A. T. (2024). The contribution of microorganisms to sustainable development: Towards a green future through synthetic biology and systems biology. *Journal of Umm Al-Qura University for Applied Sciences*, 1–17.

Radzun, K. A., Agha, H. M., Abdullah, N. F. F., Ahmad, M. I., Ivanovski, I., Mohammed, A. A., & Alkamil, A. A. (2024). Media optimization techniques for microalgae through technological advancements: A mini review. *AUIQ Complementary Biological System*, *1*(1), 7.

Raghunath, B., Bin, W. A. N. G., Pattnaik, P. R. I. Y. A. B. R. A. T. A., & Janssens, J. E. R. O. E. N. (2012). Best practices for optimization and scale-up of microfiltration TFF processes. *Bioprocess. J*, *11*(1), 30–40.

Rahalkar, H., Cetintas, H. C., & Salek, S. (2018). Quality, non-clinical and clinical considerations for biosimilar monoclonal antibody development: EU, WHO, USA, Canada, and BRICS-TM regulatory guidelines. *Frontiers in Pharmacology*, *9*, 1079. DOI: 10.3389/fphar.2018.01079 PMID: 30364154

Rahalkar, H., Sheppard, A., Santos, G. M. L., Dasgupta, C., Perez-Tapia, S. M., Lopez-Morales, C. A., & Salek, S. (2021). Current Regulatory Requirements for Biosimilars in Six Member Countries of BRICS-TM: Challenges and Opportunities. *Frontiers in Medicine*, *8*, 726660. DOI: 10.3389/fmed.2021.726660 PMID: 34568384

Rahman, A. M., Rahman, T. T., Pei, Z., Ufodike, C. O., Lee, J., & Elwany, A. (2023). Additive Manufacturing Using Agriculturally Derived Biowastes: A Systematic Literature Review. *Bioengineering (Basel, Switzerland), 10*(7), 845. DOI: 10.3390/bioengineering10070845 PMID: 37508872

Rahman, A., & Bhoi, P. R. (2021). An overview of non-biodegradable bioplastics. *Journal of Cleaner Production, 294*, 126218. DOI: 10.1016/j.jclepro.2021.126218

Raj, A. E., & Karanth, N. G. (2005). 03 Fermentation Technology and Bioreactor Design. In *Food Biotechnology* (pp. 60–113). CRC Press.

Rajaeifar, M. A., Ghadimi, P., Raugei, M., Wu, Y., & Heidrich, O. (2022). Challenges and recent developments in supply and value chains of electric vehicle batteries: A sustainability perspective. *Resources, Conservation and Recycling, 180*, 106144. DOI: 10.1016/j.resconrec.2021.106144

Ramos, F. D., Delpivo, C., & Borsarelli, C. D. (2019). Polyhydroxyalkanoates (PHAs): Production, applications, and end-of-life strategies. *Biotechnology Advances, 42*, 107582. DOI: 10.1016/j.biotechadv.2019.107582

Ramos, P. E., Cerqueira, M. A., Teixeira, J. A., & Vicente, A. A. (2018). Physiological protection of probiotic microcapsules by coatings. *Critical Reviews in Food Science and Nutrition, 58*(11), 1864–1877.

Rangel, A. E., Gómez Ramírez, J. M., & Gonzalez Barrios, A. F. (2020). From industrial by-products to value-added compounds: The design of efficient microbial cell factories by coupling systems metabolic engineering and bioprocesses. *Biofuels, Bioproducts & Biorefining, 14*(6), 1228–1238.

Rantanen, J., & Khinast, J. (2015). The future of pharmaceutical manufacturing sciences. *Journal of Pharmaceutical Sciences, 104*(11), 3612–3638. PMID: 26280993

Rasala, B. A., & Mayfield, S. P. (2015). Photosynthetic biomanufacturing in green algae; production of recombinant proteins for industrial, nutritional, and medical uses. *Photosynthesis Research, 123*(3), 227–239. DOI: 10.1007/s11120-014-9994-7

Rath, K. C., Khang, A., Rath, S. K., Satapathy, N., Satapathy, S. K., & Kar, S. (2024). Artificial intelligence (AI)-enabled technology in medicine-advancing holistic healthcare monitoring and control systems. In *Computer Vision and AI-Integrated IoT Technologies in the Medical Ecosystem* (pp. 87–108). CRC Press.

Rathore, A. S. (2009). Roadmap for implementation of quality by design (QbD) for biotechnology products. *Trends in Biotechnology, 27*(9), 546–553. PMID: 19647883

Rathore, A. S., Agarwal, H., & Sharma, A. (2018). Energy-efficient and sustainable bioprocessing strategies. *Current Opinion in Chemical Engineering, 22*, 42–48.

Rathore, A. S., Agarwal, H., Sharma, A. K., Pathak, M., & Muthukumar, S. J. P. B. (2015). Continuous processing for production of biopharmaceuticals. *Preparative Biochemistry & Biotechnology, 45*(8), 836–849. PMID: 25674930

Rathore, A. S., & Jesubalan, N. G. (2022). Perspectives on Process Analytical Technology. *Biopharm International, 35*(5), 31–35.

Rathore, A. S., & Kapoor, G. (2015). Analytical characterization of protein aggregates. *Biopharm International, 28*(5), 28–34.

Rathore, A. S., Kumar, D., & Kateja, N. (2018). Recent developments in chromatographic purification of biopharmaceuticals. *Biotechnology Letters, 40*(6), 895–905. PMID: 29700726

Rathore, A. S., Mishra, S., Nikita, S., & Priyanka, P. (2021). Bioprocess control: Current progress and future perspectives. *Life (Chicago, Ill.), 11*(6), 557. Advance online publication. DOI: 10.3390/life11060557

Rathore, A. S., Nikita, S., & Jesubalan, N. G. (2022). Digitization in bioprocessing: The role of soft sensors in monitoring and control of downstream processing for production of biotherapeutic products. *Biosensors & Bioelectronics: X, 12*, 100263.

Rathore, A. S., & Rajan, R. S. (2008). Current perspectives on validation of protein purification processes. *Biotechnology Progress, 24*(5), 1090–1098. PMID: 19194918

Rathore, A. S., & Saxena, N. (2023). Digitalization: The Route to Biopharma 4.0. *Biopharm International, 36*(11), 25–29.

Rathore, A. S., & Winkle, H. (2009). Quality by design for biopharmaceuticals. *Nature Biotechnology, 27*(1), 26–34. DOI: 10.1038/nbt0109-26

Rathore, A. S., & Winkle, H. (2009). Quality by Design for Biopharmaceuticals. *Nature Biotechnology, 27*(1), 26–34. PMID: 19131992

Rathore, A., & Shereef, F. (2022). Innovating manufacturing technology in emerging economies. *Nature Biotechnology, 40*(12), 1714–1716. DOI: 10.1038/s41587-022-01499-5 PMID: 36171278

Ravindran, R., Hassan, S. S., Williams, G. A., & Jaiswal, A. K. (2018). A review on bioconversion of agro-industrial wastes to industrially important enzymes. *Bioengineering (Basel, Switzerland), 5*(4), 93.

Raybould, A., & Pillai, S. P. (2023). Insights in Biosafety and Biosecurity: Current Challenges and Future Perspectives. *Frontiers in Bioengineering and Biotechnology, 11*, 1118506. DOI: 10.3389/fbioe.2022.1118506 PMID: 36714616

Ray, R. C., Paramithiotis, S., Thekkangil, A., Nethravathy, V., Rai, A. K., & Martin, J. G. P. (2024). Food fermentation and its relevance in the human history. In *Trending topics on fermented foods* (pp. 1–57). Springer.

Rayung, M., Aung, M. M., Azhar, S. C., & Suait, M. S. (2020). Bio-based polymer electrolytes for electrochemical devices: Insight into the ionic conductivity performance. *Materials (Basel), 13*(4), 838. DOI: 10.3390/ma13040838 PMID: 32059600

Raza, A. (2024). Advances in Biotechnological Innovations: Bridging the Gap Between Laboratory Discoveries and Industrial Applications. *Agricultural and Biotechnological Reflections, 1*(02), 84–97.

Razzak, M. T., Darwis, D., & Zainuddin, S. (2017). Irradiation of polyvinyl alcohol and polyvinyl pyrrolidone blended hydrogel for wound dressing. *Radiation Physics and Chemistry, 140*, 96–100. DOI: 10.1016/j.radphyschem.2017.02.046

Reddy, K. R., & Cameselle, C. (2009). *Electrochemical remediation technologies for polluted soils, sediments and groundwater*. John Wiley & Sons., DOI: 10.1002/9780470523650

Reisman, H. B. (1993). Problems in scale-up of biotechnology production processes. *Critical Reviews in Biotechnology, 13*(3), 195–253. PMID: 8221898

Remmers, I. M., Hidalgo-Ulloa, A., Brandt, B. P., Evers, W. A. C., Wijffels, R. H., & Lamers, P. P. (2017). Continuous versus batch production of lipids in the microalgae Acutodesmus obliquus. *Bioresource Technology, 244*, 1384–1392. DOI: 10.1016/j.biortech.2017.04.093

Restelli, V., Wang, M. D., Huzel, N., & Butler, M. (2006). The effect of enhanced oxygenation on the metabolic profile and productivity of recombinant CHO cells. *Biotechnology and Bioengineering, 94*(4), 679–687. DOI: 10.1002/bit.20899

Reyes, S. J., Durocher, Y., Pham, P. L., & Henry, O. (2022). Modern sensor tools and techniques for monitoring, controlling, and improving cell culture processes. *Processes (Basel, Switzerland), 10*(2), 189.

Rhee, S., Lee, J.-E., & Lee, C.-H. (2011). Importance of lactic acid bacteria in Asian fermented foods. *Microbial Cell Factories, 10*(Suppl 1), S5. DOI: 10.1186/1475-2859-10-S1-S5

Ro, D.-K., Paradise, E. M., Ouellet, M., Fisher, K. J., Newman, K. L., Ndungu, J. M., Ho, K. A., Eachus, R. A., Ham, T. S., Kirby, J., Chang, M. C. Y., Withers, S. T., Shiba, Y., Sarpong, R., & Keasling, J. D. (2006). Production of the antimalarial drug precursor artemisinic acid in engineered yeast. *Nature, 440*(7086), 940–943. DOI: 10.1038/nature04640

Rodríguez, J., Rubio, L., Celemín, M., & Alonso-Almeida, M. (2019). Analysis of the relations between circular economy and sustainable development goals. *International Journal of Sustainable Development and World Ecology, 26*(1), 1–13. DOI: 10.1080/13504509.2019.1666754

Roeva, O., & Slavov, T. (2012). PID controller tuning based on metaheuristic algorithms for bioprocess control. *Biotechnology, Biotechnological Equipment, 26*(5), 3267–3277.

Rogers, L., & Jensen, K. F. (2019). Continuous manufacturing–the Green Chemistry promise? *Green Chemistry, 21*(13), 3481–3498.

Rojas, L., Yepes, V., & Garcia, J. (2025). Complex Dynamics and Intelligent Control: Advances, Challenges, and Applications in Mining and Industrial Processes. *Mathematics, 13*(6), 961.

Rojek, I., Jasiulewicz-Kaczmarek, M., Piechowski, M., & Mikołajewski, D. (2023). An artificial intelligence approach for improving maintenance to supervise machine failures and support their repair. *Applied Sciences (Basel, Switzerland), 13*(8), 4971.

Rolinger, L., Rüdt, M., & Hubbuch, J. (2020). A critical review of recent trends, and a future perspective of optical spectroscopy as PAT in biopharmaceutical downstream processing. *Analytical and Bioanalytical Chemistry, 412*, 2047–2064. PMID: 32146498

Rollin, J. A., Tam, T. K., & Zhang, Y.-H. P. (2013). New biotechnology paradigm: Cell-free biosystems for biomanufacturing. *Green Chemistry, 15*(7), 1708–1719.

Roman, M. D., & Muresan, M. V. (2015). Process optimization of aeration in the biological treatment using fine bubble diffusers. In *Proc., 6th Int. Conf. on Modern Power System.* Cluj-napoca, Romania: EBSCO Information Services.

Romero-García, J. M., Niño, L., Martínez-Patiño, C., Ruiz, E., Romero, I., & Castro, E. (2016). Bioethanol production from olive tree biomass. *Renewable Energy, 86*, 1067–1073. DOI: 10.1016/j.renene.2015.09.043

Romyasamit, C., Saengsuwan, P., Boonserm, P., Thamjarongwong, B., & Singkhamanan, K. (2022). Optimization of cryoprotectants for freeze-dried potential probiotic Enterococcus faecalis and evaluation of its storage stability. *Drying Technology, 40*(11), 2283–2292.

Ronda, C., Pedersen, L. E., Hansen, H. G., Kallehauge, T. B., Betenbaugh, M. J., & Kildegaard, H. F. (2014). Accelerating genome editing in CHO cells using CRISPR Cas9 and CRISPy, a web-based target finding tool. *Biotechnology and Bioengineering, 111*(8), 1604–1616. PMID: 24827782

Roque, A. C. A., Lowe, C. R., & Taipa, M. A. (2004). Antibodies and genetically engineered related molecules: Production and purification. *Biotechnology Progress, 20*(3), 639–654. PMID: 15176864

Rosenboom, J. G., Langer, R., & Traverso, G. (2022). Bioplastics for a circular economy. *Nature Reviews. Materials, 7*(2), 117–137. DOI: 10.1038/s41578-021-00407-8 PMID: 35075395

Rösner, L. S., Walter, F., Ude, C., John, G. T., & Beutel, S. (2022). Sensors and techniques for on-line determination of cell viability in bioprocess monitoring. *Bioengineering (Basel, Switzerland), 9*(12), 762. PMID: 36550968

Rossi, C., Shen, L., Junginger, M., & Wicke, B. (2024). Sustainability certification of bio-based products: Systematic literature review of socio-economic impacts along the supply chain. *Journal of Cleaner Production*, •••, 143079.

Rossi, M., Martini, E., & Kolte, A. (2021). The role of venture capitalists in an organised innovation ecosystem: Evidence from the USA. *International Journal of Business Environment, 12*(3), 265–286.

Ross, R. P., Morgan, S., & Hill, C. (2002). Preservation and fermentation: Past, present and future. *International Journal of Food Microbiology, 79*(1-2), 3–16. DOI: 10.1016/S0168-1605(02)00174-5 PMID: 12382680

Rout, P., & Chakraborty, C. (2020). The commercial application of biosensors as an analytical device. *International Journal of Current Microbiology and Applied Sciences, 9*(5), 864–880.

Rowe, J. D., Amijee, F., Brody, S. D., Wandrey, G. G., & Dreyer, C. C. (2012). The globalization of agricultural biotechnology: implications for regulatory compliance, stewardship and stakeholder engagement. In *Regulation of Agricultural Biotechnology: The United States and Canada* (pp. 335-375). Springer.

Roy, S., Mandal, B., & Das, B. K. (2025). Quality Assurance in Laboratory Practices and Equipment Maintenance: Ensuring Precision, Reliability, and Compliance. In *Laboratory Techniques for Fish Disease Diagnosis* (pp. 79-103). Springer.

Rueda, E., García-Galán, M. J., & Ortiz, A. (2023). Life cycle assessment of polyhydroxybutyrate production from *Synechocystis* sp. PCC 6803. *Algal Research, 69*, 102929. DOI: 10.1016/j.algal.2022.102929

Rydz, J., Sikorska, W., Kyulavska, M., & Christova, D. (2015). Polyester-based (bio)degradable polymers as environmentally friendly materials for sustainable development. *International Journal of Molecular Sciences, 16*(1), 564–596. DOI: 10.3390/ijms16010564 PMID: 25551604

Sabaté, J.-M., & Iglicki, F. (2022). Effect of Bifidobacterium longum 35624 on disease severity and quality of life in patients with irritable bowel syndrome. *World Journal of Gastroenterology, 28*(7), 732.

Sablayrolles, J. M., & Mouret, J. R. (2022). Nitrogen management during fermentation. In *White Wine Technology* (pp. 143–154). Academic Press., DOI: 10.1016/B978-0-12-823497-6.00027-2

Saeed, M. U., Hussain, N., Sumrin, A., Shahbaz, A., Noor, S., Bilal, M., & Iqbal, H. M. (2022). Microbial bioremediation strategies with wastewater treatment potentialities–A review. *The Science of the Total Environment, 818*, 151754. PMID: 34800451

Sahoo, N., Choudhury, K., & Manchikanti, P. (2009). Manufacturing of Biodrugs: Need for Harmonization in Regulatory Standards. *BioDrugs, 23*(1), 1–9. DOI: 10.2165/11317110-000000000-00000 PMID: 19697964

Sahu, L., & Panda, S. K. (2018). Innovative technologies and implications in fermented food and beverage industries: an overview. *Innovations in technologies for fermented food and beverage industries*, 1-23.

Sahu, L., & Panda, S. K. (2018). Innovative technologies and implications in fermented food and beverage industries: an overview. *Innovations in technologies for fermented food and beverage industries*, 1-23. https://doi.org/DOI: 10.1007/978-3-319-74820-7_1

Sain, M. (2020). Production of bioplastics and sustainable packaging materials from rice straw to eradicate stubble burning: A Mini-Review. *Environment Conservation Journal, 21*(3), 1–5. DOI: 10.36953/ECJ.2020.21301

Sakuma, T., Hattori, T., & Deshusses, M. A. (2006). Comparison of different packing materials for the biofiltration of air toxics. Journal of the Air & Waste Management Association (1995), 56(11), 1567–1575. https://doi.org/DOI: 10.1080/10473289.2006.10464564

Salazar-Fontana, L. I. (2022). A regulatory risk-based approach to ATMP/CGT development: Integrating scientific challenges with current regulatory expectations. *Frontiers in Medicine, 9*, 855100. PMID: 35646952

Salim, A., & Lim, S. (2018). Review of recent metamaterial microfluidic sensors. *Sensors (Basel), 18*(1), 232. PMID: 29342953

Samaras, J. J., Micheletti, M., & Ding, W. (2022). Transformation of biopharmaceutical manufacturing through single-use technologies: Current state, remaining challenges, and future development. *Annual Review of Chemical and Biomolecular Engineering, 13*, 73–97. DOI: 10.1146/annurev-chembioeng-092220-120343

Sammut, S. M. (2021). The role of the biotechnology industry in addressing health inequities in Africa: Strengthening the entire health care value chain. *Journal of Commercial Biotechnology*, *26*(4).

Samoraj, M., Çalış, D., Trzaska, K., Mironiuk, M., & Chojnacka, K. (2024). Advancements in algal biorefineries for sustainable agriculture: Biofuels, high-value products, and environmental solutions. *Biocatalysis and Agricultural Biotechnology*, *58*, 103224. DOI: 10.1016/j.bcab.2024.103224

Sánchez-Castro, I., Martínez-Rodríguez, P., Abad, M. M., Descostes, M., & Merroun, M. L. (2021). Uranium removal from complex mining waters by alginate beads doped with cells of Stenotrophomonas sp. Br8: Novel perspectives for metal bioremediation. *Journal of Environmental Management*, *296*, 113411. DOI: 10.1016/j.jenvman.2021.113411 PMID: 34351286

Sander, J. D., & Joung, J. K. (2014). CRISPR-Cas systems for editing, regulating and targeting genomes. *Nature Biotechnology*, *32*(4), 347–355. DOI: 10.1038/nbt.2842 PMID: 24584096

Sandle, T. (2012). Environmental monitoring: A practical approach. In *Environmental monitoring: A comprehensive handbook* (Vol. 6, pp. 29–54). Oxford University Press.

Sangavi, C. (2023). *Regulatory Requirements for the New Drug Approval Process in Different Countries*. International Journal Of Drug Regulatory Affairs. https://www.researchgate.net/publication/372914168

Sangavi, C. (2023). *Regulatory Requirements for the New Drug Approval Process in Different Countries*. International Journal of Drug Regulatory Affairs. ResearchGate.

Sano, C. (2009). History of glutamate production. *The American Journal of Clinical Nutrition*, *90*(3), 728S–732S. DOI: 10.3945/ajcn.2009.27462F

Sanofi. (2020). *Digital Factory of the Future*. Retrieved from https://www.sanofi.com/en/our-stories/our-people/our-digital-factory-of-the-future

Santos, A. G., de Albuquerque, T. L., Ribeiro, B. D., & Coelho, M. A. Z. (2021). In situ product recovery techniques aiming to obtain biotechnological products: A glance to current knowledge. *Biotechnology and Applied Biochemistry*, *68*(5), 1044–1057.

Santos, A. J., Carvalho, F., Oliveira, C. S., & Fortunato, E. (2020). Bioplastics from agro-waste for food packaging applications. *Food Packaging and Shelf Life*, *25*, 100523. DOI: 10.1016/j.fpsl.2020.100523

Saranya, S., Thamanna, L., & Chellapandi, P. (2024). Unveiling the potential of systems biology in biotechnology and biomedical research. *Systems Microbiology and Biomanufacturing*, *4*(4), 1217–1238. DOI: 10.1007/s43393-024-00286-4

Sarma, S., Sharma, S., Rudakiya, D., Upadhyay, J., Rathod, V., Patel, A., & Narra, M. (2021). Valorization of microalgae biomass into bioproducts promoting circular bioeconomy: a holistic approach of bioremediation and biorefinery. *3 Biotech*, *11*(8), 378.

Sarnaik, A., Liu, A., Nielsen, D., & Varman, A. M. (2020). High-throughput screening for efficient microbial biotechnology. *Current Opinion in Biotechnology*, *64*, 141–150. PMID: 32302926

Sartorius. (2020). *Sustainable Biomanufacturing: Environmental Footprint Assessment of Bioprocesses.* White Paper. Retrieved from https://www.sartorius.com

Šašinková, D., Serbruyns, L., & Julinová, M., FayyazBakhsh, A., De Wilde, B., & Koutný, M. (2022). Evaluation of the biodegradation of polymeric materials in the freshwater environment—An attempt to prolong and accelerate the biodegradation experiment. *Polymer Degradation & Stability, 203*, 110085. DOI: 10.1016/j.polymdegradstab.2022.110085

Satari, L., Iglesias, A., & Porcar, M. (2023). The microbiome of things: Appliances, machines, and devices hosting artificial niche-adapted microbial communities. *Microorganisms, 11*(6), 1507.

Sawarkar, S., & Bapat, A. (2022). Global Regulatory Frameworks and Quality Standards for Stem Cells Therapy and Regenerative Medicines. In *Stem Cell Production: Processes, Practices and Regulations* (pp. 69-111). Springer.

Scavone, P., Miyoshi, A., Rial, A., Chabalgoity, A., Langella, P., Azevedo, V., & Zunino, P. (2007). Intranasal immunisation with recombinant Lactococcus lactis displaying either anchored or secreted forms of Proteus mirabilis MrpA fimbrial protein confers specific immune response and induces a significant reduction of kidney bacterial colonisation in mice. *Microbes and Infection, 9*(7), 821–828. DOI: 10.1016/j.micinf.2007.02.023

SCBD. (2000). *Cartagena Protocol on Biosafety to the Convention on Biological Diversity.* https://bch.cbd.int/protocol

SCBD. (2011). *Nagoya Protocol on Access and Benefit-Sharing.* https://www.cbd.int/abs/

Schirmer, C., Maschke, R. W., Pörtner, R., & Eibl, D. (2021). An overview of drive systems and sealing types in stirred bioreactors used in biotechnological processes. *Applied Microbiology and Biotechnology, 105*, 2225–2242. DOI: 10.1007/s00253-021-11180-7 PMID: 33649923

Schladt, T., Engelmann, N., Kubaczka, E., Hochberger, C., & Koeppl, H. (2021). Automated design of robust genetic circuits: Structural variants and parameter uncertainty. *ACS Synthetic Biology, 10*(6), 1393–1405. DOI: 10.1021/acssynbio.0c00608 PMID: 34807573

Schmitt, R. H., Ochs, J., & Moutsatsou, P. (2019). Automation in cell and gene therapy manufacturing: From past to future. *Biotechnology Letters, 41*(10), 1179–1190. https://link.springer.com/article/10.1007/s10529-019-02732-z PMID: 31541330

Schneider, A., Herlevi, L. M., Guo, Y., & Fernandez Lahore, H. M. (2022). Perspectives on adsorption technology as an effective strategy for continuous downstream bioprocessing. *Journal of Chemical Technology and Biotechnology, 97*(9), 2305–2316.

Schwaiger, N., Feiner, R., & Wimmer, B. (2011). Bioplastics from renewable resources: The role of life cycle assessment in the development of new products. *The International Journal of Life Cycle Assessment, 16*(7), 675–676. DOI: 10.1007/s11367-011-0315-5

Sebastián Serna Loaiza, Miltner, A., & Miltner, M. (2022). Microbial utilization of next generation feedstocks for biomanufacturing. *Frontiers in Bioengineering and Biotechnology, 10*, 874612. Advance online publication. DOI: 10.3389/fbioe.2022.874612 PMID: 35480982

Seenivasagan, R., & Babalola, O. O. (2021). Utilization of microbial consortia as biofertilizers and biopesticides for the production of feasible agricultural product. *Biology (Basel), 10*(11), 1111. Advance online publication. DOI: 10.3390/biology10111111

Segall-Shapiro, T. H., Meyer, A. J., Ellington, A. D., Sontag, E. D., & Voigt, C. A. (2014). A 'resource allocator' for transcription based on a highly fragmented T7 <scp>RNA</scp> polymerase. *Molecular Systems Biology, 10*(7). Advance online publication. DOI: 10.15252/msb.20145299

Selvarajan, G. (2021). Leveraging AI-enhanced analytics for industry-specific optimization: A strategic approach to transforming data-driven decision-making. *International Journal of Enhanced Research in Science Technology and Engineering, 10*, 78–84.

Serna Loaiza, S., Miltner, A., Miltner, M., & Friedl, A. (2019). A review on the feedstocks for the sustainable production of bioactive compounds in biorefineries. *Sustainability, 11*(23), 6765. DOI: 10.3390/su11236765

Sevda, S., & Kumar, S. (2024). Introduction of bioreactor. In *Bioreactor design concepts for viral vaccine production* (pp. 1–34). Academic Press., DOI: 10.1016/B978-0-443-15378-5.00001-2

Sewsynker-Sukai, Y., Faloye, F., & Kana, E. B. G. (2017). Artificial neural networks: An efficient tool for modelling and optimization of biofuel production (a mini review). *Biotechnology, Biotechnological Equipment, 31*(2), 221–235.

Shahab, M. A., Destro, F., & Braatz, R. D. (2025). Digital twins in biopharmaceutical manufacturing: Review & human-machine collaborative intelligence. arXiv. http://dx.doi.org//arXiv.2504.00286DOI: 10.48550

Shahcheraghi, N., Golchin, H., Sadri, Z., Tabari, Y., Borhanifar, F., & Makani, S. (2022). Nanobiotechnology, an applicable approach for sustainable future. *3 Biotech, 12*(3), 65. https://doi.org/DOI: 10.1007/s13205-021-03108-9

Shalaby, E. A. (2013). Biofuel: sources, extraction and determination. In Liquid, Gaseous and Solid Biofuels - Conversion Techniques, 18, 451-478. DOI: https://doi.org/DOI: 10.5772/51943

Shankar, A., Saini, S., & Sharma, K. K. (2024). Fungal-integrated second-generation lignocellulosic biorefinery: Utilization of agricultural biomass for co-production of lignocellulolytic enzymes, mushroom, fungal polysaccharides, and bioethanol. *Biomass Conversion and Biorefinery, 14*(1), 1117–1131.

Sharma, S., Rabbani, S. A., & Sharma, R. (2022). *Regulatory Affairs in the Pharmaceutical Industry*. Elsevier. https://www.sciencedirect.com/science/article/pii/B9780128222119000058

Sharma, B., Dangi, A. K., & Shukla, P. (2018). Contemporary enzyme based technologies for bioremediation: A review. *Journal of Environmental Management, 210*, 10–22. DOI: 10.1016/j.jenvman.2017.12.075 PMID: 29329004

Sharma, P., Bano, A., Singh, S. P., Dubey, N. K., Chandra, R., & Iqbal, H. (2022). Recent advancements in microbial-assisted remediation strategies for toxic contaminants. *Cleaner Chemical Engineering, 2*, 100020. DOI: 10.1016/j.clce.2022.100020

Sharma, P., Bano, A., Verma, K., Yadav, M., Varjani, S., Singh, S. P., & Tong, Y. W. (2023). Food waste digestate as biofertilizer and their direct applications in agriculture. *Bioresource Technology Reports*, *23*, 101515.

Sharma, P., Gaur, V. K., Sirohi, R., Varjani, S., Kim, S. H., & Wong, J. W. (2021). Sustainable processing of food waste for production of bio-based products for circular bioeconomy. *Bioresource Technology*, *325*, 124684.

Sharma, S., Monga, A., Jamwal, P., & Kaur, A. (2025). Biosimilars: A Critical Review of Development, Regulatory Landscape, and Clinical Implications. *AAPS PharmSciTech*. Advance online publication. DOI: 10.1208/s12249-025-03038-2 PMID: 39870890

Sharma, S., Pathania, S., Bhagta, S., Kaushal, N., Bhardwaj, S., Bhatia, R. K., & Walia, A. (2024). Microbial remediation of polluted environment by using recombinant E. coli: A review. *Biotechnology for the Environment*, *1*(1), 8. DOI: 10.1186/s44314-024-00008-z

Sheikh, H., Anand, G. G., & Shivanna, G. B. (2024). Fermentation: A Potential Strategy for Microbial Metabolite Production. https://doi.org/DOI: 10.5772/intechopen.114814

Sheikholeslami, Z., Mahfouzi, M., Karimi, M., & Ghiafehdavoodi, M. (2021). Modification of dough characteristics and baking quality based on whole wheat flour by enzymes and emulsifiers supplementation. *Lebensmittel-Wissenschaft + Technologie*, *139*, 110794.

Sheldon, R. A., & Brady, D. (2022). Green chemistry, biocatalysis, and the chemical industry of the future. *ChemSusChem*, *15*(9), e202102628. PMID: 35026060

Sheldon, R. A., & Brady, D. (2022). The limits to biocatalysis: Pushing the envelope. *Chemical Science (Cambridge)*, *13*(12), 3232–3245. DOI: 10.1039/D1SC05620A

Shen, C. R., Lan, E. I., Dekishima, Y., Baez, A., Cho, K. M., & Liao, J. C. (2011). Driving forces enable high-titer anaerobic 1-butanol synthesis in *Escherichia coli*. *Applied and Environmental Microbiology*, *77*(9), 2905–2915. DOI: 10.1128/AEM.03003-10 PMID: 21398484

Shen, Y., Yuan, W., Pei, Z., & Mao, E. (2009). Microalgae mass production methods. *Transactions of the ASABE*, *52*(4), 1275–1287. DOI: 10.13031/2013.27771

Shetranjiwalla, S., & Ononiwu, A. (2025). Identifying barriers to scaled-up production and commercialization of chitin and chitosan using green technologies: A review and quantitative green chemistry assessment. *International Journal of Biological Macromolecules*, •••, 305.

Shetty, K., & Sarkar, D. (2020). *Functional Foods and Biotechnology: Biotransformation and analysis of functional foods and ingredients*. CRC Press.

Shiio, I., & Nakamori, S. (1969). Microbial production of L-threonine part I. Production by *Escherichia coli* mutant resistant to α-amino-β-hydroxyvaleric acid. *Agricultural and Biological Chemistry*, *33*(8), 1152–1160. DOI: 10.1080/00021369.1969.10859439

Shintani, H. (2016). Inactivation of bacterial spore, endotoxin, lipid A, normal prion and abnormal prion by exposures to several sorts of gases plasma. *Biocontrol Science*, *21*(1), 1–12. DOI: 10.4265/bio.21.1

Shi, S., Liang, Y., Zhang, M. M., Ang, E. L., & Zhao, H. (2016). A highly efficient single-step, markerless strategy for multi-copy chromosomal integration of large biochemical pathways in *Saccharomyces cerevisiae*. *Metabolic Engineering*, *33*, 19–27. DOI: 10.1016/j.ymben.2015.10.011 PMID: 26546089

Shokoohi, M., & Attar, T. (2024). Biomanufacturing for a sustainable future: Unleashing the potential of biotechnology in pharmaceutical raw material production. [IJHES]. *International Journal of New Findings in Health and Educational Sciences*, *2*(2), 142–153.

Shori, A. B., & Al Zahrani, A. J. (2021). Non-dairy plant-based milk products as alternatives to conventional dairy products for delivering probiotics. *Food Science and Technology (Campinas)*, *42*, e101321.

Shukla, A. A., & Gottschalk, U. (2013). Single-use disposable technologies for biopharmaceutical manufacturing. *Trends in Biotechnology*, *31*(3), 147–154. DOI: 10.1016/j.tibtech.2012.10.004

Shukla, A. A., & Hinckley, P. (2008). Host cell protein clearance during protein A chromatography: Development of an improved column wash step. *Biotechnology Progress*, *24*(5), 1115–1121. DOI: 10.1002/btpr.50

Shukla, A. A., & Thömmes, J. (2010). Recent advances in large-scale production of monoclonal antibodies and related proteins. *Trends in Biotechnology*, *28*(5), 253–261. DOI: 10.1016/j.tibtech.2010.02.001

Shukla, A. A., Wolfe, L. S., Mostafa, S. S., & Norman, C. (2017). Evolving trends in biopharmaceutical process development and manufacturing. *Bioengineering & Translational Medicine*, *2*(1), 58–69. DOI: 10.1002/btm2.10049 PMID: 29313024

Siegel, J. B., Smith, A. L., Poust, S., Wargacki, A. J., Bar-Even, A., Louw, C., Shen, B. W., Eiben, C. B., Tran, H. M., Noor, E., Gallaher, J. L., Bale, J., Yoshikuni, Y., Gelb, M. H., Keasling, J. D., Stoddard, B. L., Lidstrom, M. E., & Baker, D. (2015). Computational protein design enables a novel one-carbon assimilation pathway. *Proceedings of the National Academy of Sciences of the United States of America*, *112*(12), 3704–3709. DOI: 10.1073/pnas.1500545112

Siegel, J. B., Zanghellini, A., Lovick, H. M., Kiss, G., Lambert, A. R., St.Clair, J. L., Gallaher, J. L., Hilvert, D., Gelb, M. H., Stoddard, B. L., Houk, K. N., Michael, F. E., & Baker, D. (2010). Computational Design of an Enzyme Catalyst for a Stereoselective Bimolecular Diels-Alder Reaction. *Science*, *329*(5986), 309–313. 1190239

Siegfried, T. (2005). In Praise of Hard Questions. *Science*, *309*(5731), 76–77. DOI: 10.1126/science.309.5731.76

Siegrist, M., & Hartmann, C. (2020). Perceived naturalness, disgust, trust and food neophobia as predictors of cultured meat acceptance in ten countries. *Appetite*, *155*, 104814.

Silva, A. P. S. e, Araújo, N. M. da F. T. de S., Oliveira, M. D. S. de, Chagas, S. C. S., Marques, F. R. V., Britto, L. P. da S., … Nascimento, A. V. S. do. (2024). Industry 4.0 and Biotechnology: Strategies For Innovation snd Sustainability. Revista De Gestão - RGSA, 18(10), e08998. https://doi.org/DOI: 10.24857/rgsa.v18n10-094

Silva, S. O., Mafra, A. K. C., Pelissari, F. M., Rodrigues de Lemos, L., & Molina, G. (2025). Biotechnology in Agro-Industry: Valorization of Agricultural Wastes, By-Products and Sustainable Practices. *Microorganisms, 13*(8), 1789.

Silverman, A. D., & Karim, A. S. (2020). Cell-free gene expression: An expanded repertoire of applications. *Nature Reviews. Genetics, 21*(3), 151–170. DOI: 10.1038/s41576-019-0185-8 PMID: 31780816

Simon, B., Nomellini, J., Chiou, P., Bingle, W., Thornton, J., Smit, J., & Leong, J. (2001). Recombinant vaccines against infectious hematopoietic necrosis virus: Production by the Caulobacter crescentus S-layer protein secretion system and evaluation in laboratory trials. *Diseases of Aquatic Organisms, 44*, 17–27. DOI: 10.3354/dao044017

Simpson, R., & Sastry, S. K. (2013). Scale-up in chemical and bioprocess engineering. In *Chemical and bioprocess engineering: Fundamental concepts for first-year students* (pp. 261–275). Springer., DOI: 10.1007/978-1-4614-9126-2_11

Sims, R. E., Mabee, W., Saddler, J. N., & Taylor, M. (2010). An overview of second generation biofuel technologies. *Bioresource Technology, 101*(6), 1570–1580. DOI: 10.1016/j.biortech.2009.11.046 PMID: 19963372

Simutis, R., & Lübbert, A. (2015). Bioreactor control improves bioprocess performance. *Biotechnology Journal, 10*(8), 1115–1130. PMID: 26228573

Sindhi, K., Pingili, R. B., Beldar, V., Bhattacharya, S., Rahaman, J., & Mukherjee, D. (2025). The role of biomaterials-based scaffolds in advancing skin tissue construct. *Journal of Tissue Viability, 34*(2), 100858. DOI: 10.1016/j.jtv.2025.100858

Singh, A., & Negi, P. S. (2025). Biotechnological application of health-promising bioactive compounds. In *Biotechnological Intervention in Production of Bioactive Compounds: Biosynthesis, Characterization and Applications* (pp. 73-94). Springer.

Singh, A. K., Pal, P., Pandey, B., Goksen, G., Sahoo, U. K., Lorenzo, J. M., & Sarangi, P. K. (2023). Development of "Smart Foods" for health by nanoencapsulation: Novel technologies and challenges. *Food Chemistry: X, 20*, 100910. DOI: 10.1016/j.fochx.2023.100910

Singh, A., & Kumar, S. (2025). Exploring the Functionality of Microbes in Fermented Foods: Technological Advancements and Future Directions. *Fermentation (Basel, Switzerland), 11*(6), 300.

Singh, B. P. (2025). Harnessing probiotic fermentation for the generation of food-derived bioactive peptides: Current status and prospects. *European Food Research and Technology*, •••, 1–16.

Singh, J. S., Abhilash, P. C., Singh, H. B., Singh, R. P., & Singh, D. P. (2011). Genetically engineered bacteria: An emerging tool for environmental remediation and future research perspectives. *Gene, 480*(1-2), 1–9. DOI: 10.1016/j.gene.2011.03.001 PMID: 21402131

Singh, N., Malik, S., Gupta, A., & Srivastava, K. R. (2021). Revolutionizing enzyme engineering through artificial intelligence and machine learning. *Emerging Topics in Life Sciences, 5*(1), 113–125.

Singh, N., Ogunseitan, O. A., Wong, M. H., & Tang, Y. (2022). Sustainable materials alternative to petrochemical plastics pollution: A review analysis. *Sustainable Horizons*, *2*, 100016. DOI: 10.1016/j.horiz.2022.100016

Singh, P., & Kumar, S. (2019). Microbial enzyme in food biotechnology. In *Enzymes in food biotechnology* (pp. 19–28). Elsevier.

Singh, P., Shukla, S., & Misra, G. (2024). Good Manufacturing Practices in Quality Control. In *Quality Control and Regulatory Aspects for Biologicals* (pp. 100–118). CRC Press.

Singh, S., Raj, D., Mathur, A., Mani, N., & Kumar, D. (2025). Current approaches in CRISPR-Cas systems for hereditary diseases. *Progress in Molecular Biology and Translational Science*, *210*, 205–229. DOI: 10.1016/bs.pmbts.2024.07.002

Singh, V. (Ed.). (2021). *Microbial cell factories engineering for production of biomolecules*. Academic Press.

Singh, V., Haque, S., Niwas, R., Srivastava, A., Pasupuleti, M., & Tripathi, C. (2017). Strategies for fermentation medium optimization: An in-depth review. *Frontiers in Microbiology*, *7*, 2087. PMID: 28111566

Singla, P. (2020). Plant synthetic biology: A paradigm shift targeting stress mitigation, reduction of ecological footprints and sustainable transformation in agriculture. *Plant Stress Biology: Strategies and Trends*, 435–489.

Sinhmar, D., & Purohit, R. (2025). Patenting Life: Global Perspectives on Intellectual Property in Genetic and Biotechnological Innovation Amidst Ethical and Legal Challenges. *Journal on Development of Intellectual Property and Research*, *1*(1), 29–40. https://journal.cdipr.ac.in/index.php/jdipr/article/view/5

Sinner, P., Herwig, C., & Kager, J. (2020). Time scale analysis and optimization of a continuous microbial bioprocess. *Computer-Aided Chemical Engineering*, *48*, 1603–1608.

Sinreih, M., Zukunft, S., Sosič, I., Cesar, J., Gobec, S., Adamski, J., & Lanišnik Rižner, T. (2015). Combined application of *in silico* and *in vitro* screening for AKR1B10 inhibitors. *PLoS One*, *10*(2), e0117984. DOI: 10.1371/journal.pone.0117984 PMID: 25680188

Skrzypczak, K., Teterycz, D., Gustaw, W., Domagała, D., Mielczarek, P., & Kasprzyk-Pochopień, J. (2024). The possibility of using Lactobacillus plantarum 299v to reinforce the bioactive properties of legume-derived beverages. *Applied Sciences (Basel, Switzerland)*, *14*(12), 5187.

Smith, H. O., Hutchison, C. A., Pfannkoch, C., & Venter, J. C. (2003). Generating a synthetic genome by whole genome assembly: PhiX174 bacteriophage from synthetic oligonucleotides. *Proceedings of the National Academy of Sciences of the United States of America*, *100*(26), 15440–15445. DOI: 10.1073/pnas.2237126100 PMID: 14657399

Smith, K. M., Cho, K. M., & Liao, J. C. (2010). Engineering *Corynebacterium glutamicum* for isobutanol production. *Applied Microbiology and Biotechnology*, *87*(3), 1045–1055. DOI: 10.1007/s00253-010-2522-6 PMID: 20376637

Smuda, M. (2004). Bioplastics: A growing trend. *Packaging Technology & Science*, *17*(5), 255–261. DOI: 10.1002/pts.663

Sochaj, A. M., Świderska, K. W., & Otlewski, J. (2015). Current methods for the synthesis of homogeneous antibody–drug conjugates. *Biotechnology Advances, 33*(6), 775–784. DOI: 10.1016/j.biotechadv.2015.05.001

Somero, G. N. (2020). The cellular stress response and temperature: Function, regulation, and evolution. *Journal of Experimental Zoology. Part A, Ecological and Integrative Physiology, 333*(6), 379–397. PMID: 31944627

Song, A. A.-L., In, L. L. A., Lim, S. H. E., & Rahim, R. A. (2017). A review on Lactococcus lactis: From food to factory. *Microbial Cell Factories, 16*(1), 55. DOI: 10.1186/s12934-017-0669-x

Song, M., Fisher, R., & Kwoh, Y. (2019). Technological challenges of green innovation and sustainable resource management with large scale data. *Technological Forecasting and Social Change, 144*, 361–368.

Soonsanga, S., Rungrod, A., Utamatho, M., Trakulnaleamsai, C., Paenpong, P., Pootakham, W., Phaonakrop, N., Roytrakul, S., & Promdonkoy, B. (2025). Integrated genomic and proteomic analysis of local Bacillus thuringiensis isolates for targeted insect pest control and functional insight. *Archives of Microbiology, 207*(9), 1–12.

Sorooshian, S. (2024). The sustainable development goals of the United Nations: A comparative midterm research review. *Journal of Cleaner Production, 142272*. Advance online publication. DOI: 10.1016/j.jclepro.2024.142272

Srai, J. S.. (2020). Digitalisation in pharmaceutical manufacturing: State-of-the-art review and future perspectives. *Computers in Industry, 117*, 103213.

Srai, J. S., & Kumar, M. (2019). Supply network configuration for distributed manufacturing: Case studies in the biopharmaceutical industry. *International Journal of Production Research, 57*(8), 2436–2453.

Srivastav, A. K., & Das, P. (2025). Green Finance and Investment in IoT–Biotechnology Synergies. In *Biotechnology and IoT in Agriculture and Food Production: Green Innovation* (pp. 153-160). Berkeley, CA: Apress. https://doi.org/DOI: 10.1007/979-8-8688-1469-3_17

Srivastav, A. K., & Das, P. (2025). *Artificial Intelligence in the Production of Biotherapeutics: Principles, Practices and Standards*. CRC Press.

Srivastav, A. K., Das, P., & Srivastava, A. K. (2024). Future Trends, Innovations, and Global Collaboration. In *Biotech and IoT: An Introduction Using Cloud-Driven Labs* (pp. 309–398). Springer.

Stana, A., Rista, A., Mukli, L., & Xhaferra, E. (2024). The Role of the Academic Incubator as an Acceleration Tool to Foster Entrepreneurship and Academic-Industry Connections. *Interdisciplinary Journal of Research and Development, 11*(3), 104–104.

Stazi, A., & Jovine, R. (2022). Food traceability in Europe, the US and China: comparative law and regulatory technology. *BioLaw Journal*(2).

Steen, E. J., Chan, R., Prasad, N., Myers, S., Petzold, C. J., Redding, A., Ouellet, M., & Keasling, J. D. (2008). Metabolic engineering of *Saccharomyces cerevisiae* for the production of n-butanol. *Microbial Cell Factories, 7*, 36. DOI: 10.1186/1475-2859-7-36 PMID: 19055772

Steen, E. J., Kang, Y., Bokinsky, G., Hu, Z., Schirmer, A., McClure, A., Del Cardayre, S. B., & Keasling, J. D. (2010). Microbial production of fatty-acid-derived fuels and chemicals from plant biomass. *Nature*, *463*(7280), 559–562.

Steinegger, A., Wolfbeis, O. S., & Borisov, S. M. (2020). Optical sensing and imaging of pH values: Spectroscopies, materials, and applications. *Chemical Reviews*, *120*(22), 12357–12489. PMID: 33147405

Stephanopoulos, G. (2012). Synthetic biology and metabolic engineering. *ACS Synthetic Biology*, *1*(11), 514–525. DOI: 10.1021/sb300094q PMID: 23656228

Stephen, M. D. (2021). China's new multilateral institutions: A framework and research agenda. *International Studies Review*, *23*(3), 807–834. DOI: 10.1093/isr/viaa076

Stern, E. K., & Brenner, D. M. (2018). Gut microbiota-based therapies for irritable bowel syndrome. *Clinical and Translational Gastroenterology*, *9*(2), e134.

Straathof, A. J., Wahl, S. A., Benjamin, K. R., Takors, R., Wierckx, N., & Noorman, H. J. (2019). Grand research challenges for sustainable industrial biotechnology. *Trends in Biotechnology*, *37*(10), 1042–1050. PMID: 31054854

Subramanian, M. R., Suvarna, T., & Christopher, L. P. (2015). Production of lactic acid using a new homofermentative *Enterococcus faecalis* isolate. *Microbial Biotechnology*, *8*(2), 221–229. DOI: 10.1111/1751-7915.12133

Sudhakar, M., Priya, M., & Dharani, G. (2024). A review on the environmental impacts of microplastics and its remediation techniques. *Environmental Science and Pollution Research International*, *31*(11), 15927–15951. DOI: 10.1007/s11356-024-32151-1

Suganthi, P., Usharani, B., Venkateswari, R., & Muthuraj, M. (2023). Biosafety Practices in Mycobacteriology Laboratory. *Research Advances in Microbiology and Biotechnology*, *3*(3), 1–39.

Suhail, M., Shao, Y.-F., Vu, Q. L., & Wu, P.-C. (2022). Designing of pH-sensitive hydrogels for colon targeted drug delivery; characterization and in vitro evaluation. *Gels (Basel, Switzerland)*, *8*(3), 155.

Sundaram, J. (2025). Analysis of TRIPS Agreement and the justification of international IP rights protection in the WTO's multilateral trading system, with particular reference to pharmaceutical patents. *Information & Communications Technology Law*, *24*(2), 121–163. DOI: 10.1080/13600834.2015.1004244

Sun, T., Song, J., Wang, M., Zhao, C., & Zhang, W. (2022). Challenges and recent progress in the governance of biosecurity risks in the era of synthetic biology. *Journal of Biosafety and Biosecurity*, *4*(1), 59–67. PMID: 35005525

Süntar, I., Çetinkaya, S., Haydaroğlu, Ü. S., & Habtemariam, S. (2021). Bioproduction process of natural products and biopharmaceuticals: Biotechnological aspects. *Biotechnology Advances*, *50*, 107768. PMID: 33974980

Sun, W., Shahrajabian, M. H., & Lin, M. (2022). Research progress of fermented functional foods and protein factory-microbial fermentation technology. *Fermentation (Basel, Switzerland)*, *8*(12), 688.

Sun, X., Liu, H., Wang, P., Wang, Y., & Lu, L. (2019). Construction of a novel MK-4 biosynthetic pathway in *Pichia pastoris* through heterologous expression of HsUBIAD1. *Microbial Cell Factories*, *18*, 169. DOI: 10.1186/s12934-019-1215-9 PMID: 31601211

Sun, Y., & Jung, H. (2024). Machine Learning (ML) Modeling, IoT, and Optimizing Organizational Operations through Integrated Strategies: The Role of Technology and Human Resource Management. *Sustainability*, *16*(16), 6751.

Sun, Y.-Q., Shen, J.-T., Yan, L., Zhou, J.-J., Jiang, L.-L., Chen, Y., Yuan, J.-L., Feng, E., & Xiu, Z.-L. (2018). Advances in bioconversion of glycerol to 1,3-propanediol: Prospects and challenges. *Process Biochemistry*, *71*, 134–146. DOI: 10.1016/j.procbio.2018.05.009

Sun, Z., Wu, B., Ren, Y., Wang, Z., Zhao, C., Hai, M., Weitz, D. A., & Chen, D. (2021). Diverse Particle Carriers Prepared by Co-Precipitation and Phase Separation: Formation and Applications. *ChemPlusChem*, *86*(1), 49–58. DOI: 10.1002/cplu.202000497

Su, Q., Ganesh, S., Moreno, M., Bommireddy, Y., Gonzalez, M., Reklaitis, G. V., & Nagy, Z. K. (2019). A perspective on Quality-by-Control (QbC) in pharmaceutical continuous manufacturing. *Computers & Chemical Engineering*, *125*, 216–231. PMID: 36845965

Su, R., Ting, W., Taidong, B., Ningyun, C., Meng, Y., Chen, W., & Hao, J., Huadong, & P., Ning, C. (2023). Enhanced production of d-pantothenic acid in *Corynebacterium glutamicum* using an efficient CRISPR–Cpf1 genome editing method. *Microbial Cell Factories*, *22*, 3. DOI: 10.1186/s12934-023-02017-1

Suri, G. S., Kaur, G., & Shinde, D. (2024). Beyond boundaries: Exploring the transformative power of AI in pharmaceuticals. *Discover Artificial Intelligence*, *4*(1), 82.

Suzette, T., Gaylan, E. G., Taneo, J. K. B., Bercero, G. I. M. R., Piloton-Narca, M., & Marchee, T. (2024). Challenges in teaching biotechnology in the Philippine STE program. *International Journal of Learning. Teaching and Educational Research*, *23*(3), 367–389.

Swaminaathan, P., Saravanan, A., & Thamarai, P. (2024). Utilization of bioresources for high-value bioproducts production: Sustainability and perspectives in circular bioeconomy. *Sustainable Energy Technologies and Assessments*, *63*, 103672. DOI: 10.1016/j.seta.2024.103672

Swartz, J. R. (2012). Transforming biochemical engineering with cell-free biology. *AIChE Journal. American Institute of Chemical Engineers*, *58*(1), 5–13. DOI: 10.1002/aic.13701

Taghavi, N., Singhal, N., Zhuang, W. Q., & Baroutian, S. (2021). Degradation of plastic waste using stimulated and naturally occurring microbial strains. *Chemosphere*, *263*, 127975. DOI: 10.1016/j.chemosphere.2020.127975 PMID: 32828061

Taha, B. A., Abbas, E. M., Kadhim, A. C., Azzahrani, A. S., Haider, A. J., Chaudhary, V., & Arsad, N. (2024). Needle scattered light guided chiplets-interfaced with AI for advanced biomedical application. *Microelectronic Engineering*, *292*, 112228.

Taheri-Kafrani, A., Kharazmi, S., Nasrollahzadeh, M., Soozanipour, A., Ejeian, F., Etedali, P., Mansouri-Tehrani, H.-A., Razmjou, A., Yek, S. M.-G., & Varma, R. S. (2021). Recent developments in enzyme immobilization technology for high-throughput processing in food industries. *Critical Reviews in Food Science and Nutrition*, *61*(19), 3160–3196.

Tamborini, L., Fernandes, P., Paradisi, F., & Molinari, F. (2018). Flow bioreactors as complementary tools for biocatalytic process intensification. *Trends in Biotechnology*, *36*(1), 73–88. PMID: 29054312

Tamime, A. Y. (2009). *Dairy powders and concentrated products.* Wiley-Blackwell., DOI: 10.1002/9781444322729

Tan, D., Wu, Q., Chen, J.-C., & Chen, G.-Q. (2014). Engineering Halomonas TD01 for the low-cost production of polyhydroxyalkanoates. *Metabolic Engineering*, *26*, 34–47. DOI: 10.1016/j.ymben.2014.09.001

Tang, C., Wang, L., Zang, L., Wang, Q., Qi, D., & Dai, Z. (2023). On-demand biomanufacturing through synthetic biology approach. *Materials Today. Bio*, *18*, 100518. DOI: 10.1016/j.mtbio.2022.100518

Tang, D. Y. Y., Ooi, C., & Show, P. L. (2025). Blue bioeconomy and biotechnology: Towards a sustainably growing microalgae industry. *Blue Biotechnology*, *2*, 13. DOI: 10.1186/s44315-025-00036-8

Tang, D. Y. Y., Yew, G. Y., Koyande, A. K., Chew, K. W., Vo, D. V. N., & Show, P. L. (2020). Green technology for the industrial production of biofuels and bioproducts from microalgae: A review. *Environmental Chemistry Letters*, *18*(6), 1967–1985.

Tang, H. H., & Ahmad, N. S. (2024). Fuzzy logic approach for controlling uncertain and nonlinear systems: A comprehensive review of applications and advances. *Systems Science & Control Engineering*, *12*(1), 2394429.

Tang, H., Xiang, G., Xiao, W., Yang, Z., & Zhao, B. (2024). Microbial mediated remediation of heavy metals toxicity: Mechanisms and future prospects. *Frontiers in Plant Science*, *15*, 1420408. DOI: 10.3389/fpls.2024.1420408 PMID: 39100088

Tangyu, M., Muller, J., Bolten, C. J., & Wittmann, C. (2019). Fermentation of plant-based milk alternatives for improved flavour and nutritional value. *Applied Microbiology and Biotechnology*, *103*(23), 9263–9275. DOI: 10.1007/s00253-019-10175-9

Tan, S.-I., & Ng, I.-S. (2020). New Insight into Plasmid-Driven T7 RNA Polymerase in *Escherichia coli* and Use as a Genetic Amplifier for a Biosensor. *ACS Synthetic Biology*, *9*(3), 613–622. DOI: 10.1021/acssynbio.9b00466

Tao, F.. (2019). Digital twin in industry: State-of-the-art. *IEEE Transactions on Industrial Informatics*, *15*(4), 2405–2415.

Tao, F., Qi, Q., Liu, A., & Kusiak, A. (2018). Data-driven smart manufacturing. *Journal of Manufacturing Systems*, *48*, 157–169.

Tao, J., Aamir, M., Shoaib, M., Yasir, N., & Babar, M. (2025). Bridging the Gap Between Supply Chain Risk and Organizational Performance Conditioning to Demand Uncertainty. *Sustainability*, *17*(6), 2462. DOI: 10.3390/su17062462

Tarafdar, A., Pandey, A., Sirohi, R., Soccol, C. R., & Dussap, C.-G. (2022). *Current Developments in Biotechnology and Bioengineering: Advances in Food Engineering*. Elsevier.

Tarfeen, N., Nisa, K. U., Hamid, B., Bashir, Z., Yatoo, A. M., Dar, M. A., Mohiddin, F. A., Amin, Z., Ahmad, R. A., & Sayyed, R. Z. (2022). Microbial Remediation: A Promising Tool for Reclamation of Contaminated Sites with Special Emphasis on Heavy Metal and Pesticide Pollution: A Review. *Processes (Basel, Switzerland)*, *10*(7), 1358. DOI: 10.3390/pr10071358

Tawade, M., & Pandya, S. (2023). *Optimizing Pharmaceutical Quality Audits: Enhancing Compliance and Performance through Best Practices*. ResearchGate.

Tawo, O. E., & Mbamalu, M. I. (2025). Advancing waste valorization techniques for sustainable industrial operations and improved environmental safety. *International Journal of Scientific Research Archive*, *14*(2), 127–149. DOI: 10.30574/ijsra.2025.14.2.0282

Tekere, M. (2019). Microbial bioremediation and different bioreactors designs applied. In *Biotechnology and bioengineering*. IntechOpen., DOI: 10.5772/intechopen.83661

Terpou, A., Papadaki, A., Lappa, I. K., Kachrimanidou, V., Bosnea, L. A., & Kopsahelis, N. (2019). Probiotics in food systems: Significance and emerging strategies towards improved viability and delivery of enhanced beneficial value. *Nutrients*, *11*(7), 1591.

Teusink, B., Bachmann, H., & Molenaar, D. (2011). Systems biology of lactic acid bacteria: A critical review. *Microbial Cell Factories*, *10*(Suppl 1), S11. DOI: 10.1186/1475-2859-10-S1-S11

Thakur, S., Chaudhary, J., Sharma, B., Verma, A., Tamulevicius, S., & Thakur, V. K. (2018). Sustainability of bioplastics: Opportunities and challenges. *Current Opinion in Green and Sustainable Chemistry*, *13*, 68–75. DOI: 10.1016/j.cogsc.2018.04.013

Thon, J. N., Dykstra, B. J., & Beaulieu, L. M. (2017). Platelet bioreactor: Accelerated evolution of design and manufacture. *Platelets*, *28*(5), 472–477. DOI: 10.1080/09537104.2016.1265922 PMID: 28112988

Tiquia-Arashiro, S. M., & Rodrigues, D. F. (2016). *Bioremediation and biotechnology: Sustainable approaches to pollution degradation*. Springer International Publishing., DOI: 10.1007/978-3-030-35691-0

Tišma, S., & Škrtić, M. M. (2023). Integrating Bioeconomy Principles in Bionic Production: Enhancing Sustainability and Environmental Performance. *Journal of Risk and Financial Management*, *16*(10), 437.

Tobias, J. Erb., Patrik, Jones, R., & Bar-Even, A. (2017). Synthetic metabolism: Metabolic engineering meets enzyme design. *Current Opinion in Chemical Biology*, *37*, 56–62. DOI: 10.1016/j.cbpa.2016.12.023

Tokunaga, H., Arakawa, T., & Tokunaga, M. (2010). Novel soluble expression technologies derived from unique properties of halophilic proteins. *Applied Microbiology and Biotechnology*, *88*(6), 1223–1231. DOI: 10.1007/s00253-010-2832-8

Tomczak, W., & Gryta, M. (2022). The application of cellulose acetate membranes for separation of fermentation broths by the reverse osmosis: A feasibility study. *International Journal of Molecular Sciences*, *23*(19), 11738. PMID: 36233037

Tomczyk, P., Wdowczyk, A., Wiatkowska, B., & Szymańska-Pulikowska, A. (2023). Assessment of heavy metal contamination of agricultural soils in Poland using contamination indicators. *Ecological Indicators, 156*, 111161. DOI: 10.1016/j.ecolind.2023.111161

Toromade, A. S., Soyombo, D. A., Kupa, E., & Ijomah, T. I. (2024). Reviewing the impact of climate change on global food security: Challenges and solutions. *International journal of applied research in social sciences, 6*(7), 1403-1416.

Torrorey-Sawe, R. (2025). *Global Bioethics: Addressing Current Challenges.* Innovations, and the Needs of Underserved Populations.

Tounekti, O., Prior, S., Wassmer, S., Xu, J., Wong, A., Fang, X., Sonderegger, I., Smeraglia, J., Huleatt, J., & Loo, L. (2025). 2024 White Paper on Recent Issues in Bioanalysis: Evolution of Immunogenicity Assessment beyond ADA/NAb; Regulated Genomic/NGS Assays; Hypersensitivity Reactions; Minimum Noise Reduction; False Positive Range; Modernized Vaccine Approaches; NAb/TAb Correlation (PART 3A–Recommendations on Advanced Strategies for Molecular Assays and Immunogenicity of Gene Therapy, Cell Therapy, Vaccine; Biotherapeutics Immunogenicity Assessment & Clinical Relevance PART 3B–Regulatory Agencies' Input on Immunogenicity/Technologies of Biotherapeutics, Gene, Cell & Vaccine Therapies). *Bioanalysis, 17*(3), 105–149. PMID: 39862111

Toy, J. Y. H., Lu, Y., Huang, D., Matsumura, K., & Liu, S.-Q. (2022). Enzymatic treatment, unfermented and fermented fruit-based products: Current state of knowledge. *Critical Reviews in Food Science and Nutrition, 62*(7), 1890–1911.

Trabucco, B., Geng, X., Kumar, A., & Levine, S. (2022, June). Design-bench: Benchmarks for data-driven offline model-based optimization. In *International Conference on Machine Learning* (pp. 21658-21676). PMLR.

Trejo-Solís, C., Serrano-García, N., Castillo-Rodríguez, R. A., Robledo-Cadena, D. X., Jimenez-Farfan, D., Marín-Hernández, Á., Silva-Adaya, D., Rodríguez-Pérez, C. E., & Gallardo-Pérez, J. C. (2024). Metabolic dysregulation of tricarboxylic acid cycle and oxidative phosphorylation in glioblastoma. *Reviews in the Neurosciences, 35*(7), 813–838. DOI: 10.1515/revneuro-2024-0022

Tripathi, N. K., & Shrivastava, A. (2019). Recent Developments in Bioprocessing of Recombinant Proteins: Expression Hosts and Process Development. *Frontiers in Bioengineering and Biotechnology, 7*. Advance online publication. DOI: 10.3389/fbioe.2019.00420

Tristan, C. A., Ormanoglu, P., Slamecka, J., Malley, C., Chu, P.-H., Jovanovic, V. M., Gedik, Y., Jethmalani, Y., Bonney, C., Barnaeva, E., Braisted, J., Mallanna, S. K., Dorjsuren, D., Iannotti, M. J., Voss, T. C., Michael, S., Simeonov, A., & Singeç, I. (2021). Robotic high-throughput biomanufacturing and functional differentiation of human pluripotent stem cells. *Stem Cell Reports, 16*(12), 3076–3092. DOI: 10.1016/j.stemcr.2021.11.004

Trump, B., Cummings, C., Klasa, K., Galaitsi, S., & Linkov, I. (2023). Governing biotechnology to provide safety and security and address ethical, legal, and social implications. *Frontiers in Genetics, 13*, 1052371.

Tsakalova, M., Onorato, C., Karathanasis, A. Z., & Deligkiozi, I. (2024). A circular economy framework for the assessment of bio-based value chains. *Sustainable Chemistry for the Environment, 6*, 100099. DOI: 10.1016/j.scenv.2024.100099

Tsydenova, O., & Bengtsson, M. (2011). Chemical hazards associated with treatment of waste electrical and electronic equipment. *Waste Management (New York, N.Y.), 31*(1), 45–58. DOI: 10.1016/j.wasman.2010.08.014 PMID: 20869229

Turanli, B., Gulfidan, G., Aydogan, O. O., Kula, C., Selvaraj, G., & Arga, K. Y. (2024). Genome-scale metabolic models in translational medicine: The current status and potential of machine learning in improving the effectiveness of the models. *Molecular Omics, 20*(4), 234–247. DOI: 10.1039/D3MO00239A

Tusé, D., Nandi, S., McDonald, K. A., & Buyel, J. F. (2020). The emergency response capacity of plant-based biopharmaceutical manufacturing-what it is and what it could be. *Frontiers in Plant Science, 11*, 594019. DOI: 10.3389/fpls.2020.594019 PMID: 33193552

Udayan, A., Sirohi, R., Sreekumar, N., Sang, B. I., & Sim, S. J. (2022). Mass cultivation and harvesting of microalgal biomass: Current trends and future perspectives. *Bioresource Technology, 344*, 126406. PMID: 34826565

Udugama, I. A., Lopez, P. C., Gargalo, C. L., Li, X., Bayer, C., & Gernaey, K. V. (2021). Digital Twin in biomanufacturing: Challenges and opportunities towards its implementation. *Systems Microbiology and Biomanufacturing, 1*(3), 257–274.

Ulber, R., Frerichs, J. G., & Beutel, S. (2003). Optical sensor systems for bioprocess monitoring. *Analytical and Bioanalytical Chemistry, 376*(3), 342–348. PMID: 12728296

Ullah, R., Ahmad, H., Rehman, F. U., & Fawad, A. (2023). Green innovation and Sustainable Development Goals in SMEs: The moderating role of government incentives. *Journal of Economic and Administrative Sciences, 39*(4), 830–846. DOI: 10.1108/JEAS-07-2022-0168

Umoga, U. J., Sodiya, E. O., Ugwuanyi, E. D., Jacks, B. S., Lottu, O. A., Daraojimba, O. D., & Obaigbena, A. (2024). Exploring the potential of AI-driven optimization in enhancing network performance and efficiency. *Magna Scientia Advanced Research and Reviews, 10*(1), 368–378.

Union, A. (2020). The digital transformation strategy for Africa (2020-30). http://www.au.int/

Valverde, J. M., & Avilés-Palacios, C. (2021). Circular economy as a catalyst for progress towards the sustainable development goals: A positive relationship between two self-sufficient variables. *Sustainability, 13*(22), 12652. DOI: 10.3390/su132212652

Van Dijl, J., & Hecker, M. (2013). *Bacillus subtilis*: From soil bacterium to super-secreting cell factory. *Microbial Cell Factories, 12*, 3. Advance online publication. DOI: 10.1186/1475-2859-12-3

van Heerden, C. D., & Nicol, W. (2013). Continuous and batch cultures of Escherichia coli KJ134 for succinic acid fermentation: Metabolic flux distributions and production characteristics. *Microbial Cell Factories, 12*(1), 80. DOI: 10.1186/1475-2859-12-80

Vandenberghe, L., Valladares-Diestra, K., Bittencourt, G. A., Torres, L. Z., Vieira, S., Karp, S. G., Sydney, E., de Carvalho, J. C., Soccol, V. T., & Soccol, C. R. (2022). Beyond sugar and ethanol: The future of sugarcane biorefineries in Brazil. *Renewable & Sustainable Energy Reviews, 167*, 112721.

Vasic-Racki, D. (2006). *History of Industrial Biotransformations-Dreams and Realities.*

Vasilakis, P., Pyrgakis, K., Psycha, M., Biundo, A., & Kokossis, A. (2023). A novel industrial biotechnology approach to valorize fatty acids to bioplastics: Scope for scale-up and process efficiency using an integrated approach. [). Elsevier.]. *Computer-Aided Chemical Engineering, 52*, 2563–2568.

Vasile, C., Baican, M., & Darie-Ni ă, R. N. (2019). Emerging and advanced technologies in bioplastics. *Journal of Cellular Plastics, 55*(3), 251–277. DOI: 10.1177/0021955X19833637

Vees, C. A., Neuendorf, C. S., & Pflügl, S. (2020). Towards continuous industrial bioprocessing with solventogenic and acetogenic clostridia: Challenges, progress and perspectives. *Journal of Industrial Microbiology & Biotechnology, 47*(9–10), 753–787. DOI: 10.1007/s10295-020-02296-2

Vegineni, G. C. (2025). Sustainable tech development: Integrating AI, XR, and CI/CD pipelines for a greener future. In *Exploring the impact of extended reality (XR) technologies on promoting environmental sustainability* (pp. 267–293). Springer., DOI: 10.1007/978-3-031-72904-1_14

Verma, D., Sharma, R., & Sharma, A. (2021). Digital twins in biopharmaceutical manufacturing: A transformative approach for smart production. *Biotechnology Advances, 49*, 107764.

Vigentini, I., Merico, A., Tutino, M. L., Compagno, C., & Marino, G. (2006). Optimization of recombinant human nerve growth factor production in the psychrophilic Pseudoalteromonas haloplanktis. *Journal of Biotechnology, 127*(1), 141–150. DOI: 10.1016/j.jbiotec.2006.05.019

Vilkhovoy, M., Adhikari, A., Vadhin, S., & Varner, J. D. (2020). The evolution of cell free biomanufacturing. *Processes (Basel, Switzerland), 8*(6), 675.

Vinderola, G., Ouwehand, A., Salminen, S., & von Wright, A. (2019). *Lactic acid bacteria: microbiological and functional aspects.* Crc Press.

Vinicius De Melo Pereira, G., De Carvalho Neto, D. P., Junqueira, A. C. D. O., Karp, S. G., Letti, L. A., Magalhães Júnior, A. I., & Soccol, C. R. (2020). A review of selection criteria for starter culture development in the food fermentation industry. *Food Reviews International, 36*(2), 135–167.

Voeikova, T., Zhuravliova, O., & Debabov, V. (2020). Comparative analysis of legal regulation of industrial use of genetic-engineering-modified microorganisms in the united states, European Union, and Russian Federation. *Molecular Genetics, Microbiology and Virology, 35*(2), 69–77.

Voidarou, C., Antoniadou, M., Rozos, G., Tzora, A., Skoufos, I., Varzakas, T., Lagiou, A., & Bezirtzoglou, E. (2020). Fermentative foods: Microbiology, biochemistry, potential human health benefits and public health issues. *Foods, 10*(1), 69.

Vojdani, F., & Gerhard, L. (2019). Plant-based expression systems for biopharmaceuticals: Developments and challenges. *Frontiers in Plant Science, 10*, 1276.

von Stosch, M., Oliveira, R., & Peres, J. (2021). Digital Twins in Bioprocessing: Applications and Challenges. *Current Opinion in Chemical Engineering, 34*, 100735. DOI: 10.1016/j.coche.2021.100735

Vrchota, J., Pech, M., Rolinek, L., & Bednář, J. (2020). Sustainability outcomes of green processes in relation to industry 4.0 in manufacturing: Systematic review. *Sustainability, 12*(15), 5968.

Vučurović, D., Bajić, B., Trivunović, Z., Dodić, J., Zeljko, M., Jevtić-Mučibabić, R., & Dodić, S. (2024). Biotechnological Utilization of Agro-Industrial Residues and By-Products—Sustainable Production of Biosurfactants. *Foods, 13*(5), 711. DOI: 10.3390/foods13050711 PMID: 38472824

Wahab, W. A. A. (2025). Review of research progress in immobilization and chemical modification of microbial enzymes and their application. *Microbial Cell Factories, 24*(1), 167. DOI: 10.1186/s12934-025-02791-0

Waksman, S. A., Reilly, H. C., & Johnstone, D. B. (1946). Isolation of Streptomycin-producing Strains of Streptomyces griseus. *Journal of Bacteriology, 52*(3), 393–397.

Walsh, G. (2013). *Biopharmaceuticals: Biochemistry and biotechnology* (2nd ed.). John Wiley & Sons.

Walsh, G. (2018). Biopharmaceutical benchmarks 2018. *Nature Biotechnology, 36*(12), 1136–1145. DOI: 10.1038/nbt.4305

Walsh, G. (2018). *Biopharmaceuticals: Biochemistry and Biotechnology* (3rd ed.). Wiley-Blackwell.

Walsh, G., & Walsh, E. (2022). Biopharmaceutical benchmarks 2022. *Nature Biotechnology, 40*(12), 1722–1760. PMID: 36471135

Wang, G., Mohsin, A., Chu, J., Zhuang, Y., & Zhang, S. (2024). Advances and prospects for advanced biomanufacturing. *Scale-up and Chemical Process for Microbial Production of Plant-Derived Bioactive Compounds*, 1-16.

Wang, G., Mohsin, A., Chu, J., Zhuang, Y., & Zhang, S. (2024). Advances and prospects for advanced biomanufacturing. *Scale-up and Chemical Process for Microbial Production of Plant-Derived Bioactive Compounds*, 1–16.

Wang, A., & Zhong, Q. (2024). Drying of probiotics to enhance the viability during preparation, storage, food application, and digestion: A review. *Comprehensive Reviews in Food Science and Food Safety, 23*(1), e13287.

Wang, B., Wang, Z., Chen, T., & Zhao, X. (2020). Development of novel bioreactor control systems based on smart sensors and actuators. *Frontiers in Bioengineering and Biotechnology, 8*, 7. DOI: 10.3389/fbioe.2020.00007 PMID: 32117906

Wang, C., Fu, L., Ametefe, D. S., Wang, S., & John, D. (2025). E-textiles in healthcare: A systematic literature review of wearable technologies for monitoring and enhancing human health. *Neural Computing & Applications, 37*(4), 2089–2111.

Wang, D., Lin, J., Lin, J., Wang, W., & Li, S. (2019). Biodegradation of Petroleum Hydrocarbons by Bacillus subtilis BL-27, a Strain with Weak Hydrophobicity. *Molecules (Basel, Switzerland), 24*(17), 3021. DOI: 10.3390/molecules24173021 PMID: 31438460

Wang, F., Bi, Y., Diao, J., Lv, M., Cui, J., Chen, L., & Zhang, W. (2019). Metabolic engineering to enhance biosynthesis of both docosahexaenoic acid and odd-chain fatty acids in Schizochytrium sp. S31. *Biotechnology for Biofuels, 12*(1), 141.

Wang, G., Xie, L., Huang, Z., & Xie, J. (2024). Recent advances in polysaccharide biomodification by microbial fermentation: Production, properties, bioactivities, and mechanisms. *Critical Reviews in Food Science and Nutrition, 64*(33), 12999–13023. DOI: 10.1080/10408398.2023.2259461 PMID: 37740706

Wang, H., Chen, Y., Wang, L., Liu, Q., Yang, S., & Wang, C. (2023). Advancing herbal medicine: Enhancing product quality and safety through robust quality control practices. *Frontiers in Pharmacology, 14*, 1265178. PMID: 37818188

Wang, L., Ju, C., Han, C., Yu, Z., Bai, M. Y., & Wang, C. (2025). The interaction of nutrient uptake with biotic and abiotic stresses in plants. *Journal of Integrative Plant Biology, 67*(3), 455–487. DOI: 10.1111/jipb.13613

Wang, L., Zhang, B., & Xiao, J. (2022). Carrageenan-based films and coatings for food packaging applications: A review. *Trends in Food Science & Technology, 119*, 257–273. DOI: 10.1016/j.tifs.2021.12.015

Wang, Y., Chan, K.-L., Abdel-Rahman, M. A., Sonomoto, K., & Leu, S.-Y. (2020). Dynamic simulation of continuous mixed sugar fermentation with increasing cell retention time for lactic acid production using Enterococcus mundtii QU 25. *Biotechnology for Biofuels, 13*(1), 112. DOI: 10.1186/s13068-020-01752-6

Wang, Z., Chen, T., Ma, X., Shen, Z., & Zhao, X. (2011). Enhancement of riboflavin production with Bacillus subtilis by expression and site-directed mutagenesis of zwf and gnd gene from Corynebacterium glutamicum. *Bioresource Technology, 102*(4), 3934–3940. DOI: 10.1016/j.biortech.2010.11.120

Wang, Z., Zeng, D., Zhu, Y., Zhou, M., Kondo, A., Hasunuma, T., & Zhao, X. (2025). Fermentation design and process optimization strategy based on machine learning ML-BASED FERMENTATION DESIGN AND OPTIMIZATION. *Biodesign Research*, •••, 100002.

Warda, M., Tekin, S., Khafaga, N., Sengul, E., Çelebi, F., & Laçin, B. B. (2025). *Comprehensive Insights Into Genetically Modified Foods: Technological Advances, Nutritional Benefits, Therapeutic Applications, and Health Implications*. Food Safety and Health.

Warnock, J. N., Bratch, K., & Al-Rubeai, M. (2005). Packed bed bioreactors. In *Bioreactors for Tissue Engineering: Principles, Design and Operation* (pp. 87–113). Springer Netherlands., DOI: 10.1007/1-4020-3741-4

Wasalathanthri, D. P., Feroz, H., Puri, N., Hung, J., Lane, G., Holstein, M., & Li, Z. J. (2020). Real-time monitoring of quality attributes by in-line Fourier transform infrared spectroscopic sensors at ultrafiltration and diafiltration of bioprocess. *Biotechnology and Bioengineering, 117*(12), 3766–3774. PMID: 32776504

Wasalathanthri, D. P., Rehmann, M. S., Song, Y., Gu, Y., Mi, L., Shao, C., Chemmalil, L., Lee, J., Ghose, S., & Borys, M. C. (2020). Technology outlook for real-time quality attribute and process parameter monitoring in biopharmaceutical development—A review. *Biotechnology and Bioengineering, 117*(10), 3182–3198. PMID: 32946122

Waśko, A., Kordowska-Wiater, M., Podleśny, M., Polak-Berecka, M., Targoński, Z., & Kubik-Komar, A. (2010). The Plackett-Burman design in optimization of media components for biomass production of Lactobacillus rhamnosus OXY. *Acta Biologica Hungarica, 61*(3), 344–355. PMID: 20724280

Wasli, A. S., Salleh, M. M., Abd-Aziz, S., Hassan, O., & Mahadi, N. M. (2009). Medium optimization for chitinase production from Trichoderma virens using central composite design. *Biotechnology and Bioprocess Engineering; BBE, 14*(6), 781–787.

Watanabe, S., Ito, M., & Kigawa, T. (2021). DiRect: Site-directed mutagenesis method for protein engineering by rational design. *Biochemical and Biophysical Research Communications, 551*, 107–113.

Way, J. C., Collins, J. J., Keasling, J. D., & Silver, P. A. (2014). Integrating biological redesign: Where synthetic biology came from and where it needs to go. *Cell, 157*(1), 151–161. DOI: 10.1016/j.cell.2014.02.039 PMID: 24679533

Weber, E., Engler, C., Gruetzner, R., Werner, S., & Marillonnet, S. (2011). A modular cloning system for standardized assembly of multigene constructs. *PLoS One, 6*(2), e16765. DOI: 10.1371/journal.pone.0016765 PMID: 21364738

Wen, L., Yang, L., Chen, C., Li, J., Fu, J., Liu, G., Kan, Q., Ho, C.-T., Huang, Q., & Lan, Y. (2024). Applications of multi-omics techniques to unravel the fermentation process and the flavor formation mechanism in fermented foods. *Critical Reviews in Food Science and Nutrition, 64*(23), 8367–8383.

Westfall, P. J., Pitera, D. J., Lenihan, J. R., Eng, D., Woolard, F. X., Regentin, R., & Renninger, N. S. (2012). Production of Amorphadiene in yeast, and its conversion to dihydroartemisinic acid, precursor to the antimalarial agent artemisinin. *Proceedings of the National Academy of Sciences of the United States of America, 109*(3), E111–E118. DOI: 10.1073/pnas.1110740109 PMID: 22247290

Whitaker, W. B., Jones, J. A., Bennett, R. K., Gonzalez, J. E., Vernacchio, V. R., Collins, S. M., Palmer, M. A., Schmidt, S., Antoniewicz, M. R., & Koffas, M. A.. (2017). Engineering the biological conversion of methanol to specialty chemicals in Escherichia coli. *Metabolic Engineering, 39*, 49–59.

Whitford, B., Jones, D., & Kinnane, S. (2022). Biomanufacturing design: Reducing the environmental burden. *Current Opinion in Biotechnology, 76*, 102717. DOI: 10.1016/j.copbio.2022.102717 PMID: 35439701

WHO. (2004). *Laboratory Biosafety Manual* (3rd ed.). https://www.who.int/publications/i/item/9241546506

Whomsley, R., Palmi Reig, V., & Hidalgo-Simon, A. (2021). Environmental risk assessment of advanced therapies containing genetically modified organisms in the EU. *British Journal of Clinical Pharmacology, 87*(6), 2450–2458. PMID: 33600022

Wichard, T., Charrier, B., & Potin, P. (2015). Green algae as model organisms for biological fluid dynamics. *Annual Review of Fluid Mechanics, 47*, 343–375. DOI: 10.1146/annurev-fluid-010313-141426 PMID: 26594068

Wijekoon, W., Priyashantha, H., Gajanayake, P., Manage, P., Liyanage, C., Jayarathna, S., & Kumarasinghe, U. (2025). Review and prospects of phytoremediation: Harnessing biofuel-producing plants for environmental remediation. *Sustainability, 17*(3), 822. DOI: 10.3390/su17030822

Wijffels, R. H., Barbosa, M. J., & Eppink, M. H. M. (2016). Microalgae for the production of bulk chemicals and biofuels. *Biofuels, Bioproducts & Biorefining, 4*(3), 287–295. DOI: 10.1002/bbb.215

Willett, A., & Hajduk, M. (2024). Perspectives for using CO_2 as a feedstock for biomanufacturing. *Bioengineering (Basel, Switzerland), 10*(12), 1357. Advance online publication. DOI: 10.3390/bioengineering10121357 PMID: 38135948

Williams, T., Kalinka, K., Sanches, R., Blanchard-Emmerson, G., Watts, S., Davies, L., & Dikicioglu, D. (2023). Machine learning and metabolic modelling assisted implementation of a novel process analytical technology in cell and gene therapy manufacturing. *Scientific Reports, 13*(1), 834. PMID: 36646795

Wilson, S., Steele, S., & Adeli, K. (2022). Innovative technological advancements in laboratory medicine: Predicting the lab of the future. *Biotechnology & Biotechnological Equipment, 36*(sup1), S9–S21. https://doi.org/DOI: 10.1080/13102818.2021.2011413

Winkler, T., Ulz, A., Knöbl, W., & Lercher, H. (2020). Frugal innovation in developed markets–Adaption of a criteria-based evaluation model. *Journal of Innovation & Knowledge, 5*(4), 251–259. DOI: 10.1016/j.jik.2019.11.004

Worrell, E., Bernstein, L., Roy, J., Price, L., & Harnisch, J. (2018). Industrial energy efficiency and climate change mitigation. In *Renewable energy* (p. Vol1_548-Vol1_568). Routledge.

Woteki, C. E., Buckley, G. J., & National Academies of Sciences, Engineering, and Medicine. (2020). Global Efforts to Strengthen Regulatory Systems. In *Stronger Food and Drug Regulatory Systems Abroad*. National Academies Press (US).

Woźniak, E., Tyczewska, A., & Twardowski, T. (2021). Bioeconomy development factors in the European Union and Poland. *New Biotechnology, 60*, 2–8. PMID: 32835869

Wu, G., Fanzo, J., Miller, D. D., Pingali, P., Post, M., Steiner, J. L., & Thalacker-Mercer, A. E. (2014). Production and supply of high-quality food protein for human consumption: Sustainability, challenges, and innovations. *Annals of the New York Academy of Sciences, 1321*(1), 1–19.

Wurm, F. M. (2004). Production of recombinant protein therapeutics in cultivated mammalian cells. *Nature Biotechnology, 22*(11), 1393–1398. PMID: 15529164

Wurm, F. M. (2013). CHO quasispecies—Implications for manufacturing processes. *Processes (Basel, Switzerland), 1*(3), 296–311.

Wu, S., Snajdrova, R., Moore, J. C., Baldenius, K., & Bornscheuer, U. T. (2021). Biocatalysis: Enzymatic synthesis for industrial applications. *Angewandte Chemie International Edition*, *60*(1), 88–119. PMID: 32558088

Wu, Y., Jha, R., Li, A., Liu, H., Zhang, Z., Zhang, C., Zhai, Q., & Zhang, J. (2022). Probiotics (Lactobacillus plantarum HNU082) supplementation relieves ulcerative colitis by affecting intestinal barrier functions, immunity-related gene expression, gut microbiota, and metabolic pathways in mice. *Microbiology Spectrum*, *10*(6), e01651–e01622.

Wyma, A., Martin-Alarcon, L., Walsh, T., Schmidt, T. A., Gates, I. D., & Kallos, M. S. (2018). Non-Newtonian rheology in suspension cell cultures significantly impacts bioreactor shear stress quantification. *Biotechnology and Bioengineering*, *115*(8), 2101–2113. DOI: 10.1002/bit.26723 PMID: 29704461

Xian, Z. N., Yin, C. F., Zheng, L., Zhou, N. Y., & Xu, Y. (2023). Biodegradation of additive-free polypropylene by bacterial consortia enriched from the ocean and from the gut of Tenebrio molitor larvae. *The Science of the Total Environment*, *892*, 164721. DOI: 10.1016/j.scitotenv.2023.164721 PMID: 37301383

Xiao, X., Cheng, Y., & Zhang, Y. (2024). Sustainable Innovation in the Biopharmaceutical Industry: An Analysis of the Impact of Policy Configuration. *Sustainability*, *16*(6), 2339. DOI: 10.3390/su16062339

Xie, D. (2022). Continuous biomanufacturing with microbes—Upstream progresses and challenges. *Current Opinion in Biotechnology*, *78*, 102793. DOI: 10.1016/j.copbio.2022.102793 PMID: 36088736

Xie, D., Jackson, E. N., & Zhu, Q. (2015). Sustainable source of omega-3 eicosapentaenoic acid from metabolically engineered Yarrowia lipolytica: From fundamental research to commercial production. *Applied Microbiology and Biotechnology*, *99*(4), 1599–1610. DOI: 10.1007/s00253-014-6318-y

Xie, D., Miller, E., Sharpe, P., Jackson, E., & Zhu, Q. (2017). Omega-3 production by fermentation of *Yarrowia lipolytica* : From fed-batch to continuous. *Biotechnology and Bioengineering*, *114*(4), 798–812. DOI: 10.1002/bit.26216

Xie, L., Gao, J., & Zhou, Y. J. (2024). Synthetic biology for Taxol biosynthesis and sustainable production. *Trends in Biotechnology*, *42*(6), 674–676. DOI: 10.1016/j.tibtech.2024.04.001 PMID: 38609783

Xie, L., & Wang, D. I. C. (1996). High cell density and high monoclonal antibody production through medium design and rational feeding in a fed-batch culture of hybridoma cells. *Biotechnology and Bioengineering*, *51*(6), 725–729. PMID: 18629840

Xu, D., & Wang, J. (2015). Strategic emerging industries in China: Literature review and research prospect. *American Journal of Industrial and Business Management*, *5*(07), 486. DOI: 10.4236/ajibm.2015.57049

Xu, F., Su, L., Gao, H., Wang, Y., Ben, R., Hu, K., & Tian, X. (2025). Harnessing near-infrared and Raman spectral sensing and artificial intelligence for real-time monitoring and precision control of bioprocess. *Bioresource Technology*, •••, 132204. PMID: 39923859

Xu, S., & Zydney, A. L. (2023). Strategies for integration of perfusion-based upstream with continuous downstream purification. *Frontiers in Bioengineering and Biotechnology, 11*, 1211410.

Xu, X., Zuo, Y., Chen, S., Hatami, A., & Gu, H. (2024). Advancements in brain research: The in vivo/in vitro electrochemical detection of neurochemicals. *Biosensors (Basel), 14*(3), 125. PMID: 38534232

Xu, Y., Chen, C., Hellwarth, P. B., & Bao, X. (2019). Biomaterials for stem cell engineering and biomanufacturing. *Bioactive Materials, 4*, 366–379. DOI: 10.1016/j.bioactmat.2019.11.002

Yaashikaa, P. R., Senthil Kumar, P., & Varjani, S. (2022). Valorization of agro-industrial wastes for biorefinery process and circular bioeconomy: A critical review. *Bioresource Technology, 343*, 126126. DOI: 10.1016/j.biortech.2021.126126 PMID: 34673193

Yadav, D. K., Singh, A., Agrawal, V., & Yadav, N. (2021). Algal Biomass: A Natural Resource of High-Value Biomolecules. *Bioprospecting of Plant Biodiversity for Industrial Molecules*, 303–334.

Yadwad, V. B., Wilson, S., & Ward, O. P. (1994). Production of human epidermal growth factor by an ampicillin resistant recombinant Escherichia coli strain. *Biotechnology Letters, 16*(9), 885–890. DOI: 10.1007/BF00128619

Yamada, Y., & Yukphan, P. (2008). Genera and species in acetic acid bacteria. *International Journal of Food Microbiology, 125*(1), 15–24. DOI: 10.1016/j.ijfoodmicro.2007.11.077

Yan, B., Wrenn, B. A., Basak, S., Biswas, P., & Giammar, D. E. (2008). Microbial reduction of Fe(III) in hematite nanoparticles by Geobacter sulfurreducens. *Environmental Science & Technology, 42*(17), 6526–6531. DOI: 10.1021/es800620f PMID: 18800525

Yang, H., Cai, G., Lu, J., & Gómez Plaza, E. (2021). The production and application of enzymes related to the quality of fruit wine. *Critical Reviews in Food Science and Nutrition, 61*(10), 1605–1615.

Yang, L., Shakeel, Q., Xu, X., Ali, L., Chen, Z., Mubeen, M., Sohail, M. A., Iftikhar, Y., Kumar, A., Solanki, M. K., & Zhou, Y. (2024). Optimized submerged batch fermentation for metabolic switching in *Streptomyces yanglinensis* 3–10 providing platform for reveromycin A and B biosynthesis, engineering, and production. *Frontiers in Microbiology, 15*, 1378834. Advance online publication. DOI: 10.3389/fmicb.2024.1378834

Yang, L., Wang, X.-C., Dai, M., Chen, B., Qiao, Y., Deng, H., Zhang, D., Zhang, Y., de Almeida, C. M. V. B., & Chiu, A. S. (2021). Shifting from fossil-based economy to bio-based economy: Status quo, challenges, and prospects. *Energy, 228*, 120533.

Yang, M., Zhang, W., Ji, S., Cao, P., Chen, Y., & Zhao, X. (2013). Generation of an Artificial Double Promoter for Protein Expression in Bacillus subtilis through a Promoter Trap System. *PLoS One, 8*(2), e56321. DOI: 10.1371/journal.pone.0056321

Yang, S., Fei, Q., Zhang, Y., Contreras, L. M., Utturkar, S. M., Brown, S. D., Himmel, M. E., & Zhang, M. (2016). *Zymomonas mobilis* as a model system for production of biofuels and biochemicals. *Microbial Biotechnology, 9*(6), 699–717. DOI: 10.1111/1751-7915.12408

Yang, S., Mohagheghi, A., Franden, M. A., Chou, Y. C., Chen, X., & Zhang, M. (2016). Metabolic engineering of *Zymomonas mobilis* for 2,3-butanediol production from lignocellulosic biomass sugars. *Biotechnology for Biofuels*, *9*(1), 1–15. DOI: 10.1186/s13068-016-0606-y PMID: 27594916

Yang, S.-T., Wang, G., & Qin, Z. (2023). A perspective in future biomanufacturing: Challenges in industrial fermentation—understanding and controlling microbial lifespan and aging. *Synthetic Biology and Engineering*, *1*(3), 10019. DOI: 10.35534/sbe.2023.10019

Yap, J. X., Chan, Y. H., & Tshai, K. Y. (2023). A review on the degradation of poly(lactic acid) blends. *Polymer Degradation & Stability*, *208*, 110256. DOI: 10.1016/j.polymdegradstab.2023.110256

Yari, K., Fatemi, S. S.-A., & Tavallaei, M. (2012). High level expression of recombinant BoNT/A-Hc by high cell density cultivation of Escherichia coli. *Bioprocess and Biosystems Engineering*, *35*(3), 407–414. DOI: 10.1007/s00449-011-0579-y

Yasarla, L. R., & Ramarao, B. V. (2012). Dynamics of flocculation of lignocellulosic hydrolyzates by polymers. *Industrial & Engineering Chemistry Research*, *51*(19), 6847–6861.

Yazdi, M. (2024). Augmented reality (AR) and virtual reality (VR) in maintenance training. In *Advances in Computational Mathematics for Industrial System Reliability and Maintainability* (pp. 169–183). Springer Nature Switzerland.

Yee, C. S., Zahia-Azizan, N. A., Abd Rahim, M. H., Mohd Zaini, N. A., Raja-Razali, R. B., Ushidee-Radzi, M. A., Ilham, Z., & Wan-Mohtar, W. A. A. Q. I. (2025). Smart Fermentation Technologies: Microbial Process Control in Traditional Fermented Foods. *Fermentation (Basel, Switzerland)*, *11*(6), 323.

Ye, Z., Li, S., Hennigan, J. N., Lebeau, J., Moreb, E. A., Wolf, J., & Lynch, M. D. (2021). Two-stage dynamic deregulation of metabolism improves process robustness & scalability in engineered E. coli. *Metabolic Engineering*, *68*, 106–118. DOI: 10.1016/j.ymben.2021.09.009

Yigzaw, Y., Piper, R., Tran, M., & Shukla, A. A. (2006). Exploiting the adsorptive properties of depth filters for host cell protein removal during monoclonal antibody purification processes. *Biotechnology Progress*, *22*(1), 288–296. PMID: 16454522

Yim, H., Haselbeck, R., Niu, W., Pujol-Baxley, C., Burgard, A., Boldt, J., Khandurina, J., Trawick, J. D., Osterhout, R. E., Stephen, R., Estadilla, J., Teisan, S., Schreyer, H. B., Andrae, S., Yang, T. H., Lee, S. Y., Burk, M. J., & Van Dien, S. (2011). Metabolic engineering of Escherichia coli for direct production of 1,4-butanediol. *Nature Chemical Biology*, *7*(7), 445–452. DOI: 10.1038/nchembio.580

Yin, J., Li, G., Liu, Y., & Wang, J. (2021). Application of SCADA Systems in Biopharmaceutical Manufacturing. *Journal of Biotechnology Advances*, *39*(5), 210–225. DOI: 10.1016/j.biotechadv.2021.107581

Yi, W., Hu, S., Qian, X., Yan, W., & Li, Y. (2025). Synthetic Biology-Based Engineering Cells for Drug Delivery. *Exploration*, *5*(2). Advance online publication. DOI: 10.1002/EXP.20240095

Yoha, K., Nida, S., Dutta, S., Moses, J., & Anandharamakrishnan, C. (2022). Targeted delivery of probiotics: Perspectives on research and commercialization. *Probiotics and Antimicrobial Proteins*, *14*(1), 15–48.

Ytterberg, A. J., Zubarev, R. A., & Baumgarten, T. (2019). Posttranslational Targeting of a Recombinant Protein Promotes Its Efficient Secretion into the Escherichia coli Periplasm. *Applied and Environmental Microbiology*, *85*(13). Advance online publication. DOI: 10.1128/AEM.00671-19

Yue, D., You, F., & Snyder, S. W. (2014). Biomass-to-bioenergy and biofuel supply chain optimization: Overview, key issues and challenges. *Computers & Chemical Engineering*, *66*, 36–56.

Yuk, I. H., Baskar, D., Duffy, P. H., Hsiung, J., Leung, S., & Lin, A. A. (2011). Overcoming challenges in WAVE bioreactors without feedback controls for pH and dissolved oxygen. *Biotechnology Progress*, *27*(5), 1397–1406. PMID: 21987370

Yusuf, A., Almotairy, A. R. Z., Henidi, H., Alshehri, O. Y., & Aldughaim, M. S. (2023). Nanoparticles as Drug Delivery Systems: A Review of the Implication of Nanoparticles' Physicochemical Properties on Responses in Biological Systems. *Polymers*, *15*(7), 1596. DOI: 10.3390/polym15071596

Zainurin, S. N., Wan Ismail, W. Z., Mahamud, S. N. I., Ismail, I., Jamaludin, J., Ariffin, K. N. Z., & Wan Ahmad Kamil, W. M. (2022). Advancements in monitoring water quality based on various sensing methods: A systematic review. *International Journal of Environmental Research and Public Health*, *19*(21), 14080. PMID: 36360992

Zala, S. P., Patel, K. P., Patel, K. S., Parmar, J. P., Sen, D. J., Parmar, J. P., & Scopus, C. (2012). Laboratory techniques of purification and isolation. *Int. J. Drug Dev. Res*, *4*(2), 41–55.

Zeng, A. P., & Sabra, W. (2011). Microbial production of diols as platform chemicals: Recent progresses. *Current Opinion in Biotechnology*, *22*(6), 749–757. DOI: 10.1016/j.copbio.2011.05.005

Zeng, Y., Hong, Y., Azi, F., Liu, Y., Chen, Y., Guo, C., Lin, D., Wu, Z., Chen, W., & Xu, P. (2022). Advanced genome-editing technologies enable rapid and large-scale generation of genetic variants for strain engineering and synthetic biology. *Current Opinion in Microbiology*, *69*, 102175. PMID: 35809388

Zhang, J. (2010). Mammalian cell culture for biopharmaceutical production. *Manual of industrial microbiology and biotechnology*, 157-178.

Zhang, J., Bilal, M., Liu, S., Zhang, J., Lu, H., Luo, H., Luo, C., Shi, H., Iqbal, H. M., & Zhao, Y. (2020). Isolation, identification and antimicrobial evaluation of bactericides secreting *Bacillus subtilis* Natto as a biocontrol agent. *Processes (Basel, Switzerland)*, *8*(3), 259. Advance online publication. DOI: 10.3390/pr8030259

Zhang, P., Zhang, D. F., Zhou, W., Wang, Q., Zhang, Y., & Li, Y. (2024). Network pharmacology: Towards the artificial intelligence-based precision traditional Chinese medicine. *Briefings in Bioinformatics*, *25*(1), bbad518. Advance online publication. DOI: 10.1093/bib/bbad518 PMID: 38197310

Zhang, S., Guo, F., Yan, W., Dai, Z., Dong, W., Zhou, J., Zhang, W., Xin, F., & Jiang, M. (2020). Recent Advances of CRISPR/Cas9-Based Genetic Engineering and Transcriptional Regulation in Industrial Biology. *Frontiers in Bioengineering and Biotechnology*, *7*. Advance online publication. DOI: 10.3389/fbioe.2019.00459

Zhang, X., Luo, W., & Xiang, D. (2025). Strategic emerging industries and innovation: Evidence from China. *International Review of Economics & Finance*, *98*, 103858. DOI: 10.1016/j.iref.2025.103858

Zhang, X., Zhao, C., Shao, M. W., Chen, Y. L., Liu, P., & Chen, G. Q. (2022). The roadmap of bioeconomy in China. *Engineering Biology*, *6*(4), 71–81. DOI: 10.1049/enb2.12026 PMID: 36968339

Zhang, Y.-H. P. (2013). Next generation biorefineries will solve the food, biofuels, and environmental trilemma in the energy–food–water nexus. *Energy Science & Engineering*, *1*(1), 27–41. DOI: 10.1002/ese3.2

Zhang, Y.-H. P. (2015). Production of biofuels and biochemicals by in vitro synthetic biosystems: Opportunities and challenges. *Biotechnology Advances*, *33*(7), 1467–1483. DOI: 10.1016/j.biotechadv.2014.10.009

Zhang, Y.-H. P., Sun, J., & Ma, Y. (2017). Biomanufacturing: History and perspective. *Journal of Industrial Microbiology & Biotechnology*, *44*(4–5), 773–784. DOI: 10.1007/s10295-016-1863-2

Zhang, Y., Peng, J., Zhao, H., & Shi, S. (2021). Engineering oleaginous yeast Rhodotorula toruloides for overproduction of fatty acid ethyl esters. *Biotechnology for Biofuels*, *14*(1), 115. DOI: 10.1186/s13068-021-01965-3

Zhang, Y., Zhu, X., Wang, N., Liu, X., Wang, L., & Ning, K. (2025). Synergy of traditional practices and modern technology: Advancing the understanding and applications of microbial resources and processes in fermented foods. *Trends in Food Science & Technology*, •••, 104891.

Zhan, Y., Shi, J., Xiao, Y., Zhou, F., Wang, H., Xu, H., Li, Z., Yang, S., Cai, D., & Chen, S. (2022). Multilevel metabolic engineering of Bacillus licheniformis for de novo biosynthesis of 2-phenylethanol. *Metabolic Engineering*, *70*, 43–54. DOI: 10.1016/j.ymben.2022.01.007

Zhao, J., Li, Q., Sun, T., Zhu, X., Xu, H., Tang, J., Zhang, X., & Ma, Y. (2013). Engineering central metabolic modules of Escherichia coli for improving β-carotene production. *Metabolic Engineering*, *17*, 42–50.

Zhao, M., Ma, J., Zhang, L., Huang, Y., Zhang, Y., & Yu, R. (2024). Engineering strategies for enhanced heterologous protein production by *Saccharomyces cerevisiae*. *Microbial Cell Factories*, *23*, 32. DOI: 10.1186/s12934-024-02299-z PMID: 38247006

Zhao, X., Sun, Y., Li, Y., Jia, N., & Xu, J. (2024). Applications of machine learning in real-time control systems: A review. *Measurement Science & Technology*. Advance online publication. DOI: 10.1088/1361-6501/ad8f85

Zhao, Y., Wang, H., Dong, W., Chang, Y., Yan, G., Chu, Z., & Li, C. (2020). Nitrogen removal and microbial community for the treatment of rural domestic sewage with low C/N ratio by A/O biofilter with Arundo donax as carbon source and filter media. *Journal of Water Process Engineering*, *37*, 101509. DOI: 10.1016/j.jwpe.2020.101509

Zheng, C., Gao, L., Sun, H., Zhao, X.-Y., Gao, Z., Liu, J., & Guo, W. (2024). Advancements in enzymatic reaction-mediated microbial transformation. *Heliyon*, *10*(19), e38187. DOI: 10.1016/j.heliyon.2024.e38187

Zhou, S., Zhuang, Y., & Li, Y. (2021). Engineering microbial cell factories for sustainable production of chemicals. *Biotechnology Advances*, *51*, 107733. DOI: 10.1016/j.biotechadv.2021.107733

Zhou, X., Tang, J., Jacobs, T. L., & Saguy, I. S. (2025). Transforming Food Supply Chains Through Digital Tracking and Monitoring Technologies. *Trends in Food Science & Technology*, •••, 105142.

Zhu, C., Ji, Z., Ma, J., Ding, Z., Shen, J., & Wang, Q. (2021). Recent Advances of Nanotechnology-Facilitated Bacteria-Based Drug and Gene Delivery Systems for Cancer Treatment. *Pharmaceutics*, *13*(7), 940. DOI: 10.3390/pharmaceutics13070940

Zhu, C., Mu, J., & Liang, L. (2024). Nanocarriers for intracellular delivery of proteins in biomedical applications: Strategies and recent advances. *Journal of Nanobiotechnology*, *22*(1), 688. DOI: 10.1186/s12951-024-02969-5

Zhu, J., Li, J., Kong, Y., Dong, M., Li, Y., & Zou, M. (2025). Study on the high-speed penetration and shear failure mechanism of beach sand. *Materials (Basel)*, *18*(9), 1922. Advance online publication. DOI: 10.3390/ma18091922

Zhu, M., Zheng, J., Xie, J., Zhao, D., Qiao, Z.-W., Huang, D., & Luo, H.-B. (2022). Effects of environmental factors on the microbial community changes during medium-high temperature Daqu manufacturing. *Food Research International*, *153*, 110955.

Zhu, Q., & Jackson, E. N. (2015). Metabolic engineering of *Yarrowia lipolytica* for industrial applications. *Current Opinion in Biotechnology*, *36*, 65–72. DOI: 10.1016/j.copbio.2015.08.010

Zhu, X., Rehman, K. U., Wang, B., & Shahzad, M. (2020). Modern soft-sensing modeling methods for fermentation processes. *Sensors (Basel)*, *20*(6), 1771. PMID: 32210053

Zia, S., Paris, F., & Alviano, F. (2024). *Emerging technologies for quality control of cell-based ATMPs. Journal of Pharmaceutical and Biomedical Analysis*. https://www.sciencedirect.com/science/article/pii/S073170852400222X

Zydney, A. L. (2016). Continuous downstream processing for high value biological products: A review. *Biotechnology and Bioengineering*, *113*(3), 465–475. PMID: 26153056

Zydney, A. L. (2016). Continuous downstream processing for high value biologics: A review. *Biotechnology and Bioengineering*, *113*(3), 465–475. PMID: 26153056

About the Contributors

Ayush Madan is an Assistant Professor in the Department of Biotechnology at People's University and a Graduate Research Assistant at Universiti Malaysia Terengganu. He holds an M.Tech. in Biotechnology from Graphic Era University and has extensive expertise in microbial technology and environmental bioremediation. He has also completed his Ph.D. work in the field of Nanobiotechnology where he has studied the cytotoxic effects of silver and gold nanoparticles on human cells with special reference to chromosomal aberrations. He has published numerous research and review articles in national and international journals and has presented his work at various conferences. He has also served as an editor in 14 books in prestigious publishing house including Taylor and Francis, CABI, Cambridge Scholars, Wiley Scrivener, etc. Previously, he was an Assistant Professor at Shobhit Institute of Engineering and Technology and completed a six-month internship at Biocon Research Limited. His current research involves integrated microalgae-shrimp cultivation for wastewater treatment and shrimp growth enhancement.

Mohd. Tariq is now employed as an Assistant Registrar (Academics) in the Department of Academics at the Sumandeep Vidyapeeth Deemed to be University in Vadodara, Gujarat, India. Dr. Tariq earned his Ph.D. in Biotechnology from Kumaun University, Nainital, India, in 2018. His research was focused on biotechnological and ecological approaches for the conservation of Paris polyphylla Smith, a medicinally important herb of the Indian Himalayan region. He holds an M.Sc. in Biotechnology from Graphic Era University, Dehradun, and a B.Sc. in Zoology (Honors) from Ramjas College, University of Delhi. Dr. Tariq's academic contributions include extensive research in the fields of conservation biology, medicinal plant biotechnology, and ecological modeling. He has published numerous research articles in reputed journals, authored book chapters, and presented his work at national and international conferences. His areas of expertise include tissue culture, molecular biology techniques, ecological assessment, and habitat distribution modeling. He has also guided over 65 undergraduate and postgraduate students and is supervising three Ph.D. candidates. With a strong commitment to academic excellence, Dr. Tariq has received several accolades, including the Research Excellenece Award (2025) and the Young Scientist Award (2019) and Emerging Scientist Award (2020). His contributions to academia and research reflect his dedication to advancing scientific knowledge and fostering the next generation of scholars.

Mantosh Kumar Satapathy, is a Research Scientist at Taipei Medical University (TMU), Taiwan. He holds a Ph.D. in Biomedical Materials and Tissue Engineering from TMU, a M.Tech. in Industrial Biotechnology, and a B.Pharm from India. His research spans biomedical and environmental challenges, includes the development of smart stimuli-responsive nanocomposite biomaterials for controlled drug delivery, non-thermal cold microplasma–based biomaterial fabrication, stem cell–driven technologies, and biomaterial scaffold design for regenerative medicine, and tissue engineering applications. He has been recognized with the Outstanding Postdoctoral Award from TMU, and involved in Taiwan government–funded projects under the NHRI and the NSTC. He served as an Assistant Professor at NIET, NIMS University, Jaipur, Rajasthan, and received appreciation for the academic excellence. He has commitments to advancing biomedical innovation and translating scientific discoveries into future therapeutics.

Yousef Rasmi holds his PhD degree in Clinical Biochemistry from Tarbiat Modarres University (TMU), Tehran, Iran, in 2006. Short visiting scholar training/2006 in the Department Of Pathology at the JCU, Townsville, Australia. Appointed as an Assistant Professor/2006 at the Department of Biochemistry, Urmia University of Medical Sciences (UMSU), Urmia, Iran. In 2014, granted the degree of Professor. Currently, works on nano-medicine, inflammation, CSX, endothelial function, and signaling pathways.

***

Banzeer Ahsan Abbasi received her graduate degree in Botany from Quaid-i-Azam University, Islamabad, Pakistan. Dr. Banzeer is currently working as an Assistant Professor at Department of Botany, Rawalpindi Women University, Rawalpindi, Pakistan. She has published more than 60 research articles in various international journals and 10 chapters in reputed publishers (ELSIEVER, RSC and SPRINGER). Currently, she is supervising 2 Ph.D, 6 MPhil and 6 BS students. She has expertise in the synthesis of novel nanomaterials from medicinal plants and their multiple biological and envirnemental applications. Her research is also focusing on phytochemistry, natural products of medicinal plants and Phylogenetics. She has a very decent research background with research published in well-reputed journals with H-index 28, i-10 index 44 and overall citations 3317.

Muhammad Anas is a plant scientist and nanobiotechnology researcher with expertise in stress physiology, ionomics, phytochemistry, and nano-enabled solutions for sustainable agriculture. His research focuses on the green synthesis and application of metal-based and quantum dot nanomaterials for plant growth enhancement, environmental detoxification, and biomedical relevance. He has authored over 30 peer-reviewed articles in leading journals, including more than 20 in Q1 category, with a cumulative impact factor exceeding 115. He currently serves as editor for two international scientific books focused on nanotechnology and microbial-plant interactions. His methodological strength spans antioxidant assays, nanoparticle characterization, plant-metal interaction studies, and omics integration. Anas is committed to translating fundamental research into innovative tools for food security, environmental safety, and health applications.

Muhammad Anas is a plant scientist specializing in wheat and environmental agricultural studies, with a strong focus on nanotechnology-driven stress mitigation, heavy metal tolerance, ionomics, histology, antioxidant systems, and cultivar-specific resilience. Earning his PhD in Plant Sciences from Quaid-i-Azam University, Islamabad, he developed biogenic quantum dots and manganese-based nanomaterials to alleviate cadmium and chromium toxicity in wheat, and is currently a TÜBİTAK–TWAS Research Fellow at Selçuk University, Türkiye, where he explores miRNAomics in wheat under heavy metal stress . With more than 30 peer-reviewed publications, contributions to international book chapters, and editorial roles in upcoming volumes on soil health and plant–microbe interactions, his work bridges plant physiology, nanotechnology, and environmental sustainability. His expertise extends to omics-based approaches, phenotyping, crop stress physiology, and rhizosphere microbiome studies, offering innovative solutions for enhancing crop resilience and safeguarding global food security.

Nibedita Bardhan is a senior surgeon (Urology), Specialist in MIS, PCNL, URSL.

Mukul Machhindra Barwant is Dean of Research and Innovation, Assistant Professor, Department of Botany Sanjivani Arts, Commerce, and Science College, Kopargaon, Ahilyanagar, Maharashtra, India. He is an accomplished botanist, researcher, and academic leader, currently serving as the Dean of Research and Innovation and Assistant Professor in the Department of Botany at Sanjivani Arts, Commerce, and Science College, Kopargaon, Ahilyanagar, Maharashtra, India. With over five years of teaching experience, he is deeply committed to advancing education, scientific research, and innovation in botany and allied fields.In addition to academia, he has hands-on industry experience as the Production In-Charge at Ashvamedh Pvt. Ltd., a herbal medicine company in Kopargaon, Ahilyanagar. His expertise lies in phycology, nutraceuticals, pharmacology of seaweeds, and herbal biotechnology.In 2018, he qualified for the Ph.D. Entrance Test (PET) at Shivaji University, Kolhapur, securing the 6th rank. He has successfully completed his Ph.D. in Phycology (Nutraceutical and Pharmacology of Seaweeds) from Yashwantrao Chavan Institute of Science, Satara, Maharashtra, affiliated with Shivaji University, Kolhapur Academic.

Shourya Bodla is currently pursuing a Bachelor of Technology in Biotechnology at Parul University. With a passion for the intersection of technology and biological sciences, Shourya is dedicated to advancing knowledge and skills in this dynamic field.

Zohre Elaysi is currently pursuing a Master's degree in Medical Biotechnology, with ongoing research in a laboratory specializing in biomaterials. He previously earned both his Bachelor's and Master's degrees in Pharmacy from Rajiv Gandhi University of Health Sciences, India. His academic journey bridges pharmaceutical sciences with innovative biomedical research.

Erdogan Esref Hakki was born in Greece in 1968. After completing his Biology degree at Ankara University's Faculty of Science, he completed his master's and doctoral studies in Biotechnology at Middle East Technical University in Ankara. Since 2002, he has been pursuing his academic career at Selçuk University's Faculty of Agriculture. He runs the Biotechnology laboratory, which he founded, within the Faculty of Agriculture and participates in numerous national and international projects.

|Sameel Hassan - Contributing Author|Researcher

Vinay Jain is a highly accomplished academic and administrative professional, currently serving as the Principal of ShriRam College of Pharmacy. He holds an M. Pharm and Ph.D. in Pharmacognosy, and has amassed 20 years of experience in teaching and administration. He has made significant contributions to the field through his research and publications, including 18 peer-reviewed articles, edited and indexed books, and guidance for over 20 research scholars. Dr. Jain completed his M. Pharm in Pharmacognosy from Barkatullah University in 2007 and began his professional career as Assistant Professor at ShriRam College of Pharmacy, Banmore. In 2017, he successfully defended his Ph.D. thesis entitled "Phytochemical and Pharmacological investigation of Arisaema leschenaultii from Berhampur University, Odisha. In addition to his academic pursuits, Dr. Jain has been an active member of the pharmacy community, serving as Co-convener of the Indo-Caribbean conference and Organizing Secretary of the national conference on "The Future Prospect in Pharma-Marketing". He is also a lifetime member of the Indian Society of Pharmacognosy, and has been recognized for his leadership and mentorship in the field. Dr. Jain has been a strong advocate for the holistic development of society and individuals, and has been actively involved in Corporate Social Responsibility initiatives such as health checkup camps, cloth donation drives, and social awareness drives. He has also filed 2 patents and published 50+ papers in international and national journals. In recognition of his excellence, Dr. Jain has received various awards and honors, including the Dhanvantari Awarded during SRIJAN 2021, and has been granted an allowance of INR 2.5 lac for conducting an international conference by AICTE and a grant of INR 8.5 lac by AICTE under ModRob Scheme for laboratory upgradation. He has also been invited as a guest of honor at several conferences and workshops held in MP. Furthermore, his efforts in training and placement have been unmatched and he has been able to invite Pharma giants like MacLeod's and Akums for campus placement. His recent achievements include Best Principal award in 2022 by INSC publishers and Pharma Rising Star Award in 2022, which he received at New Delhi Overall, Dr. Vinay Jain is an exceptional leader and a valued member of the pharmacy community, dedicated to the development of both individuals and society as a whole.

Deepak Kumar Jha, M. Pharm, Ph.D., currently serves as a QA/QC Officer at iCREST Biotechnologies and Associate Professor at Karnataka College of Pharmacy. He specializes in preclinical and clinical research, stem cell applications, clinical and preclinical protocol development, and regulatory compliance. I committed to advancing pharmaceutical research and education through quality-driven practices and translational innovation.

Waseem Ahmed Khattak is a researcher from Pakistan, specializing in plant sciences, particularly plant physiology and mycology. He holds an MPhil degree in Plant Sciences from Quaid-i-Azam University, Islamabad. With a strong research focus on sustainable agriculture and nanobiotechnology, Waseem has published numerous papers in esteemed journals. His work is recognized for its potential to contribute significantly to agricultural research and innovation.

Rahul Kumar has research interests of Antimicrobial Resistance, Medical, Microbiology, Pathology, Bacteriology, Healthcare, Parasitology and Biotechnology, Neuroscience, (Agriculture and Environmental Effects on Healthcare)

Debasis Mitra, Fellow of SASS and IOASD Society, India, is currently serving as Assistant Professor, Department of Microbiology, Graphic Era (Deemed to be University), Dehradun, Uttarakhand, India. Dr. Mitra is distinguished for his extensive contributions to the practical application and formulation of beneficial plant growth-promoting microorganisms, both in laboratory settings and field environments, aimed at fostering sustainable crop production, protection, and development. He earned his Ph.D. in Microbiology from Raiganj University, Raiganj, West Bengal, India and ICAR-National Rice Research Institute (NRRI), Cuttack, Odisha, India. Dr. Mitra holds M.Sc. in Biotechnology from Graphic Era (Deemed to be University), India, and B.Sc. in Biotechnology from Oriental Institute of Science and Technology, Vidyasagar University, India. He is an esteemed alumnus researcher of the Division of Soil Science & Agricultural Chemistry at ICAR- Indian Institute of Horticultural Research, India. Dr. Mitra further expanded his academic horizons through a virtual doctoral internship at the Agroenvironmental and Health Biotechnology Laboratory, Universidad de Santander, Colombia.

P. Saranraj, Head, PG and Research Department of Microbiology, Sacred Heart College (Autonomous), Tirupattur – 635 601, Tamil Nadu, India

Nethikunta Aashrith Patel is an enthusiastic and goal-oriented student currently pursuing a Bachelor of Technology (B.Tech) in Biotechnology at Parul University. His academic journey is fueled by a strong interest in the dynamic and ever-evolving field of biotechnology, particularly in areas related to genetic engineering, molecular biology, and environmental applications. Aashrith is passionate about exploring innovative solutions through science and is keen on bridging the gap between theoretical knowledge and practical implementation.

Samhita Kumar Polavarapu is a final year student pursuing B.Tech Biotechnology at Parul University. With an international academic experience and hands-on industrial exposure in pharmaceutical production and bioinformatics, she seeks opportunities to apply and expand her skills in a dynamic biotech environment with a strong interest in the field of 3D bioprinting.

Bollapu Rohini Reddy is a dedicated and aspiring biotechnology professional currently pursuing a Bachelor of Technology (B.Tech) in Biotechnology at Parul University. With a strong academic foundation and a passion for scientific research, she is keenly interested in exploring the diverse applications of biotechnology in healthcare, agriculture, and environmental sustainability.

Archana S is currently pursuing part time doctoral work in the field of regenerative medicine at Ahmedabad University. More explicitly, their work narrows down in understanding the role of stem cell derived extracellular vesicles in the treatment of arthritis. At the same time, being placed in a pharmaceutical company, they also focus on developing therapeutic products for the treatment of a variety of diseases on a large scale basis. Therefore, they are rooted with both academic and industrial field.

Rakesh Sahu is an aspiring pharmaceutical researcher with a strong academic foundation and hands-on expertise in pharmacology and neurodegenerative research. His journey into pharmacy began with a Bachelor of Pharmacy (B.Pharm) from Chhattisgarh Swami Vivekanand Technical University, where he conducted a project on polymeric microspheres for controlled drug release. His passion for pharmaceutical sciences deepened during his Master's in Pharmacology at Punjab Technical University, where his research focused on exploring neuroprotective therapies for amyotrophic lateral sclerosis (ALS) specifically investigating cellular and molecular biomarkers, neurotransmitter alterations, and neuroinflammatory responses. Rakesh expanded his skill set through multiple research projects at esteemed institutions such as the Council of Scientific and Industrial Research-North East Institute of Science and Technology, Jorhat, Assam (CSIR-NEIST, Jorhat) and the National Institute of Pharmaceutical Education and Research (NIPER-Ahmedabad). His work in these settings spanned immunomodulatory research on nutraceuticals, cell culture, and molecular biology techniques, as well as advanced nanoparticle-based drug delivery systems. He gained proficiency in lipid-based nanoparticle platforms, gene expression analysis, and the design of microRNA mimics or inhibitors. Currently, Rakesh is dedicated to advancing pharmaceutical research with a focus on unraveling the molecular mechanisms underlying neurodegenerative disorders. He aims to contribute to biomarker/drug target discovery and the development of novel therapeutic strategies for motor neuron diseases. His technical expertise encompasses neurochemical analysis, animal models, molecular biology, and drug delivery systems, providing him with a robust foundation to pursue innovations in neurodegenerative drug discovery. In recognition of his scientific contributions, Rakesh also serves as a peer reviewer for reputed journals published by Elsevier and Wiley and as a review board member at Acta Scientific Pharmacology.

Rajan Singh is core hearted Geneticist and Molecular Biologist having more than 12 years of experience in the field of Human Molecular Genetics, Computational Biology, Genomics and Proteomics.

Index

A

B

C

D

E

F

G

I

L

M

O

P

Q

R

S

T

U

V

W

www.ingramcontent.com/pod-product-compliance
Lightning Source LLC
LaVergne TN
LVHW061533290926
849162LV00004B/776